Marihuana: Chemistry, Biochemistry, and Cellular Effects

MARIHUANA

Chemistry, Biochemistry, and Cellular Effects

EDITOR:

Gabriel G. Nahas

CO-EDITORS:

William D. M. Paton and
Juhana E. Idänpään-Heikkilä

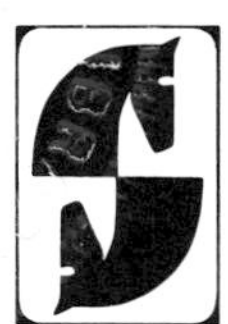

Springer-Verlag

NEW YORK HEIDELBERG BERLIN

1976

Proceedings of The Satellite Symposium on Marihuana (Matinkylä, Finland) of the Sixth International Congress of Pharmacology held July 26–27, 1975 in Helsinki, Finland.

GABRIEL G. NAHAS, M.D., Ph.D., Research Professor of Anesthesiology, College of Physicians & Surgeons of Columbia University, 630 West 168th Street, New York, New York 10032

WILLIAM D. M. PATON, M.D., Ph.D., Professor of Pharmacology, University of Oxford, Oxford, England

JUHANA E. IDÄNPÄÄN-HEIKKILÄ, M.D., D.M.Sc., Docent, Chief Medical Officer for Pharmacology, National Board of Health, Helsinki, 53, Finland

Library of Congress Cataloging in Publication Data

Helsinki Symposium on Marihuana, 1975.
Marihuana: chemistry, biochemistry, and cellular effects.

Organized under the aegis of the 6th International Congress of Pharmacology, Helsinki, 1975.
Includes index.
1. Marihuana—Physiological effect—Congresses. I. Nahas, Gabriel G., 1920– II. Paton, William Drummond Macdonald. III. Idänpään-Heikkilä, Juhana E., 1937– IV. International Congress of Pharmacology, 6th, Helsinki, 1975. V. Title.

Library of Congress Cataloging in Publication Data

QP981.C14H44 1975 615′.782 75-37724

Printed in the United States of America.

ISBN 0-387-07554-2 Springer-Verlag New York

ISBN 3-540-07554-2 Springer-Verlag Berlin Heidelberg

Cover illustration by A. Cohn
Macrophage microphoto by Dr. Marcel Bessis

Preface: Why Another Monograph on Marihuana?

Hasn't this subject been exhausted over the past 6 years by the publication of the dozen volumes that preceded the present one? After numerous investigations on the acute effects of marihuana smoking in man described in hundreds of papers, what is left to know? Following the studies of chronic users performed in Boston, Los Angeles, Jamaica, and Greece, hasn't the marihuana question been settled?

Shouldn't we now consider marihuana a "soft drug" to be used for recreational purposes, like alcohol or tobacco, with minimal danger to the user and little damage to society? A number of scientists have already given an affirmative answer to these questions, and their opinions, amplified by the media, seem to be shared by a large section of the lay public. On the other hand, some investigators claim that old empirical observations confirmed by recent scientific evidence indicate that marihuana is a harmful drug. As a result, a great marihuana debate is now raging in the scientific and lay press of the United States. Let us hope that it will not linger as long as the tobacco debate, which was settled only a decade ago.

Meanwhile, the use of marihuana, especially by adolescents, has been spreading exponentially in countries where it was nearly unknown 20 years ago (see figure on the following page). It even seems possible that some countries are prepared to give a new legal status to this drug, thereby eliminating the social stigma attached to its use: Marihuana would no longer be considered a "stupefying drug," like opium or coca leaf derivatives, the Single Convention Treaty on Stupefying Drugs would be bypassed, and marihuana products would be made commercially available.

It is against this background that the Helsinki Symposium on Marihuana, which is recorded in this monograph, was organized under the aegis of the Sixth International Congress of Pharmacology. This symposium was called to discuss the biochemical and cellular effects of marihuana products in the general perspective of their long-term use.

Following the work of Agurell, Paton, Lemberger, and Axelrod, investigators established that the fat-soluble cannabinoids remain in tissues for days and weeks. However, routine pharmacological studies

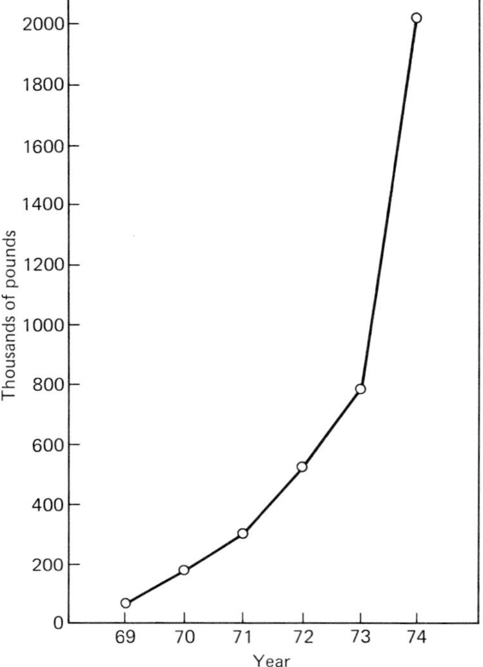

Removals of marihuana by USA federal authorities (domestic and foreign cooperative). (In order to roughly estimate the amounts consumed, the amounts removed are usually multiplied by six.)

From "Hearings of the U.S. Senate Committee on the Judiciary (Subcommittee on Internal Security): Marihuana-Hashish Epidemic, Part II, The Continuing Escalation, May 8, 1975," U.S. Government Printing Office, Washington, D.C., 1975.

then indicated that accumulation of these foreign molecules did not seem to affect permanently any of the vital functions over weeks and months as "tolerance" to their use developed.

At the same time, studies by several cell biologists were published in close succession: Zimmerman, the Leuchtenbergers, Jakubovic, McGeer, Succiu-Foca, Armand, Nahas, and Morishima all had independently investigated the effects of marihuana products on cellular anabolism and cell division. A common conclusion emerged from their studies, which employed widely different models: cannabinoids in concentrations of 10^{-6} to 10^{-4} M inhibit the synthesis of DNA, RNA, and proteins in replicating eukaryote cells. Mechoulam's Δ^9-THC and all natural cannabinoids tested—whether psychoactive or not—as well as their metabolites which accumulated in tissues, inhibited cell anabolism.

These *in vitro* observations were confirmed *in vivo* by Rosenkranz: Rodents given marihuana by ingestion or by inhalation exhibited impairment of growth, spermatogenesis, and the immunity system.

A number of investigators reported the inhibitory effect of marihuana in man on pulmonary macrophages, lymphocyte function, and sperm production.

Although these results await additional confirmation, all of the present experimental evidence tends to corroborate the early *in vitro* observations which reported an impairment of cellular anabolism by cannabinoids.

Only longitudinal epidemiological studies of marihuana-smoking populations may document the pathologic effects of long-term cannabis usage. To my knowledge the literature does not contain a single autopsy report on a long-term chronic marihuana smoker. Therefore the human pathology of marihuana cannot be written before two or three decades. (It took sixty years for investigators to establish the pathology of tobacco smoking.) Meanwhile, on the basis of their present short-term observations and past experience with other drugs, biologists and physicians can only make certain predictions about what this pathology might be.

The papers contained in this monograph, inasmuch as they describe some of the interactions between the biologically active molecules contained in marihuana and the basic components and processes of living cells, might help the biologist and the physician assess the long-term effects of marihuana use on reproduction, embryological development, learning, and growth, as well as on the integrity of physiological functions.

Gabriel G. Nahas
Helsinki, July 1975

Participants/Contributors

S. AGURELL, Department of Pharmocology, University of Uppsala, and Astra Läkemedel, Södertälje, Sweden

A. BARTOVA, Department of Psychiatry, Allen Memorial Institute of Psychiatry, McGill University, Montreal, Canada

J. S. BECKNER, Department of Pharmacology, Medical College of Virginia, Richmond, Virginia

M. BINDER, Institute of Physiological Chemistry, Ruhr-University, Bochum, Germany

M. K. BIRMINGHAM, Department of Biochemistry, Allen Memorial Institute of Psychiatry, McGill University, Montreal, Quebec, Canada

R. D. BLEVINS, Department of Health Sciences, East Tennessee University, Johnson City, Tennessee

R. BOURDON, School of Pharmacy, Université René Descartes, Paris, France

P. BRACHET, Unité de Génétique Moléculaire, Département de Biologie Moléculaire, Institut Pasteur, Paris, France

S. BRAM, Unité de Génétique Moléculaire, Département de Biologie Moléculaire, Institut Pasteur, Paris, France

M. BRAUDE, National Institute on Drug Abuse, Rockville, Maryland

D. R. BRINE, Department of Chemistry and Life Sciences, Research Triangle Institute, Research Triangle Park, North Carolina

R. CAPEK, Department of Pharmacology and Therapeutics, McGill University, Montreal, Quebec, Canada

R. A. CARCHMAN, Department of Pharmacology, Medical College of Virginia, Virginia Commonwealth University, Richmond, Virginia

A. CHARI-BITRON, Department of Biochemistry, Israel Institute for Biological Research, Tel-Aviv University Medical School, Ness-Ziona, Israel

J. CHILOW, Division of Narcotic Drugs, United Nations, Geneva, Switzerland

T. L. CHRUSCIEL, Mental Health Office, World Health Organization, Geneva, Switzerland

J. DALLMER, Department of Pharmacology, University of Copenhagen, Copenhagen, Denmark

K. H. DAVIS, Department of Psychiatry, University of North Carolina, Chapel Hill, North Carolina

B. DESOIZE, Department of Anesthesiology, Columbia University, New

York City, New York, and Unité de Toxicologie Expérimentale, Institut National de la Santé et de la Recherche Médicale, Hôpital Fernand Widal, Paris, France

W. L. DEWEY, Department of Pharmacology, Medical College of Virginia, Virginia Commonwealth University, Richmond, Virginia

E. DOMINO, Department of Pharmacology, University of Michigan, Ann Arbor, Michigan

G. ERDMAN, Max-Planck-Institut für Hirnforschung, Frankfurt, West Germany

B. ESPLIN, Department of Pharmacology and Therapeutics, McGill University, Montreal, Quebec, Canada

V. S. ESTEVEZ, Texas Research Institute of Mental Sciences, Houston, Texas

K. A. FEHR, Department of Pharmacology, University of Toronto, Toronto, Ontario, Canada

K. FONSEKA, Biomedical Center, Uppsala University, Uppsala, Sweden

E. FOURNIER, Unité de Toxicologie Expérimentale, Institut National de la Santé et de la Recherche Médicale, Hôpital Fernand Widal, Paris, France

A. L. GOUGH, School of Pharmacology, University of Bradford, Bradford, Great Britain

J. R. GRAHAM, Queen Elizabeth Hospital, Woodville, South Australia

R. N. GROVE, Department of Pharmacology, Faculty of Medicine, Laval University, Quebec City, Quebec, Canada

K. W. HADLEY, Research Institute of Pharmaceutical Sciences, University of Mississippi, Mississippi

R. D. HARBISON, Department of Pharmacology and Biochemistry, Vanderbilt University, Nashville, Tennessee

N. HARDY, Unité de Toxicologie Expérimentale, Institut National de la Santé et de la Recherche Médicale, Hôpital Fernand Widal, Paris, France

L. S. HARRIS, Department of Pharmacology, Medical College of Virginia, Virginia Commonwealth University, Richmond, Virginia

J. HARTELIUS, Karolinska Institute, Stockholm, Sweden

D. J. HARVEY, Department of Pharmacology, University of Oxford, Oxford, England

R. G. HEATH, Department of Psychiatry and Neurology, Tulane University, New Orleans, Louisiana

W. HEMBREE III, Departments of Medicine, and Obstetrics–Gynecology, College of Physicians and Suregons, Columbia University, New York City, New York

R. HENRICH, Department of Pediatrics, Columbia University, New York City, New York

B. HO, Department of Neurochemistry and Neuropharmacology, Texas Research Institute for Mental Sciences, Houston, Texas

L. E. HOLLISTER, Veterans Administration Hospital, Palo Alto, California

J. F. HOWES, Department of Pharmacology, Sharps Associates, Cambridge, Massachusetts

J. HSU, Department of Anesthesiology, Columbia University, New York City, New York

J. HUOT, Department of Pharmacology, Université Laval, Quebec City, Quebec, Canada

S. HUSAIN, Stanford Research Institute, Menlo Park, California

J. IDÄNPÄÄN-HEIKKILÄ, National Board of Health, Helsinki, Finland

M. ISSIDORIDES, Department of Psychiatry, University of Athens, Athens, Greece

A. JAKUBOVIC, Department of Psychiatry, Kinsmen Laboratory of Neurological Research, University of British Columbia, Vancouver, B.C., Canada

K. M. JOHNSON, Department of Pharmacology, Medical College of Virginia, Virginia Commonwealth University, Richmond, Virginia

S. JOU, Department of Pediatrics, Columbia University, New York City, New York

W. JUST, Max-Planck Institute für Hirnforschung, Frankfurt, West Germany

H. KALANT, Department of Pharmacology, University of Toronto, Toronto, Ontario, Canada

S. KAYMAKCALAN, Tip Fakultesi, Pharmacological Institute, Ankara, Turkey

T. A. KEPHALAS, Department of Biological Chemistry, University of Athens, Athens, Greece

J. KIBURIS, Department of Physiological Chemistry, University of Athens, Athens, Greece

G. L. KIMMEL, Department of Psychiatry, University of North Carolina, Chapel Hill, North Carolina

L. J. KING, Department of Biochemistry, University of Surrey, Guildford, United Kingdom

G. V. KNOX, Department of Pharmacology, University of Toronto, Toronto, Ontario, Canada

N. LANDER, Hebrew University Pharmacy School, Jerusalem, Israel

K. LEANDER, Astra Läkemedel, Södertälje, Sweden

A. E. LeBLANC, Department of Pharmacology, University of Toronto, and Alcoholism and Drug Addiction Research Foundation, Toronto, Ontario, Canada

L. LEMBERGER, Department of Clinical Pharmacology, Lilly Laboratories for Clinical Research, and Departments of Pharmacology and Medicine, Indiana University School of Medicine, Indianapolis, Indiana

C. LEUCHTENBERGER, Department of Cytochemistry, Swiss Institute for Experimental Cancer Research, Lausanne, Switzerland

R. LEUCHTENBERGER, Department of Cytochemistry, Swiss Institute for Experimental Cancer Research, Lausanne, Switzerland

S. LEVY, School of Pharmacy, Hebrew University, Jerusalem, Israel

J. E. LINDGREN, Astra Läkemedel, Södertälje, Sweden

F. MAGNAN, Department of Pharmacology, Laval University, Quebec City, Quebec, Canada

B. MANTILLA-PLATA, Department of Pharmacology, Vanderbilt University, Nashville, Tennessee

V. MARKS, Department of Biochemistry, University of Surrey, Guildford, England

B. MARTIN, Department of Pharmacy, Biomedical Center, University of Uppsala, Uppsala, Sweden

B. R. MARTIN, Department of Pharmacology, Medical College of Virginia, Virginia Commonwealth University, Richmond, Virginia

D. MARTIN, United States Senate Subcommittee on Internal Security, Washington, D.C.

T. MAUGH, American Association for the Advancement of Science, Washington, D.C.

N. McCALLUM, Hebrew University Pharmacy School, Jerusalem, Israel

P. L. McGEER, Department of Psychiatry, University of British Columbia, Vancouver, Canada

R. MECHOULAM, Department of Natural Products, School of Pharmacy, Hebrew University, Jerusalem, Israel

A. MELLORS, Department of Chemistry, University of Guelph, Ontario, Canada

C. M. MICHAEL, Department of Biological Chemistry, University of Athens, Athens, Greece

C. MIRAS, Department of Biochemistry, University of Athens, Athens, Greece

A. MORISHIMA, Department of Pediatrics, Columbia University, New York City, New York

G. NAHAS, Department of Anesthesiology, College of Physicians and Surgeons, Columbia University, New York City, New York, and Institut National de la Santé et de la Recherche Médicale, Paris, France

I. M. NILSSON, Astra Läkemedel, Södertälje, Sweden

I. NIR, Department of Applied Pharmacology, School of Pharmacy, Hebrew University, Jerusalem, Israel

M. NORDQVIST, Biomedical Center, University of Uppsala, Uppsala, Sweden

A. OHLSSON, Astra Läkemedel, Södertälje, Sweden

H. OKSANEN, Mantypaadentie, Helsinki, Finland

J. E. OLLEY, University of Bradford, Bradford, England

P. F. OSGOOD, Department of Pharmacology, Sharps Associates, Cambridge, Massachusetts

D. P. PAPADAKIS, Department of Biological Chemistry, University of Athens, Athens, Greece

K. J. PARKS, Department of Obstetrics and Gynecology, University of Utah Medical Center, Salt Lake City, Utah

W. D. M. PATON, Department of Pharmacology, University of Oxford, Oxford, England

M. PEREZ-REYES, Department of Psychiatry, School of Medicine, University of North Carolina, Chapel Hill, North Carolina

S. RADUCO-THOMAS, Department of Pharmacology, Universite Laval, Quebec City, Quebec, Canada

J. D. REGAN, Biology Division, Oak Ridge National Laboratory, Oak Ridge, Tennessee

S. ROSELL, Department of Pharmacology, Karolinska Institute, Stockholm, and Department of Pharmacy, University of Uppsala, Uppsala, Sweden

E. ROSENBERG, Unité de Toxicologie Expérimentale, Institut National de la Santé et de la Recherche Médicale, Hôpital Fernand Widal, Paris, France

J. ROSENFELD, Department of Pathology, McMaster University, Hamilton, Ontario, Canada

H. ROSENKRANZ, Department of Biology, Clark University and the Mason Research Institute, Worcester, Massachusetts

C. A. SALEMINK, Department of Organic Chemistry, State University of Utrecht, Utrecht, Netherlands

F. SANDBERG, Biomedical Center, University of Uppsala, Uppsala, Sweden

E. SCHLEH, Department of Cytochemistry, Swiss Institute for Experimental Cancer Research, Lausanne, Switzerland

J. C. SCHOOLAR, Texas Research Institute of Mental Sciences, Houston, Texas

J. SCHOU, Department of Pharmacology, University of Copenhagen, Copenhagen, Denmark

J. SIMMONS, Department of Psychiatry, University of North Carolina, Chapel Hill, North Carolina

C. STEFANIS, Department of Psychiatry, University of Athens, Greece

P. R. SRINIVASAN, Department of Biochemistry, College of Physicians and Surgeons, Columbia University, New York City, New York

M. A. STENCHEVER, Department of Obstetrics and Gynecology, University of Utah Medical Center, Salt Lake City, Utah

M. R. STENCHEVER, Department of Obstetrics and Gynecology, University of Utah Medical Center, Salt Lake City, Utah

C. STEFANIS, Department of Psychiatry, Athens University Medical School, Athens, Greece

J. D. TEALE, Department of Biochemistry, University of Surrey, Guildford, United Kingdom

M. TEN HAM, National Institute of Public Health, Utrecht, Netherlands.

S. THEL, Max-Planck-Institut für Hirnforschung, Frankfurt, West Germany

G. TOPP, Department of Pharmacology, University of Copenhagen, Copenhagen, Denmark

C. E. TURNER, School of Pharmacy, University of Mississippi, Oxford, Mississippi

VAN NOORDWUK, National Institute of Public Health, Utrecht, Netherlands

M. WALL, Department of Chemistry and Life Sciences, Research Triangle Institute, Research Triangle Park, North Carolina

C. WALLER, School of Pharmacy, University of Mississippi, Oxford, Mississippi

W. WARNER, Department of Pharmacology, Medical College of Virginia, Virginia Commonwealth University, Richmond, Virginia

G. WERNER, Max-Planck-Institut für Hirnforschung, Frankfurt, West Germany

A. C. WHITE, Department of Pharmacology, Medical College of Virginia, Virginia Commonwealth University, Richmond, Virginia

M. WIDMAN, Biomedical Center, University of Uppsala, Uppsala, Sweden

M. WEICHMANN, Max-Planck-Institut für Hirnforschung, Frankfurt, West Germany

J. ZBINDEN, Department of Cytochemistry, Swiss Institute for Experimental Cancer Research, Lausanne, Switzerland

P. ZEIDENBERG, Department of Psychiatry, College of Physicians and Surgeons, Columbia University, New York City, New York

A. M. ZIMMERMAN, Department of Zoology, University of Toronto, Toronto, Canada

S. B. ZIMMERMAN, Glendon College, York University, Toronto, Canada

Contents

II

Marihuana: Biochemical and Cellular Effects

Interactions with Neurotransmitters

II

Marihuana: Biochemical and Cellular Effects

Organic and Developmental Effects

I

Marihuana Chemistry

Detection and Identification of Cannabinoids and Their Metabolites

1

Cannabinoid Chemistry: An Overview

R. MECHOULAM, N. MCCALLUM, S. LEVY,
AND N. LANDER

Every now and then we should reevaluate our scientific efforts: Are we doing more of the same? Is our work still relevant to the problem? Are we just mopping up or are we trying to open new vistas? In cannabinoid research, such a reevaluation is particularly important in view of the concerted efforts by numerous groups.

We shall try to analyze the situation in several areas of cannabinoid research. Some of our views may be somewhat radical; we hope that they may generate a dialog and thus help clarify the relevant problems and aims of research.

Isolation and Elucidation of the Structures of New Natural Cannabinoids

Thirty-seven cannabinoids have been isolated so far from the plant *Cannabis sativa* or its preparations (marihuana, hashish, etc.) [8,21,23]. This number excludes the metabolites and the pyrolysis products formed during smoking.

Is it worthwhile initiating new projects aimed at isolating additional natural cannabinoids? We are skeptical on this point. One may be able to isolate a few new variations on an old theme: a new methyl ether of a cannabinoid with a propyl side; the carboxylic acid derivatives of the "methyl" cannabinoids—cannabiorcol, cannabidiorcol, etc. Will these new components add to our understanding or just to our catalogs?

On the other hand, dimeric, trimeric, and polymeric cannabinoids are barely known, although they undoubtedly exist [31] in the yet uninvestigated "polymeric" fraction remaining as a residue after the extraction of hashish or marihuana with various solvents. On extraction with most solvents (petroleum ether, chloroform), some "polymeric" material is invariably taken up. By analogy to other related natural products, such as tanins, cannabinoids, which possess

Marihuana: Chemistry, Biochemistry, and Cellular Effects, edited by Gabriel G. Nahas,

carboxylic and phenolic groups, can be expected to form dimeric or higher polymeric structures. These may be of interest not only as such, but may be relevant to cannabis activity, as on smoking they will be expected to form (at least in part) potentially active monomers.

Noncannabinoid Constituents in Cannabis Sativa

Every plant contains hundreds of secondary constituents. If one tries hard enough, one can isolate many of these; triterpenes and steroids, carbohydrates and cyclitols, phenols, carboxylic acids, alkanes, monoterpenes, sesquiterpenes, alkaloids, amines, and other constituents have been isolated and identified [23]. It is doubtful whether these compounds are of any significance to cannabinoid activity [4]. We consider any further work specifically aimed at isolating additional noncannabinoid components of cannabis not of major interest. However, if some of the various pharmacological activities of cannabis cannot be accounted for by the activity of the cannabinoids (alone or together), it may be worthwhile to look for additional substances. Such an investigation should be closely monitored by pharmacological tests. Otherwise, the final result may be again a catalog of unexciting molecules.

From a chemical (rather than a pharmacological) viewpoint, it may be of interest to continue investigating the alkaloids in *C. sativa,* as they may yield novel structures. Many botanical families contain specific alkaloid types; until now the Cannabinaceae have not been thoroughly investigated.

Cannabinoids in Cannabis Smoke

Most of the work reported has indicated that Δ^1-tetrahydrocannabinol (Δ^1-THC) goes into the body as such, although part of it is destroyed on smoking or forms cannabinol ([15,21]; Kinzer *et al.* found an unknown material with a GLC RT equal to that of Δ^1-THC. It is probably cannabielsoin, a product of the oxidative cyclization of cannabidiol [16,29]). Cannabidiol is apparently converted in part to new compounds (such as cannabielsoin [16,29]; see Figure 1.1); however, most of the material enters the body unchanged. Cannabielsoin is inactive in the "ring test" for CNS ac-

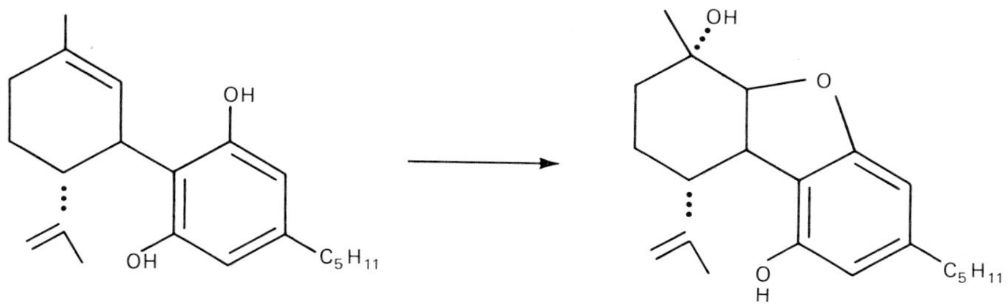

Figure 1.1. Conversion of cannabidiol.

tivity up to 10 mg/kg in mice (Segal, M., S. Dikstein, and R. Mechoulam, unpublished data).

Little is known about the fate of cannabichromene and other constituents on smoking. Hence, it should be of considerable interest to continue work in this area. Unfortunately, it is not simple to reproduce exactly human smoking conditions. Although most groups working in the field consider their own smoking experiments to be relevant to actual smoking, it is difficult to establish this point beyond doubt.

Syntheses of natural plant cannabinoids

This field was extremely active during the late 1960s, but interest has waned in the last few years [21,23]. The reason is simple: most cannabinoids are readily available by the methods fully described in the literature. Any further research is worthwhile only if a truly new route is investigated which may open a path to types of otherwise inaccessible cannabinoid analogs.

Syntheses of metabolites

Most known cannabinoid metabolites can be prepared rather simply [21,23]. Indeed, this simplicity of the synthetic approach makes it the method of choice for identifying new metabolites: the structure of a metabolite is tentatively suggested on the basis of a limited amount of information available (frequently only mass spectrum). The few most obvious structural possibilities are then synthesized, and the structure of the metabolite is unequivocally shown by direct comparison. In this manner recently 6α- and 6β-hydroxy-cannabidiol were shown to be metabolites of cannabidiol [17].

We achieved [18] a new high-yield synthesis of 7-OH-Δ^6-THC

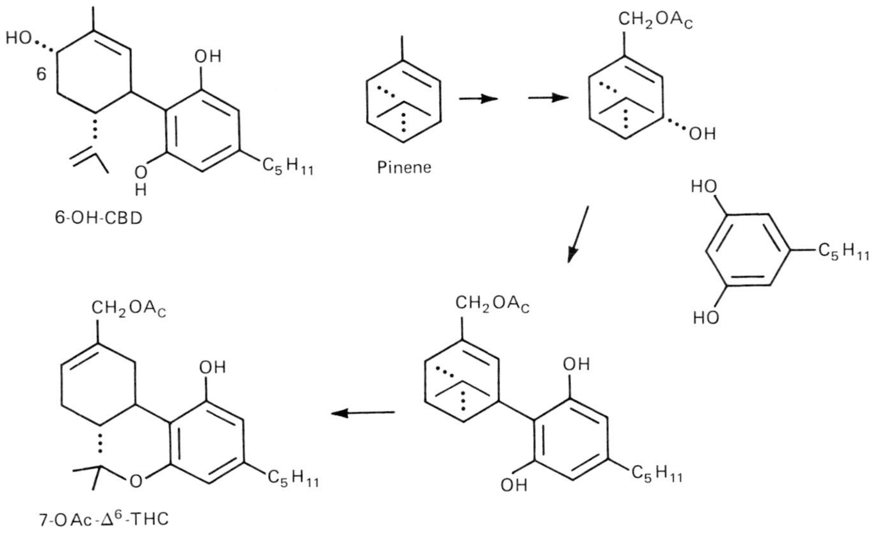

Figure 1.2. High-yield synthesis of 7-OH-Δ^6-THC.

(Figure 1.2). This synthesis may represent the method of choice for preparing this metabolite.

Novel routes leading to new types of labeled cannabinoids are of considerable importance and will undoubtedly be explored further.

Analytical Aspects of Cannabis Chemistry

Well-established chromatographic methods for analyzing and isolating the many cannabinoid and noncannabinoid constituents of *C. sativa* have served the natural product chemist well, but until recently pharmacologists, toxicologists, and forensic scientists have been severely handicapped by the lack of sufficiently sensitive and specific techniques. New developments have changed this situation, and we may expect to see further advances in these fields soon. Even the well-established chromatographic methods of thin-layer chromatography (TLC), gas-liquid chromatography (GLC), and column chromatography have been refined considerably, and the introduction of mass spectrometry (MS) has revolutionized recent investigations of the minor constituents of cannabis.

The identification and quantification of cannabinoids in plant material do not represent a major problem today; however, the quantification of cannabinoids in biological fluids is still of major importance, and because of the small amounts involved it has posed the biggest challenge.

Good resolution of cannabinoids by TLC is difficult to achieve because of their structural similarity, and only two types of thin-layer systems have been found to give good results. The first of these is based on modifying the absorbant properties of Silica Gel by the presence of bases (dimethylformamide or diethylamine) and elution with nonpolar solvents (cyclohexane for the former, and toluene for the latter; [2]), or pyridine, hexane, methanol (18:75:7) [26]. Silver nitrate has also been used to modify cannabinoid separations by Silica Gel to good effect. In this case silver nitrate can complex with molecular double bonds, and a good resolution can be achieved when the chromatogram is eluted with a solvent such as toluene [12]. Still, the most widely used method for detecting cannabinoids on these thin-layer chromatograms is spraying with a freshly prepared solution of di-*o*-anisidine tetrazolium chloride (fast blue salt B), which offers both excellent sensitivity of detection (to approximately 50 ng) and different color reactions for different components. The need for even more sensitive TLC techniques led to the method of Forrest *et al.* [7], in which the cannabinoids are converted to 1-dimethylaminonaphthalene sulfonates and separated by TLC. By virtue of their strong fluorescence under ultraviolet light, the compounds may be detected down to levels of 0.5 ng. These derivatives have also been found useful in high-pressure liquid chromatography; by this technique standard mixtures of cannabinoids were separated and detected with subnanogram sensitivity [1].

It is doubtful whether major advances can be expected by further development of TLC techniques.

Gas-liquid chromatography is the method of choice for rapid qualitative and quantitative identifications. A large variety of stationary phases have been found to provide excellent separations of the cannabinoids on packed columns, and the use of capillary columns has been found to improve separations by an order of magnitude. In the few reports on capillary column separation of cannabinoids, the separations achieved were little short of spectacular [8,24]. Capillary columns will probably be much more widely used in the next few years.

The development of more sensitive gas chromatographic techniques has also been the subject of considerable interest. Flame ionization detection, normally used with GLC, gives a maximum sensitivity of approximately 50 ng. The formation of trimethylsilyl derivatives increases the maximum sensitivity of detection to about 10 ng [27].

The use of electron capture detection for suitably derivatized cannabinoids has improved detection sensitivity. Schou *et al.* report that the use of chloroacetyl derivatives gives maximum sensitivities of approximately 0.04 ng, and later work successfully applied this to urinalysis [28]. Garrett and Hunt demonstrate a maximum sensitivity of detection of approximately 5 pg for Δ^1-THC pentafluorobenzoate [10], whereas 1 pg of Δ^1-THC heptafluorobutyrate can be detected when a capillary column and low-volume coaxial electron capture detector are used [6]. However, pentafluorobenzoates have been shown to give a greater sensitivity of detection than other phenol derivatives under identical conditions [6,19]. They should be considered as an alternative to heptafluorobutyrates. Working with these small amounts of compounds in biological extracts presents considerable problems for purification, which Fenimore *et al.* solved using a dual-column system [6]. The derivatized extract is first injected into a packed column, and at the appropriate retention time (RT) a small fraction of the eluent gas is trapped and subjected to further GLC on a capillary column. This appears to be an effective and relatively rapid clean-up procedure which could be applied to many other toxicological and pharmacological problems.

Even the development of such a sensitive technique does not ensure a successful method. At the low levels of detection needed (less than 2 ng/ml blood), many compounds in biological samples may interfere with the analysis, and to a large extent, these depend on the method of detection chosen. For example, the electron capture methods [6,10] detect all strongly electron-capturing compounds plus any others (e.g., having hydroxy or amino groups) extracted from the plasma and capable of reacting with the derivatizing agents used.

Analytical selectivity, then, is as big a problem as analytical sensitivity. For adequate selectivity, a preliminary purification is generally necessary before the final analysis. However, such a process can be costly in terms of time, material, and equipment.

To overcome the necessity of purification, McCallum has developed a method of analysis for phenols involving GLC with flame photometric detection of their phosphate esters [19]. The flame photometric detection of cannabinoids gives a maximum sensitivity of 0.5 ng per injection, which is not as good as electron capture detection. On the other hand, perfectly stable base line and sensitivity are obtained, and detection is so specific that preliminary clean-up procedures are unnecessary, so that analysis time is shortened considerably [19].

The mass fragmentometric method is one of high sensitivity and specificity. Agurell *et al.* report that a preliminary purification of the extract from human plasma by chromatography on Sephadex LH-20 provides adequate clean-up for subsequent quantification of the Δ^1-THC by mass fragmentometry [2]. Their method has been found suitable for measuring Δ^1-THC down to levels of 0.3 ng/ml when fragmentograms of the 299 and 314 mass fragments (at 50 eV) are used. Here mass fragmentometry provides what is in effect a highly specific GLC detector. The more mass fragments monitored, the more certain one can be that a peak at a given RT is the one of interest. On the other hand, the more of these minor fragments used, the less sensitive is the detection. Also, because many cannabinoids have common mass fragments, when analyzing blood of cannabis smokers with the method of Agurell *et al.,* one still has to be sure that the cannabinoid to be measured has a GLC retention time discrete from those of the other cannabinoids. Confirmatory analyses on another column are still advisable, especially when cannabis smoking rather than Δ^1-THC smoking is involved.

Rosenfeld *et al.* [25] have reported an MS method requiring no preliminary column purification. A factor limiting the sensitivity of the assay is a background corresponding to 300 pg of the internal standard. Further developments in this area are eagerly awaited.

Some of the major future advances seem to be in the field of immunoassay methods. A number of laboratories are indeed developing such assays, but as yet none of the methods can be applied to the quantification of Δ^1-THC in human plasma. One method [30] is reported to have a detection limit of 5 ng/ml. It is capable of analyzing for the cannabinoids as a group and could thus provide the basis for a facile screening procedure. Another method (detection limit 25–50 ng/ml) can be used to estimate cannabinoids in chronic marihuana users, but probably not in occasional users [13]. Cais *et al.* [5] have developed a free-radical immunoassay (comparable to the one available for morphine). Preliminary free-radical immunoassay experiments with extracts from human urines collected from both casual and habitual hashish smokers indicate a positive, significant increase in the ESR signal. The sensitivity of this method does not seem to be high enough to allow direct screening of urine samples rather than extracts. Further work in this direction is certainly indicated.

Metabolites and Metabolism

Through the concerted efforts of many groups in the United States, Sweden, England, Switzerland, and Israel, metabolites of Δ^1- and Δ^6-THC, cannabidiol, and cannabinol have been isolated and identified *in vitro,* as well as in many species including man [21,23]. Exact quantification is as yet missing in most cases, but the picture seems to be more or less complete: the cannabinoid is first oxygenated to an alcohol (allylic or on the side chain); further oxidation leads to formation of acids, which may also contain additional hydroxyl groups in various positions of the molecule [3,22]. There are also variations on this theme, such as dehydrogenation of Δ^1- or Δ^6-THC to cannabinol [20]. Further metabolites will certainly continue to be identified. As mentioned above, it is doubtful whether a major effort toward this goal is really worthwhile.

We believe that the chemical trends in this area will be in three major directions. The first is determination of the ultimate fate of metabolites, i.e., isolation and elucidation of the structure of the cannabinoid "conjugates" present in urine and possibly in blood.

Most of the cannabinoid metabolites seem to be excreted as water-soluble metabolites, which apparently are not only (if at all) glucuronides or sulfates; they may be mostly amides of amino acids [3]. In this respect they may resemble the "bile salts" (amides of bile acids with amino acids or taurine). These are metabolites of the bile acids, a group of natural steroids which resemble in their lipid solubility and general chemical nature (planarity of molecule, molecular weight) the THC acids.

We have synthesized several of the simplest possible "cannabis salts" (Figure 1.3), and these are being compared by Agurell with the natural conjugates.

The second chemical trend we predict is quantification of and rate studies on metabolites and natural products in body fluids and in body tissues.

Very few data are available on the exact amounts and ratios of the various natural cannabinoids and metabolites present at a given time in blood, urine, or tissues [14]. This information is necessary if we want to discuss intelligently the problem of the magnitude of the binding of the active substances to the "active site." The modifications of THC action by other cannabinoids (or drugs) cannot be explained (and hence channeled into a desired direction) if these basic quantitative data are missing. As Gillette [11] has pointed out, "the magnitude of covalent binding [of drugs to body tissues] depends on the rate of formation of the reactive metabolite,

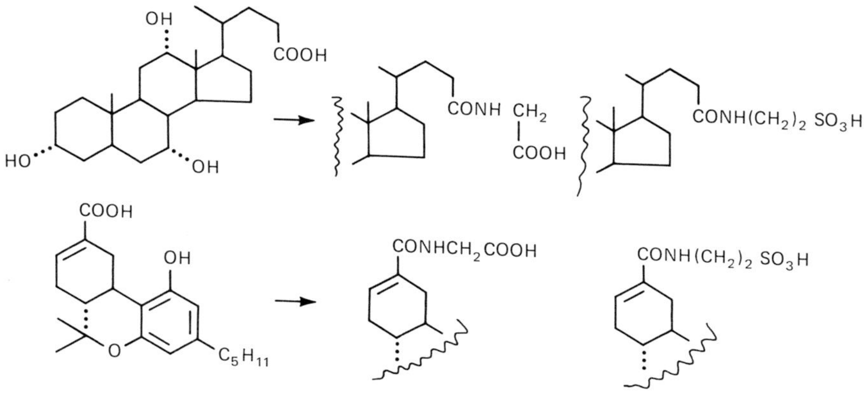

Figure 1.3. Synthesis of "cannabis conjugates."

on the rate at which the parent drug is eliminated from the body by other processes, on the rate at which the reactive metabolite is covalently bound, and on the rate at which it is inactivated by other processes."

The third chemical trend will probably be identification of the "target macromolecules" with which cannabinoids and metabolites combine.

In recent years major advances have been reported on the binding of morphine to a natural receptor. This research and the recent identification of a natural "pain killer" in the brain have opened the way to an understanding of the molecular basis of opiate action.

Do "cannabis receptors" exist? In view of the high stereochemical specificity of THC, one is inclined to accept such a possibility tentatively. No work in this direction has yet been reported with any cannabinoid. We expect this area to be fruitful.

We have tried to indicate those directions in which it is worthwhile to spend more of our efforts as well as those where, in our opinion, the law of diminishing returns is in force. Nevertheless, new discoveries or new ideas may change the whole picture.

REFERENCES

1. Abbott, S. R., A. Abu-Shymays, K. O. Loeffler, and I. S. Forrest (1975) High pressure liquid chromatography of cannabinoids as their fluorescent dansyl derivatives. *Res. Commun. Chem. Pathol. Pharmacol. 10:*9.
2. Agurell, S., B. Gustafsson, B. Holmstedt, K. Leander, J. Lindgren, I. M. Nilsson, F. Sandberg, and M. Asberg (1973) Quantitation of

Δ^1-tetrahydrocannabinol in plasma from cannabis smokers. *J. Pharm. Pharmacol. 25:*554.

3. Burstein, S., J. Rosenfeld, and T. Wittstruck (1972) Isolation and characterization of two major urinary metabolites of Δ^1-tetrahydrocannabinol. *Science 176:*422.
4. Burstein, S., C. Varanelli, and L. T. Slade (1975) Prostaglandins and cannabis. III. Inhibition of biosynthesis by essential oil components of marihuana. *Biochem. Pharmacol. 24:*1053.
5. Cais, M., S. Dani, Y. Josephy, A. Modiano, L. Snarsky, H. Gershon, and R. Mechoulam (1975) A free-radical immunoassay for cannabinoid metabolites. *FEBS Lett. 55:*257.
6. Fenimore, D. C., R. R. Freeman, and P. R. Loy (1973) Determination of Δ^9-tetrahydrocannabinol in blood by electron capture gas chromatography. Anal. Chem. *45:*2331.
7. Forrest, I. S., D. E. Green, S. D. Rose, G. C. Skinner, and D. M. Torres (1971) Fluorescent-labelled cannabinoids. *Res. Commun. Chem. Pathol. Pharmacol. 2:*787.
8. Friedrich-Fiechtl, J. and G. Spiteller (1975) Neue cannabinoide. *Tetrahedron 31:*479.
9. Galanter, M., H. Weingartner, F. B. Vaughan, W. T. Roth, and R. J. Wyatt (1973) Δ^9-Trans-tetrahydrocannabinol and natural marihuana. The controlled comparison. *Arch. Gen. Psychiatry 28:*278.
10. Garrett, E. R. and C. A. Hunt (1973) Picogram analysis of tetrahydrocannabinol and its application to biological fluids. *J. Pharm. Sci. 62:*1211.
11. Gillette, J. R. (1975) Formation of reactive drug metabolites as a basis of drug action and toxicity. Abstracts, The 25th IUPAC Congress, Jerusalem, p. 217.
12. Grlić L. (1970) A simple thin-layer chromatography of cannabinoids by means of silica gel sheets treated with amines. *J. Chromatogr. 48:*562.
13. Gross, S. J., J. R. Soares, S. L. R. Wong, and R. E. Schuster (1974) Marihuana metabolites measured by a radioimmune technique. *Nature 252:*581.
14. Jones, G., R. G. Pertwee, E. W. Gill, W. D. M. Paton, I. M. Nilsson, M. Widman, and S. Agurell (1974) Relative pharmacological potency in mice of optical isomers of Δ^1-tetrahydrocannabinol. *Biochem. Pharmacol. 23:*439.
15. Kinzer, G. W., R. L. Foltz, R. I. Mitchell, and E. B. Truit (1974) The fate of the cannabinoid components of marihuana during smoking. *Bull. Narc. 26*(3):41.
16. Küppers, F. J. E. M., C. A. L. Bercht, C. A. Salemink, R. J. J. Ch. Lousberg, J. K. Terlouw, and W. Heerma (1976) Pyrolysis of cannabidiol. Structure elucidation of four pyrolytic products. *Tetrahedron. 31:*15–13.
17. Lander, N., Z. Ben-Zvi, R. Mechoulam, B. Martin, M. Nordqvist, and S. Agurell (1976) Total syntheses of cannabidiol and Δ^1-tetrahydrocannabinol metabolites. *J. Chem. Soc. Perkin I 8.*
18. Lander, N. (1976) The synthesis of new monoterpenes and their use in the synthesis of cannabinoid metabolites. Ph.D. Thesis, Jerusalem: Hebrew University.

2

Detection and Identification of Compounds in Cannabis

COY W. WALLER, KATHY W. HADLEY, AND CARLTON E. TURNER

The discussion in this chapter is restricted to three categories:

1. basic analytical developments applicable to synthetic cannabinoids and extracts from cannabis preparations;
2. application of electron voltage–mass fragment graphs as a potential tool in identifying cannabinoids and their metabolites in body fluids and fermentation processes;
3. new alkaloids that have been isolated and identified from *C. sativa* L.

Gas-liquid Chromatography Methodology

Chemical analytical data obtained from preparations are routinely reported as dry weight analyses determined by gas-liquid chromatography (GLC). When needed, thin-layer chromatography (TLC) and gas-liquid chromatography–mass spectrometry (GLC–MS) are used as supportive analytical tools.

Since the basic GLC procedure recommended by a working group sponsored by the United Nations [12] was developed in our laboratories, we will discuss this procedure first and then detail the recent advancements in quantitating the cannabinoids.

GLC analysis

The extraction procedure is basically that described by Lerner [8] with minor modifications [13,14]. Three 1-gm samples are extracted simultaneously with 40 ml of spectrograde chloroform. The resulting solutions are allowed to sit at an ambient temperature without agitation for 1 hr; the marc (plant material, hashish, etc.) is then removed by filtration, and the filtrate concentrated *in vacuo* at an ambient temperature to a greenish paste void of solvent.

At this point, 1.5 ml of an ethanolic solution containing 10 mg/ml of androst-4-ene-3,17-dione[1] is added as the internal standard. Continuous vibration from an ultrasonic vibrator is then applied until all resin is in solution. Usually, 15 mg of the internal standard is adequate. Routinely, 0.2 μl of the resulting solution is injected with 0.2 μl of ethanol as a flush solvent. In our laboratories, this method provides excellent results [15]. A dilute sample must be prepared by adding 11 parts alcohol to 1 part extract when an automatic sampler is used. The inject volume must also be increased to 0.5 μl. No detector overload has been observed at this inject volume with the dilute sample.

Analyses are performed using Beckman (GC-45, GC-72-5, GC-65) chromatographs equipped with hydrogen flame-ionization detectors and operated isothermally at 210°C. Inlet and detector temperatures are 240 and 260°C, respectively. Glass columns, 0.64 cm OD and 2 mm ID by 2.43 meters packed with 2 percent OV-17 (high-purity polar phenylmethyl silicone; approximately 30,000 MW) on 100–120 mesh Chromosorb WHP are used. Nitrogen is the carrier gas at a flow rate of 10–30 ml/min, depending upon separation and instrument requirements. Head pressure is usually between 26 and 40 psi.

Peak area measurements are made with a Digital PDP-8 computer. Peak area, measured in millivolts, is compared with peak area of the internal standard. Relative response factors obtained from synthetic and/or natural cannabinoids are prerequisites for reproducibility and accuracy.

Discussion of GLC column developments

Figure 2.1, a chromatogram of an Indian[2] variant grown in Mississippi, illustrates routine separations obtained with a 2 percent OV-17 column, which gives good analytical results for some cannabinoids. Propyl homologs in this variant and labeled on the chromatogram have been reported previously [5]. Cannabidivarin (CBDV) is adequately separated, but (-)-Δ^9-*trans*-tetrahydrocannabivarin (Δ^9-THCV) is located under the same peak as cannabicyclol (CBL). Cannabidiol (CBD) and cannabichromene (CBC) are also under a single peak. (-)-Δ^9-*Trans*-tetrahydrocannabinol (Δ^9-THC), cannabigerol (CBG), cannabinol (CBN), and C_{29} hydrocarbon are separated and can be quantitated. (-)-Δ^8-*Trans*-

[1] First used by Davis, K. H., N. H. Martin, C. G. Pitt, J. W. Wildes, and M. E. Wall (1970). *Lloydia, 33*(4):453–60.

[2] Seeds obtained from Dr. C. K. Atal of the Regional Research Lab., Jammutawi, India.

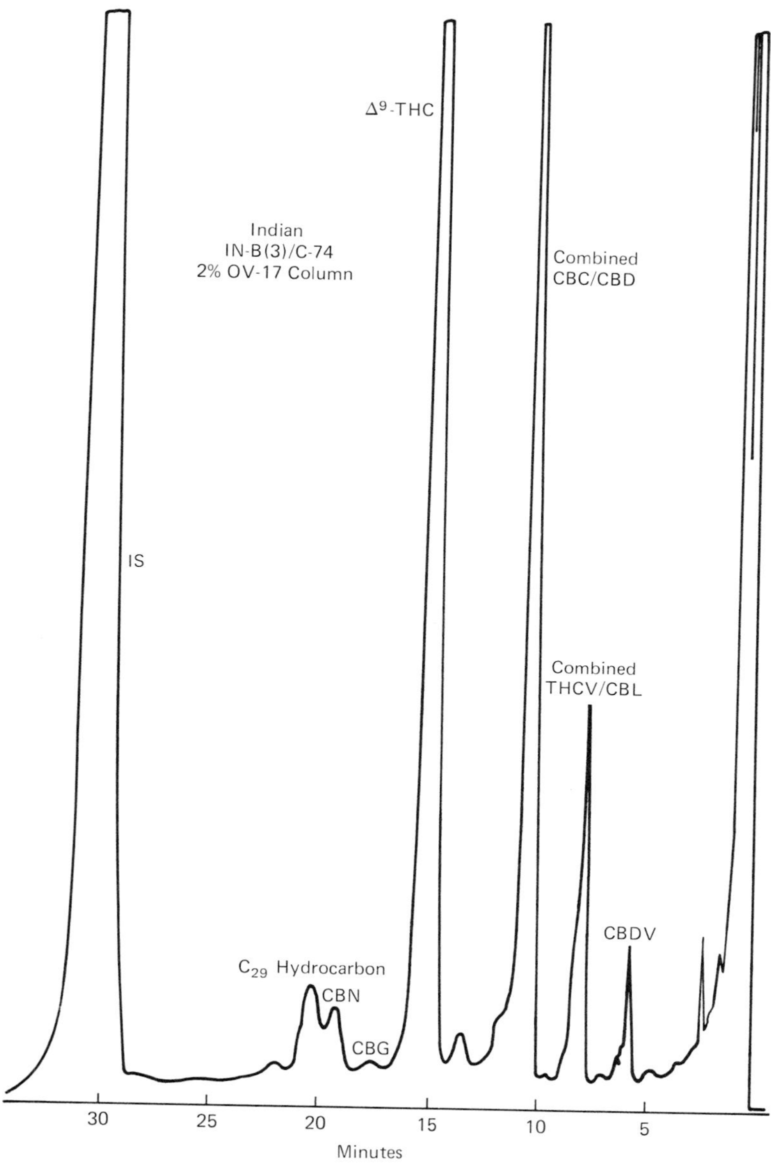

Figure 2.1. Chromatogram of an Indian variant. Column temperature was 210°C.

Table 2.1 Relative retention times of underivatized cannabinoids and other components found in cannabis using the 2% OV-17 column

Olivetol	0.04
Dimethylether CBD (DMCBD)	0.15
Cannabidivarin (CBDV)	0.18
Monomethyl ether CBD (MMCBD)	0.21
Δ^9-Tetrahydrocannabivarin (Δ^9-THCV)	0.26
Cannabicyclol (CBL)	0.26
Methyl ether Δ^9-THC (M-Δ^9-THC)	0.30
Cannabichromene (CBC)	0.34
Cannabivarin (CBV)	0.34
Cannabidiol (CBD)	0.34
Hexahydrocannabinol (HHC)	0.37
Cannabigerol monomethyl ether (CBGM)	0.38
Methyl ether CBN (MCBN)	0.39
$\Delta^{9,11}$-Tetrahydrocannabinol (ETHC; $\Delta^{9,11}$-THC)	0.41
Δ^8-Tetrahydrocannabinol (Δ^8-THC)	0.44
Cannabielsoin (CBE)	0.48
Δ^9-Tetrahydrocannabinol (Δ^9-THC)	0.49
Cannabigerol (CBG)	0.57
Cannabinol (CBN)	0.63
C_{29} Hydrocarbon	0.67
Androst-4-ene-3,17-dione (Δ^4-dione)	1.00

tetrahydrocannabinol (Δ^8-THC) is not found in this sample, but the peak which appears just before Δ^9-THC at approximately 13.5 min and which has a relative RT of 0.42 is usually mislabeled Δ^8-THC. In fact, Δ^8-THC is probably an artifact since it is not present in fresh plant samples when good analytical techniques are used [16].

Although the 2 percent OV-17 column is adequate for certain cannabinoids, it does not separate CBD from CBC and Δ^9-THCV from CBL,[3] which presents some problems in pharmacological studies.

Recent works by Carlini and associates [7] and others [1] have shown interactions between cannabinoids in cannabis preparations. Thus, for detailed pharmacological studies, investigators needed a refined technique for separating and quantitating CBC and CBD as well as CBL and Δ^9-THCV. These problems were solved by using a silyl procedure [15]. In our laboratories, the silyl pro-

[3] See Table 2.1 for relative RTs of cannabinoids using the 2 percent OV-17 column.

cedure provides excellent reproducibility in quantitating all cannabinoids when responsible analytical procedures are followed. Cannabinoid acids can also be quantitated with this procedure [4,15]. (-)-Δ^9-*Trans*-tetrahydrocannabinolic acids A and B can be separated and quantitated using this procedure when the column temperature is 190°C [15]. Nevertheless, incomplete silylation because of insufficient reaction time, too weak a silylating reagent, and/or insufficient amounts of silylating reagent may diminish reproducibility. Response factors for all silyl derivatives are also needed for quantitation [16]. In view of these potential problems, our group investigated the possibility of developing a procedure for separating and quantitating CBC and CBD, and Δ^9-THCV and CBL without the potential problems of the silyl procedure.

Different GLC columns prepared with methyl silicone and phenylmethyl silicones as well as other liquid phases and operated isothermally between 200 and 250°C provided no separation of the desired cannabinoids (see Table 2.2). Column parameters reported in the literature for separating CBD and CBC were also investigated [2]. None gave positive results; but we discovered that when CBC was present under the peak routinely labeled CBD, a peak preceding the CBC + CBD peak representing CBL was almost always erroneously reported as CBC in the literature.

By experimenting with column temperatures and working between 180 and 200°C, we finally had some columns that did separate or began to separate CBC and CBD. Ultimately, the column of choice was one prepared from 6 percent OV-1 and operated at 180°C. This column affords a clear and concise separation of CBD and CBC, as can be seen in Figure 2.2. Also CBL and Δ^9-THCV are separated.

Thus, by using the 2 percent OV-17 column to obtain a dry weight analysis and employing the 6 percent OV-1 to obtain normalized analyses for CBD, CBC, CBL, and Δ^9-THCV, one can quantitate these cannabinoids routinely.

The 6 percent OV-1 column does, however, have some limitations. For example, a dry weight analysis is not easily accomplished since CBG, CBN, and the C_{29} hydrocarbon elute under the internal standard peak (see Figure 2.2). Although combining the OV-17 and OV-1 columns did eliminate negative factors associated with the silyl procedure, the prolonged analysis time (70 min per analysis) led us to continue our research and development program for a single column which would:

1. separate CBC and CBD;
2. separate Δ^9-THCV and CBL;

Table 2.2 GC columns and conditions for the separation of a mixture of cannabichromene and cannabidiol[a]

			Separation		
Liquid phase	*Percentage*	*Oven temp. (C)*	*No*	*Nq*[b]	*q*[c]
OV-1	3	180°		X	
OV-1	3	200°	X		
OV-1	6	180°			X
OV-1	6	200°	X		
OV-1	8	180°			X
OV-1	8	190°		X	
OV-3	3	180°			X
OV-7	3	180°		X	
OV-7	3	200°	X		
OV-7	6	180°		X	
OV-11	3	200°	X		
OV-17	2	180°	X		
OV-17	2	210°	X		
OV-17	3	180°	X		
OV-17	3	210°	X		
OV-17	5	250°[d]	X		
OV-17	5	210°	X		
OV-25	2	210°	X		
OV-25	2	210°	X		
QF-1	3	210°	X		

[a] The mixture can be natural and/or synthetic.

[b] Quantitation is possible using a GC-computer system.

[c] Quantitative without computer.

[d] 80–100 mesh and 4-mm ID 6-ft column used.

3. remove CBN, CBG, and the C_{29} hydrocarbon from under the I S peak;
4. provide reproducible results comparable with those of the combined 2 percent OV-17 and 6 percent OV-1 columns;
5. shorten analysis time.

6.5 Percent phenylmethyl silicone column

Since temperature was critical in separating CBD and CBC on the OV-1 column, several columns containing various phenyl to methyl silicone ratios were prepared and operated between 180 and 190°C. A 5 percent phenyl to methyl silicone ratio liquid phase at 4 percent on 100–120 mesh Gas Chrom Q provided most separations desired, but no base line separation between CBN and the

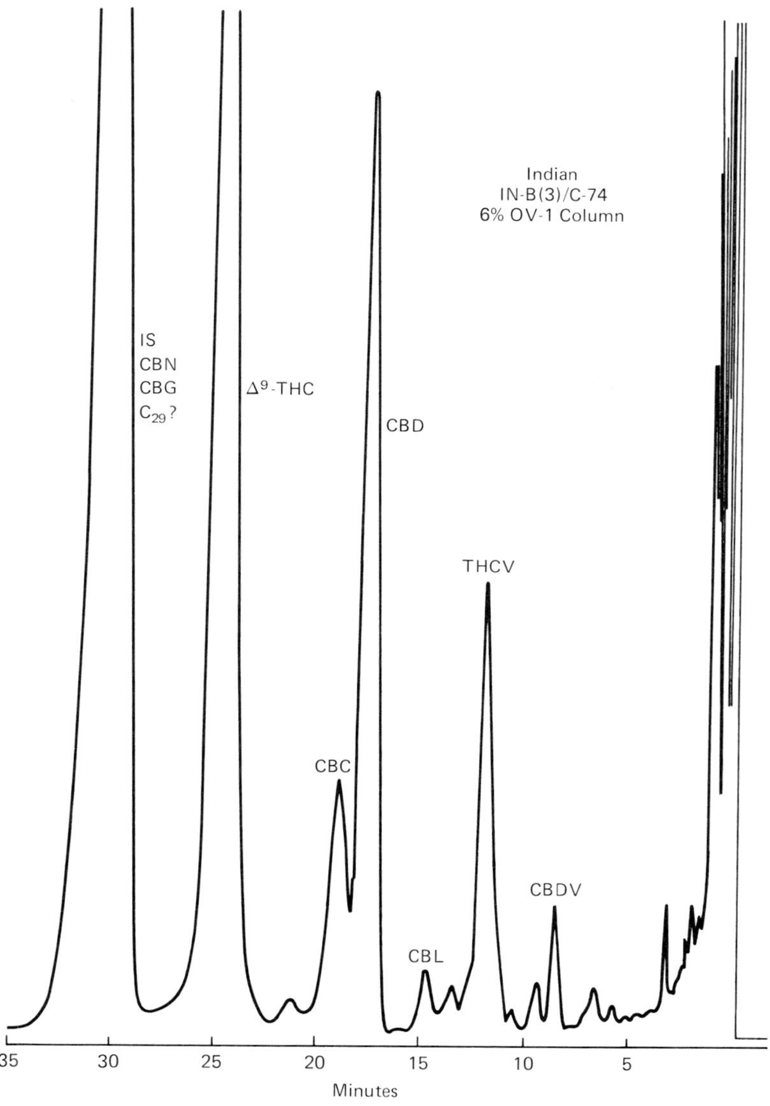

Figure 2.2. Chromatogram of the same Indian variant as shown in Figure 2.1 produced on the 6% OV-1 column at 180°C.

internal standard was obtained. Columns with nuances of polarity differences were then prepared. The polarity of a 6.5 percent phenyl to methyl silicone ratio column (4 percent on 100–120 Gas Chrom Q) ultimately provided acceptable and reproducible results (see Figure 2.3).

Figure 2.3. Chromatogram of the same Indian variant as shown in Figures 2.1 and 2.2 produced on a column at 190°C.

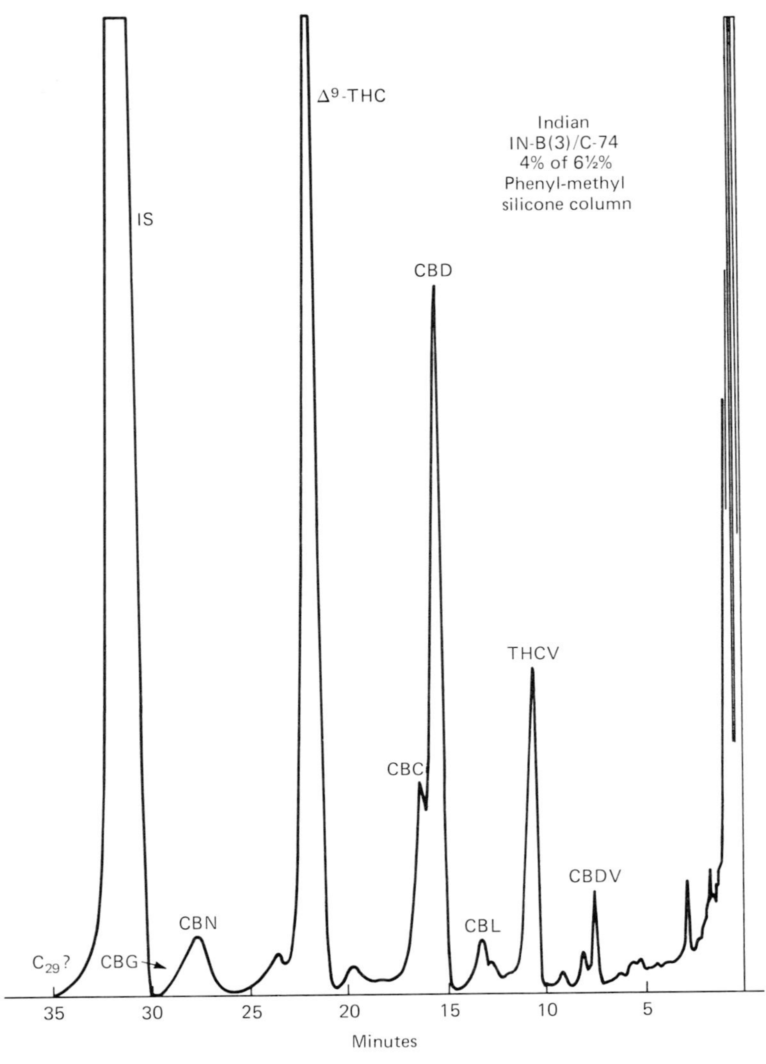

Table 2.3 Comparison of OV-1, OV-17, and 6.5% phenylmethyl columns

Sample	*Column*	*CBDV*	*THCV*	*CBL*	*CBD*	*CBC*	*Δ⁹-THC*	*CBN*[a]
Indian IN-B(3) C-74	2% OV-17 and 6% OV-1[b]	0.02	0.11	t	0.30	0.09	0.62	0.03
	4% of 6.5% phenylmethyl silicone	0.02	0.11	0.01	0.30	0.09	0.60	0.60

[a] Other cannabinoids such as CBGM, Δ^8-THC, and CBG can be calculated.

[b] The ratio from the OV-1 column was applied to the original OV-17 analyses to obtain the THCV-CBL and CBD-CBC concentrations.

When operated isothermally at 190°C (see Figure 2.3), the 6.5 percent phenylmethyl silicone column gives adequate separation of CBD, CBC, Δ^9-THCV, and CBL, and removes CBN, CBD, and the C_{29} hydrocarbon from under the internal standard peak. It also reduces analysis time by 50 percent and provides analytical data within experimental error to data obtained by using both the 6 percent OV-1 and 2 percent OV-17 columns (see Table 2.3). Moreover, a previously unobserved peak in the chromatogram is shifted from under the Δ^9-THC peak. This peak is the one between Δ^9-THC and CBN and is not labeled in Figure 2.3. This cannabinoid has not been positively identified.

Electron Voltage–Mass Fragment Graphs

Mass spectra data are often used to identify and/or confirm structural features of molecules by providing the molecular weights and mass fragments according to known fragmentation patterns. However, when chemical entities possessing identical molecular weights are fragmented in a "mass spec" at an ion source temperature of 250°C and an electron energy level of 70 eV, it is difficult and often impossible to obtain a mass spectrum that can be used for identification. Vree and associates [19,20] have developed a relatively simple procedure to circumvent if not to entirely negate this negative feature. By maintaining a constant ion source temperature (250°C) and scanning between 10 and 20 eV, Vree obtained several fragmentation patterns that may be related to reaction sequences whereby the line intensities of the various fragments are a direct measure of ion concentration abundance. Thus, at each electron energy–ion source setting, the energy level influences the reaction rate which, in most cases, is unique and can be related to a particular chemical moiety. Using this concept, Vree then plotted data as percent relative mass fragment abundance versus eV and called the resulting graph an electron voltage–mass fragment intensity graph. When eV–MF graphs were obtained on known cannabinoids, Vree used this method to identify previously unknown cannabinoid homologs. Using Vree's method, investigators also have successfully confirmed the presences of CBC in certain cannabis variants, whereas at 70 eV it was impossible to distinguish CBC from CBD [16].

Seeking to obtain maximum utility of Vree's method and an additional tool for structure identification, our group initiated a program to produce representative eV–MF graphs on all available cannabinoids and their metabolites. We envisioned that this data bank would allow us to ascertain whether Vree's method could provide us with additional data useful for structural identification of previously unknown cannabinoids and/or metabolites.

Since a basic feature of eV–MF graphs is similar mass fragments but differing line intensities, we decided to prepare eV–MFs of 8α- and 8β-hydroxy-Δ^9-THC. These two isomeric metabolites have nearly identical mass spectra at 70 eV; however, at lower electron energy (5.5–21 eV) the intrinsic energy of activation provided marked differences in the line intensities.

Figures 2.4 and 2.5 depict graphically data obtained from 8α- and 8β-hydroxy-Δ^9-THC, respectively. As can readily be seen, the molecular ion (M^+ 330) varies between the two isomers according to the electron energy level, but no striking differences exist for M^+ that could be used to identify either isomer. However, $m/e = 312$ and $m/e = 271$ are striking and are strongly characteristic for each isomer. In 8α-hydroxy-Δ^9-THC (see Figure 2.4), $m/e = 312$ is the most abundant mass between 5.5 and 18.5 eV; after an energy of 18.5 eV is reached, $m/e = 271$ becomes the most abundant mass. However, in 8β-hydroxy-Δ^9-THC, over the range of 5.5–21 eV, $m/e = 271$ is the most abundant with $m/e = 312$ present in relatively low abundances.

These marked differences in data between very similar isomeric compounds are also found in other isomeric cannabinoids. For example, Δ^9-THC acids A and B can be distinguished readily by this method. Moreover, we are currently doing structural work on a naturally occurring cannabinoid which was originally believed to be 9-OH-hexahydrocannabivarin on the basis of a comparison between 70-eV spectra of the unknown and synthetic 9-OH-hexahydrocannabinol. Therefore, we investigated other isomeric possibilities

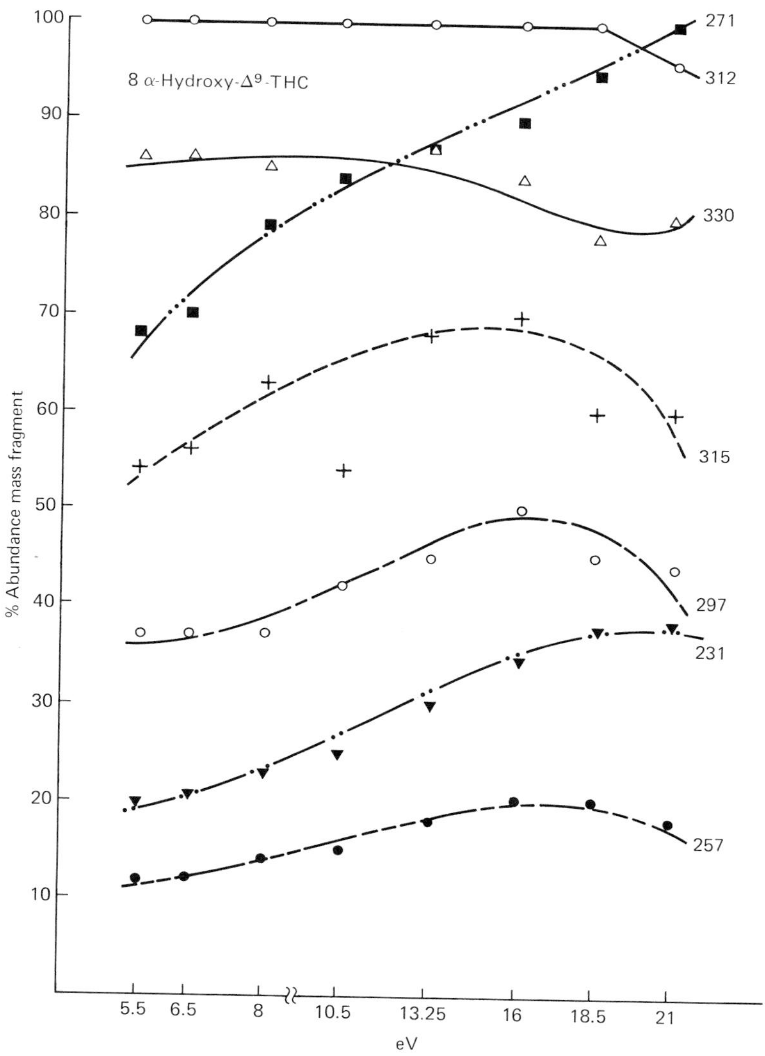

Figure 2.4. eV-MF graph of 8α-hydroxy-Δ^9-THC. Spectra obtained on Dupont 21–492.

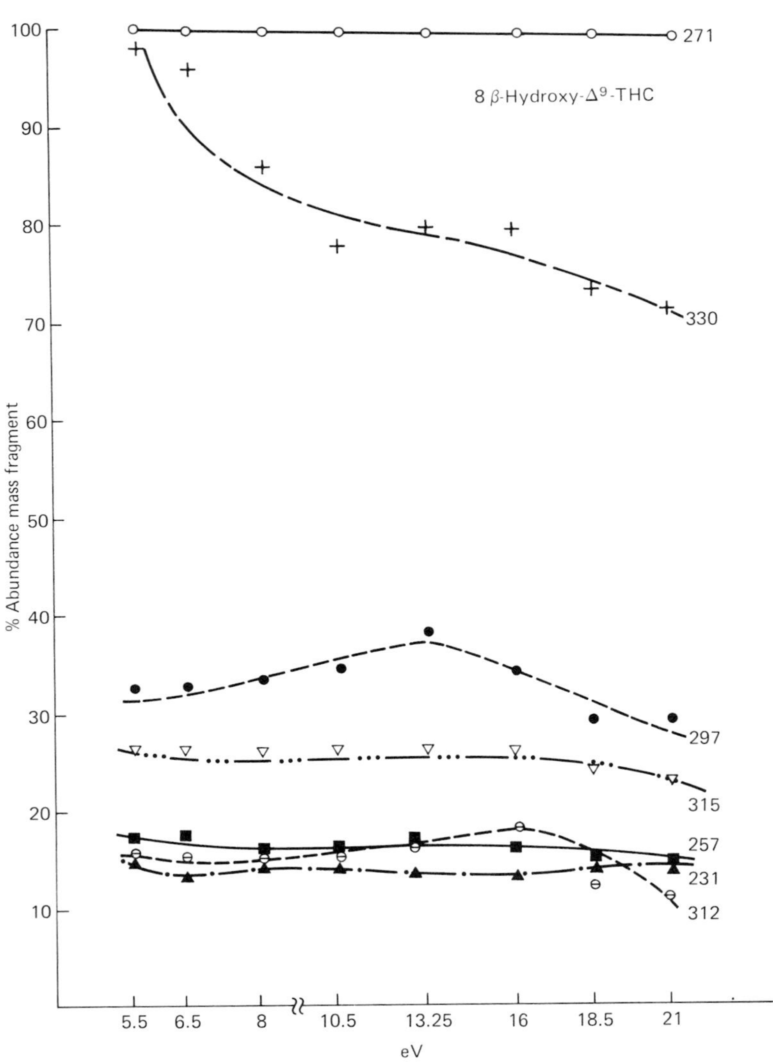

Figure 2.5. eV-MF graph of 8β-hydroxy-Δ⁹-THC. Spectra obtained on Dupont 21–492.

for the unknown, and it is definitely of a slightly different structure. Thus, to our group Vree's method is particularly useful as an additional tool for structural determinations.

Nitrogen-Containing Compounds from Cannabis

For many years, investigators searched for alkaloids in cannabis. Choline, trigonelline, and piperidine were identified, and the presence of muscarine was indicated. Recently *L*-(+)-isoleucine betaine was isolated and four alkaloids were detected. These four alkaloids were not isolated and characterized [10,11,18]. In our laboratories, *N*-(*p*-hydroxy-*β*-phenylethyl)-*p*-hydroxy-*trans*-cinnamamide, proline, and neurine have been isolated and identified [10, 18].

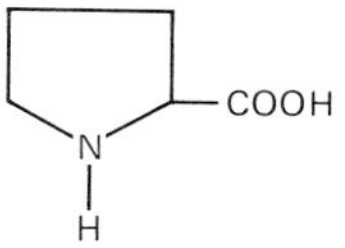

Proline

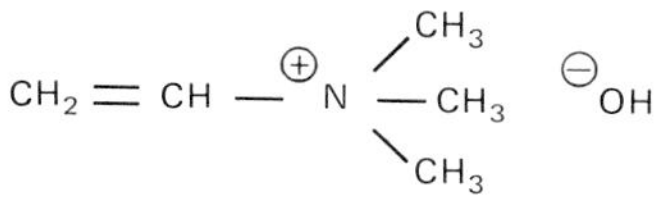

Neurine

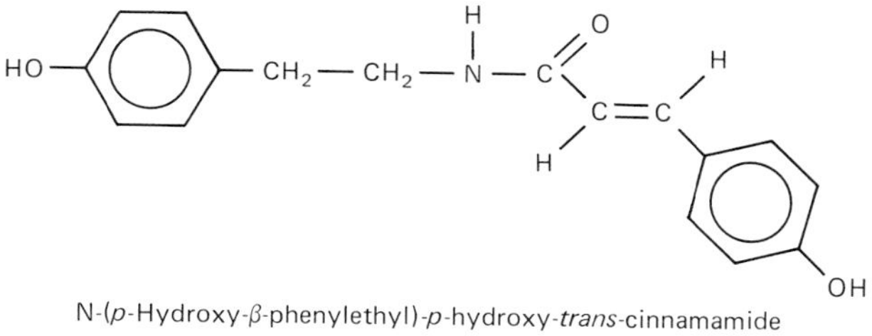

N-(*p*-Hydroxy-*β*-phenylethyl)-*p*-hydroxy-*trans*-cinnamamide

More recently, our efforts have been directed toward isolating nitrogen compounds of the *β*-arylethylamine class. To this end, we have been successful and wish to report the first isolation of a *β*-arylethylamine from cannabis: 4-(*β*-dimethylaminoethyl)-phenol or hordenine. Hordenine was isolated from the leaves of cannabis using the following procedure:

Dried leaves were ground and extracted with 95 percent alcohol at room temperature. After removing the solvent *in vacuo* at 40°C, we partitioned the residue between 2 percent citric acid solution in H_2O and $CHCl_3$.

The aqueous phase was rendered alkaline with concentrated NH_3 and extracted with $CHCl_3$. The alkaloidal fraction thus obtained was further purified by dissolving it in 1*M* HCl and extraction with $CHCl_3$ then alkalinized with concentrated NH_3 and reextracted with $CHCl_3$. This latter fraction was chromatographed on Silica Gel G and eluted with methanol-concentrated NH_3 (99:1) to provide hordenine [3].

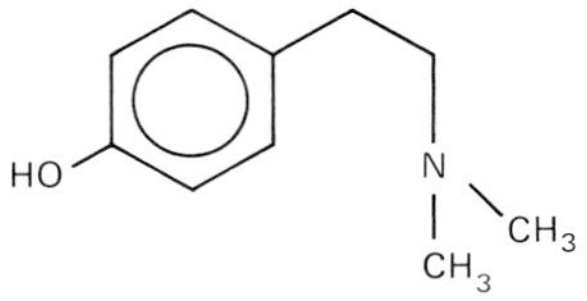

Hordenine

In a joint effort with other groups,[4] we have been investigating the presence of an unknown class of alkaloids found in cannabis. Recently, one of these alkaloids was isolated from the roots of a Mexican variant of cannabis. The alkaloid has been identified as belonging to the spermidine class, and to our knowledge this is the first report of isolating a nonquaternary alkaloid from the roots of *C. sativa* L. The structure was determined with x-ray crystallography [9]. The chemical name is 13-(1,2-dihydroxyheptanyl)-1,4,5,6,7,8,9,10,11,13,16, 16a-dodecahydropyrido[2,1-d][1,5,9]triazacyclotridecin-2(3*H*)-one. We have named this spermidine alkaloid cannabisativine.

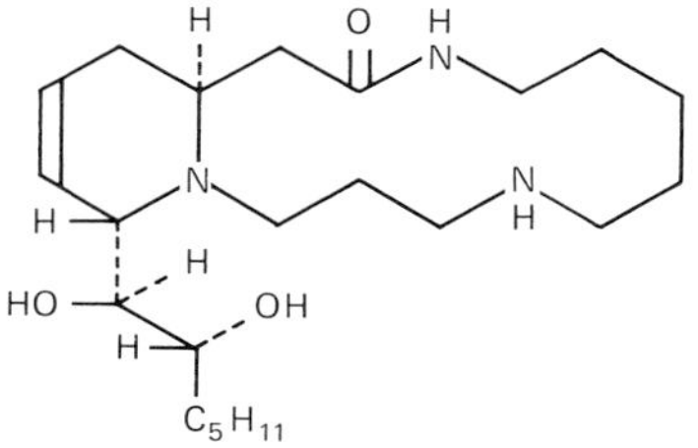

Cannabisativine

Separation of cannabisativine was basically as follows:

The dark brown syrup obtained by a methanol extraction of cannabis roots was partitioned between H_2O and chloroform. The chloroform fraction was then partitioned between petroleum ether and 10

[4] Dr. Herman L. Lotter, Max Planck, Institute for Biochemistry Munich-Martinsried, West Germany; Dr. Donald J. Abraham, Department of Medicinal Chemistry and Crystallography; and Drs. Joseph Knapp, Paul L. Schiff, Jr., and David J. Slatkin, Department of Pharmacognosy, School of Pharmacy, University of Pittsburgh, Pittsburgh, Pennsylvania 15261.

percent aqueous methanol. Subsequently, the aqueous methanol fraction was chromatographed on silicic acid. Elution with 8 percent methanol-chloroform provided a residue which on work-up with acid and base yielded cannabisativine as a white residue.

A more detailed account of the isolation procedure will be published soon [17]. Cannabisativine has been tentatively identified in the leaves of some cannabis variants. Other alkaloids of the spermidine class are present in cannabis and, as is the case with cannabinoids [6], alkaloid content varies somewhat within each cannabis variant.

Now that we know that nitrogen-containing compounds of the β-arylethylamine and spermidine classes are present in cannabis, the number of alkaloids found in cannabis will obviously increase significantly in the future.

ACKNOWLEDGMENTS

This work was supported in part by the Research Institute of Pharmaceutical Sciences, School of Pharmacy, University of Mississippi, and Grant #DA-00928-01 and contract #HSM-42-70-109 from the National Institute on Drug Abuse.

REFERENCES

1. Borgen, L. A., G. C. Lott, and W. M. Davis (1973) Cannabis induced hypothermia: a dose-effect comparison of crude marihuana extract and synthetic Δ^9-tetrahydrocannabinol in male and female rats. *Res. Commun. Chem. Pathol. Pharmac. 5:*621.
2. De Zeeuw, R. A., J. Wijsbeek, and T. H. Malingré (1973) Interference of alkanes in the gas chromatographic analysis of cannabis products. *J. Pharm. Pharmacol. 25:*21.
3. El-Feraly, F. S. and C. E. Turner (1975) Alkaloids of *Cannabis sativa* L. leaves. *Phytochem. Rep.* (in press).
4. Fetterman, P. S., N. J. Doorenbos, E. S. Keith, and M. W. Quimby (1971) A simple gas liquid chromatography procedure for determination of cannabinoidic acids in *Cannabis sativa* L. *Experientia 27:*988.
5. Fetterman, P. S. and C. E. Turner (1972) Constituents of *Cannabis sativa* L. I: Propyl homologs of cannabinoids from an Indian variant. *J. Pharm. Sci. 61*(9):1476.
6. Holley, J. H., K. W. Hadley, and C. E. Turner (1975) Constituents of *Cannabis sativa* L. XI: Cannabidiol and cannabichromene in samples of known geographical origin. *J. Pharm. Sci. 64*(5):892.
7. Karniol, I. G., I. Shirakawa, N. Kasinski, A. Pfefcrman, and E. A. Carlini (1974) Cannabidiol interferes with the effects of Δ^9-tetrahydrocannabinol in man. *Eur. J. Pharmacol. 28:*172.

8. Lerner, P. (1969) The precise determination of tetrahydrocannabinol in marihuana and hashish. *Bull. Narc. 21:*38.
9. Lotter, H. L., D. J. Abraham, C. E. Turner, J. E. Knapp, P. L. Schiff, Jr., and D. J. Slatkin (1976) Cannabisativine, a new alkaloid from *Cannabis sativa* L. root. *Tetrahedron* (in press).
10. Mole, M. L., Jr. and C. E. Turner (1974) Phytochemical screening of *Cannabis sativa* L. I: Constituents of an Indian variant. *J. Pharm. Sci. 63*(1):154.
11. Mole, M. L., Jr. and C. E. Turner (1973) Phytochemical screening of *Cannabis sativa* L. II: Choline and neurine in the roots of a Mexican variant. *Acta Pharm. Jugoslav. 23*(4):203.
12. The chemistry of cannabis and its components: report of a working group, Utrecht, 20–24 May, 1974. United Nations Document MNAR/9/74.
13. Turner, C. E. and K. Hadley (1973) Constituents of *Cannabis sativa* L. II: absence of cannabidiol in an African variant. *J. Pharm. Sci. 62*(2):251.
14. Turner, C. E., K. W. Hadley, and K. H. Davis, Jr. (1973) Constituents of *Cannabis sativa* L. V: stability of an analytical sample extracted with chloroform. *Acta Pharm. Jugoslav. 23*(2):89.
15. Turner, C. E., K. W. Hadley, J. Henry, and M. L. Mole (1974) Constituents of *Cannabis sativa* L. VII: use of silyl derivatives in routine analysis. *J. Pharm. Sci. 63*(12):1872.
16. Turner, C. E., K. W. Hadley, J. Holley, S. Billets, and M. L. Mole, Jr. (1975) Constituents of *Cannabis sativa* L. VIII: possible biological application of a new method to separate cannabidiol and cannabichromene. *J. Pharm. Sci. 64*(5):810.
17. Turner, C. E., M. H. Hsu, J. E. Knapp, P. L. Schiff, Jr., and D. J. Slatkin (1976) The isolation of cannabisativine, an alkaloid from *Cannabis sativa* L. root. *J. Pharm. Sci.* (in press).
18. Slatkin, D. J., N. J. Doorenbos, L. S. Harris, A. M. Masoud, M. W. Quimby, and P. L. Schiff, Jr. (1971) Chemical constituents of *Cannabis sativa* L. root. *J. Pharm. Sci. 60*(12):1891.
19. Vree, T. B., D. D. Breimer, C. A. M. van Ginneken, and J. M. van Rossum (1971) Identification of cannabivarins in hashish by a new method of combined gas chromatography–mass spectrometry. *Clin. Chim. Acta. 34:*365.
20. Vree, T. B., D. D. Breimer, C. A. M. van Ginneken, and J. M. van Rossum (1972) Identification in hashish of tetrahydrocannabinol, cannabidiol and cannabinol analogues with a methyl side-chain. *J. Pharm. Pharmacol. 24:*7.

3

Pyrolysis of Cannabinoids

C. A. SALEMINK

Cannabis is known to produce more immediate and stronger effects when smoked than when taken orally in similar amounts. However, insufficient data are available on the pharmacology and toxicology of cannabis smoke. It has been reported that the psychoactive effects of smoked marihuana are stronger than can be expected on the basis of the tetrahydrocannabinol (THC) content [3]. It is therefore important to investigate the pharmacology of the products obtained after smoking, rather than to concentrate only on the pharmacology of the natural products. Some factors influencing the relative ratios are the variety of seed, the region of cultivation, the type of soil, and the method of preparation and storage of the sample. Consequently, results reported for pharmacological and clinical research vary considerably. The complexity of marihuana or hashish, as indicated above, hardly allows a proper characterization of changes occurring during smoking (pyrolysis); the known pyrolytic products are given in Annex IV of a recent United Nations report [11].

Therefore, we decided to investigate first the pyrolysis of a single cannabis constituent and started with cannabidiol (CBD). Further reasons for this choice were the following:

1. Many cannabis samples are characterized as being of chemo- or phenotype 2 [2], a type which contains CBD as a main component.
2. The cannabis material cultivated from Fibrimon seeds in Holland and Turkey contained hardly any Δ^1-tetrahydrocannabinol (Δ^1-THC) and large quantities of CBD. However, when smoked by experienced users the material proved to be moderately "psychotropic."
3. The structure of CBD suggests a susceptibility for conversion into the psychotropic Δ^1-THC. This was earlier pointed out [12], in order to explain the increased pharmacological activity of a CBD preparation after smoking.
4. CBD could be isolated from the dutch hemp material in crystalline form through a simple isolation procedure.

Marihuana: Chemistry, Biochemistry, and Cellular Effects, edited by Gabriel G. Nahas,

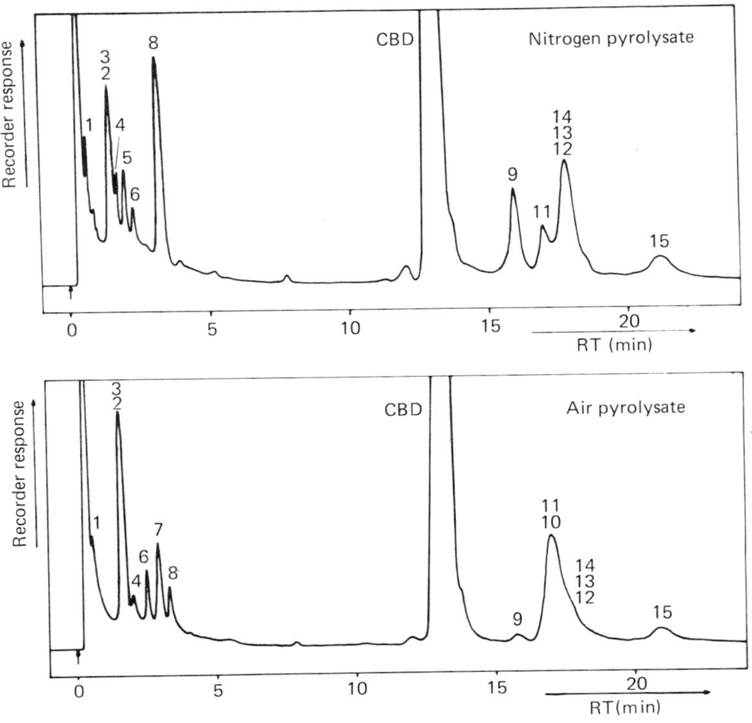

Figure 3.1. Gas chromatograms of nitrogen and air pyrolysates.

Pyrolysis under aerobic conditions of the pure isolated (-)3,4-*trans*-CBD, in the apparatus we developed, produced a mixture of products as represented in Figure 3.1a. Later, CBD was pyrolysed with both air and nitrogen as carrier gas, because it had been observed that by changing the nature of the gas phase, which was used during pyrolysis, the yield of the various components in the pyrolysate was influenced considerably.

Each of the peaks was isolated by preparative gas chromatography. Consecutive mass spectra were recorded during the slow evaporation of each sample into the ion source. The spectra indicated that most of the GLC peaks constituted a mixture of several components (see Figure 3.1b).

The peaks eluted ahead of the starting material (*in casu* CBD) can be considered as a mixture of cracked products of CBD. The cracked products—the most volatile products of the CBD pyrolysates—were separated by gas chromatography.

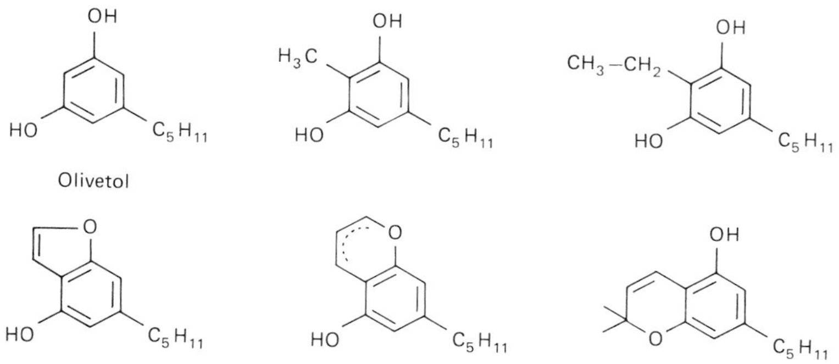

Figure 3.2. Components of CBD.

Silylation and mass spectrometric analysis revealed the molecular weight and the number of hydroxyl groups accessible for silylation. The components [6] shown in Figure 3.2 could be identified. Other "cracking" products are still to be identified.

Preliminary pharmacological assays—general screening—on the volatile constituents of the CBD pyrolysate revealed no significant effects. However, recent work by Burstein *et al.* [1] on the inhibition of prostaglandins biosynthesis by naturally occurring cannabinoids included the assay on olivetol in the tests. Olivetol showed high inhibitory activity in the assays considered. Our findings that olivetol represents a substantial amount of the volatile products formed by pyrolysis of CBD may therefore be of further pharmacological interest.

From the peaks with larger retention times (RT) than CBD in the gas chromatograms of the pyrolysate under aerobic conditions, the main one was first thought to be Δ^1-THC because of its RT relative to CBD. However, this peak too was a mixture of at least two components, the main one possessing a molecular ion $m/e = 330$ and two intense fragment ions at $m/e = 247$ and $m/e = 205$. The component's molecular formula, determined by exact mass measurement, was $C_{21}H_{30}O_3$, which suggested the incorporation of one oxygen atom in the molecule of CBD.

Through the interpretation and comparison of the spectroscopic data of the unknown component with those of the decarboxylated synthetic products of the cannabielsoic acids, first isolated by Shani and Mechoulam [9,10], the structure could be established as cannabielsoin (CBE) [8]. This cannabielsoin (Figure 3.3) is not formed by pyrolysis of CBD under nitrogen. In this respect it is noteworthy that CBE was also absent from the smoke condensate

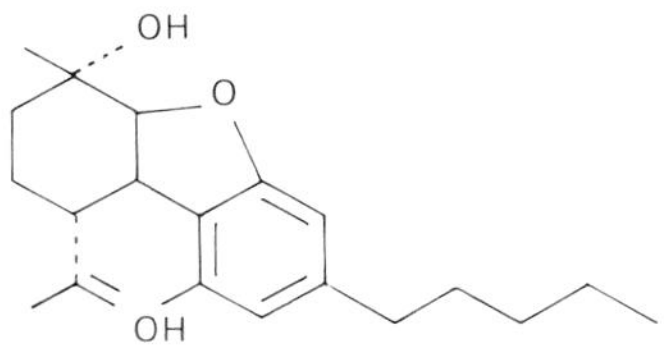

Figure 3.3. Structural formula of cannabielsoin.

obtained by Kephalas *et al.* under normal experimental conditions.

This and the fact that the oxygen content of the gas phase just behind the glowing zone in the marihuana and hashish cigarettes is practically zero provided us with additional reasons to perform our pyrolytic experiments under nitrogen.

Combined gas chromatography and mass spectrometry (GC–MS) further revealed the structural identity of most of the products in the two (under N_2 and air) pyrolysates we obtained.

We have been able to isolate and identify [7] from the so-called nitrogen pyrolysate of CBD thus far the substances given in Figure 3.4.

The formation of 314/108 from CBD can be visualized to proceed as shown in Figure 3.5.

The fragmentation upon electron impact can be visualized to take place according to the mechanism outlined in Figure 3.6.

Some pharmacological aspects of the CBD pyrolysates have been examined by Van Noordwijk, Ten Ham, *et al.* at the National Institute of Health in Utrecht.

In interpretating the following pharmacological results, remem-

Figure 3.4. Substances isolated from the "nitrogen" pyrolysate of CBD.

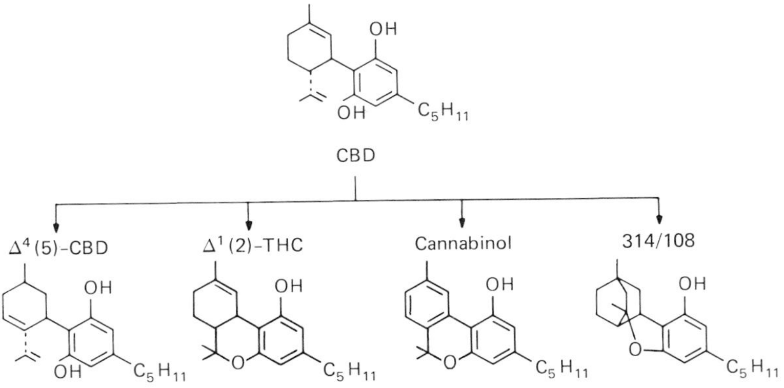

Figure 3.5. Formation of 314/108 from CBD.

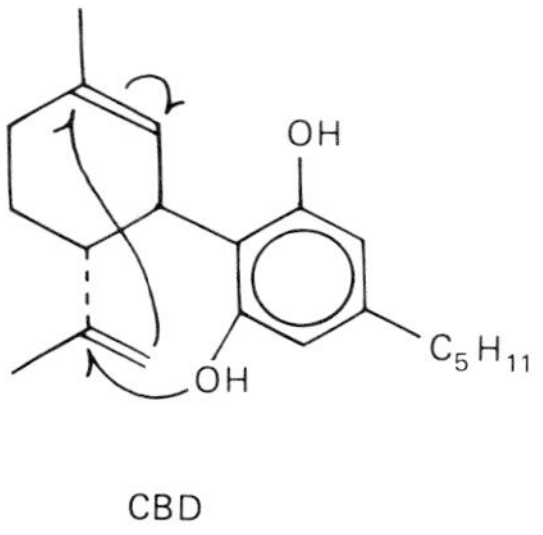

ber that the pharmacological screening could be performed only on a moderate scale because only 10–20 mg of material were available in most cases.

To obtain a first impression of eventual pharmacological activity, we used the so-called Sindroom assay on mice. This Sindroom assay, a series of experiments, was developed and executed by Van Noordwijk, Ten Ham, *et al.* (Figure 3.7).

Figure 3.6. Fragmentation of CBD upon electron impact.

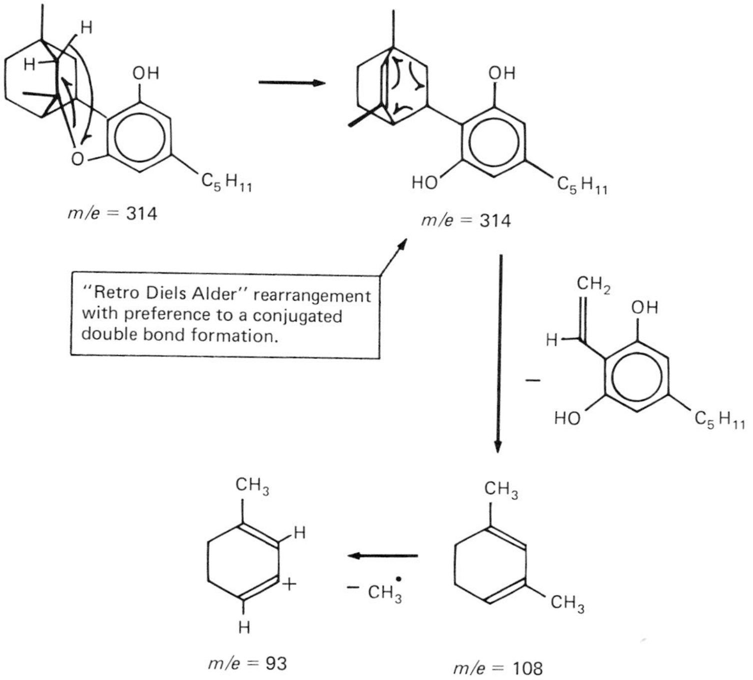

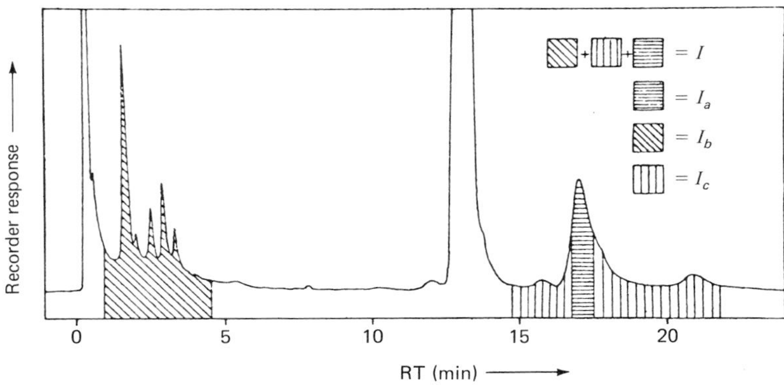

Figure 3.7. Composition of the fractions submitted to the Sindroom assay (see text).

The schematic indication of fractions, either in air or nitrogen pyrolysate, is as follows:

Ia. The air pyrolysate—without CBD—caused decreased respiration, decreased mobility, increased temperature at a dose of 50 mg/kg body weight, and decreased temperature at a dose of 100 mg/kg body weight. A weak analgesic activity could be observed.

Ib. The components from the air pyrolysate—with a shorter RT than CBD—showed hardly any pharmacological activity in the assay used; 75 and 150 mg/kg body weight caused an increase in temperature (0.5–1°C).

$I_a + I_c$. The components from the nitrogen pyrolysate with a longer RT than CBD show an activity comparable to the activity of the air pyrolysate of CBD freed of the unchanged CBD. Especially the thermal effects are alike. In I_a, *inter alia,* cannabielsoin is not active. The observed activity is partly caused by Δ^1-THC.

In summary, the pyrolysis of a single cannabinoid like CBD clearly results in a complex mixture of components. The main component in the air pyrolysate of CBD—cannabielsoin—is not active. This suggests that the distinct pharmacological activity has to be attributed to one or a combination of the compounds contained in the pyrolysate in small quantities.

The chemistry of cannabis smoke is obviously even more complicated. Analytical data from combined experiments in Athens and Utrecht have shown the presence of several new compounds in cannabis smoke after pyrolysis.

During the pyrolytic decomposition of cannabis components, a number of fragments and radicals of the original molecules are generated. Some of these are unstable and may undergo rearrangements. Stereochemical changes may also occur. Obviously, the relative compositions of the naturally occurring compounds will be changed.

ACKNOWLEDGMENTS

This research was supported by the Ministry of Public Health and Environmental Hygiene. We acknowledge collaboration with the Pharmacological Department of J. van Noordwijk and M. ten Ham; and cooperation with the Department of Mass Spectrometry of G. Dijkstra, W. Heerma, and J. K. Terlouw. The participants in our group are C. A. L. Bercht, F. J. E. M. Küppers, R. J. J. Ch. Lousberg, and H. W. A. Spronck.

REFERENCES

1. Burstein, S., E. Levin, and C. Varanelli (1973) Prostaglandines and cannabis. II. Inhibition of biosynthesis by the naturally occurring cannabinoids. *Biochem. Pharmacol. 22:*2905.
2. Fetterman, P. S., E. S. Keith, C. W. Waller, O. Guerrero, N. J. Doorenbos, and M. W. Quimby (1971) Mississippi-grown *Cannabis sativa L.:* preliminary observation on chemical definition of phenotype and variations in tetrahydrocannabinol content versus age, sex, and plant part. *J. Pharm. Sci. 60:*1246.
3. Galanter, M., H. Weingartner, F. B. Vaughan, W. T. Roth, and R. J. Wyatt (1973) Δ^9-*Trans*-tetrahydrocannabinol and natural marihuana. The controlled comparison. *Arch. Gen. Psychiatry 28:*278.
4. Karniol, I. G. and E. A. Carlini (1972) The content of $(-)\Delta^9$-*trans*-tetrahydrocannabinol (Δ^9-THC) does not explain all biological activity of some Brazilian marihuana samples. *J. Pharm. Pharmacol. 24:*833.
5. Kubena, R. K. and H. Barry, III (1972) Stimulus characteristics of marihuana components. *Nature 235:*397.
6. Küppers, F. J. E. M., C. A. L. Bercht, C. A. Salemink, and R. J. J. Ch. Lousberg (1975) Cannabis. XIV. Pyrolysis of cannabidiol—analysis of the volatile constituents. *J. Chromatogr. 108:*375.
7. Küppers, F. J. E. M., C. A. L. Bercht, C. A. Salemink, R. J. J. Ch. Lousberg, J. K. Terlouw, and W. Heerma (1975) Cannabis XV. Pyrolysis of cannabidiol—Structure elucidation of four pyrolytic products. *Tetrahedron 31:*1513.
8. Küppers, F. J. E. M., R. J. J. Ch. Lousberg, C. A. L. Bercht, C. A. Salemink, J. K. Terlouw, W. Heerma, and A. Laven (1973) Cannabis VIII. Pyrolysis of cannabidiol—Structure elucidation of the main pyrolytic product. *Tetrahedron 29:*2797.
9. Shani, A. and R. Mechoulam (1970) A new type of cannabinoid. Synthesis of cannabielsoic acid A by a novel photo-oxidative cyclisation. *Chem. Comm. 1970:*273.
10. Shani, A. and R. Mechoulam (1971) Photochemical reactions of can-

nabidiol. Cyclization to Δ^1-tetrahydrocannabinol and other *trans* formation. *Tetrahedron 27:*601.

11. The chemistry of cannabis smoke from a working group in Athens in April 1975, United Nations Division of Narcotic Drugs, Document MNAR/6/1975.
12. Waser, P. G. and F. Mikeš (1971) Marihuana components: effect of smoking on Δ^9-tetrahydrocannabinol and cannabidiol. *Science 172:*1158.

4

Some Aspects of Cannabis Smoke Chemistry

T. A. KEPHALAS, J. KIBURIS, C. M. MICHAEL,
C. J. MIRAS, AND D. P. PAPADAKIS

Introduction

In the past few years, the chemical composition of cannabis has been clarified and the class of compounds that are characteristic of the plant, i.e., the cannabinoids, has been identified. The compounds which possess a pharmacological activity similar to that observed in cannabis users have been described. The availability of the various cannabinoids in pure form has contributed to a better understanding of the pharmacology and the clinical effects of cannabis and its different preparations.

However, after nearly 10 years of intensive work, scientists investigating the chemistry or biochemistry of cannabis still face some unresolved problems. Some of these problems are due to the fact that few cannabis users take the drug orally; most of them prefer to smoke cannabis either as a cigarette or with various appliances such as pipes and water pipes. (It is now well established [1,6,8,11,13,18] that cannabis is more active and its effects are more immediate when it is smoked rather than ingested.) How do the various ways of smoking affect the chemical composition of the smoke which is absorbed through the lungs? Several investigators have dealt with the problem [1,11,13–15], but the information available is fragmentary.

In view of the fact that smoking through a water pipe is the favorite way of cannabis consumption by Greek and Middle Eastern users, we have investigated the effects of this way of smoking on the chemical composition of the resulting smoke.

Information concerning the composition of cannabis smoke, obtained under various experimental conditions simulating the actual way of smoking by the users, will be of great importance to the understanding of the pharmacological and toxicological effects of this drug on man.

Marihuana: Chemistry, Biochemistry, and Cellular Effects, edited by Gabriel G. Nahas, © 1976 by Springer-Verlag New York Inc.

Methods

Simulation of actual hashish smoking

Bearing in mind the importance of standardized experimental smoking procedures, we have tried to replicate experimentally as closely as possible the human technique of smoking cannabis through a water pipe.

Our water pipe device (Figure 4.1) is almost identical to that used by experienced Greek smokers. The pipe bowl is made from a hollowed potato which, according to the experience of chronic smokers, is easy to make. Chronic users report that smoking hashish in a potato is pleasant and eliminates the undesirable taste or smell present when hashish is smoked in a wooden pipe. A volume of water of 75–100 ml is used in conjunction with the pipe when 4 persons are smoking a known amount of cannabis and tobacco mixture. The water is changed after each pipeful. We have followed the same pattern in our experimental model.

We have carried out our experiments with a United Nations reference cannabis sample (UNC 351), which enables us to compare our results with those of other investigators. This sample was

Figure 4.1. Experimental model of cannabis and tobacco mixture smoking through water; (a) nut charcoal, (b) pipe bowl, (c) water pipe device, (d) water, (e) double-coiled condenser, (f) smoking machine.

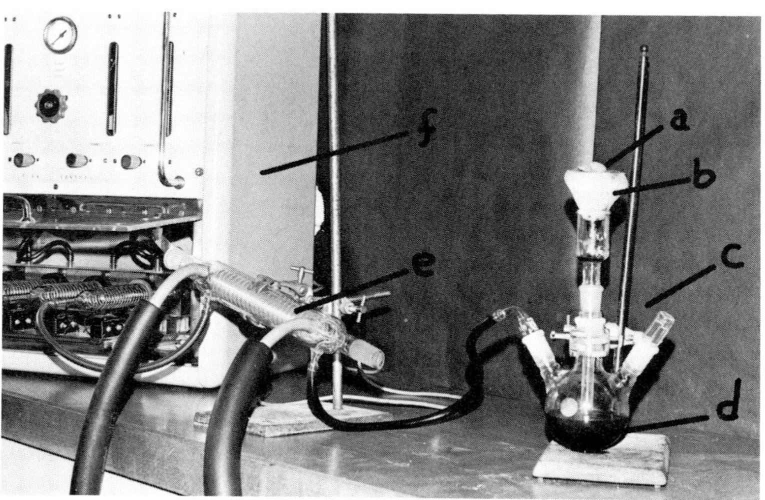

subjected to the same treatment used by actual cannabis smokers. The reference sample (approximately 10 gm) was placed in a waterproof aluminum foil wrapper, which was in turn wrapped in newspaper. The package was immersed in water and ironed several times with a hot (90°C) electric iron until the newspaper was almost dried. The resulting preparation consists of a thin solid slab of cannabis. According to chronic smokers, this is the best preparation for smoking cannabis, and it will last longer than the original powder form.

This preparation is never smoked alone but is mixed with a special variety of tobacco known as "tubeki." In our experiments, we used the same variety subjected to the same treatment used by the smokers. Dried leaves of tubeki were ground, washed repeatedly with tap water, and left to dry at room temperature for a couple of days. We used 3 gm of the cannabis slab and 4 gm of tubeki tobacco—the usual amounts for one course of smoking involving 4 persons and for the volume of water mentioned previously.

The pipe bowl is filled with successive layers of tobacco (usually three layers, one of which is always put on top of the pipe bowl) and cannabis (usually two layers). This mixture was pyrolysed by placing burning coals of walnut on top of it. According to our smokers, this is the best burning method mainly because it leaves very little ash.

In our experiments, smoking was performed by a standard tobacco smoking machine. In a recent report of a group studying the chemistry of cannabis smoke [17], it was stated that such machines should be used until suitable apparatuses are developed for cannabis. We have used an Ethel MK VII tobacco smoking machine, which provides a wide choice of puff durations and frequencies, allowing the simulation of a variety of human smoking patterns. The frequency and duration of puffs were regulated to 1 puff per min and 8 sec, respectively. Theses values were considered as best approximating the smoking pattern of chronic cannabis users.

Collection and analysis of the smoke

Under our experimental conditions, three types of material were collected. First, the particulate matter of the smoke, which was electrostatically precipitated in the glass tubes of the machine and which comprises "the sublimate." With the above-mentioned type of machine, the electrostatic precipitation of the particulate matter is almost complete. Second, we collected water-soluble components of cannabis with or without their pyrolysis products, which

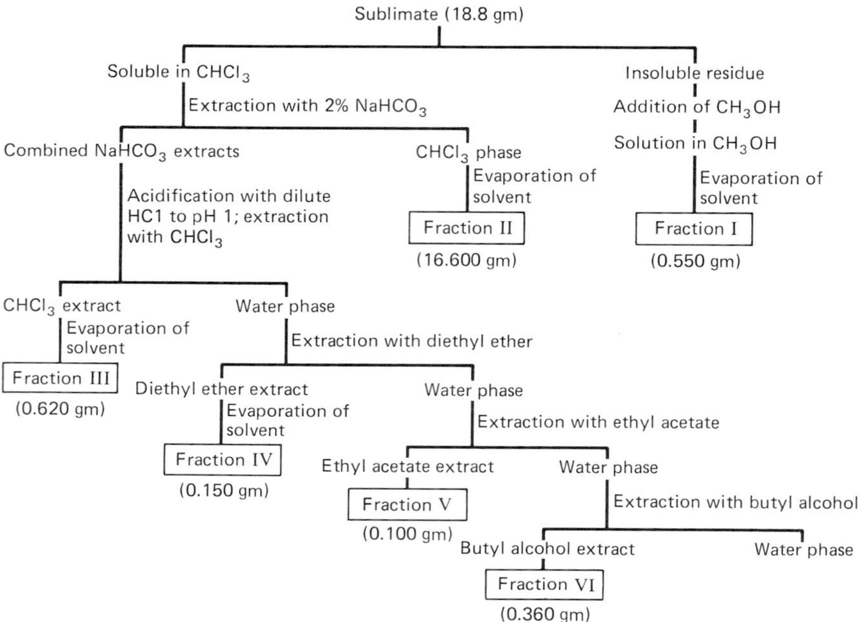

Figure 4.2. General procedure followed to extract the "sublimate."

are dissolved in the water of the pipe, as well as tobacco components with or without their pyrolysis products, which are also water soluble. Third, cannabis and tobacco components were recovered with or without their pyrolysis products, which appear as small particles on the walls of the water container and on top of the water. These are insoluble in water but they remain there due to the solidification of smoke components, with low volatility, when the smoke is passed through the water. This last type of material can be separated from the water-soluble products by filtration through a filter paper (Whatman No. 50).

For comparison, we obtained analogous types of material by smoking only tubeki tobacco and subjected these to the same analytical procedures described below for mixtures of cannabis and tubeki tobacco.

Of the three types of material described, the sublimate is what the smoker normally inhales; therefore, our analytical efforts have been concerned mainly with this type of material. We first fractionated the sublimate as indicated in Figure 4.2. Six fractions were obtained, of which the last four could be considered acidic.

Table 4.1 Column chromatography of the petrol extractable part of fraction II on Silica Gel G.

Fractions (N°)	*Solvent or solvent systems used*	
1– 150	Petroleum ether	
151– 450	Petroleum ether/ether	99: 1
451– 600	Petroleum ether/ether	98: 2
601– 750	Petroleum ether/ether	97: 3
751– 900	Petroleum ether/ether	96: 4
901–1000	Petroleum ether/ether	95: 5
1001–1250	Petroleum ether/ether	99:10
1251–1400	Petroleum ether/ether	80:20
1401–1550	Petroleum ether/ether	50:50
1551–1650	Ethyl ether	
1651–1750	Chloroform	
1751–2000	Chloroform/methanol	95: 5
2001–2100	Chloroform/methanol	80:20
2101–2300	Methanol	

Gas chromatographic analysis of each fraction indicated that only fraction II contained, among other substances, the well-known main cannabinoids. For this reason, fraction II was selected for further investigation of its chemical composition. Two grams of fraction II was extracted with petrol ether (3 × 50 ml). Under these conditions, 50 percent of fraction II is petrol ether extractable. After evaporation of the solvent, the residue was subjected to column chromatography (Silica Gel G, Merck 7734). The solvent systems used for elution and the number of fractions collected (15 ml each) are given in Table 4.1.

Monitoring of the column by thin-layer chromatography (TLC) followed by detection of the spots under UV light or by staining with fast blue B indicated that a number of substances with higher R_f values than the main cannabinoids were eluted first (fractions 430 to 450). Examination of these fractions by gas chromatography-mass spectrometry (GC–MS) revealed the presence of at least five components; their retention times (RTs) and mass spectra (MS) characteristics are given in Table 4.2. Of these, component 1 was tentatively identified as cannabinol methyl ether on the basis of its nuclear magnetic resonance (NMR) and mass spectra. The other four were not found in the reference sample and, therefore, constitute new components formed during smoking.

We attempted to isolate these products in a pure form to

Table 4.2 RRT[a] and mass spectra characteristics of cannabis smoke components present in fractions 430–450

Component	RRT	Base peak(m/e)	Mol. peak(m/e)
1	0.36	309	324
2	0.46	252	308
3	0.64	319	334
4	0.70	333	348
5	0.84	247	362

[a] OV—17: 2.5%; N_2 flow: 30 ml/min; column temperature: 250°C; injector and detector temperature: 280°C. Androst-4-ene-3,14-dione was used as internal standard.

elucidate their structure. Using repeated column chromatography (silicic acid, neutral alumina 20 percent) and preparative gas chromatography, we isolated three of these products—components 2, 3, and 5. Studies on their structure elucidation are in progress.

Fractions 451–779 contained at least 11 compounds. These were rather well separated on TLC and on the gas chromatograph, and all were colored by fast blue B. RTs and MS characteristics of these compounds obtained after subjecting fractions 451–779 to GC–MS analysis are given in Table 4.3.

Table 4.3 RRT[a] and mass spectra characteristics of cannabis smoke components present in fractions 451–779

Component	RRT	Base peak(m/e)	Mol. peak(m/e)
1	0.01	148	222
2	0.20	231	314[b]
3	0.24	231	310
4	0.21	203	286
5	0.58	325	340
6	0.79	295	310[b]
7	0.29	231	316
8	0.26	231	314[b]
9	0.44	299	314
10	0.54	295	336
11	0.28	231	319

[a] GC conditions were those described in Table 4.2.

[b] These components were also found to be present in the UNC 351 reference sample.

I

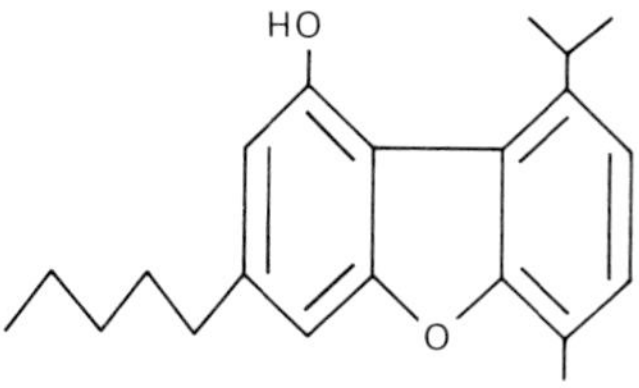

Figure 4.3. Structure of "compound 6."

Of these, compound 6, which was also found in the reference cannabis sample, has been isolated in a pure form. On the basis of its NMR and MS, the structure shown in Figure 4.3 has been assigned to this compound [9]. In a recent report, investigators assigned the same structure to a product isolated from cannabis extracts [5].

Work on elucidating the structures of the other components is in progress. The MS characteristics of some of the compounds, which have not been found in the reference sample, suggest that they have a cannabinoid-type structure.

In our experimental model, new cannabinoids (some of them known, and some perhaps not yet known) probably are formed during smoking. In contradiction to earlier reports [1,12], this conclusion has been supported by our results and by those of others [3,11] investigating the effect of smoking on individual cannabinoids.

Fractions 780–1000 contained, among other substances, the main cannabinoids: CBD, Δ^9-THC, and CBN. Quantitation of these gave the following values: CBD 3.29 percent; Δ^9-THC 7.18 percent; and CBN 25.28 percent. The corresponding values in the cannabis reference sample used were found to be 1.87 percent, 5.4 percent, and 6.54 percent, respectively.

The amount of the sublimate derived from the initial amount of cannabis smoked has also been estimated. It corresponds to 9.4 percent of the amount of cannabis smoked. Assuming that under our experimental conditions all the cannabinoid acids in the reference sample are completely decarboxylated during both smoking and the quantitation of cannabinoids by gas chromatography, it follows that approximately 24.3 percent of the main cannabinoids (i.e., CBD, Δ^9-THC, and CBN) are transferred into the sublimate.

From the above figures it also follows that the percentage of CBN in the sublimate is considerably increased in comparison to the percentage of this cannabinoid in the cannabis reference sample. This finding is in accordance with the results of similar experiments by other investigators [13]. However, the ratio of Δ^9-THC to CBD is slightly lower in the sublimate than in the reference sample. This finding seems to contradict those of other investigators [3,10,13] and of ours, which indicate that during smoking CBD is partially converted to Δ^9-THC. It is possible that during smoking, although CBD is partially converted to Δ^9-THC, the degree of pyrolysis of Δ^9-THC is greater than that of CBD.

In addition to the main cannabinoids, at least three other substances were present in fractions 781–1000. These have been isolated in a pure form by subjecting these fractions to repeated column chromatography on Sephadex LH-20 (solvent system *n*, heptane-chloroform-ethanol 10:10:1). The structures of these products are being investigated.

Very little is know about the part of fraction II which is insoluble in petrol ether, fractions III to VI and, the types (b) and (c) of material collected, as previously described.

However, some preliminary work has indicated that fraction III did not contain any detectable amounts of cannabinoid acids. As one can conclude from Figure 4.1, the presence of cannabinoid acids surviving decarboxylation during smoking would be expected in fraction III. However, column chromatography of this fraction on silicic acid (biosyl H, elution with increasing amounts of ethyl acetate in benzene), followed by TLC monitoring of the various fractions, indicated the presence of only two substances which could be colored by fast blue B. Both substances have been isolated in pure form. However, the available information is not indicative of a cannabinoid type of structure.

Type b of material collected seems to be devoid of known "neutral" cannabinoids. This has been found by lyophilization of the water phase, followed by dissolving the lyophilized material in methanol and subjecting the methanolic solution to TLC (Silica Gel GF_{254}, elution with petrol ether-ether 4:1). Except for a mixture of substances migrating nearly at the origin of the plate, no other spot migrating at positions of the plate expected for known cannabinoids could be detected by fast blue B. The possibility that some of the substances migrating at the origin might correspond to cannabinoid acids has also been tested. Thus, TLC of the methanolic solution of the lyophilized material, using a solvent system that we have found particularly useful for TLC analysis of cannabinoid acids, indicated the presence of at least three substances which could be colored with fast blue B (Figure 4.4). We cannot say whether or not these substances correspond to known cannabinoid acids.

Figure 4.4. Thin-layer chromatogram (Silica Gel GF_{254}, Merck, solvent system:ethyl acetate-dioxan-hexane 10:20:70) of type b of material collected (i.e., the water phase). T—tobacco sample (tubeki); T + H—tobacco and cannabis mixture.

The effect of smoking through a water pipe on individual cannabinoids

The effect of smoking on various cannabinoids in a pure form has been the subject of several investigations [4,11,13,16].

We carried out similar investigations with cannabidiol in our experimental model. We followed the same procedure described for smoking cannabis and tubeki tobacco mixtures: The material smoked consisted of tubeki tobacco impregnated with a solution of CBD in chloroform, which had been left at room temperature for the solvent to evaporate. Materials similar to those described previously were collected. The sublimate was fractionated as for the cannabis and tubeki tobacco mixture. A fraction analogous to the previously described fraction II was obtained. Subjection of the petrol ether–extractable part of this fraction to column chromatography, followed by GC–MS analysis of the fractions obtained, revealed the presence of at least nine substances other than CBD. (A full report on their chemical composition will be published elsewhere [7].) Three of these substances have been tentatively identified as Δ^8-THC, Δ^9-THC, and CBN on the basis of their GC and MS characteristics. Therefore, during smoking CBD seems to be partially converted to THC and CBN. This finding is in agreement with observations reported by other investigators [3,10,13]. The MS characteristics of some of the above-mentioned substances strongly suggest a cannabinoid structure. All of our findings, as well as the results obtained by other investigators [3,10], leave little doubt that new cannabinoids or compounds with a cannabinoidlike structure are formed when cannabis is smoked.

ACKNOWLEDGMENTS

This work has been carried out in close collaboration with Professor Salamink *et al.,* Department of Organic Chemistry of Natural Products, University of Utrecht. We thank the United Nations Narcotics Laboratory for their support in carrying out this work and for the opportunity to perform part of this study in Geneva.

The technical assistance of Mr. S. Logakis, Miss A. Tsiapara, and Miss S. Papageorgiou is also acknowledged.

REFERENCES

1. Agurell, S. and K. Leander (1971) Stability, transfer and absorption of cannabinoid constituents of cannabis (hashish) during smoking. *Acta. Pharm. Suec. 8:*391.
2. Coutselinis, A. S. and C. J. Miras (1970) The effects of the smoking process on cannabinols. United Nations Document ST/SOA/SERS/24.
3. Dahl, C. (1975) Data presented at the meeting of the working group on the chemistry of cannabis smoke, Athens, April 21–25.
4. El-Darawy, Z. I., A. M. Rizk, F. M. Hammoud, and Z. M. Mobarak (1972) Studies on hashish. II. Effect of heat on cannabinols. *Indian J. Appl. Chem. 35*(1):9.
5. Friedrich-Fiechtl, J. and G. Spiteller (1975) Neue cannabinoide. *Tetrahedron 31:*479.
6. Grinspoon, L. (1969) Marihuana. *Sci. Am. 221*(6):17.
7. Heerma, W., R. J. J. Ch. Lousberg, C. A. Salemink, H. J. W. Spronck, T. A. Kephalas, J. Kiburis, C. Michael, and D. Papadakis (1975) (unpublished data).
8. Isbell, H., C. W. Gorodetzsky, D. Jasinski, F. Clausen, v. Spulak, and F. Korte (1967) Effects of $(-)$-Δ^9-trans-tetrahydrocannabinol in man. *Psychopharmacologia 11:*184.
9. Kephalas, T. A., J. Kiburis, C. Michael, D. Papadakis, W. Heerma, R. J. J. Ch. Lousberg, C. A. Salemink, and H. J. W. Spronck (1975) (unpublished data).
10. Küppers, F. J. E. M., C. A. L. Bercht, H. J. W. Spronck, C. A. Salemink, R. J. J. Ch. Lousberg, J. K. Terlouw, and W. Heerma (unpublished results).
11. Küppers, F. J. E. M., R. J. J. Ch. Lousberg, C. A. L. Bercht, C. A. Salemink, J. K. Terlouw, W. Heerma, and A. Laven (1973) Cannabis. VIII. Pyrolysis of cannabidiol. Structure elucidation of the main pyrolytic product. *Tetrahedron 29:*2797.
12. Merkus, F. W. H. M., M. G. L. Jaspers von Wouw, and J. F. C. Roovers-Bollen (1972) Introduction to the analysis of cannabis constituents especially in smoke and body fluids. *Pharm. Weekbl. 107:*98.

13. Mikes, F., and P. G. Waser (1971) Marihuana components: effects of smoking on Δ^9-tetrahydrocannabinol and cannabidiol. *Science 172:*1158.
14. Miras, C., S. Simos, and J. Kiburis (1964) Comparative assay of the constituents from the sublimate of smoked cannabis with that from ordinary cannabis. *Bull. Narc. 16*(1):13.
15. O'Brien Fehr, K. and H. Kalant (1972) Analysis of cannabis smoke obtained under different combustion conditions. *Can. Physiol. Pharmacol. 50:*761.
16. Shoyama, Y., A. Yamaguchi, T. Sato, T. Yamauchi, and I. Nishioka (1969) Cannabis. IV. Smoking test. *Yakugaku Zasshi. 89*(6):842.
17. The chemistry of cannabis smoke: report of a working group (Athens 21–25 April 1975): United Nations Division of Narcotic Drugs MNAR/6/1975 GE 75–5104.
18. Weil, A. T. (1969) Cannabis. *Science Journal 5A*(3):36.

5

Identification of Cannabinoids and Metabolites in Biological Materials by Combined Gas-Liquid Chromatography–Mass Spectrometry

MONROE E. WALL AND DOLORES R. BRINE

Studies from several research groups have shown that Δ^9-tetrahydrocannabinol (Δ^9-THC) and related cannabinoids, such as cannabidiol and cannabinol, are extensively metabolized by liver microsomal enzymes (cf. Mechoulam [2] and Paton and Crown [3] for recent reviews). Studies from our laboratories have shown that the major metabolic route involves rapid hydroxylation at carbon 11 followed by further oxidation to the carboxylic acids [4–7]. Minor routes involve hydroxylation at the 8α or 8β positions, or in the side chain singly or in combination with the major routes. The sites of hydroxylation in the THC molecule are shown in Figure 5.1.

The identification of these metabolites in biological material is of major importance. We will present a systematic procedure by which combined gas-liquid chromatography (GLC) and mass spectrometry (MS) can be used to identify many of the metabolites found as a result of *in vitro* metabolism by the liver microsomal fraction or in blood, urine, or feces obtained after administering cannabinoids to animals or human volunteers.[1]

Materials and Methods

Extraction and preliminary concentration of cannabinoids

Table 5.1 presents an extraction scheme which we have used for extracting Δ^9-THC in a variety of microsomal metabolites from a monkey liver 10,000×g supernatant. The method is based on separating crude extract into neutral and acidic fractions. Usually the

[1] A preliminary report on a portion of these studies was presented by M. E. Wall and D. R. Brine at the International Symposium on Mass Spectrometry in Biochemistry and Medicine, Milan, Italy, May 7–9, 1973.

Marihuana: Chemistry, Biochemistry, and Cellular Effects, edited by Gabriel G. Nahas,

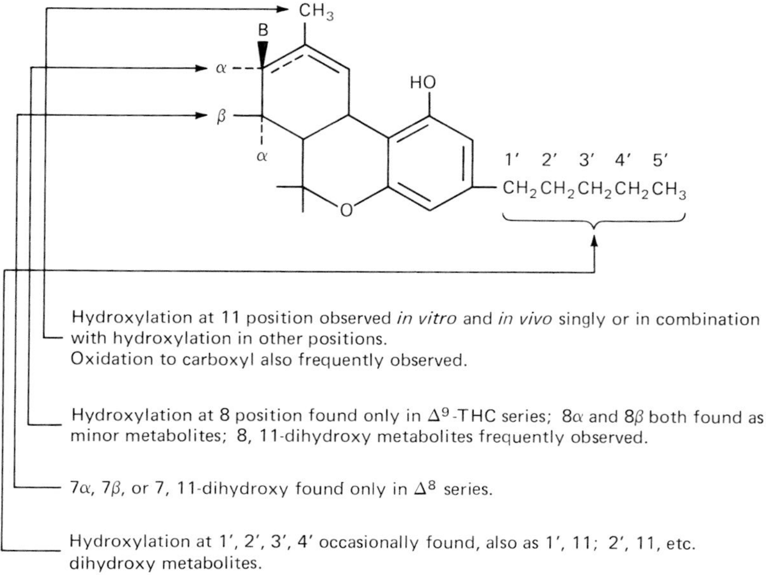

Figure 5.1. Hydroxylation sites of cannabinoids observed *in vitro* or *in vivo.*

neutral fraction was sufficiently concentrated so that further purification was not required before analysis. The acidic compounds required additional column chromatography on Sephadex LH-20, and in some cases, further purification by means of a Silica Gel chromatography under high-pressure conditions. Analogous methodology was used for the extraction and preliminary concentration of various cannabinoids and their metabolites in the blood, urine, or feces of animals or human volunteers.

Derivatization and gas chromatography conditions

Due to the polarity of the hydroxylated cannabinoids and their 9-carboxylic acid derivatives, it was necessary to convert the various cannabinoid reference compounds or the crude extracts to the corresponding trimethylsilyl derivatives. For this purpose the solvent solutions were evaporated *in vacuo,* and the residue converted to the trimethylsilyl (TMS) derivatives using the reagent N,O-bis(TMS)-trifluoroacetamide (BSTFA), which contains 1 percent of trimethylchlorosilane (TMCS). This reagent converted both hindered and nonhindered hydroxyl groups and also the 9-carboxylic acid to the corresponding TMS derivatives. After the reaction was

Table 5.1 *In vitro* incubation of Δ^9-THC with rhesus monkey liver microsomes

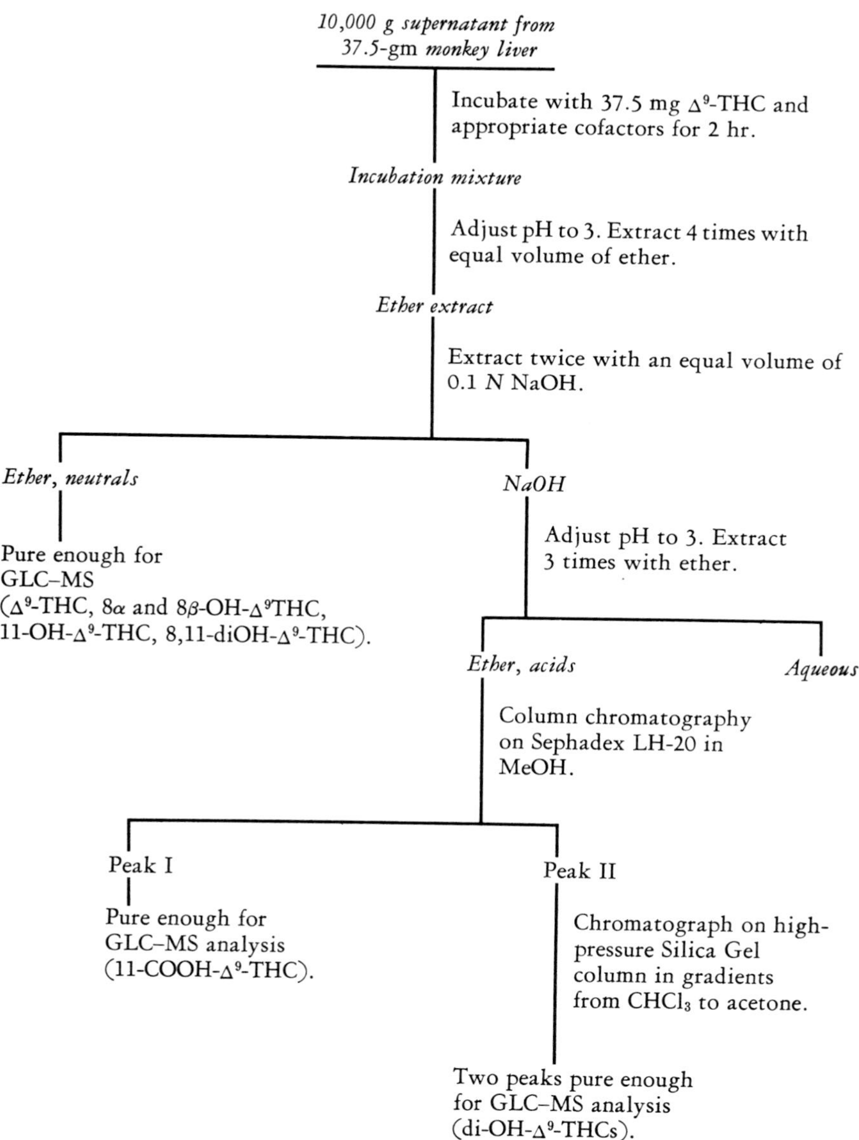

completed (sample plus 100 μl of reagent heated at 100°C for 3 hr), the excess silylating reagent was removed *in vacuo* and the residue dissolved in a small volume of hexane. An aliquot of the hexane solution was injected directly into the gas chromatograph system of the GLC–MS.

The gas chromatography column used 1 percent OV-17 on a support of chromosorb W 100/200 mesh and was normally operated isothermally at a temperature of 230°C. We used two GLC–MS instruments in our studies. The LKB 9000 instrumentation was used when the retention times (RTs) of the various compounds were sufficiently different to yield reasonable separations; alternatively, we used the Varian CH-7 GLC–MS equipped with a computer system. With this latter instrument all of the data could be accumulated on tapes, which later could be used to generate the mass spectra. The computer techniques and programs available in many cases permitted resolution of mixtures and identification of compounds of these mixtures that had been poorly resolved in the gas chromatographic column. We used the following reference compounds in our studies, all of them of synthetic origin: Δ^9-THC; Δ^8-THC; 8α- and 8β-hydroxy-Δ^9-THC; 11-hydroxy-Δ^9-THC; 8α,11-, 8β,11-dihydroxy-Δ^9-THC; 11-carboxy-Δ^8-THC; 11-carboxy-Δ^9-THC; 1′-hydroxy-, 2′-hydroxy-, 3′-hydroxy-, 4′-hydroxy-, and 5′-hydroxy-Δ^8-THC.

Results

Separation of Δ^9-THC and metabolites by GLC

Tables 5.2 and 5.3 present the RTs for a number of hydroxylated analogs of Δ^9- or Δ^8-THC. The double bond isomerism has little effect on RT values. As a result, data presented for the Δ^8-series (which is more available from synthetic routes) would also hold for the Δ^9-series, and vice versa. In general, RT values for the TMS ethers of various hydroxy-THC metabolites are significantly affected by their position in the THC molecule. Thus, whereas the 8α- and 8β-hydroxy epimers cannot be separated from each other, these compounds have significantly different RT values from both Δ^9-THC and 11-OH-Δ^9-THC, the latter having the longest RT. Adding a second hydroxyl group, such as in the 8,11-diOH-Δ^9-THC, results in an increase in the RT values. In this case, 8α,11- and 8β,11-TMS ethers differ markedly, the latter having a much longer RT.

Table 5.2 GLC retention times of Δ^9-THC and metabolites, TMS ethers

Neutrals		
TMS ethers of	*RT (min) at 220°C on 1% OV-17, 6 ft*	*RT (min) at 210–230°C on 1% OV-17, 6 ft*
Δ^9-THC	2.7	8
1′-OH-Δ^8-THC	3.3	9.3
8α-OH-Δ^9-THC	5.3	13.4
8β-OH-Δ^9-THC	5.4	13.5
3′-OH-Δ^8-THC	5.6	13.8
11-OH-Δ^9-THC	7.0	16.1
8α,11-diOH-Δ^9-THC	7.8	17.8
8β,11-diOH-Δ^9-THC	10.0	20.7
Acids		
TMS ethers of	*RT (min) at 247°C on 1% OV-17, 6 ft*	*RT (min) at 240°C on 1% OV-17, 6 ft*
11-COOH-Δ^9-THC	4.5	6.0
11-COOH, ξ-OH-Δ^9-THC	8.5	10.8
11-COOH, 8β-OH-Δ^9-THC	6.4	8.6

Table 5.3 Comparison of GLC retention times of TMS Ethers of Δ^8-THC hydroxylated in side chain

TMS ethers of	*RT (min) at 230°C on 2% OV-17 on Supelcoport (110/120 mesh), 6 ft*
1′-OH-Δ^8-THC	3
2′-OH-Δ^8-THC	4
3′-OH-Δ^8-THC	5.2
4′-OH-Δ^8-THC	5.4
5′-OH-Δ^8-THC	7.4

Position on the side chain also affects RT values. As shown in Table 5.3, the RT values increase progressively from the 1′ to the 5′ positions. Table 5.4, which gives RT values for a number of Δ^9-THC metabolites produced *in vitro* from rhesus monkey liver microsomal preparations, shows similar results. In this case the 1′-, 2′-, and 3′,11-diTMS ethers of Δ^9-THC showed progressively

Table 5.4 GLC retention times of TMS ethers of monkey liver metabolites

Compound identified	RT (min) at 230°C on 2% OV-17
Δ^9-THC	2.5
8α- and 8β-OH-Δ^9-THC	4.5
11-OH-Δ^9-THC	5.5
11-COOH-Δ^9-THC	10.0
8α,11-diOH-Δ^9-THC	7.0
1′,11-diOH-Δ^9-THC	6.5
2′,11-diOH-Δ^9-THC	8.0
3′,11-diOH-Δ^9-THC	10.5
ε,11-diOH-Δ^9-THC	11.5

Table 5.5 Mass spectral diagnostic peaks for TMS derivatives of Δ^9-THC and its metabolites

Compound	Hydroxyl and/or carboxyl groups (no.)	Parent ion m/e	Base peak or diagnostic peak (D) m/e
Δ^9-THC	1	386	386 371 (D)
Δ^8-THC	1	386	386 303 (D)
8β-OH-Δ^9-THC	2	474	343 (M-131)
8α-OH-Δ^9-THC	2	474	384 (M-90) M-[$OHSi(CH_3)_3$]
11-OH-Δ^9-THC	2	474	371 (M-103) M-[$CH_2OSi(CH_3)_3$]
1′-OH-Δ^8-THC	2	474	417 (M-57) M-C_4H_9
2′-OH-Δ^8-THC	2	474	145
3′-OH-Δ^8-THC	2	474	330 (M-144) 445 (D) M-29, M-C_2H_5
4′-OH-Δ^8-THC	2	474	474, 391 (D) (M-83), 330 (D) (M-144)
5′-OH-Δ^8-THC	2	474	474, 391 (D) (M-83) 330 (D) M-144
8α,11-diOH-Δ^9-THC	3	562	472 (M-90) 459 (D) M-103
8β,11-diOH-Δ^9-THC	3	562	369 (M-103-90)
11-COOH-Δ^9-THC	2	488	371 (M-117) M-$COOSi(CH_3)_3$

Table 5.6 Mass spectral diagnostic peaks for TMS derivatives of metabolite mixture obtained by incubation of Δ^9-THC with rhesus monkey liver microsomal preparation

Compound identified (TMS ether)	*RT (min)*	*Number of OH or COOH groups*	*Parent ion m/e*	*Base peak or diagnostic peak (D) m/e*
Δ^9-THC	2.5	1	386	386, 371 (D)
8α-OH-Δ^9-THC	4.5	2	474	384
8β-OH-Δ^9-THC	4.5	2	474	343
11-OH-Δ^9-THC	5.5	2	474	371
11-COOH-Δ^9-THC	10.0	1 OH, 1 COOH	488	371
8α,11-diOH-Δ^9-THC	7.0	3	562	472, 459[a]
1′,11-diOH-Δ^9-THC	6.5	3	562	459, 505
2′,11-diOH-Δ^9-THC	8.0	3	562	459, 145
3′,11-diOH-Δ^9-THC	10.5	3	562	459, 418[a]
4′,11-diOH-Δ^9-THC	11.5	3	562	459, 418

[a] Very strong peak; almost as intense as base peak.

longer RTs. A compound shown as ε,11-diOH-Δ^9-THC may actually be the 4′ analog. The RT value found would be in accord with this assignment. In this table, in agreement with the data in Table 5.2, RT values increased progressively with the number of additional hydroxyl groups formed.

Characteristic mass special fragmentation patterns

Table 5.5 is a compilation of the most important MS peaks of a number of synthetic analogs of Δ^9- or Δ^8-THC. Most of them have been shown to be *in vivo* or *in vitro* metabolites of Δ^9- or Δ^8-THC or of cannabinol [1,4–9]. Table 5.5 gives for each compound the *m/e* of the parent ion of the TMS ether derivative. For each additional hydroxyl group (Δ^9- and Δ^8-THC have 1 hydroxyl group), there is an increase of 88 mass units. In addition, Table 5.5 gives the *m/e* value of the strongest fragment, the base peak, which most frequently is not the parent ion but some fragment. In some cases the *m/e* values for other peaks which may be diagnostically useful are presented. In conjunction with RT values given earlier, this information can frequently characterize partially purified metabolite mixtures of cannabinoids found in biological material. Table 5.6 presents mass fragmentation data for a metabolite mixture obtained by the action of a rhesus liver microsomal preparation on Δ^9-THC.

Discussion

In recent years, the complex pattern of metabolic hydroxylation of Δ^9- or Δ^8-THC and other cannabinoids in the liver or lungs has been elucidated [2–9]. It is now apparent that the THC molecule (cf. Figure 5.1) is readily hydroxylated allylic to the double bond in Δ^9-THC or Δ^8-THC. We will restrict our discussion to the former, which is the naturally occurring bond isomer. The 11-methyl group of Δ^9-THC is most rapidly hydroxylated to give the 11-hydroxyl, which is then further oxidized to the carboxyl [7]. This latter, acidic form is the main cannabinoid excreted in the urine in man [7]. Similar results have been found for cannabinol and cannabidiol [7]. Secondary hydroxylation occurs more slowly in the 8α and 8β positions and on almost all the carbon atoms in the side chain [4–9]. The secondary and primary hydroxylations often occur sequentially. For example 8,11-diOH-cannabinoids are frequently found when Δ^9-THC is metabolized. Since many of these metabolites are found in minor quantities and isolation in pure form is frequently impractical, the application of combined GLC–MS is an ideal solution. Although many MS peaks of modest intensity are useful for diagnostic purposes when working with pure compounds, such a practice would be dangerous with metabolic mixtures obtained from biological sources.

We use only high molecular weight fragments with m/e greater than 300 for identification. This eliminates many possibilities for interference by endogenous substances. The only exception is the fragment at $m/e = 145$ found for the TMS ether of 2′-OH-cannabinoids, which has very strong intensity. Fortunately, as indicated in Table 5.5, many strong peaks are available. The most useful strong fragments are 8α-OH (M^+-90), 8β-OH (M^+-131), 11-OH (M^+-103), and 11-COOH (M^+-117). Usually, the combination of 8 and 11 hydroxylations gives strong fragments for both functions. Another striking usage of the combined techniques lies in recognizing the location of side chain hydroxylation by the combined GLC–MS technique [1,4,6]. As shown in Table 5.5, the 1′-, 2′-, and 3′-TMS ethers show strong fragments, respectively, at M-57, a strong fragment at $m/e = 145$, and at M-144. The 4′- and 5′-TMS ethers also show the M-144 fragment but much less intense than the 3′ metabolite. Since there is reason to believe that all of the side chain metabolites are separable by GLC techniques (cf. Tables 5.2, 5.3, and 5.5), the comparative RTs are useful in identification, and combined with the characteristic fragmentation patterns permit unequivocal identification.

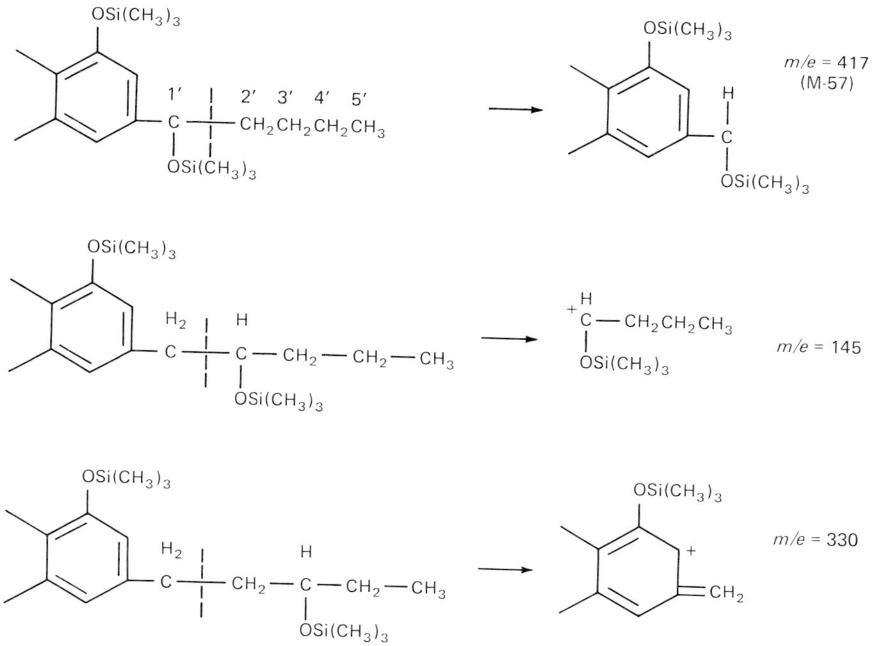

Figure 5.2. Mass spectral fragmentation of Δ^8-THC-TMS ethers at various positions in side chain.

Mechanism of side chain fragmentation

The mechanism of the side chain fragmentation of TMS ethers is shown in Figure 5.2. Interestingly, each of the side chain cleavages involves fission between the C-1′ and C-2′ carbons. When the TMS ether is located on the benzylic C-1′ carbon, the charge remains on C-1′ and a neutral C_4H_9 fragment is lost (M-57). With the silyl ether on the 2′ position, the charge remains on this carbon, and we note a strong fragment at $m/e = 145$. When the TMS ether is at 3′, 4′, or 5′, a neutral 4-carbon moiety containing the silyl group is lost, and a very strong charged fragment is seen, depicted in Figure 5.2 at $m/e = 330$. The mechanism for C-4′ and C-5′ resembles that of C-3′, but this fragmentation does not predominate to the extent found for C-3′.

Application of method to biological systems

The application of these mass fragmentation patterns to biological systems will now be briefly discussed. Incubation of Δ^9-THC with a microsomal rhesus monkey liver preparation followed by extraction and partial purification as shown in Table 5.1 gave a metabolite mixture with GLC retention behavior shown in Tables 5.4 and 5.6. A number of cannabinoids were readily identified in the neutral fraction: unmetabolized Δ^9-THC, 11-hydroxy- and 11-carboxy-Δ^9-THC (11-nor-Δ^9-THC-9-carboxylic acid). This was the first time that the carboxylic acid was noted in *in vitro* metabolism. The above compounds were readily identified by their characteristic fragmentation patterns and GLC retention times. The 8α- and 8β-hydroxy metabolites could not be separated by GLC. However, by obtaining sequential spectra over the entire THC peak in which the 8-hydroxy metabolite mixture was found, we achieved sufficient resolution so that the characteristic M-90 and M-131 fragments of the 8α- and 8β-TMS ethers were obtained.

A number of dihydroxy metabolites were obtained. These included the well-known metabolite 8α,11-diOH-Δ^9-THC [4,5], easily recognized by strong M-90 and M-103 fragments (cf. Table 5.6). A group of novel metabolites, found for the first time, included the 1′,11-, 2′,11-, and 3′,11-diOH-Δ^9-THC. These were separable by GLC and were readily recognized since the mass fragmentation patterns in each case showed characteristic fragments for M-103, diagnostic for the TMS-ether of the 11-OH group. In addition, the characteristic C-1′-, C-2′-, and C-3′-TMS fragments (Table 5.6) were noted in each case.

A typical spectrum shown in Figure 5.3 illustrates the mass spectra of the TMS ether of 3′,11-diOH-Δ^9-THC identified in the monkey liver microsomal extract. There was also some evidence for the presence of 4′,11-diOH-Δ^9-THC, but clear-cut differentiation from the 5′-OH possibility was not obtained. No monohydroxy side chain metabolites were found, although Widman *et al.* [8] noted that the 3′- and 4′-OH-Δ^9-THC were major metabolites in an *in vitro* perfused dog lung metabolism experiment, and Wall [4] noted the 2′-OH metabolite of cannabinol, as well as the 2′,11-diOH metabolite, when cannabinol was incubated with a rat liver microsomal preparation. Obviously, species, substrate, and experimental conditions (cofactors, organ, microsomal preparation, perfusion, or *in vivo* factors) will all affect metabolite composition. The key point is that the methodology described in this paper (a preliminary report was made in 1973) [6] and the similar but independent studies of Binder, Agurell, *et al.* [1] are more than adequate to identify most of the hydroxylated metabolites produced under *in vitro* and *in vivo* conditions. Moreover, excellent quantitation can be obtained by mass fragmentography techniques using deuterated internal standards.

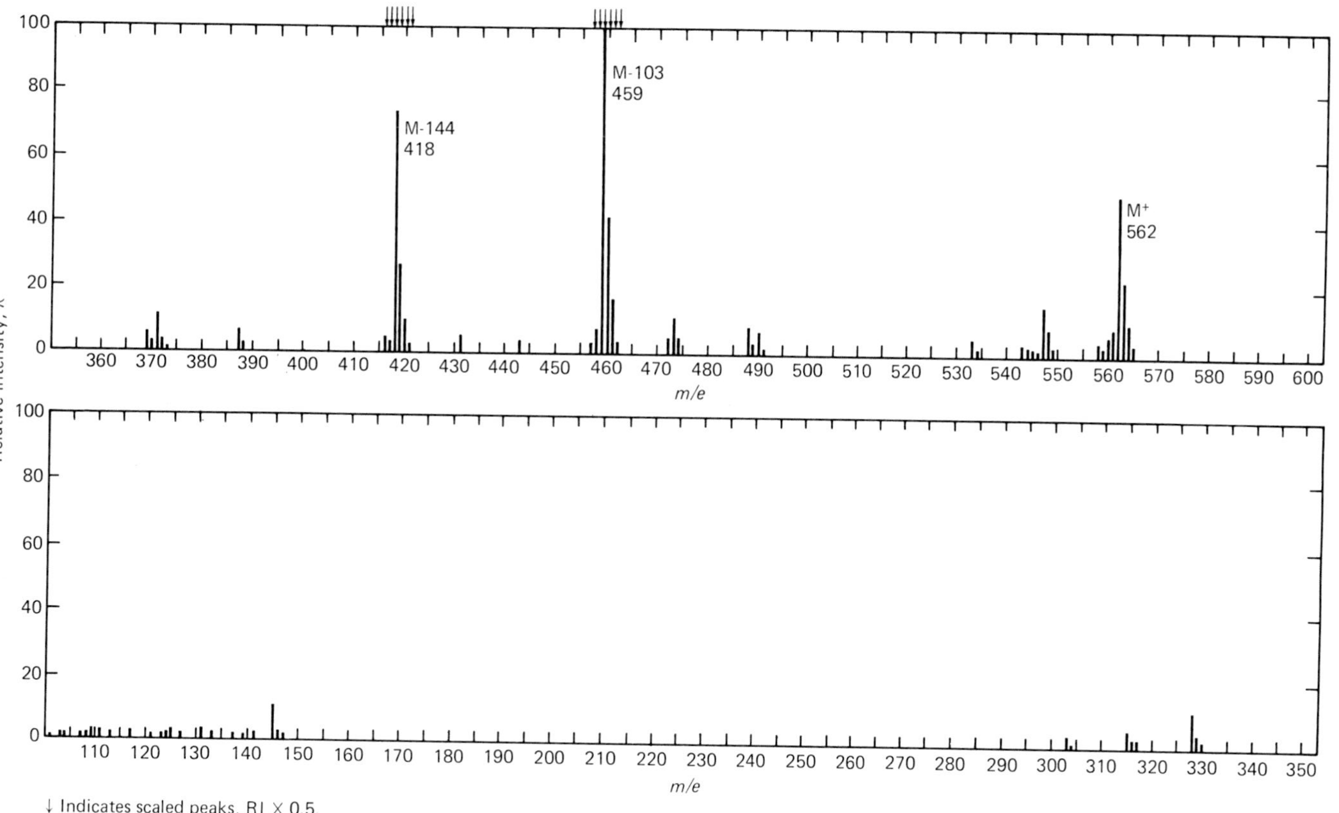

Figure 5.3. Mass spectrum of 3′,11-diOH-Δ^9-THC, TMS derivative (from monkey liver incubation).

ACKNOWLEDGMENTS

The studies described in the paper were supported under Contract No. HSM-42-71-95 with the National Institute on Drug Abuse (formerly National Institute of Mental Health), Division of Biomedical Research, Biomedical Research Branch. We should like to thank Drs. M. Braude and S. Szara, Scientific Project Officers, NIDA, for their encouragement of these studies. We are indebted to Dr. Joan Bursey and J. M. Taylor for technical assistance in mass spectral determinations. We wish to thank Professor S. Agurell, Astra Läkemedel AB, Sweden, for sending us recent and unpublished information concerning the research being conducted in his group.

REFERENCES

1. Binder, M., S. Agurell, K. Leander, and J. E. Lindgren (1974) Zur identification potentieller metabolite von cannabis-inhaltstoffen: kernresonanz- und massenspektroskopische untersuchungen an seitenkettenhydroxylierten cannabinoiden. *Helv. Chim. Acta 57*:1626.
2. Mechoulam, R. (ed.) (1973) *Marihuana.* New York: Academic Press.
3. Paton, W. D. and J. Crown (eds.) (1972) *Cannabis and Its Derivatives.* London: Oxford University Press.
4. Wall, M. E. (1971) The *in vitro* and *in vivo* metabolism of tetrahydrocannabinol (THC). *Ann. N.Y. Acad. Sci. 191*:23.
5. Wall, M. E., D. R. Brine, C. G. Pitt, and M. Perez-Reyes (1972) Identification of Δ^9-tetrahydrocannabinol and metabolites in man. *J. Amer. Chem. Soc. 94*:8579.
6. Wall, M. E. and D. R. Brine (1973) Applications of mass spectrometry to structure of metabolites of Δ^9-tetrahydrocannabinol (THC). Presented the International Symposium on Mass Spectrometry in Biochemistry and Medicine, Milan, Italy.
7. Wall, M. E. and D. R. Brine (1976) Metabolism of cannabinoids in man. *Pharmacology of Marihuana* (M. Braude and S. Szara, eds.). New York: Raven Press.
8. Widman, M., M. Nordqvist, C. T. Dollery, and R. H. Briant (1975) Metabolism of Δ^1-tetrahydrocannabinol in the dog. *J. Pharm. Pharmacol.* (in press).
9. Widman, M., J. Dalmen, K. Leander, and K. Peterson (1975) *In vitro* metabolism of cannabinol in rat and rabbit liver (unpublished data).

6

Comparison of Various Solvent Extractions for the Chromatographic Analysis of Δ^9-THC and Its Metabolites

JOSEPH C. SCHOOLAR, BENG T. HO, AND VICENTE S. ESTEVEZ

Introduction

Great progress has been made in recent years in elucidating the metabolism of Δ^9-tetrahydrocannabinol (Δ^9-THC), the major psychoactive constituent of marihuana. The main metabolites of Δ^9-THC, resulting from the liver microsomal oxidase reactions, have been identified as 11-hydroxy-Δ^9-THC (11-OH-Δ^9-THC) and 8,11-diOH-Δ^9-THC [1,3,20]. In addition, the formation of acidic metabolites has been proven [4,17,21]. Treatment of rats with SKF-525-A before administering Δ^9-THC resulted in a substantial reduction of all three metabolites [7]. Some reports indicate that the monohydroxylated metabolite is as active as Δ^9-THC behaviorally and pharmacologically [8,12,19,20], although others imply that unchanged Δ^9-THC is responsible for certain effects of marihuana [13,18]. The dihydroxylated product is behaviorally inactive [5,19,20].

The lipophilicity of cannabinoids [11] has led most investigators to use nonpolar or slightly polar solvents to extract Δ^9-THC and its metabolites from tissues and fluids [2,14–16]. However, several of these reports have pointed out the presence in tissues of some metabolites that are not extractable by the solvents used.

In our laboratories, we have studied the metabolism of Δ^9-THC [7,9,10] and other cannabinoids [6,11] in rats and monkeys and have used methanol to extract cannabinoids from tissues completely before chromatographic separation of metabolites [9]. In the present study, we have compared the extraction efficiency of two of the most commonly used solvent systems with methanol.

Marihuana: Chemistry, Biochemistry, and Cellular Effects, edited by Gabriel G. Nahas,

Methods

Male Sprague-Dawley rats (175–200 gm) were injected intravenously via the tail vein with 5 mg/kg of ^{3}H-Δ^{9}-THC (46 mCi/mM) in 4 percent Tween 80-saline suspension. Half of the animals were placed in metabolic cages for collection of urine and feces during a 24 hr period. The other half were sacrificed by decapitation under ether anesthesia at 30 min postinjection. Blood was collected by exsanguination, and the brain and liver were removed. Tissues and feces were homogenized in 9 volumes of water.

Urine and aliquots of the homogenates were assayed for tritium by liquid scintillation spectrometry [9]. Fifty microliters of blood or fecal homogenate was placed in counting vials and decolorized with 1 ml of 10 percent hydrogen peroxide in methanol. The solvent was evaporated overnight under a hood, and the residue was treated with 1 ml of 1.0 *N* aqueous sodium hydroxide. After heating at 75 °C for 2 hr in an incubator shaker, 0.2 ml of ethyl hexanoic acid was added to neutralize the basic medium. Radioactivity was determined after adding 10 ml of Insta-Gel.

Methanol extraction

Lyzed blood or homogenate in 1-ml aliquots was extracted with 5 volumes of methanol, followed by two more extractions with 90 percent methanol in water. All extracts, containing from 91–98 percent of the original radioactivity, were pooled, the combined volume measured, and the radioactivity assayed.

n-Heptane-*i*-amyl alcohol, ether extraction

A set of samples of urine, blood, and homogenates was mixed with 1 ml of 0.2 *M* phosphate buffer, pH 7.4, and extracted three times with 5 volumes of 1.5 percent *i*-amyl alcohol in *n*-heptane. The solvent extracts were pooled, then the aqueous solution was extracted three times with 5 volumes of diethyl ether, and the extracts were again pooled. The remaining compounds in the final aqueous medium were then extracted with methanol.

Petroleum ether, diethyl ether extraction

Another set of samples was extracted three times with 5 volumes of petroleum ether. Subsequent extractions were made with diethyl ether and methanol.

Chromatography

All extracts were evaporated to dryness, and the residues were redissolved in 0.1–0.2 ml of methanol. After centrifugation, the supernatant was chromatographed on Silica Gel G precoated plates and developed, along with reference compounds, in the solvent system chloroform-acetone (4:1) [9]. The distribution of radioactivity in the chromatograms was determined by scraping sections of silica and assaying for tritium. The percentage of each metabolite was calculated by a mapping technique which involved plotting the percent of radioactivity in each section versus R_f values. The 11-OH-Δ^9-THC, 8,11-diOH-Δ^9-THC, and 11-nor-Δ^9-THC-carboxylic acid used as reference standards were furnished by the National Institute of Drug Abuse, U.S. Public Health Service.

Results and Discussion

In Table 6.1 the efficiency of the three solvent systems for extracting radioactivity from various rat tissues and fluids is compared. The proportions of unchanged Δ^9-THC to its metabolites in each extract as determined by thin-layer chromatography are shown in Tables 6.2–6.5.

Table 6.1 Extraction of radioactivity from various tissues and fluids by three solvent systems

		Percent radioactivity extracted[a]				
Procedure	*Solvent*	*Brain*	*Liver*	*Blood*	*Urine*	*Feces*
A	Methanol	95.6	98.0	90.9	98.3	92.5
B	*n*-Heptane-*i*-amyl alcohol	88.9	32.5	15.4	7.1	—
	Ethyl ether	5.1	17.7	29.3	28.2	—
	Methanol	2.2	36.8	47.7	59.8	—
		(96.2)[b]	(87.0)	(92.4)	(95.1)	—
C	Petroleum ether	71.0	16.8	7.9	1.9	—
	Ethyl ether	13.7	21.1	36.2	25.4	—
	Methanol	10.1	50.2	49.8	63.6	—
		(94.8)	(88.1)	(93.9)	(90.9)	—

[a] Each value represents the mean from 5 animals.

[b] Values in parentheses are the combined total percentages of radioactivity extracted by all the solvents of the same system.

Table 6.2 Extraction of Δ⁹-THC and metabolites from brain homogenates using the three solvent systems

Procedure	Solvent	Percent radio-activity extracted	Percent distribution of metabolites		
			Δ⁹ (0.94)[a]	11-OH (0.59)	Acid[b] (0)
A	Methanol	95.6	71.8	15.6	7.8
B	*n*-Heptane-*i*-amyl alcohol	88.9	71.6	13.1	3.7
	Ethyl ether	5.1	—	2.3	2.7
	Methanol	2.2	—	0.3	1.8
C	Petroleum ether	71.0	69.6	—	1.4
	Ethyl ether	13.7	0.7	12.1	0.8
	Methanol	10.1	1.2	3.5	5.4

[a] Numbers in parentheses represent R_f values on Silica Gel G plates developed in chloroform-acetone (4:1).

[b] A possible contamination by other metabolites.

Table 6.3 Extraction of Δ⁹-THC and metabolites from liver homogenates using the three solvent systems

Procedure	Solvent	Percent radio-activity extracted	Percent distribution of metabolites				
			Δ⁹ (0.94)	11-OH (0.59)	Un-known (0.30)	8,11-di OH (0.14)	Acid (0)
A	Methanol	98.0	11.0	18.7	12.1	15.3	39.8
B	*n*-Heptane-*i*-amyl alcohol	32.5	9.5	12.4	—	1.3	9.1
	Ethyl ether	17.7	0.2	4.8	—	5.9	6.7
	Methanol	36.8	—	1.0	10.2	7.4	17.7
C	Petroleum ether	16.8	9.8	—	—	—	6.4
	Ethyl ether	21.1	1.8	16.1	—	1.0	2.1
	Methanol	50.2	—	2.0	11.0	12.3	23.5

The use of methanol (solvent 1) yields a 91–98 percent extraction of Δ⁹-THC and metabolites from all samples, and the extracts are ready for chromatographic separation. Neither solvent system 2 (*n*-heptane-*i*-amyl alcohol followed by ethyl ether) nor solvent system 3 (petroleum ether followed by ethyl ether) gave quantitative extraction of Δ⁹-THC and its metabolites from all

Table 6.4 Extraction of Δ^9-THC and metabolites from urine using the three solvent systems

			Percent distribution of metabolites				
Procedure	*Solvent*	*Percent radio-activity extracted*	Δ^9 (0.94)	*11-OH* (0.59)	*Un-known* (0.30)	*8,11-di OH* (0.14)	*Acid* (0)
A	Methanol	98.3	1.1	2.4	5.5	7.9	76.2
B	*n*-Heptane-*i*-amyl alcohol	7.1	0.9	0.2	0.1	—	5.7
	Ethyl ether	28.2	—	1.9	1.2	2.0	22.4
	Methanol	59.8	—	0.1	4.2	5.5	47.5
C	Petroleum ether	1.9	1.0	0.2	—	—	0.6
	Ethyl ether	25.9	—	2.0	1.7	1.9	19.3
	Methanol	63.6	—	—	3.7	5.7	53.5

Table 6.5 Extraction of Δ^9-THC and metabolites from blood using the three solvent systems

			Percent distribution of metabolites				
Procedure	*Solvent*	*Percent radio-activity extracted*	Δ^9 (0.94)	*11-OH* (0.59)	*Un-known* (0.30)	*8,11-diOH* (0.14)	*Acid* (0)
A	Methanol	90.9	12.0	14.4	10.7	8.3	45.0
B	*n*-Heptane-*i*-amyl alcohol	15.4	9.6	2.8	0.2	1.2	1.1
	Ethyl ether	29.3	2.3	8.4	0.6	2.5	15.1
	Methanol	47.7	—	3.5	10.3	4.5	28.5
C	Petroleum ether	7.9	7.6	0.2	—	—	—
	Ethyl ether	36.2	4.5	11.9	0.4	1.9	17.0
	Methanol	49.8	—	2.0	10.5	6.9	26.7

samples; furthermore, these solvents left substantial amounts (ranging from 37–63 percent of unextracted polar metabolites.

Although both *n*-heptane-*i*-amyl alcohol and petroleum ether extract as much unchanged Δ^9-THC from brain (Table 6.2) and urine (Table 6.4), the two solvents do not give quantitative recoveries of Δ^9-THC from liver (Table 6.3) and blood (Table 6.5). This is extremely important, especially in measuring the drug concentration in blood for pharmacokinetic studies in humans and animals and for correlation of tolerance development with metabolism. Another disadvantage of using *n*-heptane-*i*-amyl alcohol is that it extracts a considerable amount of 11-OH-Δ^9-THC from all tissues along with the unchanged Δ^9-THC.

Unchanged Δ^9-THC can be recovered completely from tissue homogenates by a two-step extraction; namely, the use of either *n*-heptane-*i*-amyl alcohol or petroleum ether followed by ethyl ether. The two-step extraction method, however, is less satisfactory in extracting 11-OH-Δ^9-THC; the recovery from blood is particularly poor. Furthermore, the two-step method shows lower extractability for recovering the more polar metabolites, such as 8,11-diOH-Δ^9-THC and acidic metabolites.

Therefore, using a combination of solvents for extraction, such as solvent systems 2 and 3 mentioned above, does not appear to provide a clear-cut extraction method in the metabolic study of THC, especially when the data are based only on the solvent used without separating overlapping metabolites. The extraction procedure involving the use of methanol would seem to be the system of choice when total recovery of Δ^9-THC metabolites is desired.

REFERENCES

1. Agurell, S., I. M. Nilsson, A. Ohlsson, and F. Sandberg (1969) Elimination of tritium-labelled cannabinols in the rat with special reference to the development of tests for the identification of cannabis users. *Biochem. Pharmacol. 18:*1195.
2. Agurell, S., I. M. Nilsson, A. Ohlsson, and F. Sandberg (1970) On the metabolism of tritium-labelled Δ^1-tetrahydrocannabinol in the rabbit. *Biochem. Pharmacol. 19:*1333.
3. Ben-Zvi, Z., R. Mechoulam, and S. Burstein (1970) Identification through synthesis of an active $\Delta^{1(6)}$-tetrahydrocannabinol metabolite. *J. Am. Chem. Soc. 92:*3468.
4. Burstein, S., J. Rosenfeld, and T. Wittstruck (1972) Isolation and characterization of two major metabolites of Δ^1-tetrahydrocannabinol. *Science 176:*422.
5. Christensen, H. D., R. I. Freudenthal, J. R. Gidley, R. Rosenfeld, G. Boegli, L. Testino, D. R. Brine, C. G. Pitt, and M. E. Wall (1971) Activity of Δ^8- and Δ^9-tetrahydrocannabinol and related compounds in the mouse. *Science 172:*165.
6. Estevez, V. S., L. F. Englert, and B. T. Ho (1973) A new metabolite of (-)-11-hydroxy-Δ^8-tetrahydrocannabinol in rats. *Res. Commun. Chem. Pathol. Pharmacol. 6:*821.
7. Estevez, V. S., L. F. Englert, and B. T. Ho (1974) Effect of SKF-525-A on the metabolism of (-)-Δ^9-tetrahydrocannabinol in the rat brain and liver. *Res. Commun. Chem. Pathol. Pharmacol. 8:*389.
8. Gill, E. W. and G. Jones (1972) Brain levels of Δ^1-tetrahydrocannabinol and its metabolites in mice—correlation with behavior, and

the effect of the metabolic inhibitor SKF-525-A, and piperonyl butoxide. *Biochem. Pharmacol. 21:*2237.

9. Ho, B. T., V. S. Estevez, L. F. Englert, and W. M. McIsaac (1972) Δ^9-Tetrahydrocannabinol and its metabolites in monkey brains. *J. Pharm. Pharmacol. 24:*414.
10. Ho, B. T., V. S. Estevez, and L. F. Englert (1973) Effect of repeated administration on the metabolism of (-)-Δ^9-tetrahydrocannabinol in rats. *Res. Commun. Chem. Pathol. Pharmacol. 5:*215.
11. Ho, B. T., V. S. Estevez, and L. F. Englert (1973) The uptake and metabolic fate of cannabinoids in rat brains. *J. Pharm. Pharmacol. 25:*490.
12. Irwin, S. (1968) Comprehensive observation assessment: 1A. A systematic, quantitative procedure for assessing the behavioral and physiological state of the mouse. *Psychopharmacologia 13:*222.
13. Kubena, R. K. and H. Barry, III (1970) Interactions of Δ^1-tetrahydrocannabinol with barbiturates and methamphetamine. *J. Pharmacol. Exp. Ther. 173:*94.
14. Lemberger, L., S. Silberstein, J. Axelrod, and I. Kopin (1970) Marihuana: studies on the disposition and metabolism of delta-9-tetrahydrocannabinol in man. *Science 170:*1320.
15. Lemberger, L., N. Tamarkin, J. Axelrod, and I. Kopin (1971) Delta-9-tetrahydrocannabinol—metabolism and disposition in long-term marihuana smokers. *Science 173:*72.
16. Mikes, F., A. Hoffman, and P. G. Waser (1971) Identification of (-)-Δ^9-6a,10a-trans-tetrahydrocannabinol and two of its metabolites in rats by use of combination gas chromatography–mass spectrometry and mass fragmentography. *Biochem. Pharmacol. 20:*2469.
17. Nordqvist, M., S. Agurell, M. Binder, and J. M. Nilsson (1974) Structure of an acidic metabolite of Δ^1-tetrahydrocannabinol isolated from rabbit urine. *J. Pharm. Pharmacol. 26:*471.
18. Sofia, R. D. and H. Barry, III (1970) Depressant effect of Δ^1-tetrahydrocannabinol enhanced by inhibition of its metabolism. *Eur. J. Pharmacol. 13:*134.
19. Truitt, E. B. (1970) Pharmacological activity in a metabolite of *l*-trans-Δ^8-tetrahydrocannabinol. *Fed. Proc. 29:*619.
20. Wall, M. E., O. R. Brine, G. A. Brine, C. G. Pitt, R. I. Freudenthal, and H. D. Christensen (1970) Isolation, structure and biological activity of several metabolites of delta-9-tetrahydrocannabinol. *J. Am. Chem. Soc. 92:*3466.
21. Wall, M. E., O. R. Brine, and M. Pérez-Reyes (1973) Studies on the *in vitro* and *in vivo* metabolism of Δ^9-tetrahydrocannabinol. Abstracts 33rd International Congress of Pharmaceutical Sciences, Stockholm, p. 258.

7

Radioimmunoassay of Cannabis Products in Blood and Urine

VINCENT MARKS, J. D. TEALE,
AND L. J. KING

Introduction

The introduction of radioimmunoassay (RIA) by Yalow and Berson 15 years ago, for measuring first the insulin levels in plasma [18] and later those of other polypeptide hormones, led to its gradual application to almost every type of compound in biological fluids. Its use for measuring drugs has recently been reviewed [3, 4,9].

The main advantage of RIA over conventional analytical techniques is its exquisite sensitivity enabling many compounds—including drugs—to be measured at subpicomole concentrations. As with all immunoassay techniques, the most important single factor in the development of a practicable RIA procedure is the production of a high-avidity, monospecific antibody, preferably of high titer so that a large number of assays can be performed with the same antibody. Other important considerations in the development of an RIA are the availability of a high specific activity radiolabel and a pure standard, and definition of the conditions under which the assay can be performed.

In this paper the technique we have used to produce high-avidity antisera against Δ^9-tetrahydrocannabinol (Δ^9-THC) in sheep and their application to a radioimmunoassay sensitive enough to measure cannabinoids in blood and urine will be described. Because the assay we have developed for routine use is not specific for THC, we refer to the material measured in biological fluids as THC cross-reacting cannabinoids (THC–CRC). Some practical applications of the assay, including the detection of cannabis use, will also be mentioned.

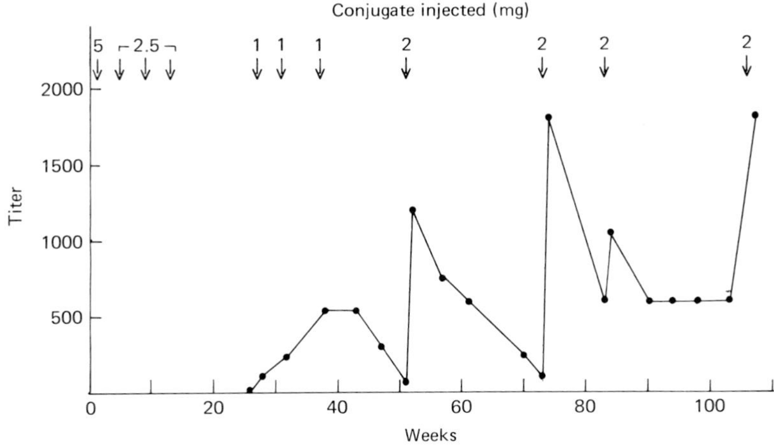

Figure 7.1. Immunization schedule and antibody titer in sheep 133Y. THC-semisuccinate BSA was injected IM in the amounts shown. Titer is defined as the reciprocal of the dilution of antiserum that bound 50% of the ^{3}H–THC label. Antiserum 133Y/25/4 was collected on week 52.

Radioimmunoassay

The general principles of radioimmunoassay are too well known to need reiteration [5,8,17,19]. The details of our own radioimmunoassay technique for THC–CRC have already been described [15] and will be briefly summarized here.

Antibody production

A THC-hemisuccinate bovine serum albumin (BSA) conjugate containing an average of 25 THC residues per molecule of protein was prepared using ethyl-(dimethylaminopropyl)-carbodiimide and injected into the leg muscles of a sheep, suspended in a modified form of Freund's complete adjuvant (B. Morris, unpublished observations), which, unlike the original material, does not cause tissue necrosis or ulceration. Booster doses containing varying amounts of conjugate emulsified in modified incomplete Freund's adjuvant were given intramuscularly at irregular intervals. The animals were bled from time to time, and the serum was tested for its capacity to bind radiolabeled THC displaceably. Each bleed was coded separately and treated as unique.

Antibodies capable of binding tritiated THC (^{3}H–THC) first ap-

Table 7.1 Immunogenicity of THC conjugates in sheep

Data represent the proportion of sheep immunized responding by production of ^{3}H-THC binding antibodies irrespective of titers

THC derivative (conjugated to BSA)	*Number responding / Number immunized*
Chlorocarbonate (1-C link through hydroxyl)	2/3
Hemisuccinate (4-C link through hydroxyl)	4/10
Hemiadipate (6-C link through hydroxyl)	1/3
Hemisebacate (10-C link through hydroxyl)	0/3
Azo-PABA (Phenyl link *para* to hydroxyl)	0/5
Mannich (1-C link *para* to hydroxyl)	0/1
Acid (1-C link *para* to hydroxyl)	1/2
Valerate (5-C link *para* to hydroxyl)	0/2
Total	8/29 (27%)

peared 6–9 months after primary immunization (Figure 7.1) but did not achieve useful titers until after a year or more. Of the 10 sheep originally immunized with the THC-hemisuccinate-BSA conjugate, 4 produced a usable antibody (Table 7.1). Most of the investigations reported here were carried out using the antiserum coded 133Y/25/4, but other antiserum bleeds have also been shown to behave similarly.

Reimmunizations were normally carried out when the antiserum titer (defined as the reciprocal of the dilution of antiserum that bound 50 percent of ^{3}H–THC label) had fallen to a low level. Before adopting the present immunization procedure, we used a number of other THC-protein conjugates as immunogens [12,13]. Aside from those produced by conjugation of chlorocarbonate derivatives of THC to BSA using the Schotten–Bauman reaction, which were the source of our first usable anti-THC antibody, none proved as immunogenic as the THC-hemisuccinate–BSA conjugate (Table 7.1).

Rabbits immunized with a variety of THC protein conjugates produced antibodies capable of binding avidly, and at high titer, a radioiodine-labeled conjugate of THC hemisuccinate and a synthetic polymer containing glutamic acid, lysine, alanine, and tyrosine (GLAT). But whereas the ^{125}I–THC–GLAT was readily displaced from antibody by "cold" THC–GLAT, it was not displaced by native THC. Consequently, it could not be used in an RIA. For reasons that are not clear, none of the antibodies raised in rabbits bound significant amounts of ^{3}H–THC.

Tracer label

During our work, high specific activity ^{3}H–THC (26 μCi/mg) became available commercially. This is now used in our standard assay. (Earlier we had used ^{3}H–THC generously given to us by Dr. E. W. Gill of Oxford.) As already mentioned, early attempts to use ^{125}I-labeled THC–GLAT as tracer in a radioimmunoassay were uniformly unsuccessful, but we have not reinvestigated it using the newer, high-titer sheep antisera now available. Nor have we attempted to use enzyme or other nonisotope labels in our THC immunoassay.

Assay conditions

Because of interference in the assay by proteins, especially lipoproteins, THC–CRC had to be extracted from the plasma before analysis. This could most conveniently be achieved by adding 2 volumes of ethanol to 1 of plasma. In this way, the proteins were precipitated but the THC–CRC remained in solution. Moreover, we found that if a sufficiently small amount of ethanolic extract of plasma was used, it could be added directly to the assay reaction mixture without interfering materially with the subsequent immunoreaction. Urine could be assayed without pretreatment. Nevertheless, because of the extreme insolubility of THC in water, a detergent had to be added to the assay mixture to keep the THC in solution. Of the many detergents examined, only Triton X-405 was satisfactory. Antibody-bound THC was separated from free THC by use of dextran-coated charcoal. A second antibody procedure might increase the sensitivity of the assay as it would reduce the effect of nonspecific protein binding of the ^{3}H–THC label. Glass tubes must be used throughout the assay because 35 percent of the ^{3}H–THC label is adsorbed by plastic.

The RIA currently in use in our laboratory is sensitive to 50 pg THC per assay tube and can be used reliably to measure THC–CRC equivalent to 7.5 ng/ml of plasma or 1 ng/ml in urine (15). Recovery of pure THC added to plasma is virtually complete over the range 5–50 ng/ml, although at the lower level the coefficient of variation is 40 percent. At plasma THC–CRC levels in excess of 25 ng/ml, the coefficient of variation is about 15 percent. This compares favorably with most RIA procedures.

Specificity

The specificity of antiserum 133Y/25/4 and of the assay derived from it have been tested in several ways. A wide range of natural and synthetic compounds was examined in the assay system *in vitro.* With the exception of certain cannabinoids—all of which possessed a closed three-ring cannabinoid nucleus, none of the compounds tested displaced ^{3}H–THC from the antibody or competed with it for binding, even at high concentrations. Among the closed three-ring cannabinoids which did cross-react, some—notably Δ^{8}-THC, 11-OH-Δ^{8}-THC, cannabinol, and 11-OH-Δ^{9}-THC (a major metabolite of THC)—behaved indistinguishably from Δ^{9}-THC (Table 7.2). However, most of the cannabinoids that were tested, showed either a much lower binding affinity for the antibody (Table 7.3) or none at all (Table 7.4).

Figure 7.2. Standard curves constructed using ^{3}H–THC as label. (a) Comparison of displacement of label by increasing amounts of SPA-80; SP-1, and THC, respectively. (b) Displacement of label by SPA-80 and SP-1 in large amounts.

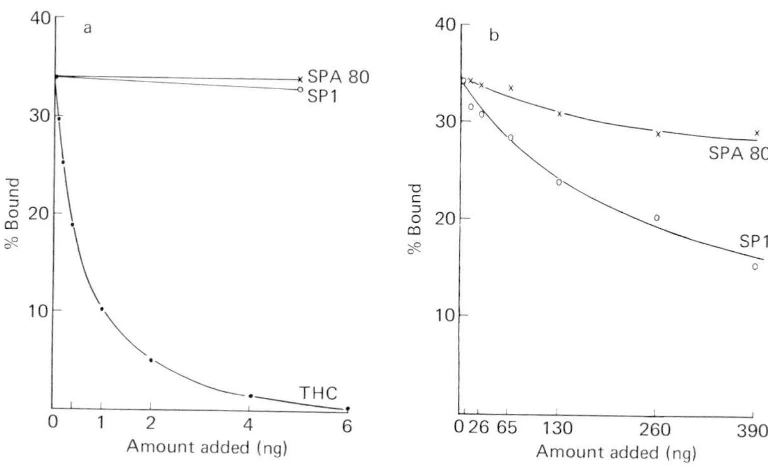

Table 7.2 Naturally occurring cannabinoids exhibiting reaction with antiserum under assay conditions

The avidity constant of each reaction and the amount of each compound required to reduce the binding of ^{3}H-THC to antiserum by 50%

Cannabinoid		*Avidity constant liters/ mole)*	*Amount reducing label binding by 50% (ng)*
OH, C_5H_{11}	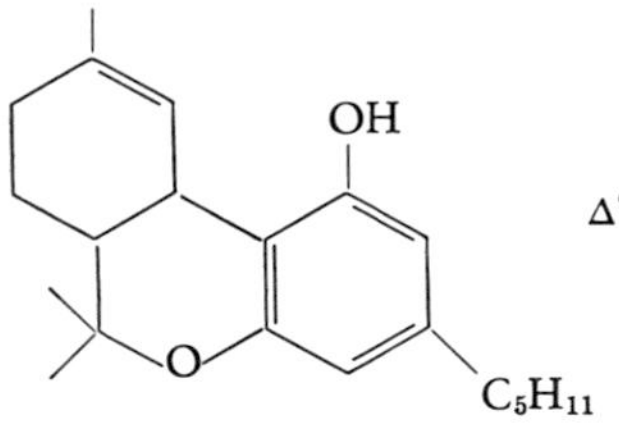 Δ^9-THC	6.0×10^9	0.4
OH, C_5H_{11}	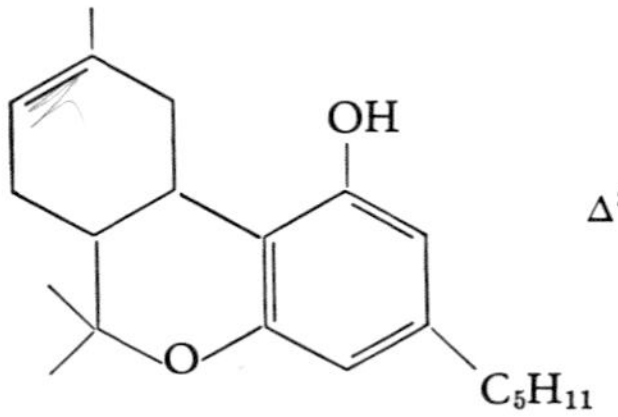 Δ^8-THC	6.0×10^9	0.4
CH_2OH, OH, C_5H_{11}	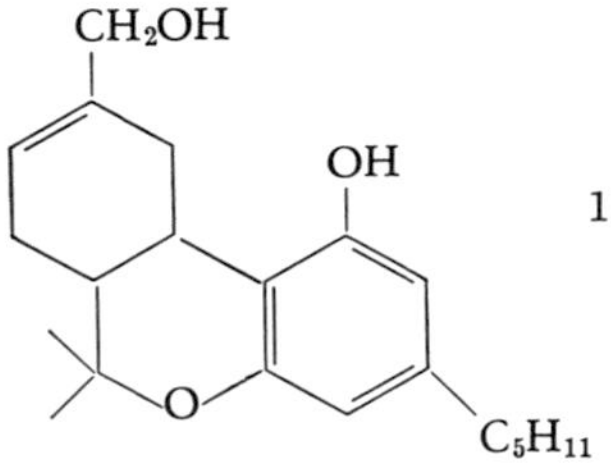 11-OH-Δ^8-THC	6.0×10^9	0.4
OH, C_5H_{11}	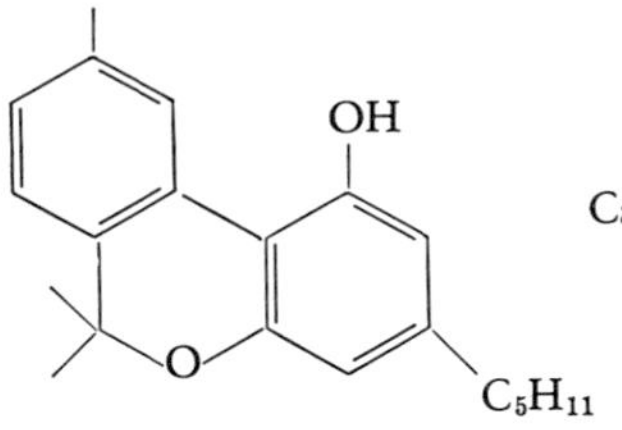 Cannabinol	6.0×10^9	0.4
CH_2OH, OH, C_5H_{11}	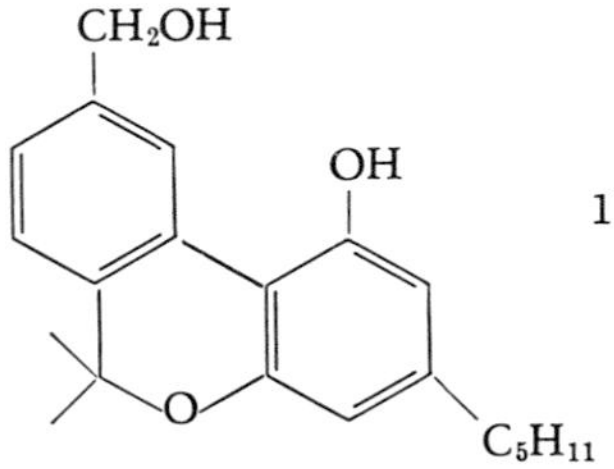 11-OH-cannabinol	2.2×10^7	35.0

Table 7.3 Synthetic cannabinoids exhibiting reaction with antiserum under assay conditions

The avidity constant of each reaction and the amount of each compound required to reduce the binding of ^{3}H-THC to antiserum by 50%

Cannabinoid		*Avidity constant (liters/mole)*	*Amount reducing label binding by 50% (ng)*
HO, OH, C_5H_{11}	8α-OH-HHC[a]	6.0×10^9	0.4
CHO, $OCOCH_3$, C_5H_{11}	Cannabinol-11-al acetate	6.0×10^9	0.4
$COOCH_3$, OH, C_5H_{11}	Δ8-THC-11-oic acid methyl ester	6.0×10^5	> 100
COOH, OCH_3, C_5H_{11}	Δ8-THC-11-oic acid methyl ether	9.8×10^6	> 100
CH_3COO, OH, OH, C_5H_{11}	8-Acetoxy-9-OH-HHC	8.8×10^5	> 100

[a] HHC—hexahydrocannabinol.

Table 7.4 Cannabinoids exhibiting no reaction with antiserum when present in the assay in amounts up to 1 μg

Structure	*Cannabinoid*
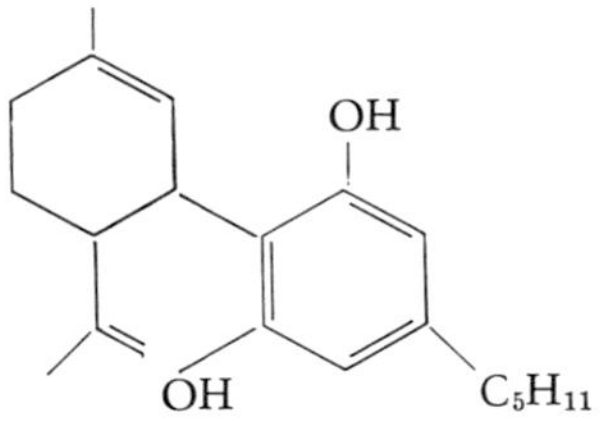 OH; OH; C_5H_{11}	Cannabidiol
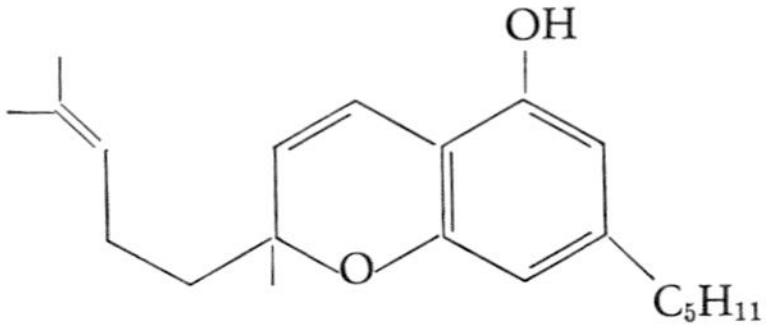 OH; O; C_5H_{11}	Cannabichromene
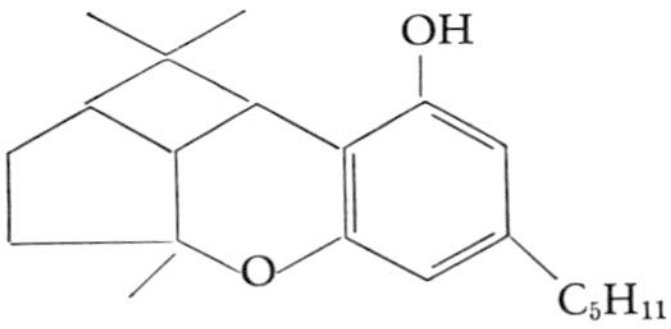 OH; O; C_5H_{11}	Cannabicyclol
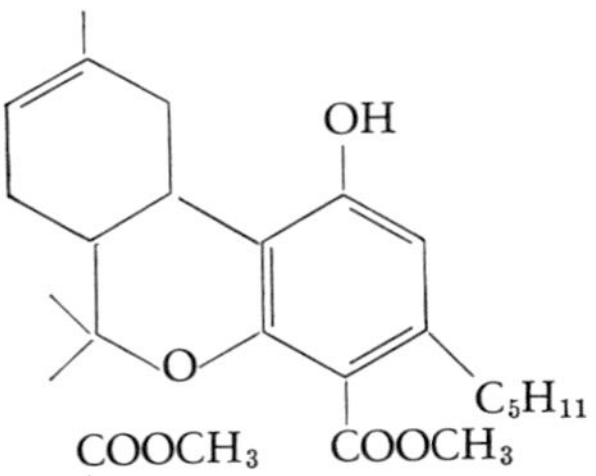 OH; O; C_5H_{11}; $COOCH_3$	4-Carbomethoxy-Δ[8]-THC[a]
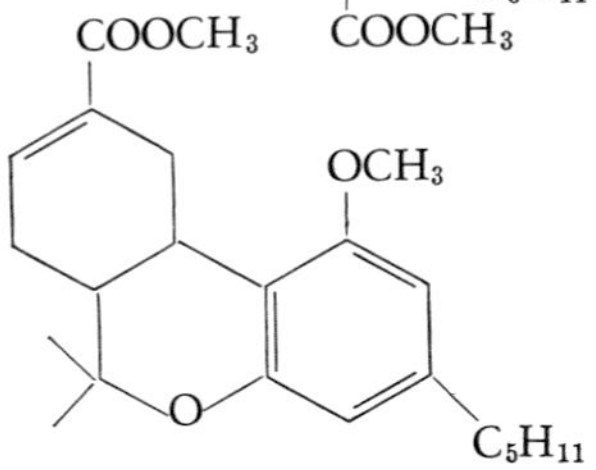 $COOCH_3$; OCH_3; O; C_5H_{11}	Δ[8]-THC-11-oic acid methyl ester[a]

[a] Synthetic.

Two synthetic cannabis derivatives of the so-called Sharp series have also been studied. Both showed minimal but definite cross-reactivity with antiserum 133Y/25/4, which, in the case of SP-1, was sufficiently strong to form the basis of a relatively insensitive radioimmunoassay (Figure 7.2). An antibody raised specifically against SP-1 would undoubtedly increase the sensitivity of the RIA immensely.

Blood samples collected from scores of normal healthy subjects and from over 100 hospital inpatients receiving treatment with various noncannabinoid drugs were examined for THC–CRC content. In no case did the results obtained differ significantly from zero. Urine samples from 50 normal healthy subjects and from 82 hospital inpatients known not to be taking cannabis in any form were also examined; in no case did the THC–CRC value exceed 5 ng/ml.

Clinical and Experimental Application of the RIA

The RIA for THC–CRC has been used to study the pharmacokinetics [16] of THC in a small number of volunteers [14] and to detect cannabis use among known or suspected drug users [10]. An ongoing study is concerned with the prevalence of cannabis use among young offenders admitted to a remand home.

Plasma THC–CRC levels were measured in 4 subjects after they had smoked a cigarette impregnated with 5 mg pure THC. The results are shown in Figure 7.3. The wide range of plasma THC–CRC values observed was more likely to have been due to differences in the volunteers' smoking patterns than to differences in absorption and metabolic disposition. Urinary excretion data obtained in these subjects revealed that use of as little as 5 mg of pure THC could be detected for up to 24–48 hours by urinalysis.

The results of urinalysis in 82 control and 393 known or suspected drug users of one type or another are shown in Figure 7.4. Although a small portion of urine specimens contained only trace amounts of THC–CRC, the results could mainly be classified as definitely negative or overtly positive. The proportion of urine specimens positive for cannabinoids in patients from two hospital (A and B) and one independent (C) narcotic drug treatment clinics are shown in Figure 7.5. In clinic C methadone was used sparingly, in contrast to the other two clinics where it was used almost routinely.

In 32 of the subjects, three or more urine specimens were ex-

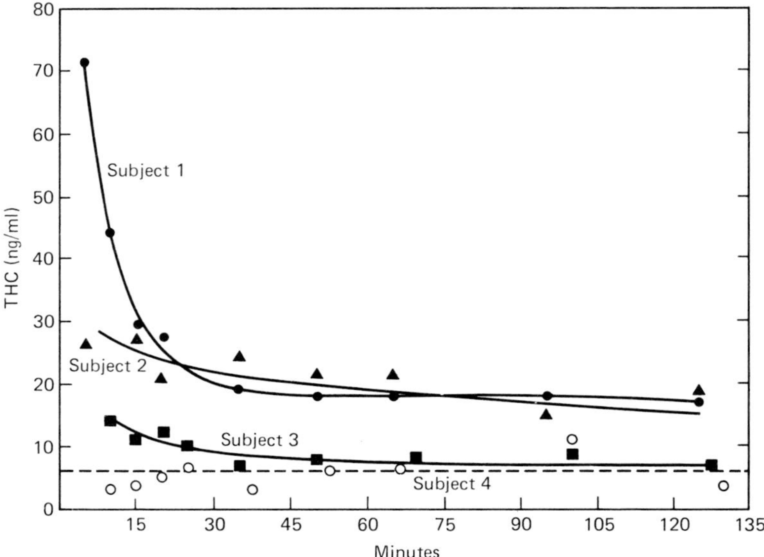

Figure 7.3. Plasma THC–CRC in 4 healthy volunteers who began smoking a cigarette impregnated with 5 mg THC at zero time. Subject 1 was a heavy cigarette smoker; subject 2 a moderate cigarette smoker; subject 3 a cigar smoker; and subject 4 a pipe smoker.

(Reproduced with permission from *The Lancet* 2:554, 1974.)

amined over 2 months. In 15 of the subjects, all of the urine samples tested were negative for cannabis. In the remaining 17, however, most or all of the urine specimens contained significant amounts of THC–CRC, suggesting that those individuals were using cannabis more or less regularly (Figure 7.6).

Discussion

Radioimmunoassay has several advantages over older conventional analytical techniques for detecting drugs in biological fluids. First, the sensitivity of RIA enables assays to be carried out on small samples containing normal pharmacological rather than toxic amounts of the drug. Second, RIA is potentially applicable to any drug or compound with a molecular weight of over 150. Third, it is usually group specific for a small class of chemically closely related substances, although like most other analytical techniques, it

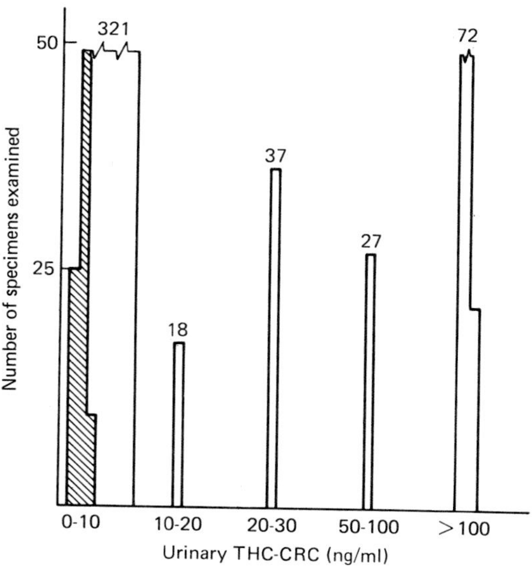

Figure 7.4. THC–CRC in 475 urine specimens. Hatched area—control urine samples from 82 hospital inpatients. Open columns—393 urine specimens from patients known or suspected to be taking drugs.

(Reproduced with the permission of the publishers of the *British Medical Journal* 3:348–49, 1975.)

Figure 7.5. Proportion of urine samples positive for THC–CRC according to origin. Same data as those used in Figure 7.4.

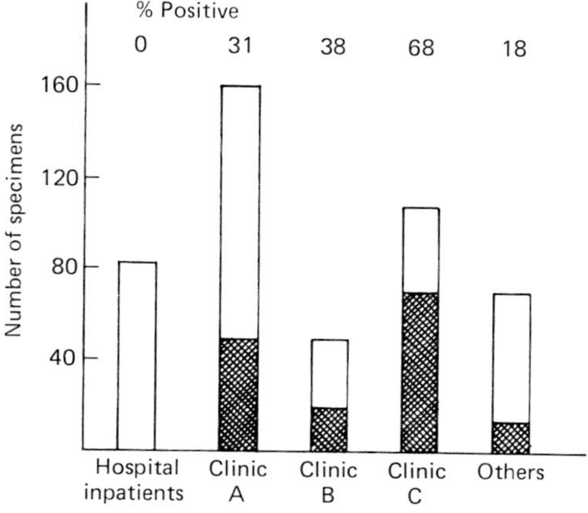

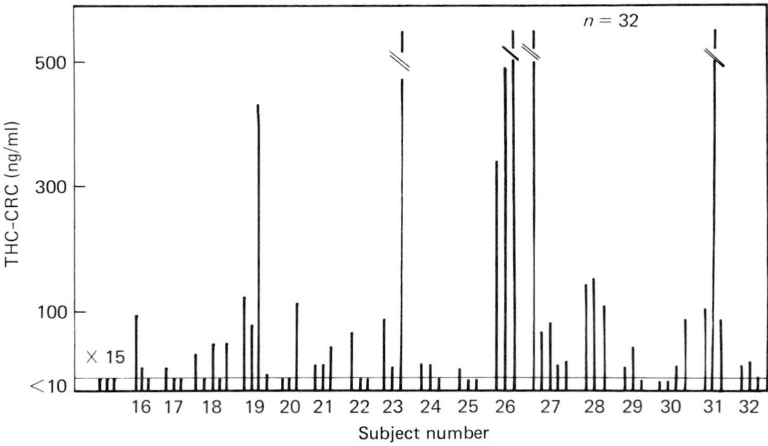

Figure 7.6. Individual random urinary THC–CRC concentrations in 32 known narcotic drug users from whom 3 or more urine specimens were received for analysis. In 15 subjects, all specimens were reported as negative (< 10 ng/ml).

is only rarely, if ever, absolutely specific for a single molecular species. This objective can often be achieved, however, merely by combining a preliminary preparative separation step, such as thin-layer chromatography, with the radioimmunoassay measurement system. Fourth, RIA can often be applied to biological fluids without prior extraction and/or purification. Finally, it is generally amenable to partial or complete automation, which makes the handling of large numbers of specimens both practicable and economic.

Disadvantages of RIA are that the key reagents—namely, high-affinity antibodies and high specific activity labels—are often extremely difficult to obtain and may be unstable. RIA is technically demanding and requires expensive radioisotope counting equipment. Disposal of radioactive waste may present problems, and much effort is currently being spent in finding other equally sensitive nonisotopic labels that can be used in immunoassay and saturation analysis procedures.

Because drugs and other low molecular weight compounds tend to evoke relatively low-titer antibody responses, it is generally necessary to use large domestic animals, rather than more conventional laboratory rodents, if sufficient amounts of antiserum from a single bleed are to be obtained for more than simple pilot studies. One liter of sheep THC antiserum used at a dilution of 1:2000 would be sufficient to perform about 2×10^6 assays allowing for wastage; this amount should be sufficient for the average institution for quite a long time.

Radioimmunoassay compares favorably in sensitivity with all other techniques for detecting and measuring cannabinoids in blood and urine although it does not possess, in its present form, the extremely high specificity of gas chromatography-mass spectrometry (GC–MS [1,2,11]). Nevertheless, apart from a few natural and synthetic closed three-ring cannabinoids, no other group or class of substances has been found to interfere in the immunoassay.

Apart from ourselves, few groups have successfully developed a usable RIA for cannabis products in biological fluids, although many have tried. Reasons for this are not altogether clear, but they undoubtedly include the low immunogenicity of THC conjugates; a seemingly marked interspecies difference with regard to the production of useful antibodies; the extreme insolubility of THC in water, and hence the necessity to solubilize it in a detergent that does not interfere with the antigen-antibody reaction; and finally the nonavailability, until recently, of a high specific activity label.

Gross *et al.* recently reported an assay for THC of slightly lesser sensitivity than our own and of different specificity [7]. Their antibody bound 11-OH–THC only half as avidly as THC itself. Since this would cause gross nonparallelism between plasma containing THC–CRC and the pure THC used in setting up a standard curve, it would prevent quantitative analysis unless a preliminary purification step was introduced. Another difference in specificity between the two antibodies is their degree of cross-reactivity with cannabidiol. Cannabidiol was totally unreactive with antiserum 133Y/25/4, but it was reported to have 0.5 percent the avidity of THC for the antiserum described by Gross and his colleagues.

The sensitivity limit of an RIA is determined by the avidity of the antiserum for the antigen [5], expressed as the avidity constant, which can be determined by analyzing the Scatchard plot. The present assay can be shown experimentally to be sensitive to the addition of 50 pg THC to the assay tube, which is well within the theoretical limits. Under the particular assay conditions adopted for analysis of blood and urine, we obtained a lower limit for acceptably precise measurements corresponding to 7.5 ng/ml THC–CRC in plasma and 1 ng/ml in urine. The sensitivity of the assay could probably be improved up to 100-fold in plasma and up to 20-fold in urine by using larger volumes of sample, adding a tracer label to compensate for losses, extracting into a suitable solvent, concentrating by evaporation, and measuring the THC–CRC in the residue. We have not pursued this line of development as it appeared to us to offer no obvious advantage over the present procedure and would be impractical for routine use.

Depending on how the assay is to be used, its specificity could be improved in one of several ways. By adding a radioactive tracer to a comparatively large volume of sample, say 10 ml or so, one could extract THC–CRC using a suitable solvent and concentrate it by evaporation. The extract could then be separated in a suitable thin-layer or column chromatographic system; the THC-containing zone could be eluted and the THC quantitated by RIA, allowing for recovery in the final calculation. This system has been successfully applied [6] to many other compounds of biological interest, and there is no reason to doubt its applicability to THC.

An alternative method of improving specificity would be to attempt to develop an antibody that did not cross-react with any cannabinoid except THC. Attractive as this idea is, such an absolutely specific antibody is in our opinion extremely unlikely to be found, especially if cross-reactivity testing is conducted thoroughly.

Because of its simplicity, rapidity, and group specificity for cannabinoids, RIA is well suited to clinical, epidemiological, and even forensic use. For example, we have used it as an aid to the differential diagnosis of cannabis-induced toxic psychosis and for investigating the prevalence of cannabis among patients [10] attending drug dependence treatment clinics as well as by newly admitted detainees at a juvenile remand center. We hope to apply it to the study of THC pharmacokinetics in man and to extend the investigations, already begun in collaboration with Professor J. Graham, into the relationship between blood levels of THC–CRC and therapeutic effectiveness.

ACKNOWLEDGMENTS

This work was carried out with financial support from the MRC under contract no. A806/5. We also thank the National Institute for Mental Health, Bethesda, Maryland, for the generous gift of THC and its analogs used in these experiments; and Abbott Laboratories for SP-1 and SPA-80.

REFERENCES

1. Agurell, S., B. Gustafsson, B. Holmstedt, K. Leander, J. E. Lindgren, I. Nilsson, F. Sandberg, and N. Asberg (1973) Quantitation of Δ^1-tetrahydrocannabinol in plasma from cannabis smokers. *J. Pharm. Pharmacol. 25:*554.

2. Agurell, S. (1974) Determination of cannabis components in blood. The poisoned patient: the role of the laboratory. *Ciba Found. Symp. 26:*125.
3. Butler, V. P., Jr. (1973) Radioimmunoassay and competitive binding radioassay methods for the measurement of drugs. *Metabolism 22:* 1145.
4. Butler, V. P., Jr. (1975) Drug immunoassays. *J. Immunol. Methods 7:*1.
5. Ekins, R. P. (1974) Basic principles and theory. *Br. Med. Bull. 30:*3.
6. English, J., J. Chakraborty, and V. Marks (1974) A competitive protein binding method for plasma prednisolone assay. *Ann. Clin. Biochem. 11:*11.
7. Gross, S. J., J. R. Soares, S-L. R. Wong, and R. E. Schuster (1974) Marijuana metabolites measured by a radioimmune technique. *Nature 252:*581.
8. Jaffe, B. M. and H. R. Behrman (1974) *Methods of Hormone Radioimmunoassays.* New York: Academic Press.
9. Marks, V., B. A. Morris, and J. D. Teale (1974) Pharmacology. *Br. Med. Bull. 30:*80.
10. Marks, V., J. D. Teale, and D. Fry (1975) Detection of cannabis products in urine by radioimmunoassay: studies in drug dependent subjects. *Br. Med. J.* (in press).
11. Rosenfeld, J. J., B. Bowins, J. Roberts, J. Perkins, and A. S. Macpherson (1974) Mass fragmentographic assay for Δ^9-tetrahydrocannabinol in plasma. *Anal. Chem. 46:*2232.
12. Teale, J. D., E. J. Forman, L. J. King, and V. Marks (1974) Production of antibodies to tetrahydrocannabinol as the basis for its radioimmunoassay. *Nature 249:*154.
13. Teale, J. D., E. J. Forman, L. J. King, and V. Marks (1974) The development of a radioimmunoassay for tetrahydrocannabinol in plasma. *Proc. Soc. Anal. Chem. 11:*219.
14. Teale, J. D., E. J. Forman, L. J. King, and V. Marks (1974) Radioimmunoassay of cannabinoids in blood and urine. *Lancet 2:*553.
15. Teale, J. D., E. J. Forman, L. J. King, E. M. Piall, and V. Marks (1975) The development of a radioimmunoassay for cannabinoids in blood and urine. *J. Pharm. Pharmacol. 27:*465.
16. Teale, J. D., J. M. Clough, E. M. Piall, L. J. King, and V. Marks (1975) Plasma cannabinoids measured by radioimmunoassay in rabbits after intravenous injection of tetrahydrocannabinol, 11-hydroxy-tetrahydrocannabinol, cannabinol and cannabidiol. *Res. Commun. Chem. Pathol. Pharmacol.* (in press).
17. Yalow, R. S. (1973) Radioimmunoassay; practice and pitfalls. *Circ. Res.* (*Suppl.*) *32:*116.
18. Yalow, R. S. and S. A. Berson (1960) Immunoassay of endogenous plasma insulin in man. *J. Clin. Invest. 39:*1157.
19. Zettner, A. (1974) Principles of competitive binding assays (saturation analyses). I. Equilibrium techniques. *Clin. Chem. 19:*699.

8

Mass Fragmentographic Assays for the Cannabinoids and Their Metabolites

J. ROSENFELD

Introduction

A prerequisite for gas chromatography assays of drugs is that appropriate compounds be available for internal standardization. If the assay is by mass fragmentography, then this usually requires synthesis of deuterated analogs. In the cannabinoid series, a synthesis of appropriately labeled Δ^9-tetrahydrocannabinol (Δ^9-THC) was described by Agurell and coworkers [1]. Burstein [2] reported labeled Δ^8-THC. Using the Δ^9-THC labeled at the 1′, 2′ positions, Agurell was the first to report an assay for Δ^9-THC in plasma [1].

An alternate approach to synthesizing deuterated analogs is the use of a derivatization that incorporates the deuterium into the derivative. The extracts are then similarly derivatized before analysis. Given the difficulties involved in synthesizing cannabinoids and their metabolites, we felt that it would be profitable to explore the derivatization route. This route could be exploited because of the presence in all cannabinoids and their metabolites of the same reactive group, which is the phenol moiety. The general philosophy would be then to synthesize the phenol perdeutero methyl ethers, and then to derivatize the extract to form the phenol methyl ether. The problem was to define a generalized chemistry that could be used in the derivatization reaction.

Assay for Δ^9-Tetrahydrocannabinol

Derivatization of Δ^9-THC

The phenol moiety is easily derivatized by methyl iodide (CH_3I) in N,N-dimethylformamide (DMF) using potassium carbonate (K_2CO_3) as a catalyst. This reaction was used to derivatize Δ^9-THC [3], 11-OH-Δ^9-THC [3], and the urinary metabolites of Δ^9-THC [4]. By using perdeutero methyl iodide (CD_3I), we were able to

Marihuana: Chemistry, Biochemistry, and Cellular Effects, edited by Gabriel G. Nahas,

synthesize Δ^9-THC-1-O-perdeutero methyl ether (Δ^9-THC-1-O-CD_3), which was our internal standard for the Δ^9-THC assay.

Once the problem of the internal standard was solved, we were faced with the task of derivatizing the sample before analysis. The $CH_3I/DMF/K_2CO_3$ reaction, although adequate for synthesis, was considered too lengthy for quantitative analysis. Therefore, another method of derivatization was sought. For Δ^9-THC, we used a solution of N,N,N-trimethyl anilinium hydroxide (TMAH) in methanol to dissolve the sample. When the resulting solution is injected, the reaction that takes place is instantaneous, quantitative, and reproducible. (The last point will be dealt with in a discussion of 11-OH-Δ^9-THC.) Using Δ^9-THC, the on-column methylating procedure, and Δ^9-THC-1-O-CD_3 as an internal standard, we obtained the linear standard curve (Figure 8.1) a 1:1 ratio between deuterated and protium forms.

Extraction of Δ^9-THC

When an appropriate quantitation technique had been established, we approached the problem of extraction from plasma and clean-up. Because Δ^9-THC and other cannabinoids are weak, highly lipophilic acids, an extract for these compounds is highly contaminated. Several workers had recognized and dealt with this problem. Fenimore [6] installed a fore-column before and in series

Figure 8.1. Standard curve for Δ^9-THC using on-column methylation and Δ^9-THC-1-O-perdeutero methyl ether as the internal standard.

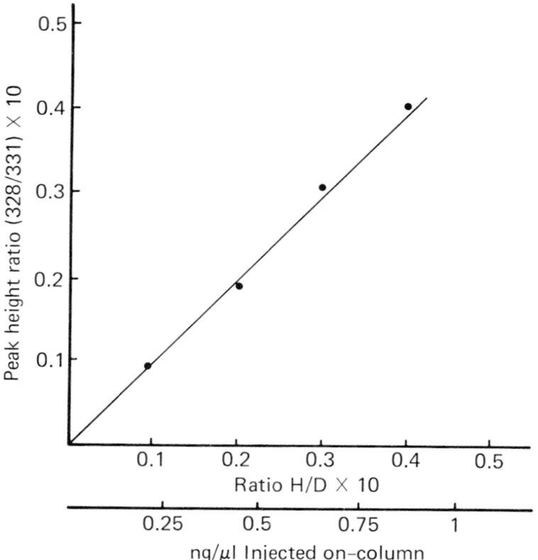

with the analytical column of the gas chromatograph. Agurell *et al.* [1] relied on a clean-up procedure using gel filtration on a column of LH-20 Sephadex. However, we felt that these procedures might be too cumbersome for the pharmacokinetic studies that we had planned.

The extraction procedure that was developed for Δ^9-THC also made use of the chemistry of the phenolic moiety. Lemberger *et al.* [7] showed that Δ^9-THC could be extracted from plasma using Brodie's solvent (1.5 percent iso amyl alcohol in heptane), but this would also extract neutral constituents in plasma. We found that a fractionation of the Brodie's extract by modified Claisens Alkali allowed for an efficient and precise extraction for the lipid phenolic fraction of plasma.

Since our original work [8], the procedure has been streamlined. A quantity of 2 ml of extracted plasma was shaken with 10 ml of Brodie's solvent for 30 min. Back extraction into 1 ml of Claisens Alkali and subsequent reextraction from the acidified Claisens phase into 8 ml Brodie's was also accomplished by shaking for 30 min. The second Brodie's phase was concentrated to dryness under a steam of N_2, and the residue was taken up in 50 μl of internal standard. This solution was ready for analysis.

Using this extraction scheme coupled with the on-column methylation procedure, we developed an assay for Δ^9-THC in human plasma and tested it in studies on human volunteers. The plasma levels reached (Figure 8.2) and the decay of these levels were similar to those reported by Agurell *et al.* [1].

Assay for 11-OH-Δ^9-THC

On-column methylation of 11-OH-Δ^9-THC

The assay for 11-OH-Δ^9-THC proved to be more difficult than that for Δ^9-THC. We proposed to use 11-OH-Δ^9-THC-1-O-perdeutero methyl ether (11-OH-Δ^9-THC-1-O-CD_3) as an internal standard and the on-column methylation just as they were used for Δ^9-THC. However, the presence of the hydroxyl group caused several problems. On-column methylation with 11-OH-Δ^9-THC resulted in the formation of two products, one of which was the dimethyl ether as evidenced by its mass spectrum (Table 8.1).

There was no attempt to identify the second product, which is possibly a pyrolysis product. If 11-OH-Δ^9-THC-1-O-CD_3 was subjected to the methylation, the same two products were formed. Therefore, it appeared that it would still be possible to develop an assay since both 11-OH-Δ^9-THC and the internal standard yielded

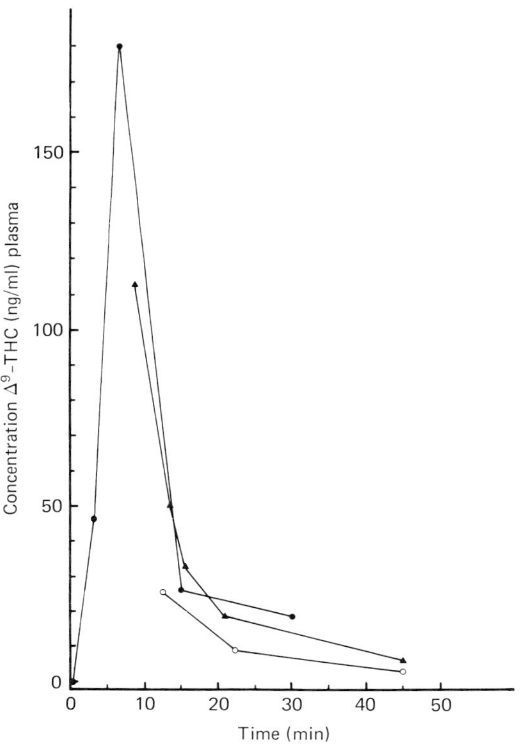

Figure 8.2. Plasma levels of Δ^9-THC in volunteers after smoking marihuana cigarettes dosed at 88 μg/kg.

the same products. But when we scrutinized the methylation reaction, we found the following detrimental points: the ratio of the two products was variable to an unacceptable degree; and the ratio of the two products for on-column methylation of 11-OH-Δ^9-THC-1-O-CD_3 and 11-OH-Δ^9-THC was different for each compound. The latter problem could have been anticipated since at least three reactions take place when 11-OH-Δ^9-THC is methylated on-column: methylation of a phenol, methylation of an allylic hydroxyl, and a "decomposition" reaction. Only methylation of a phenol and decomposition occur in the methylation of the 1-O-alkyl ether. To adjust our reaction conditions, we would have had to resolve the sequence and relative rates of the various reactions. These results indicated that either considerable effort should be spent in elucidating the on-column methylation of 11-OH-Δ^9-THC, or a different derivatization method would have to be tried. This reaction would have to be mild since it involved a relatively un-

Table 8.1 Mass spectrum of 11-OH-Δ^9-THC-1,11 dimethyl ether

m/e	*Relative intensity (%)*	*Proposed structure*
359	2.20	M + 1
358	6.8	M
314	26	$(M—CH_2OCH_3) + 1$
313	100	$M—CH_2OCH_3$
245	7.91	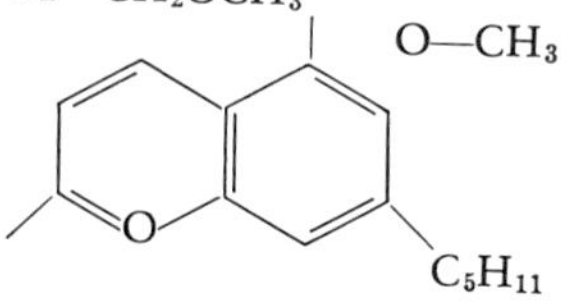 $O—CH_3$; O; C_5H_{11}

stable compound. It would also have to be simple since we intended to use it in developing an assay for pharmacokinetic studies, which require the analysis of many samples. Furthermore, we felt that this reaction should activate only one of the hydroxyls or both. The alkylative extraction technique satisfied all of our requirements.

Alkylative extraction

Alkylative extraction has been reported for a variety of compounds. The procedure involves the formation of an ion pair between the anion of a drug and a large cation (usually the tetrahexyl ammonium present in solution as its hydroxide). The ion pair so generated is lipid soluble and can easily be extracted into methylene chloride. If the methylene chloride contains an alkyl iodide, then the anion is converted to an alkyl derivative.

When the alkylative extraction procedure was tested on 11-OH-Δ^9-THC, it was found to suit our purposes admirably. The reaction takes place at room temperature using 0.5 *M* CH_3I/CH_2CI_2 and 0.1 *N* NaOH. Volumes of 10 ml CH_2CI_2, 5 ml 0.1 *N* NaOH, and 100 μm of 0.1 *M* tetrahexyl ammonium hydroxide (THAH) were found to be sufficient. The reaction time was 5 min.

Under these reaction conditions, 11-OH-Δ^9-THC is quantitatively derivatized to give the 1-O alkyl ether. At no time was the dialkyl ether observed. The concentration of NaOH or alkyl iodide did not effect any change in the reaction product. The range tested was 0.5–5 *M*, and the NaOH was 0.1–2 *N*. Reaction time likewise had no effect when shaking was continued for 30 min. When no THAH was present, only 11-OH-Δ^9-THC was recovered. Gas chromatographic data and mass spectra of the compounds were consistent with the derivatized formation of monomethylated products (Table

Table 8.2 Mass spectrum of 11-OH-Δ^9-THC-1 methyl ether

m/e	*Relative intensity (%)*	*Proposed structure*
344	15	M
326	23	M—18
314	25	($M—CH_2OH$) + 1
313	100	$M—CH_2OH$
311	15	($M—CH_2OH—2H$)
309	12	$M—CH_2OH—4H$

8.2). This reaction proved adequate in the preparative (1 mg) and the analytical (300 pg) scales.

The simplicity of reaction with both CH_3I and EtI is important. Estevez reported isolating 11-OH-Δ^9-THC-1-O-CH_3 in the central nervous system of rats treated with Δ^9-THC [5]. Thus, because the methylated metabolite might be present in plasma, it is necessary to use the pentadeutero ethyl ether as the internal standard and ethylation as the derivatization reaction [9].

REFERENCES

1. Agurell, S., B. Gustafsson, B. Holmstedt, K. Leander, J. Lindgren, I. Nilsson, F. Sandberg, and M. Asberg (1973) Quantitation and Δ^1-tetrahydrocannabinol in plasma from cannabis smokers. *J. Pharm. Pharmacol. 25:*554.
2. Burstein, S. and R. Mechoulam (1968) Stereospecifically labeled $\Delta^{1(6)}$-tetrahydrocannabinol. *J. Am. Chem. Soc. 90:*2420.
3. Burstein, S., F. Menezes, E. Williamson, and R. Mechoulam (1970) Metabolism of $\Delta^{1(6)}$-tetrahydrocannabinol, an active marihuana constituent. *Nature 225:*88.
4. Burstein, S., J. Rosenfeld, and T. Wittstruck (1972) Isolation and characterization of two major urinary metabolites of Δ^1-tetrahydrocannabinol. *Science 176:*422.
5. Estevez, V. S., L. F. Englert, and B. T. Ho (1973) A new methylated metabolite of (-)-11-hydroxy-Δ^8-tetrahydrocannabinol in rats. *Res. Commun. Chem. Pathol. Pharmacol. 6:*821.
6. Fenimore, D. C., R. R. Freeman, and P. R. Loy (1973) Determination of Δ^9-tetrahydrocannabinol in blood by electron capture gas chromatography. *Anal. Chem. 45:*2331.
7. Lemberger, L., N. R. Tamarkin, J. Axelrod, and I. J. Kopin (1971) Delta-9-tetrahydrocannabinol: metabolism and disposition in long-term marihuana smokers. *Science 173:*72.
8. Rosenfeld, J., B. Bowins, J. Roberts, J. Perkins, and A. S. Macpherson (1974) Mass fragmentographic assay for Δ^9-tetrahydrocannabinol in plasma. *Anal. Chem. 46:*2232.
9. Rosenfeld, J. and V. Taguchi (1976) Mass fragmentographic assay for 11-hydroxy-Δ^9-tetrahydrocannabinol in plasma. *Anal. Chem.* (in press).

9

Examination of the Metabolites of Δ^1-Tetrahydrocannabinol in Mouse Liver, Heart, and Lung by Combined Gas Chromatography and Mass Spectrometry

D. J. HARVEY AND W. D. M. PATON

Introduction

The distribution of Δ^1-tetrahydrocannabinol (Δ^1-THC, I) in tissues has been widely studied by radiochemical methods, and substantial accumulations have been found in certain organs, notably liver, lung, spleen, kidney, and adrenal gland [1,18,19]. Nevertheless, comparatively little is known about the nature of the accumulated material, although it is apparent that both Δ^1-THC and various metabolites are present. Differences in the relative concentrations of the metabolites in tissues, particularly lung and liver, have been recognized [16], suggesting biotransformation of Δ^1-THC at several sites. Several of the reported hydroxylated metabolites, in particular 7-OH-Δ^1-THC (II), possess pharmacological activity [9,11], and one metabolite, 1,2-epoxide (VII) [3,12], is potentially chemically active [10]. The structures of a number of metabolites are still unknown and could contribute to the overall activity of the drug (Table 9.1) [13].

The metabolism of Δ^1-THC is complex and has been studied extensively [1,6]. The primary metabolite, 7-OH-Δ^1-THC (II), is formed rapidly after administration of Δ^1-THC and can be excreted as the free compound or as a conjugate. Further biotransformation via the 7-oxo derivative (VI) [2] gives the carboxylic acid (VIII). Alternative allylic oxidation produces both the 6α- (III) and the 6β-OH-Δ^1-THC (IV), and these compounds in turn can be oxidized to 6-oxo-Δ^1-THC (V) [13]. Two other sites of attack are recognized—the Δ^1 double bond, which may be oxidized to an epoxide (VII) [3,12], and the 5′-*n*-pentyl side chain, which can be hydroxylated in several positions. Further hydroxylation of these mono-substituted metabolites has been observed with the production of 6α,7-diOH-Δ^1-THC (IX) [1,19] and the 7-acid

Marihuana: Chemistry, Biochemistry, and Cellular Effects, edited by Gabriel G. Nahas,

Table 9.1 Structure of Δ^1-THC and its metabolites

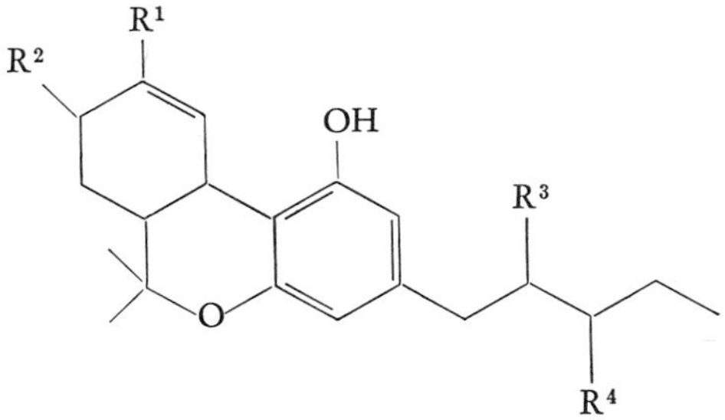

Cannabinoid (No.)	R^1	R^2	R^3	R^4
I	CH_3	H	H	H
II	CH_2OH	H	H	H
III	CH_3	α—OH	H	H
IV	CH_3	β—OH	H	H
V	CH_3	=O	H	H
VI	CHO	H	H	H
VIII	COOH	H	H	H
IX	CH_2OH	α—OH	H	H
X	COOH	OH	H	H
XI	COOH	H	OH	H
XII	COOH	H	H	OH
XIII	COOH	OH	OH	H
XIV	COOH	OH	H	OH
XVI	CH_2OH	H	OH	H
XVII	CH_2OH	H	H	OH

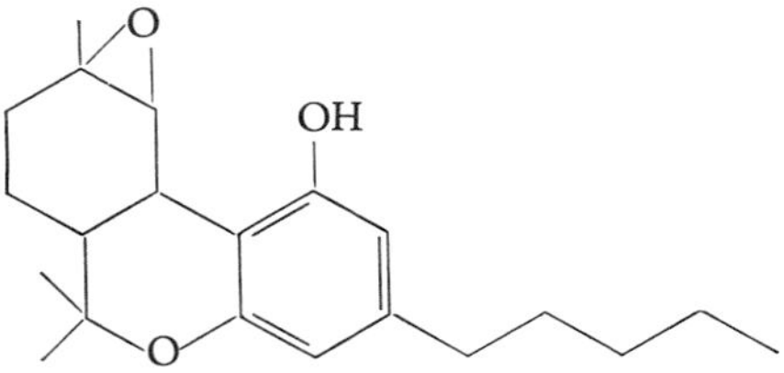

(VII)

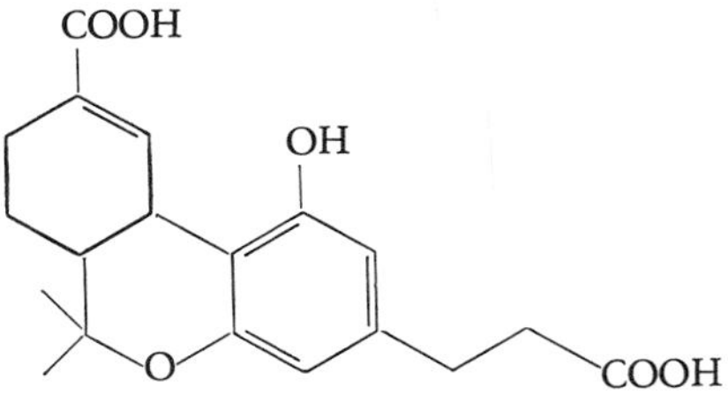

(XV)

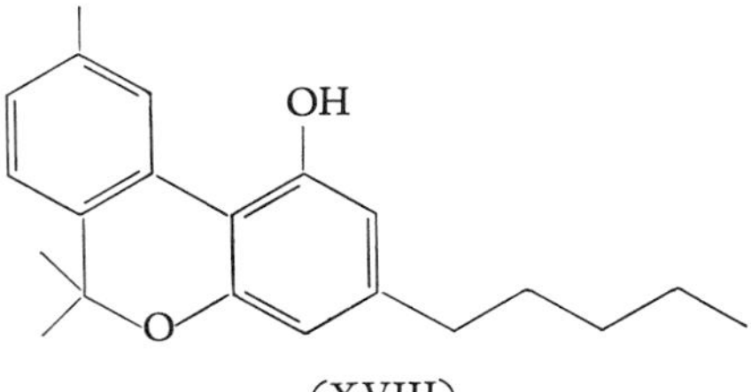

(XVIII)

substituted with hydroxyl groups in various positions, notably 1″, 2″, and 3″ of the aliphatic chain (XI, XII) [7,8]. In addition, oxidation of the 5′-pentyl side chain has been reported to give an acidic metabolite (XV) [17].

This paper describes the extraction and characterization of Δ^1-THC and several of its metabolites from mouse tissue after large intraperitoneal doses were administered. Metabolites of Δ^1-THC so far identified in mouse [13] include 6α-OH-Δ^1-THC (III), 7-OH-Δ^1-THC (II), 6α,7-diOH-Δ^1-THC (IX), 6-oxo-Δ^1-THC (V), and possibly 6β-OH-Δ^1-THC (IV).

Most published methods for examining cannabis metabolites have relied on fairly extensive thin-layer or column chromatography to separate the cannabinoids before their characterization. With high-resolution gas chromatographic columns and computer-aided processing of data collected from a combined gas-chromatograph–mass spectrometer (GC–MS), we reduced preliminary isolation stages, which lessened the possibility of degrading important but potentially reactive metabolites present in low concentration. Metabolites were characterized initially by the gas chromatographic retention time and mass spectrometric fragmentation of a number of derivatives.

Experimentation

Tissue distribution of Δ^1-THC

Four male mice (Charles Rivers CD1 strain) were treated orally with tritium-labeled (0.598 Ci/mmole) Δ^1-THC (1 mg/kg) each day for 7 days. Two animals were killed 24 hr after the final dose, and two after 15 days. Tissues were removed and the total radioactivity was determined by liquid scintillation counting after combustion in an oxygen atmosphere. Full details will be published later.

Dosage for GC–MS analysis

Two male mice (Charles Rivers CD1) were treated with Δ^1-THC (750 mg/kg IP) suspended in Tween 80 and normal saline on each of 2 successive days. Death occurred from 3–15 hr (overnight) after the second dose, and the animals were frozen until required.

Extraction and separation of cannabinoids

Samples of tissue were removed from the animal and homogenized in 10 ml of normal saline (pH 7). The cannabinoids and lipid material were extracted with three times 50 ml of ethyl

Table 9.2 Fractions eluted from LH-20 Sephadex column

Fraction	*Volume*	*Solvent*	*Contents*
1	0–13 ml	$CHCl_3$	Triglycerides
	14–17 ml	$CHCl_3$	Cholesterol
2	18–25 ml	$CHCl_3$	Δ^1-THC
3	26–36 ml	$CHCl_3$	Fatty acids
4	37–70 ml	$CHCl_3$	Monohydroxy cannabinoids
5	71–100 ml	20% MeOH—$CHCl_3$	Polar metabolites

acetate, each sample being centrifuged after extraction to ensure complete separation of the solvent from suspended cellular material. The combined extracts were dried with anhydrous magnesium sulfate, and the solvent was removed under reduced pressure. The residue was dissolved in chloroform and chromatographed on 5 gm (1 × 25 cm column) of LH-20 Sephadex, which was then eluted with chloroform followed by 20 percent methanol in chloroform. Fractions were collected as shown in Table 9.2. Fraction 1 was discarded. Fractions 2 and 3 were converted into trimethylsilyl (TMS) derivatives as described below. Eighty percent of fractions 4 and 5 from mouse liver were also converted into TMS derivatives. The remaining 20 percent was divided in two; one half was converted into D_9-TMS derivatives [15], and the other half into methyl ester–TMS derivatives. All of these fractions from the other tissue samples were converted into TMS derivatives.

Preparation of derivatives

Trimethylsilyl derivatives

Twenty microliters of a solution of acetonitrile (2 parts), *N,O*-bis(trimethylsilyl)trifluoroacetamide (BSTFA, 2 parts), and trimethylchlorosilane (TMCS, 1 part) were added to the sample in a 0.3-ml screw-capped conical vial. After agitation in a vortex mixer, the solution was allowed to stand at room temperature for 30 min to complete the formation of the derivatives. Aliquots of this solution were then examined by GLC and GC–MS.

D_9-*Trimethylsilyl derivatives*

Five microliters of D_{18}-trimethylsilylacetamide (D_{18}-BSA), 5 μl of acetonitrile, and a trace of TMCS were added to the sample in a conical vial. This was treated as described above.

Methyl ester–TMS derivatives

A solution of diazomethane in ether (200 μl) was added to a methanolic solution (50 μl) of the metabolites. After 1 min the diazomethane and solvents were removed with a nitrogen stream, and the residue was converted into TMS derivatives as described above.

Gas chromatography

Gas chromatographic data were recorded with a Varian 2400 gas chromatograph fitted with dual flame ionization detectors and two 2 m × 2 mm (ID) glass columns packed with 3 percent SE-30 on 100–120 mesh Gas-Chrom Q. Nitrogen at 30 ml/min was used as the carrier gas, and the flash heater and detector temperatures were maintained at 270° and 300°C, respectively. The column oven was temperature programmed linearly over the range 140–290°C (standard compounds) and 100–330°C (tissue extracts) at 4°C/min. Gas chromatograms were recorded with Servoscribe 1S potentiometric recorders. Methylene units are listed in Table 9.4.

Mass spectrometry

Low-resolution, electron impact-induced mass spectra were recorded with a VG Micromass 12B mass spectrometer interfaced via a glass jet separator to a Varian 2400 gas chromatograph containing an SE-30 chromatography column similar to that described above. The column oven was temperature programmed linearly at 2°C/min over the range 170–280°C with helium at 30 ml/min as the carrier gas. The injector port, GC–MS transfer line, separator, and mass spectrometer ion source temperatures were maintained at 270°C, 230°C, 230°C, and 260°C, respectively. Mass spectra were recorded at 25 eV with an ionizing current of 100 μA. The accelerating voltage was 2.5 kV, and the collector slit was adjusted to give a resolution of about 1000.

The mass spectrometer was connected to a VG Data Systems Ltd. computer system type 2040, and this was set to scan the mass spectrometer repetitively from high to low mass at 3 sec a decade with an interscan delay time of 2 sec. This resulted in 400–500 spectra in each GLC run. Normalized mass spectra and single and total ion chromatograms were examined and recorded with a Digital VT8E visual display unit and a Bryans 26,000 XY recorder.

For single-ion chromatograms recorded direct from the mass spectrometer, the slit was opened to give flat-top peaks and the magnet current was adjusted to bring the ion into focus. The resulting signal from the electron multiplier-amplifier was recorded on a Servoscribe 1S potentiometric recorder.

Results and Discussion

Gas chromatograms of typical organic solvent extracts of tissues contained high proportions of the common lipids, in particular fatty acids, cholesterol, and mono- and triglycerides. Δ^1-THC (MU = 23.50) eluted toward the upper end of the fatty acid region on 3 percent SE-30 columns and its major metabolites in the relatively clear region before cholesterol (MU = 31.10). To avoid problems with derivative preparation and column overloading while examining the Δ^1-THC metabolites, we had to remove or considerably lower the concentrations of most of this lipid material. Ethyl acetate extracts of the homogenized tissues were chromatographed on LH-20 Sephadex. The column was eluted with chloroform and chloroform/methanol mixtures. Triglycerides and cholesterol eluted rapidly, permitting complete separation from Δ^1-THC and its metabolites. Fractions were taken as shown in Table 9.2. Further separation of THC metabolites on Sephadex was not attempted, and a single fraction containing most polar metabolites was collected for examination by gas chromatography and mass spectrometry.

Radioactive studies in mice after oral administration of Δ^1-THC showed accumulation in several tissues, particularly liver, heart, and lung. Table 9.3 shows the amount found expressed in μg equivalents of Δ^1-THC per gram of tissue. On day 1 slightly higher levels were found in liver than in the other tissues, but this decayed more rapidly over a 2-week period, resulting in lower levels on day 15. Samples of tissues from mice treated with large doses of Δ^1-THC

Table 9.3 Microgram equivalents of Δ^1-THC found in mouse tissue following oral treatment with tritium-labeled (0.598 Ci/mM) Δ^1-THC

Tissue	*Day 1*	*Day 15*
Liver	0.33	0.04
Heart	0.26	0.085
Lung	0.25	0.065

were then examined by gas chromatography and mass spectrometry, the cannabinoids being extracted as described above.

Liver

Fraction 2

Fraction 2 contained small amounts of several fatty acids and Δ^1-THC, which was identified by comparing its methylene unit value and mass spectrum with those of an authentic sample (Tables 9.4 and 9.5). Quantitative measurements were not made, but levels in the region of 200 μg/gm of tissue were observed. Small amounts of cannabinol (XVIII) were also characterized; although absent from the administered Δ^1-THC, this compound could have arisen by chemical decomposition of Δ^1-THC or its metabolites, and thus may not be a true metabolite.

Fraction 3

Large amounts of carboxylic acids—mainly oleic, palmitic, and stearic—were found together with a small amount of a compound tentatively identified as 6-oxo-Δ^1-THC (V). Its TMS derivative had a molecular ion at $m/e = 400$, and its mass spectral fragmentation was similar to that of the free phenol previously reported as a metabolite of Δ^1-THC in the mouse [13].

Fractions 4 and 5

These fractions were combined. Figure 9.1 shows the total ion current chromatogram of these fractions obtained from the GC–MS computer system. The column oven was temperature programmed from 160–280°C. The compounds eluting in the early region of the chromatogram (mass spectral scans 0–150) were produced by palmitic, oleic, stearic, and related carboxylic acids. The large peaks eluting in scans 360–480 were not identified. Scans 180–350 contained a number of Δ^1-THC metabolites, many of the peaks in Figure 9.1 being produced by several components. In an attempt to deconvolute these peaks, we traced single ion chromatograms of major ions produced by Δ^1-THC metabolites across the chromatogram and then reprocessed the data using the VG Data Systems "Massmax" program. With this latter routine, a development of the program described by Biller and Biemann [4] for obtaining "reconstructed mass spectra" from total ion chromatograms, we examined every ion in each spectrum and compared its intensity with the equivalent ion in the previous spectrum. Each time an ion maximized, signalled by a decrease in its intensity in the current

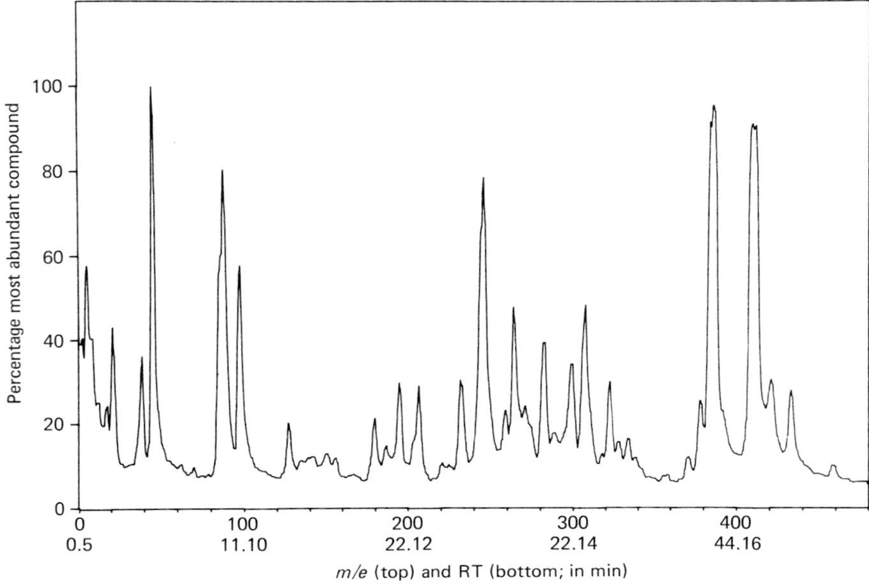

Figure 9.1. Total ion chromatogram of the metabolites of Δ^1-THC from mouse liver. Mass spectral scan numbers and RT in minutes are given on the X axis, peaks are normalized to that of the most abundant compound expressed as 100%. The conditions for the separation are given in the experimental section.

scan, it was flagged. By plotting only the flagged ions, we obtained the spectra of each component of a multicomponent peak, providing that the separation of the components was great enough for their ions to maximize in different scans. For the GLC peaks shown in Figure 9.1, about 6 scans were obtained for each peak.

Figure 9.2 shows the result of replotting the total ion chromatogram using only the flagged peaks. A considerable increase in resolution was obtained. The peaks were further enhanced by using only ions above $m/e = 210$ as Δ^1-THC metabolites did not, in general, contain many abundant ions below $m/e = 300$. Many undiagnostic ions of low mass were thus eliminated, giving a steadier base line above which the minor constituents could be seen. Figure 9.3 shows the metabolite region of Figure 9.2 on an expanded scale.

Two of the metabolites were identified by comparing their mass spectra and retention times (expressed in Table 9.4 as methylene units) with those of authentic samples recorded under identical

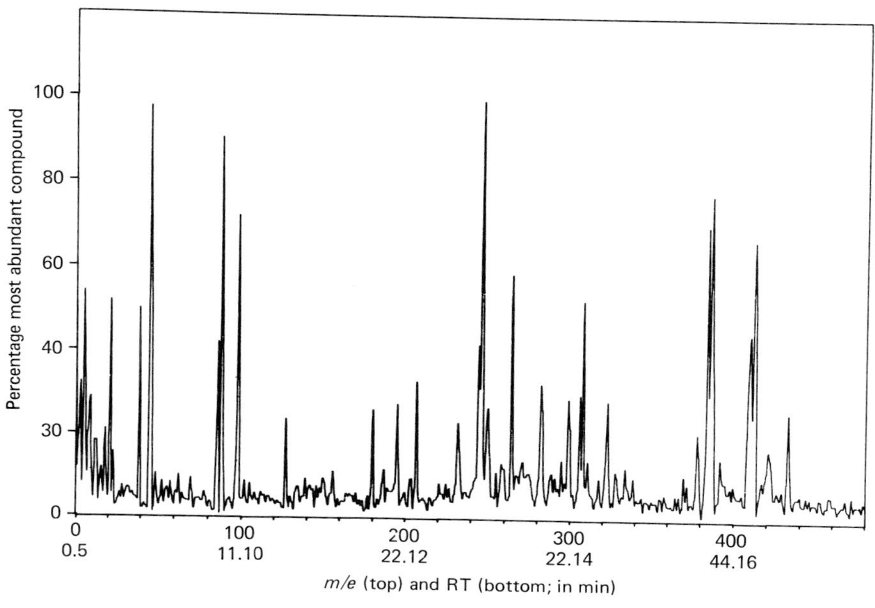

Figure 9.2. Computer processed data (Mass Max—see text) of the chromatogram shown in Figure 9.1.

Figure 9.3. Δ¹-THC metabolite region of the chromatogram shown in Figure 9.2 plotted using only the ions above $m/e = 210$.

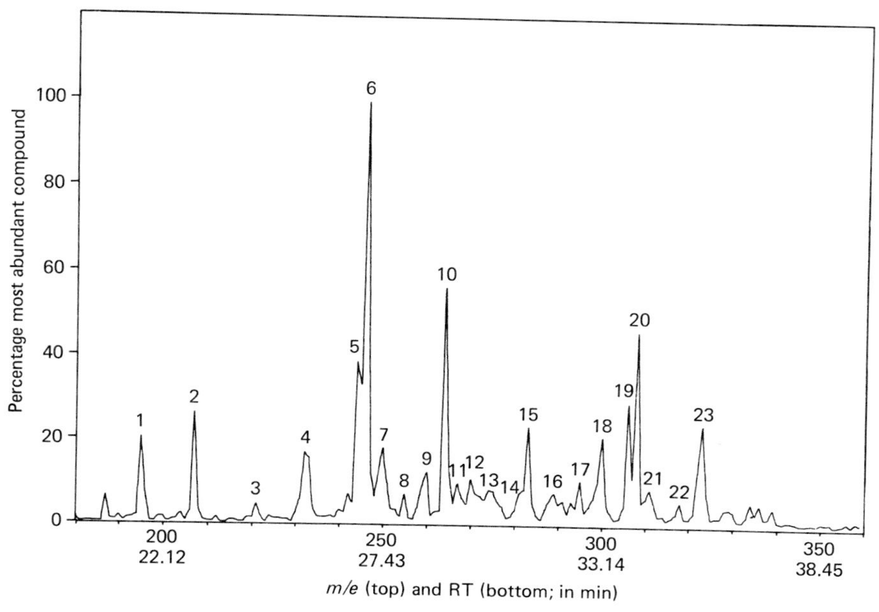

Table 9.4 Methylene unit values of the Δ^1-THC metabolites

Compound or peak (Figure 9.3)	*Structure*	mu	mu (*standard*)
Δ_1-THC	I	23.48	23.50
Cannabinol	XVIII	24.30	24.30
1	III	25.8	25.80
2	II	26.2	26.16
4	IX[a]	29.1	—
6	VIII[a]	29.56	—
7	XVI[a]	29.68	—
10	X[a]	30.24	—
13	XVII[a]	30.55	—
15	XI[a]	30.96	—
18	XIII[a]	31.61	—
20		31.9	—
23	XIV[a]	32.64	—

[a] Structural assignment not confirmed by synthesis.

conditions. Structures could be assigned to most of the other peaks on the basis of published work and by comparing their spectra with those of the identified compounds. However, these structures must remain tentative until the compounds can be synthesized and compared with the metabolites directly.

Peaks 1 and 2 were produced by 6α- (III) and 7-OH-Δ^1-THC (II), respectively, both compounds being identified by comparison with authentic samples. The presence of two hydroxyl groups was verified by the shift of the molecular ion of II by 18 (atomic mass units) in the spectra of the D_9-TMS derivatives [15], and by the shift of $[M\text{-}15]^+$ by 15 amu in III (the molecular ion was absent). The major ions in the spectra are listed in Table 9.5. The MS of 6α-OH-Δ^1-THC was characterized by elimination of the 6α-OTMS group as trimethylsilanol (90 amu) which gave the base peak at $m/e = 384$, whereas 7-OH-Δ^1-THC produced an abundant base peak at $m/e = 371$ resulting from elimination of the 7-CH_2OTMS group.

The metabolite producing peak 4 was a dihydroxy THC, $M^+ = 562$ (24 amu shift of $[M\text{-}15]^+$ in the D_9-TMS spectrum arising from the three TMS groups), and it gave a spectrum showing a base peak at $[M\text{-}90]^+$ and a second prominent ion at $[M\text{-}103]^+$. This indicated a structure containing both a 6- and a 7-hydroxy group, and in the absence of an authentic sample the compound was tentatively assigned the structure of the known 6α,7-diOH-Δ^1-THC (IX). A second diol showing a similar fragmentation (peak 7)

Table 9.5 Mass spectral data of major ions (25 eV)

Compound or GLC peak	Ion M⁺	[M-15]⁺	[M-72]⁺	[M-90]⁺	[M-103]⁺	[M-117]⁺	[M-144]⁺	m/e = 145	[a]	[b]
Δ^1-THC	386 (100)	371 (94)[a]	—	—	—	—	—	—	303 (33)	—
CBN	382 (14)	367 100	—	—	—	—	—	—	—	—
1	474 (0)	459 (4.5)	—	384 (100)	—	—	—	—	303 (4.5)	
2	474 (5.5)	459 (4.5)	—	384 (2)	371 (100)	—	—	—	303 (2)	—
4	562 (0)	547 (3)	—	472 (100)	459 (18)	—	—	—	303 (6.5)	—
6	488 (43)	473 (40)	—	398 (15.5)	—	371 (100)	—	—	303 (3)	—
10	576 (0)	561 (3)	—	486 (100)	—	—	—	—	303 (3)	—
15	576 (10)	561 (8)	504 (31)	—	—	459 (4.5)	—	145 (100)	—	391 (0.5)
18	664 (2)	649 (4.5)	502[b] (21)	574 (29)	—	547 (5.5)	—	145 (100)	—	391 (0)
19	576 (19)	561 (21)	—	—	—	—	432 (100)	—	—	391 (1)
23	664 (1)	649 (6.5)	—	574 (100)	—	547 (2)	430[c] (32)	—	—	391 (2)

[a] Relative intensities are given in parentheses.

[b] $[M\text{-}90\text{–}72]^+$.

[c] $[M\text{-}90\text{–}144]^+$.

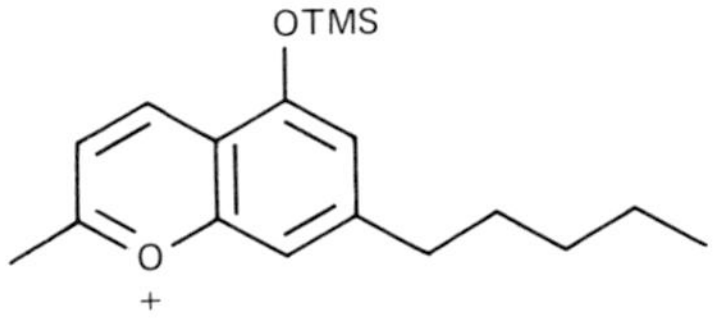

OTMS

OTMS

OTMS

O +

O +

$m/e = 303$

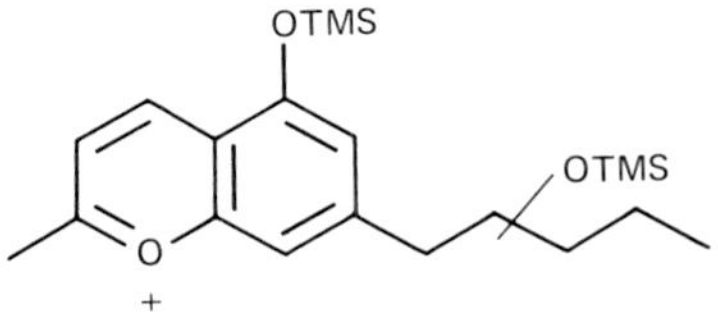

$m/e = 391$

Figure 9.4. Structures of ions *a* (left) and *b* (right).

was observed in much lower concentration but was not identified.

The major metabolite (peak 6) had a molecular ion at $m/e =$ 488, contained two TMS groups, and fragmented to give a base peak at $m/e = 371$ ($[M\text{-}117]^+$). Of the two classes of compound that fragment with loss of 117 amu, carboxylic acids (loss of COOTMS) and secondary alcohols of the type CH_3CH (OTMS)-, the latter was eliminated by the observation that the metabolite could be reacted with methylating agents such as diazomethane and must therefore be an acid. The similarity in its spectrum to that of 7-OH-Δ^1-THC and the 14 amu increase in molecular weight enables the structure Δ^1-THC-7-oic acid (VIII) to be assigned to this metabolite. The presence of an ion at $m/e = 303$ (see Figure 9.4) confirmed substitution in the terpene ring.

Most of the remaining metabolites appeared to be hydroxylated derivatives of this acid. Peak 10 had no molecular ion but a small $[M\text{-}15]^+$ ion was present, this shifted by 24 amu in the D_9-TMS spectrum indicating the presence of three TMS groups. The base peak ($m/e = 486$) was produced by eliminating TMSOH, and the spectrum resembled that of the 6α,7-diOH-Δ^1-THC with a 14 amu shift. This compound had a similar increase in methylene units from the acid (peak 6) to that of the diol (IX) over 7-OH-Δ^1-THC (peak 2) and was thus probably produced by the 6-OH acid (X).

Two other monohydroxy acids produced peaks 15 and 19, and from their fragmentations these appeared to be hydroxylated in the C_5 side chain. This was supported by the absence of ion *a* and the presence of its hydroxylated analog *b* in low abundance. In a recent paper Binder *et al.* [5] discussed the fragmentations exhibited by cannabinoids hydroxylated in each position of the side chain, and from this the two compounds appeared to be hydroxylated at positions 2″ and 3″. The spectrum of peak 15 had a molecular ion at $m/e = 576$, which shifted to $m/e = 603$ in the spectrum of the D_9-TMS derivatives. The presence of the 7-carboxyl function was indicated by the presence of the ion at $[M\text{-}117]^+$. The base peak,

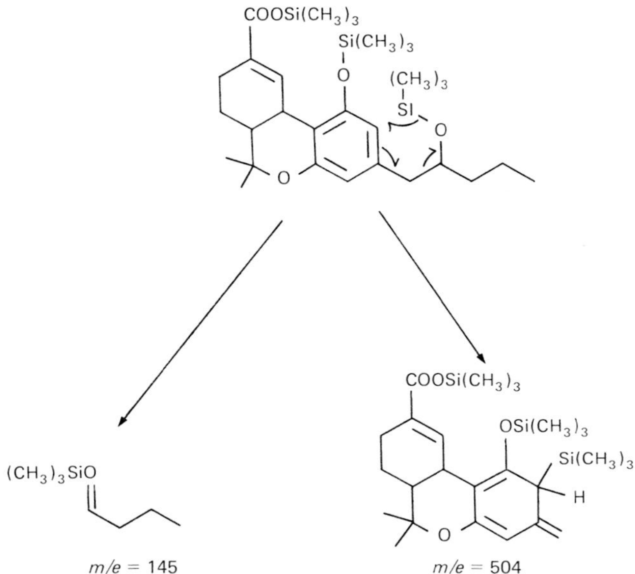

Figure 9.5. Characteristic ions produced by the fragmentation of 2″-hydroxy-Δ^1-THC-7-oic acid.

m/e = 145, was characteristic of the 2″-OTMS function (compound XI) [5,20]. A second ion (*m/e* = 504) also appeared to be characteristic of this structure (Figure 9.5); the 74 amu was eliminated without loss of a TMS group as shown by complete retention of the D_9-TMS label. [Substitution of $Si(CH_3)_3$ into the 6′ rather than the 4′ position of the benzene ring was also possible but not distinguishable on present evidence]. This rearrangement was similar to the migration of hydrogen reported [5] to produce $[M\text{-}144]^+$ in the spectrum of the 3″-OTMS metabolite.

The spectrum of the other hydroxy acid (peak 19) again showed a molecular ion at *m/e* = 576 and a small ion at *m/e* = 391 (see Figure 9.4). The base peak $[M\text{-}144]^+$ at *m/e* = 432 (450 in the D_9-TMS spectrum) was indicative of hydroxyl substitution in the 3″ position, and the compound was thus assigned the structure of the 3″-hydroxy acid XII.

Other isomeric side chain hydroxylated metabolites were not observed. This was interesting in the light of previous work which has shown 1″-hydroxylation to be common [7,8,14]. This isomer can be characterized by loss of 57 amu. (C_4H_8), but single ion chromatograms of *m/e* = 519 ($[M\text{-}57]^+$) did not reveal the presence of a hydroxy acid that fragmented in this way. Similarly, single ion chromatograms of $m/e = 117$, characteristic of 4″-hydroxy substitution, were negative.

Several trisubstituted metabolites of 664 MW indicative of dihydroxy acids were also present in this fraction. The two major compounds (peaks 18 and 23) had spectra similar to those of the side chain hydroxyl metabolites discussed above with the addition of peaks at $[M\text{-}90]^+$, suggesting 6-hydroxylation. The spectrum of peak 18 showed $[M\text{-}90]^+$ and an ion at $m/e = 502$ produced by further elimination of 72 amu (Table 9.5). This, together with the base peak at $m/e = 145$ and ion *b*, indicated 2″ substitution, and the compound was thus assigned the 6,2″-diOH-Δ^1-THC-7-oic acid structure XIII. The stereochemistry at C_6 was not determined. A second, minor metabolite (peak 21), fragmenting in a similar way, was also observed. Peak 23, the second major triol, fragmented with loss of 144 amu from $[M\text{-}90]^+$ (the base peak) and was thus probably the 6,3″-diOH-Δ^1-THC-7-oic acid (XIV). This was supported by the presence of ion *b*.

A single ion chromatogram of $m/e = 145$ showed, in addition to the 3 hydroxy acids, 2 other peaks (7 and 13) with shorter elution times. Spectra taken at the maxima of these peaks were contaminated with the spectra of other components, but both appeared to have molecular ions at $m/e = 562$, indicating that they were diols. In addition, both compounds showed prominent losses of 103 amu, suggesting 7-hydroxyl substitution. One of these probably was the 7,2″-dihydroxy metabolite (XVI). The presence of an ion at $m/e = 418$ ($[M\text{-}144]^+$ from a dihydroxy metabolite) as one of the ions in peak 13 suggests the presence of the isomeric 7,3″-diol (XVII). Similar retention increment shifts were observed between the three diol metabolites (peaks 4, 7, and 13) and the correspondingly substituted acids (peaks 10, 15, and 19).

Several of the small peaks in Figure 9.3 also appeared to be Δ^1-THC metabolites, but their mass spectra were not strong enough for structural assignments to be made.

Heart

Fraction 2

Δ^1-THC was found and identified as above. The chromatograms were contaminated with fatty acids, so quantitation was not carried out. However, levels were about $1/10$ of those found in liver. A small amount of cannabinol was also found.

Fractions 4 and 5

Analyses of these fractions as described above showed the presence of 6α-OH-Δ^1-THC, 7-OH-Δ^1-THC, 6α,7-diOH-Δ^1-THC, and Δ^1-THC-7-oic acid. The concentration of the diol was approximately equal to that in liver, whereas the 7-acid was present in about a third of the liver concentration. Much smaller quantities of the hydroxy acids were present; their spectra were too weak for positive identification, but the presence of a relatively abundant ion at $m/e = 145$ in one of these suggested the presence of the 2″-hydroxy acid (XI). Retention times were the same in each sample.

Lung

Fraction 2

Δ^1-THC was found at levels comparable to those in the heart. Cannabinol was also found.

Fractions 4 and 5

The following metabolites were found in similar concentrations to those in heart: 6α-OH-Δ^1-THC, 7-OH-Δ^1-THC, 6α,7-diOH-Δ^1-THC, and Δ^1-THC-7-oic acid.

The results discussed above indicated more rapid and extensive metabolism of Δ^1-THC by liver than in the other tissues, with the production of several di- and trisubstituted compounds. Only small quantities of the 6-monosubstituted metabolites were found, but larger amounts of the 7-monosubstituted compounds were present. The acid, VIII, was the major metabolite in liver. No metabolites substituted only in the pentyl side chain were observed, suggesting the allylic positions of the terpene ring as the major sites of metabolic attack in the mouse. The majority of the liver metabolites were acidic and contained, in addition to the 7-carboxyl group, substitution by a second hydroxyl group in either the 6 position or the 2″ and 3″ positions of the pentyl side chain. Two dihydroxy acids were found; these had hydroxyl substituents in both the 6 position and the 2″ and 3″ positions of the pentyl side chain. Concentrations of acidic metabolites were lower in both lung and heart. Δ^1-THC was identified in relatively high concentration in liver and at lower levels in heart and lung.

This method based on gas chromatography and mass spectrometry proved reasonably successful for identifying Δ^1-THC metabolites at reasonably high dose levels. For lower doses, single or preferably multiple ion detection was necessary. Although detection limits for Δ^1-THC as its TMS derivative were in the low picogram range using single-ion monitoring, in practice interference by ions from minor tissue components limited the detection limit to about 1 ng.

ACKNOWLEDGMENTS

We are indebted to Dr. M. C. Braude of the National Institute for Mental Health for supplies of Δ^1-THC and 7-OH-Δ^1-THC through the Medical Research Council. We are also grateful to Professor R. Mechoulam for a gift of 6α-OH-Δ^1-THC and to Mrs. Ann Benson and Miss Linda Salter for the results of the tritium-labeled study. Tritium-labeled Δ^1-THC was kindly supplied by Dr. E. W. Gill. We also thank the Medical Research Council for a Programme Research Grant.

REFERENCES

1. Agurell, S., J. Dahmén, B. Gustafsson, V.-B. Johansson, K. Leander, I. Nilsson, J. L. G. Nilsson, M. Nordqvist, C. H. Ramsay, A. Ryrfeldt, F. Sandberg, M. Widman (1972) Metabolic fate of tetrahydrocannabinol. *Cannabis and Its Derivatives: Pharmacology and Experimental Psychology* (W. D. M. Paton and J. Crown, eds.). London: Oxford University Press, pp. 16–36.
2. Ben-Zvi, Z. and S. Burstein (1974) 7-Oxo-Δ^1-tetrahydrocannabinol: a novel metabolite of Δ^1-tetrahydrocannabinol. *Res. Commun. Chem. Pathol. Pharmacol. 8:*223.
3. Ben-Zvi, Z. and S. Burstein (1975) Transformation of Δ^1-tetrahydrocannabinol (THC) by rabbit liver microsomes. *Biochem. Pharmacol. 24:*1130.
4. Biller, J. E. and K. Biemann (1974) Reconstructed mass spectra, a novel approach for the utilization of gas chromatograph-mass spectrometer data. *Anal. Lett.* 7*:*515.
5. Binder, M., S. Agurell, K. Leander, and J.-E. Lindgren (1974) Zur identifikation potentieller metabolite von cannabis-inhaltstoffen: kernresonanz- und massenspektroskopische untersuchungen an seitenkettenhydroxylierten cannabinoiden. *Helv. Chim. Acta 57:*1626.
6. Burstein, S. H. (1973) Labeling and metabolism of the tetrahydrocannabinols. *Marijuana: Chemistry, Pharmacology, Metabolism and Clinical Effects* (R. Mechoulam, ed.). New York: Academic Press, pp. 167–190.
7. Burstein, S. H., J. Martinez, J. Rosenfeld, and T. Wittstruck (1972) The urinary metabolites of Δ^1-THC. *Cannabis and Its Derivatives* (W. D. M. Paton and J. Crown, eds.). London: Oxford University Press, pp. 39–49.
8. Burstein, S. H., J. Rosenfeld, and T. Wittstruck (1972) Isolation and characterization of two major urinary metabolites of delta(1)-tetrahydrocannabinol. *Science 176:*422.

9. Christensen, H. D., R. I. Freudenthal, J. T. Gidley, R. Rosenfeld, G. Boegli, L. Testino, D. R. Brine, C. G. Pitt, and M. E. Wall (1971) Activity of Δ^8- and Δ^9-tetrahydrocannabinol and related compounds in the mouse. *Science 172:*165.
10. Daly, J. W., D. M. Jerina, and B. Witkop (1972) Arene oxides and the NIH shift: the metabolism, toxicity and carcinogenicity of aromatic compounds. *Experientia 28:*1129.
11. Gill, E. W., G. Jones, and D. K. Lawrence (1973) Contribution of the metabolite 7-hydroxy-Δ^1-tetrahydrocannabinol towards the pharmacological activity of Δ^1-tetrahydrocannabinol in mice. *Biochem. Pharmacol. 22:*175.
12. Gurny, O., D. E. Maynard, R. G. Pitcher, and R. W. Kierstead (1972) Metabolism of (-)-Δ^9 and (-)-Δ^8-tetrahydrocannabinol by monkey liver. *J. Am. Chem. Soc. 94:*7928.
13. Jones, G., M. Widman, S. Agurell, and J.-E. Lindgren (1974) Monohydroxylated metabolites of Δ^1-tetrahydrocannabinol in mouse brain. *Acta Pharm. Suec. 11:*283.
14. Maynard, D. E., O. Gurny, R. G. Pitcher, and R. W. Kierstead (1971) (-)-Δ^8-Tetrahydrocannabinol. Two novel *in vitro* metabolites. *Experientia 27:*1154.
15. McCloskey, J. A., R. N. Stillwell, and A. M. Lawson (1968) Use of deuterium-labeled trimethylsilyl derivatives in mass spectrometry. *Anal. Chem. 40:*233.
16. Nakazawa, K. and E. Costa (1971) Metabolism of Δ^9-tetrahydrocannabinol by lung and liver homogenates of rats treated with methylcholanthrene. *Nature 234:*48.
17. Nordqvist, M., S. Agurell, M. Binder, and I. M. Nilsson (1974) Structure of an acidic metabolite of Δ^1-tetrahydrocannabinol isolated from rabbit urine. *J. Pharm. Pharmacol. 26:*471.
18. Ryrfeldt, Å., C. H. Ramsay, I. M. Nilsson, M. Widman, and S. Agurell (1973) Whole-body autoradiography of Δ^1-tetrahydrocannabinol and $\Delta^{1(6)}$-tetrahydrocannabinol in mouse. Pharmacokinetic aspects of Δ^1-tetrahydrocannabinol and its metabolites. *Acta Pharm. Suec. 10:*13.
19. Truitt, E. B., Jr. and M. Braude (1974) *Research Advances in Alcohol and Drug Problems* (R. J. Gibbins, Y. Israel, H. Kalant, R. E. Popham, W. Schmidt, and R. G. Smart, eds.), vol. 1. New York: Wiley, p. 199.
20. Wall, M. E. (1971) The *in vitro* and *in vivo* metabolism of tetrahydrocannabinol (THC). *Ann. N.Y. Acad. Sci. 191:*23.

10

Identification and Quantification of Cannabinoids in Urine by Gallium Chelate Formation

RAYMOND BOURDON

In recent years, many papers have appeared on the identification and quantification of cannabinoids in body fluids. Most of them use ^{14}C-labeled compounds, radioimmunoassay, gas chromatography (GC) or gas chromatography–mass spectrometry (GC–MS) methods, or, more recently, a mass fragmentography method [3,7,11,12, 13,17].

Very few methods are based on a pure chemical reaction, except perhaps for the identification of dansylated compounds, followed by thin-layer chromatography [4].

The method we suggest is related to a specific reaction of most of the cannabinoid compounds: transformation in *o-o'*-dihydroxy azo compounds able to give highly fluorescent gallium chelates.

It is out of the scope of this chapter to survey the chemical structures of the cannabinoid compounds. Δ^9-THC has been extremely well studied. We now know the structures of its major metabolites, hydroxylated in different locations, i.e., 11-OH-, 8-11-diOH-side, and chain hydroxylated compounds, and so on. All these metabolites keep the general structure of Δ^9-THC [8–10,18].

The characteristic feature of all these compounds is the aromatic ring, symmetrically substituted on carbon atoms 1, 3, and 5 (dibenzopyran numbering). This structure exists in a simple compound, olivetol, which is used for the synthesis of Δ^9-THC.

Symmetrical substitutions induce a characteristic reactivity, especially toward the diazo reagents. As a classical rule, a phenol group induces electrophilic substitutions in the *para* position, and to a very small extent, in the *ortho* position(s). For example, in the case of olivetol, the two possible electrophilic substitutions each involve a carbon atom between a phenol group and the side chain; that is, with carbon atoms 4 and 6, but never with carbon atom 2 (Figure 10.1). Considering one phenol group, the first electrophilic sub-

Marihuana: Chemistry, Biochemistry, and Cellular Effects, edited by Gabriel G. Nahas,

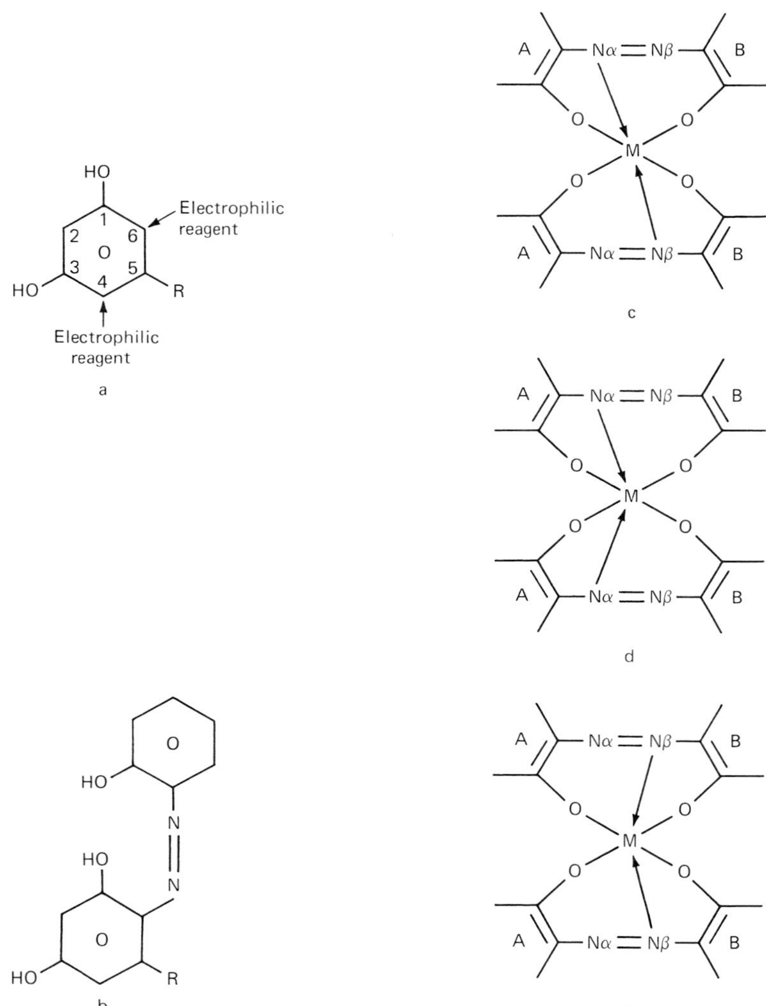

Figure 10.1. Formation and structures of gallium chelates. (a) Reactivity of symmetrical resorcinol derivatives. (b) Structure of azo compounds. (c, d, e) Structure of gallium chelates (M = Ga): type 2-I; from Pfitzner [12].

stitution enters the *para* position as usual, but as a consequence of symmetry, this substitution also enters the *ortho* position, considering the second phenol group.

Since olivetol can be considered a model not only for Δ^9-THC and its metabolites, but also for most of the cannabinoids (cannabinol, cannabidiol, cannabichromene, etc.), we used it to conduct a sensitive and as specific as possible method for identifying and quantifying the cannabinoid compounds. We proceeded from the above chemical considerations.

As early as 1956, Freeman and White [5] observed that the *o-o'*-dihydroxy azo compounds give highly fluorescent chelates with some metallic salts, particularly those of iron, indium, and gallium. To transform olivetol into an *o-o'*diOH azo compound, one can use many diazo reagents, all prepared from *o*-aminophenol derivatives. We use *o*-aminophenol, the simplest reagent, despite the low stability of its diazonium salts.

Olivetol Chelates

The *o*-aminophenol diazonium salts react in a dilute alkaline medium in molar ratio 1:1 with olivetol to give an azo compound that can be used for colorimetric measurement in a range higher than 5 μg/ml. Furthermore, this azo compound gives highly colored chelates with some metallic salts: Cu^{2+}, Ni^{2+}, Co^{2+}, Fe^{3+}, In^{3+}, Ga^{3+}, UO_2^{2+}, and Th^{4+}. Some of them are fluorescent (Fe, In, Ga). We chose gallium chelate because it is the most emissive. Moreover, its emission wavelength is in a spectral range (595 nm) where few natural products are fluorescent alone. This chelate is easily extracted from an aqueous medium by the following organic solvents: chloroform, methane dichloride, ethylacetate, and aliphatic alcohols.

Actually, we extract the chelate with *n*-amyl alcohol, for two major reasons. First, *n*-amyl alcohol provides the best compromise between solubility and extractibility. A shorter aliphatic alcohol—butanol, for example—yields a better extraction ratio, but the solubility in aqueous acidic medium is too high. On the contrary, the higher aliphatic alcohols (hexyl, heptyl, and octyl alcohols) are practically insoluble in water, but their partition coefficients are also lower. Second, and more important, dimethylformamide greatly enhances the fluorescence of the gallium chelates when added to the amyl extract. Finally, in this composite medium (dimethylformamide + *n*-amyl alcohol), it is easy to quantify more than 10 ng/ml (excitation wavelength: 515 nm; fluorescence wavelength: 595 nm).

The other chelates are equally useful, especially with the Co^{2+} and Cu^{2+} salts. The Co^{2+} chelate, stable between pH 4 and 9, is pink, easily extracted, and can be used for identification (see below). The Cu^{2+} chelate, stable in dilute alkaline medium, can be used for quantification after extraction in *n*-amyl alcohol, and measured by SAA.

Structure

The Co^{2+} and Cu^{2+} chelates are of type 2-I (one metallic atom) and the gallium chelate of type 3-I [2]. Nevertheless, very often the gallium chelates of such a structure are of type 2-I [13] (Figure 10.1).

A free phenol group is not required to form the chelates. For example, the *o*-aminophenoxy acetic diazonium salts, after copulation in *ortho-*, give metal chelates; the oxygen atom's free electrons ensure chelation. However, the highly polar phenoxyacetic group decreases solubility in organic solvents. On the other hand, Snavely *et al.* described many azo structures giving chelates [15,16]. Those with only one free phenol group should have a heteroatom with a free electron pair in the right place (e.g., pyrazolone). In the same way, we formed chelates after copulation between olivetol and the following diazonium salts: 3-amino-1,2,4-triazine, 3-amino-5-phenyl-1,2,4-triazine, and 5-amino-1,2,3,4-tetrazine. None gives better results than diazotized *o*-aminophenol.

Specificity

Diazo copulation is a common reaction of phenols. Nevertheless, because of the low reactivity of the proposed reagent and because of the chemical requirements for chelate formation, there is no reaction with most of the phenol compounds. For example, with phenol itself, as well as with thymol, 1-nitroso-2-naphthol,3,4-dimethylphenol, 4-chlorophenol, pyrocatechol, α-naphthol, β-naphthol, 2-aminoparacresol, and 3,5-dimethylphenol.

Obviously, resorcinol and its symmetrical derivatives give a positive reaction.

Cannabinoid Chelates

Resorcinol and its derivatives react easily in a dilute alkaline medium, roughly a 0.2 *N* aqueous solution of sodium hydroxide. In such a medium, Δ^9-THC does not react at all with the diazonium salt we use. Its reactivity increases with temperature and at first we used it to perform the copulation at a temperature higher than 100°C. However, reactivity is strictly dependent on the concentration of the alkaline medium (Figure 10.2) and is very low when

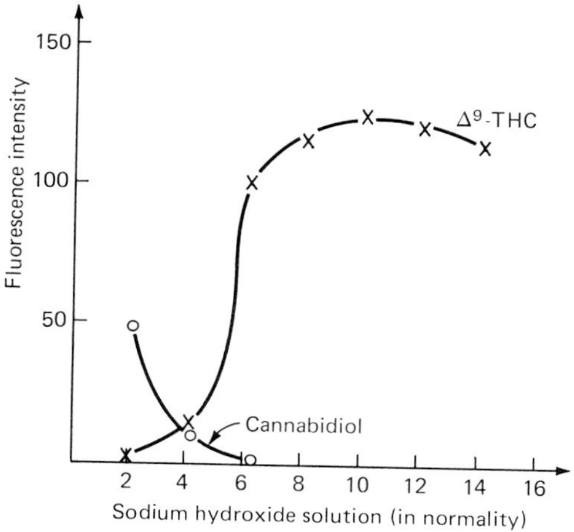

Figure 10.2. Influence of the concentration of alkaline medium on the reactivity of Δ9-THC and cannabidiol.

normality is lower than 2. At around 4 *N*, Δ9-THC begins to react and the maximum is reached at between normality 8 and 10. In the more concentrated alkaline media around 12 or 14 *N*, one observes a small decrease.

On the contrary, cannabidiol reacts better in a dilute alkaline medium, and it does not react at all in a concentrated alkaline medium (higher than 6 *N*).

For both cannabidiol and Δ9-THC, after copulation in the proper medium, chelates are obtained as usual. On pure samples, the fluorescent measurements must be easily performable in a range higher than 25 ng/ml (see Optimization).

Specificity

Basically, all the cannabinoids having a nonsubstituted carbon atom between the phenol group and the side chain are able to give gallium chelates:

Δ9-THC and its metabolites,
cannabichromene,
cannabicyclol,
cannabidiol and cannabigerol.

Nevertheless, the proper choice of a copulation medium enhances specificity. In their mixtures, Δ9-THC and cannabidiol can be specifically measured using two alkaline media: a dilute one (c #2 *N*) for cannabidiol and a concentrated one (c #10 *N*) for Δ^9-THC. Common phenols do not react in a concentrated alkaline medium.

Optimization

To improve sensitivity and reproducibility, after the copulation step, we recommend the following procedure:

1. The azo compound is extracted from the alkaline medium by *n*-amyl alcohol. Extraction in an acidic medium must be avoided in order to leave the diazo reagent excess in the water and to increase specificity.
2. The strongly alkaline amyl extract must be washed with an acetate buffer solution in order to have it in a proper pH ($3.5 < pH < 4.5$).
3. Chelate formation is slow. A 10-minute wait is required to ensure complete reaction and elimination of excess gallium salt.
4. In pure amyl alcohol, gallium chelate fluorescence is low and increases when dimethylformamide is added. The maximum is reached for a 1:1 volume: volume mixture.

Application to Urine

Cannabinoid compounds must be extracted from urine before measurement, but unfortunately, there is no satisfactory method to extract them from body fluids or tissues [8,9].

As previously described by Agurell [1], it is possible to use ether at pH around 3.8, but recovery after 5 extractions is always lower than 70 percent. The extract has to be washed with a phosphate buffer solution (pH 7.8) before being used for fluorescent measurement (pigments).

Recovery is improved with *n*-butyl alcohol as the solvent at the same pH, in the presence of ammonium chloride (salting out). But *n*-butyl alcohol is a less selective solvent than ether. After its elimination under reduced pressure, the extraction residue must be purified by chromatography on a mixture of alumina and Silica Gel. We have also successfully used formaldehyde dimethyl ether as a solvent.

In any case, for identification, the volume of the urine sample is

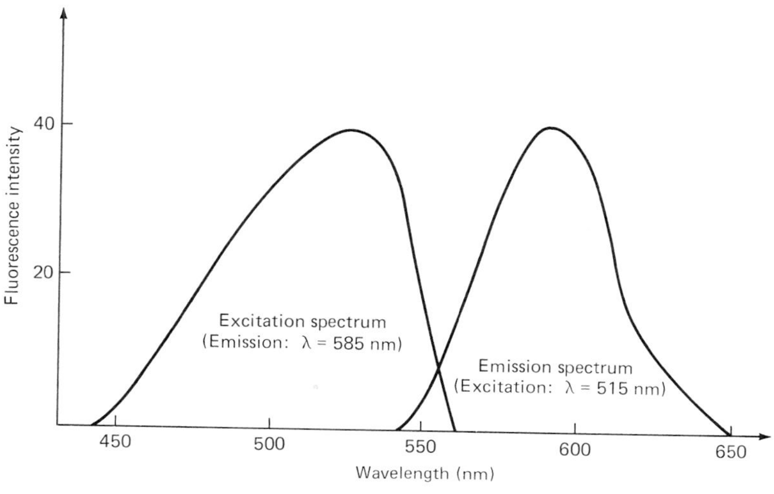

Figure 10.3. Excitation and emission spectra of gallium chelates (Δ^9-THC and olivetol).

20 ml, but it could be easily reduced during acute intoxications. After extraction, copulation, reextraction, and chelation, the emission spectrum is recorded between 530 and 700 nm (excitation wavelength: 515 nm) (Figure 10.3). Cannabinoids give a characteristic peak around 595 nm. Urine and reagent blanks give practically flat traces within the same range of spectra.

For quantification, we use the method of internal standard. Two kinds of extraction are performed on every sample: one on the sample itself, and the other on the same sample with a precise amount of Δ^9-THC (generally 1.0 μg) added.

During the last step, the two emission spectra are recorded. We explain the fluorescence intensity of both as the difference between the emissions at 595 nm and 540 nm. The Δ^9-THC concentration in the sample is calculated as a simple ratio. With this technique, we do not have to take into account either the recovery or the casual (and always low) interference of pigments.

Results

After this process, the concentrations measured are similar to those which appear in the literature [8,9]. Most of the results are lower than 30 μg/l. Nevertheless, in the course of long experimentation performed with volunteers smoking marihuana cigarettes, the concentration of cannabinoids in urine was often higher than 200 μg/l.[1]

Specificity

Except for the cannabinoids, we never observed a positive reaction with other drugs, including drugs of abuse such as barbiturates, amphetamines, tricyclic antidepressants, morphine, LSD, carbamates, salicylates, and benzodiazepines.

Note

Chelate formation can also be used to identify marihuana itself or marihuana mixed with tobacco (for example). After extraction by hexane or methanol, copulation, and reextraction by *n*-amyl alcohol, as previously described, the reaction is generally sensitive enough to form a pink cobalt chelate (pH = 8).

Experimental Materials

Reagents

Sodium nitrite, gallium chloride, ammonium chloride, ethyl ether, *n*-butyl alcohol, *n*-amyl alcohol, acetic acid, dimethylformamide, *o*-aminophenol (all reagent grade).
Dilute phosphoric acid (1/10).
Sodium hydroxide solution (c #10 *N*).
Phosphate buffer solution (1 *M*) pH 7.8.
Acetate buffer solution (acetic acid 10%, sodium acetate 3%).
Alumina (activity I–II).
Silica Gel
Diazo reagent: *o*-aminphenol ($c = 10^{-4}$ in 0.2 *N* HC1): 5 ml; sodium nitrite ($c = 10^{-3}$ in water): 0:5 ml; distilled water: 4.5 ml.

Note: All reagents are prepared in advance. The diazo reagent must be used between the 6th and 25th minutes after mixing.

Standard

Solution of Δ^9-THC (c #10^{-2} in methanol): 0.1 ml.
Methanol: 99.9 ml.
Final concentration: 10 μg/ml. (May be kept in dark refrigerator for up to 2 weeks.)

[1] We are indebted to Dr. G. Nahas (Columbia University), who kindly sent us these samples.

Extraction

With ether

To a 20-ml urine sample, add diluted phosphoric acid until pH 3.8. Extract 5 times with 20 ml ethyl ether. Collect the organic layers, wash with phosphate buffer solution (5 ml), and evaporate at low pressure.

With n-*butyl alcohol*

Saturate the sample at pH 3.8 with ammonium chloride and proceed as above for ether. After evaporation of the solvent at low pressure ($T < 50°C$), purify by chromatography with a short column of alumina (50 mg) on top and Silica Gel on the bottom (200 mg) (size 40×6 mm). Use ether as the solvent and keep all the elution phases. Evaporate.

Note: In both cases, for quantification, conduct two kinds of extraction, one on the sample itself, and the other on the same sample with an appropriate amount of Δ^9-THC added (according to the prior concentration, generally 1 μg.)

Copulation

To the evaporation residue, add 0.7 ml of concentrated hydroxide solution (c #10 N), 3 drops of n-amyl alcohol, and then the diazo reagent (0.3 ml). After waiting 10 min, extract with n-amyl alcohol (0.8 ml), mix, centrifuge, and completely reject the aqueous layer. Wash the organic phase with acetate buffer solution (1.5 ml). Centrifuge again and keep the supernatant. Add gallium chloride (0.1 ml, $c = 10^{-2}$ in acetic acid), and then dimethylformamide (0.7 ml). Mix and centrifuge after 10 min.

Measurement

Using an excitation wavelength of 515 nm, record the fluorescence spectrum between 530 and 670 nm. In order to eliminate interference due to pigments, explain the fluorescence intensity I_F as: $I_F = E_{595} - E_{540}$ (where E_{595} and E_{540} represent the measured flux at those wavelengths).

Calling I_X the fluorescence of the sample itself, and I_S the fluorescence of the sample added to 1 μg of Δ^9-THC, Q_X is the quantity of cannabinoids (in Δ^9-THC) in the sample, in μg. Use the relation

$$Q_X = \frac{I_X}{I_S - I_X} .$$

Then

$$C\,(\text{in}\,g^0/_{00}) = Q \cdot \frac{1000}{V},$$

where V is the volume of the sample in ml. Generally,

$$C = Q \cdot \frac{1000}{20} = 50\,Q.$$

REFERENCES

1. Agurell, S. and K. Leader (1971) Metabolism of cannabinoids. VIII. Stability, transfer and absorption of cannabinoid constituents of cannabis during smoking. *Acta Pharm. Suec. 8:*391.
2. Akhmedli, M. K. and E. L. Glushchenko (1961) A study of reagents for spectrophotometric determination of gallium. *Zh. Anal. Khimi 19:*556.
3. Breimer, D. D., T. B. Vree, C. M. Van Ginneken, P. Th Henderson, and J. M. Van Rossum (1972) Identification of cannabis metabolites by a new method of combined G.C.–M.S. *Proc. Int. Symp. Gas Chromotography–Mass Spectrophotometry* 87:95.
4. Forrest, I. S., D. E. Green, S. D. Rose, G. C. Skinner, and D. M. Torres (1971) Fluorescent-labelled cannabinoids. *Res. Commun. Chem. Pathol. Pharmacol. 2:*787.
5. Freeman, D. C. and C. E. White (1956) The structure and characteristics of the fluorescent metal chelates of *o-o′* dihydroxy azo compounds *J. Am. Chem. Soc. 78:*2678.
6. Gurny, O., D. E. Maynard, R. G. Pitcher, and R. W. Kierstead (1972) Metabolism of (-) Δ-9-THC. *J. Am. Chem. Soc. 94:*7928.
7. Korte, F. and H. Sieper (1964) Untersuchung von haschisch-inhaltstoffens durch dunnschicht-chromatographie. *J. Chromatogr. 13:*90.
8. Lemberger, L., L. Axelrod, and I. Kopin (1972) Metabolism and disposition of Δ-9-tetrahydrocannabinol in man. *Pharmacol. Rev. 65:*410.
9. Lemberger, L., S. D. Silberstein, L. Axelrod, and I. J. Kopin (1970) Studies on the disposition and metabolism of Δ-9-THC in man. *Science 170:*1320.
10. Mechoulam, R., H. Varconi, Z. Ben Zvi, H. Edery, and X. Grunfeld (1972) Syntheses and biological activity of five THC metabolites *J. Am. Chem. Soc. 94:*7930.
11. Paris, M. R. and R. Paris (1973) Importance de la CPG pour l'étude des constituants de *Cannabis sativa. Bull. Soc. Chim. Fr. 73:*118.
12. Pfitzner, H. (1972) Strukturisomere metallchelate unsymmetrischer *o-o′* dihydroxyverbindungen. *Angew. Chem.* [*Engl*] *8:*351.
13. Repetto, M. J. and M. Menendez (1970) Identification of cannabis from the plant, smoke and urine. *Eur. J. Toxicol. 3:*392.
14. Schou, J., A. Steentoft, K. Worm, J. Morkholo, and E. Nielsen (1971) A highly sensitive method for G.C. measurement of THC and CBN. *Acta Pharmacol. Toxicol.* (*Kbh.*) *30:*480.

15. Snavely, F. A. and B. D. Krecker (1959) Metal derivatives of aryl azo pyrazolones. III. Molarity quotients of *p.* and *m.* substituted pyrazolone dyes. *J. Am. Chem. Soc. 81:*4199.
16. Snavely, F. A. and D. A. Sweigart (1969) Metal derivatives of arylazopyrazolones. *Inorg. Chem. 8:*1659.
17. Vree, T. B., D. D. Breimer, C. A. M. Van Ginneken, J. M. Van Rossum, and N. M. M. Nibbering (1973) Gas chromatography of cannabinoids. Behavior of *cis-* and *trans*-THC and *iso*-THC. *J. Chromatogr. 79:*81.
18. Woodhouse, E. J. (1972) Confirmation of the presence of 11-hydroxy-THC. *Am. J. Public Health 62:*1394.

11

Forensic, Metabolic, and Autoradiographic Studies of Δ^8-and Δ^9-Tetrahydrocannabinol

W. W. JUST, G. ERDMANN, G. WERNER, M. WIECHMANN, AND S. THEL

To detect picomole amounts of tetrahydrocannabinol (THC) in the saliva of man after smoking a marihuana cigarette, we used fluorescence labeling of the THC molecule followed by thin-layer chromatographic (TLC) detection [5,13]. 1-Dimethylaminonaphthalene-5-sulfonyl chloride (DNS-Cl) served as a reagent to produce quantitatively the corresponding sulfonic acid esters [4]. The results suggested that the saliva of man may be used as a biological material to reveal cannabis intake after smoking.

The experiments which indicated a possible accumulation of THC in salivary glands [11,13,14] gave rise to comparative autoradiographic studies of Δ^8- and Δ^9-THC distribution in the organs of the monkey [12]. Simultaneous investigations of the metabolism of the drugs demonstrated the metabolic fate of the drugs during the incorporation periods of 30 min and 6 hr. Finally, an attempt was made to correlate the effects observed in man after cannabis use with the sites of drug accumulation in the monkey's brain [3,10]. This chapter is a synopsis of recently published results.

Materials and Methods

Male and female subjects each smoked within 10 min 400 mg of marihuana (1.5 percent Δ^9-THC) mixed with tobacco. Before smoking and at various intervals afterwards, about 1 ml of saliva was collected from each person.

Dansylation of saliva

Saliva was extracted using 5 ml portions of methylacetate-petrol ether (40–60°C), 2 : 1, in glass-stoppered centrifuge tubes. After evaporation under a stream of nitrogen, derivatization with DNS-

Cl was carried out in 1 ml of an acetone-water mixture, 2.5 : 1, adding 4 mg DNS-Cl (highly purified) and about 100 mg of solid $Na_2CO_3 \cdot 10\ H_2O$. The reaction mixture was whirled for 10 min and was left standing in the dark for another 30 min at room temperature. After the addition of proline, excess DNS-Cl was removed. The reaction mixture was then extracted three times with petrol ether (40–60 °C), and the extracts were dried under a stream of nitrogen.

Chromatography of dansylated saliva

The dried extracts were redissolved in petrol ether (40–60 °C) and TLC was performed on self-coated Silica Gel G layers in *n*-heptane–ethyl acetate, 95 : 5, by three runs in one direction in the dark. When food remnants were present in the saliva, a fourth development of the chromatograms in the opposite direction using methanol-water-acetic acid, 40 : 60 : 2, provided further cleaning of DNS–THC spots. Using a glass capillary and ethyl acetate as eluting solvent, we transferred the DNS–THC spot from the Silica Gel layer to a polyamide layer (F 1700), which was developed in acetone-water, 35 : 15.

Autoradiography

For the radiosynthesis of (2,4-^{14}C)-Δ^8- and (2,4-^{14}C)-Δ^9-THC (20 mCi/mM), we followed the methods of Petrzilka *et al.* [23] and Liebman *et al.* [19]. The drugs were purified by column chromatography at 4 °C on Silica Gel. A mixture of benzene-cyclohexane, 35 : 65, served as eluting solvent. The mass spectra of the drugs and of their DNS derivatives showed no impurities.

The drugs were injected intravenously (dissolved in 30 percent Tween 80) into four monkeys of the species *Callithrix jacchus*. The injected doses were 50 mg/kg ^{14}C- Δ^8-THC (one animal), 34 mg/kg ^{14}C- Δ^9-THC (two animals), and 25 mg/kg ^{14}C-Δ^9-THC (one animal). The animals were sacrificed 30 min or 6 hr (last animal) after the injection.

Autoradiograms were prepared from CO_2-frozen organ sections following the contact procedure of Werner *et al.* [26] using Ilford L4 emulsion and Kodak D19b developer.

Metabolic studies

The organs and body fluids were homogenized and extracted with methanol. Total radioactivities were determined by liquid scintillation counting. Following TLC of the organ extracts (Silica Gel G, benzene-methanol-acetic acid, 100 : 10 : 2), unchanged THC, 11-OH-THC and polar metabolites (R_f values lower than

Table 11.1 Specific radioactivities and ratio values of unchanged THC-11-hydroxylated metabolites (ratio 1) after administration of ^{14}C-Δ^9- and ^{14}C-Δ^8-THC in organs and body fluids of the monkey

Before sectioning, the brain was bisected by a transverse cut through the mesencephalon into brain I and brain II; the latter contained the cerebellum and exhibited a higher specific radioactivity.

	Δ^9-THC[a]				Δ^8-THC[a]		Δ^9-THC[b]	
Organs	*Spec. act. μCi/gm tissue*	*Spec. act. μCi/gm tissue*	*Ratio 1*	*Ratio 1*	*Spec. act. μCi/gm tissue*	*Ratio 1*	*Spec. act. μCi/gm tissue*	*Ratio 1*
Brain I	1.2	1.2	1.4	1.4	2.9	4.8	0.17	1.2
Brain II	2.0	1.9	1.1	1.5	2.8	4.2	0.16	1.3
Blood	1.9	1.8	3.2	2.5	1.1	7.1	0.38	0.9
Bile	110.2	113.8	—	—	28.6	—	146.0	—
Liver	9.7	10.7	2.0	1.5	12.3	6.0	0.5	1.3
Kidney	2.5	2.8	2.0	3.0	6.4	6.0	2.3	—
Stomach	1.2	1.3	2.4	2.8	2.4	6.3	0.2	1.5
Lung	1.7	1.7	1.4	1.7	3.9	5.4	0.3	0.8
Adrenal gland	9.3	9.1	3.9	3.3	—	—	0.7	2.0
Parotid gland	1.8	1.6	2.6	2.5	2.1	7.5	0.3	3.9
Pancreas	2.7	2.4	2.6	1.9	3.4	6.5	0.5	3.5

[a] Time of drug incorporation in live animal: 30 min.

[b] Time of drug incorporation in live animal: 6 hr.

those of 11-OH-THC) were determined as percentage of total radioactivities on the plates by thin-layer scanning. The calculated ratios of unchanged THC to 11-OH-THC are listed in Table 11.1 under ratio 1.

Results

The detection of Δ^9-THC in the saliva of man by fluorescence labeling of THC with DNS-Cl is shown in Figure 11.1. Synthetic Δ^9-THC labeled with the fluorophore served as a reference. Saliva was collected at intervals up to 6 hr after marihuana smoking. Two to three hours after smoking, DNS- Δ^9-THC was still detectable by Silica Gel TLC. Within that time it was possible to identify the eluted DNS-Δ^9-THC also by mass spectroscopy. For a more sensitive chromatographic detection, the DNS- Δ^9-THC spot was transferred from the Silica Gel plate to a polyamide layer by a quantitative procedure. The polyamide chromatograms obtained from three different experiments demonstrate the presence of DNS- Δ^9THC in the saliva of the subjects even 6 hr after smoking the marihuana cigarette (Figure 11.2).

Figure 11.1. Silica Gel chromatogram of saliva extracts of a subject after derivatization with DNS–Cl. Saliva samples were taken before smoking (1,2,), 10 and 30 min after (3,4), and in 1-hr intervals from 1–6 hr after having smoked (5,6,8–11). On position 7, DNS-Δ^9-THC was chromatographed as a reference. DNS-Δ^9-THC is detectable in the saliva up to 3 hr after smoking.

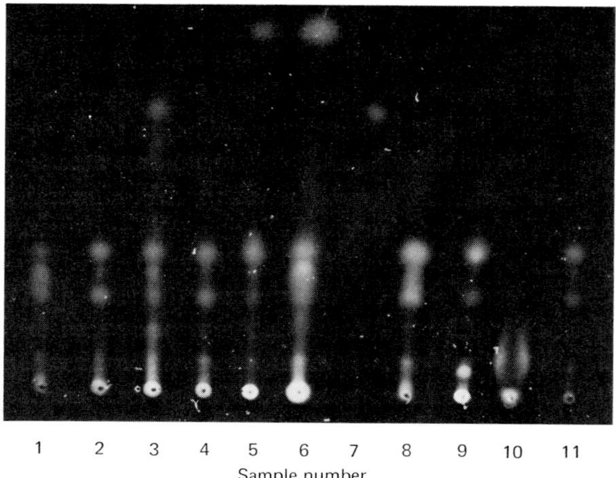

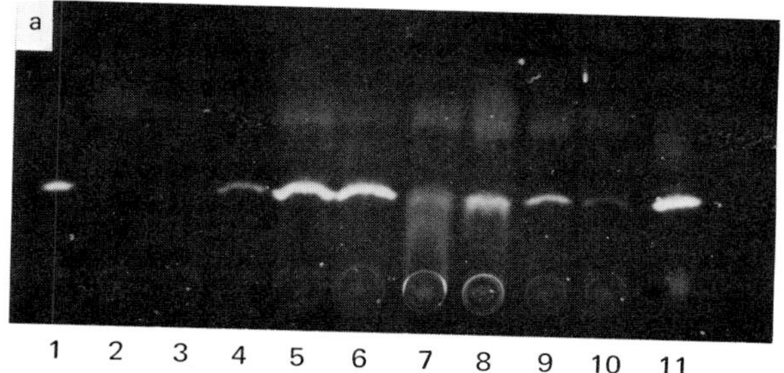

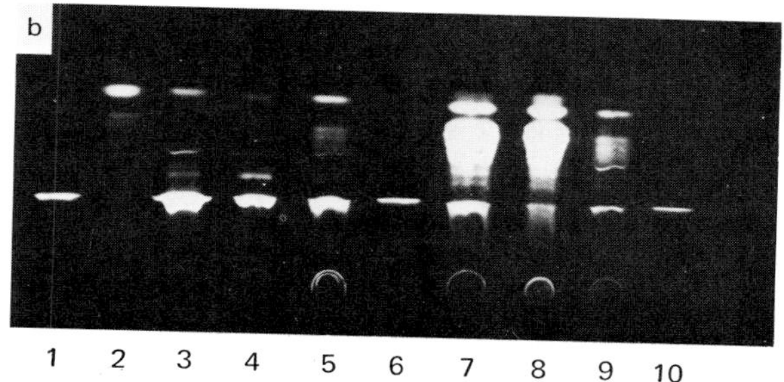

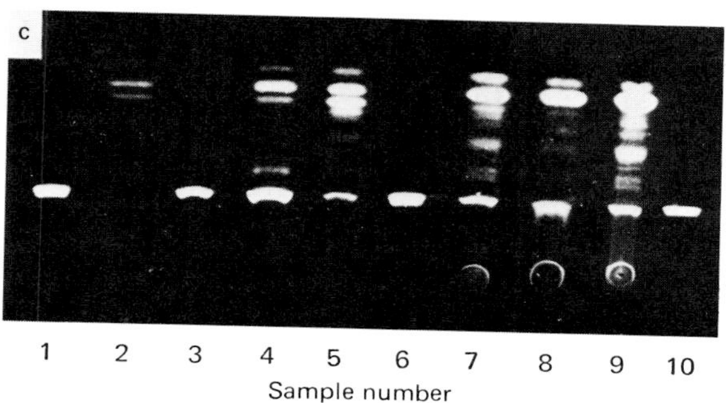

Figure 11.2 DNS-Δ^9-THC spots on the Silica Gel plates were transferred to polyamide layers. Three experiments are shown. (a) DNS-Δ^9-THC reference (1), before smoking (2,3), after 10 and 30 min (4,5), and 1–6 hr (6–11) in 1-hr intervals after smoking. (b,c) DNS-Δ^9-THC reference is placed in positions 1,6, and 10. Before smoking (2), after 10 and 30 min (3,4), and 1, 2, 4, and 6 hr after smoking (5,7,8,9). DNS-Δ^9-THC was detectable in the subjects' saliva up to 6 hr after smoking the marihuana cigarette. In some cases parts of the Silica Gel eluates were used for mass spectroscopic identification, and only the remainder was put on the polyamide layer.

Two-dimensional TLC of not fluorescent-labeled saliva extracts followed by mass spectroscopic analysis of the Δ^9-THC zone provided another possibility of detecting Δ^9-THC in the saliva of man within a 2 hr period after marihuana smoking [11].

Specific radioactivities measured in different organs and calculated values of ratio 1 are listed in Table 11.1. Thirty minutes after the injection of both Δ^8- and Δ^9-THC, the highest accumulations of radioactivity were measured in the bile, the liver, and the adrenal gland. In all organs including the brain, the values of ratio 1 were on the average two to three times higher after Δ^8-THC administration. In the frontal half of the brain, a lower specific radioactivity was measured than in the posterior half.

A prolonged incorporation period of 6 hr decreased the radioactivity in all organs save for kidney and except in bile by about 80–90 percent, whereas the values of ratio 1 were only slightly changed. Higher values of ratio 1 were found in some glandular tissues after a 6-hr incorporation of Δ^9-THC.

The different compositions of the polar metabolites of Δ^8- and Δ^9- THC are shown in the scannograms in Figures 11.3 and 11.4. Most of the polar metabolites of Δ^8-THC showed higher R_f values than that of Δ^9-THC. In brain tissue the polar metabolites were almost completely absent (Figure 11.4), although 6 hr after the drugs were administered, nearly the total radioactivity measured in the blood was attributed to them.

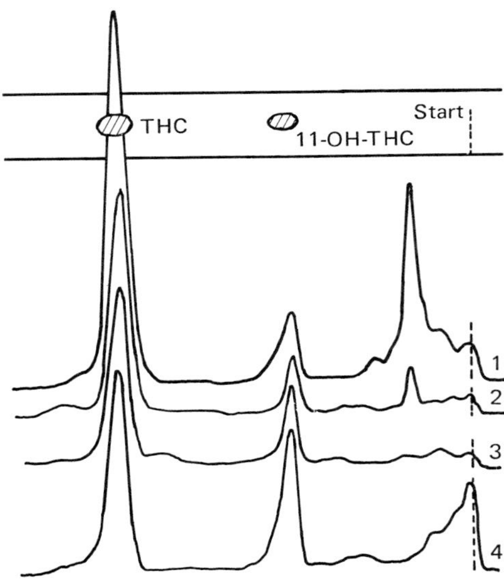

Figure 11.3. Radioscannograms of kidney (1,3) and liver (2,4) extracts after TLC. Time of incorporation of ^{14}C-Δ^8-THC (1,2) and of ^{14}C-Δ^9-THC (3,4) was 30 min. Note the ratio of the parent compounds to their 11-hydroxylated metabolites and the different compositions of the polar metabolites.

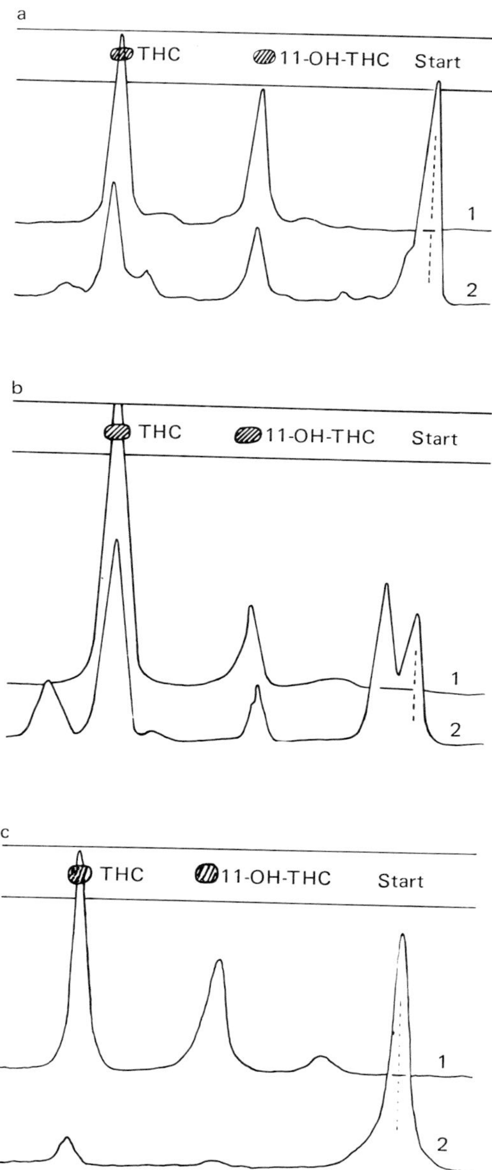

Figure 11.4. Radioscannograms of brain (1) and blood (2) extracts after TLC. Time of incorporation of ^{14}C-Δ^9-THC was 30 min (a) and 6 hr (c) and that of ^{14}C-Δ^8-THC was 30 min (b). Note the absence of polar metabolites in the brain tissue, their different compositions in the blood after Δ^9- and Δ^8-THC application, and the appearance of an unidentified substance with higher R_f-value than that of the parent Δ^8-THC (b).

In the autoradiograms, no obvious differences in label distribution were observed after the intravenous injections of ^{14}C- Δ^8- and ^{14}C- Δ^9-THC. All structures labeled by one of the drugs were also labeled by the other. Quantitative differences may exist, but they could not be demonstrated with certainty.

The localization of Δ^9-THC in the submandibular gland after a 30-min incorporation of the drug is shown in Figure 11.5. The radioactivity appeared to be distributed evenly throughout the glandular tissue, with secretory units being more or less distinctly labeled. The concentration of radioactivity was highest in the walls of the secretory ducts. The same pattern of drug distribution was also observed in the parotid and the sublingual glands [10].

Brain autoradiographs showed that gray matter was more heavily labeled than white matter. Apart from this gross distribution, however, some brain structures contained higher levels of radioactivity than gray matter in general. Most of these structures are involved in the processing of visual and acoustic information and in motor control. Brain structures and nuclei associated with motor control and demonstrating levels of radioactivity higher than those of gray matter included the subthalamic body [3], the substantia nigra, the nucleus ruber, and the nuclei controlling eye

Figure 11.5. Label distribution in the parotid gland after a 30-min incorporation. The radioactivity is highly concentrated in the ducts (d); × 16.

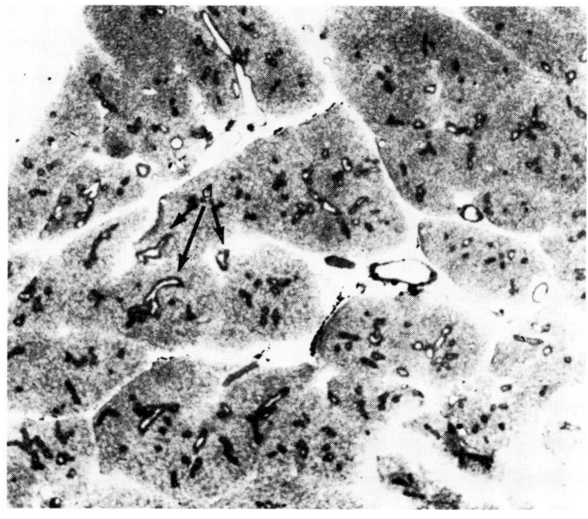

movement (Figure 11.7), as well as the inferior olive and the cerebellar and vestibular nuclei (Figure 11.9). In the caudate nucleus (Figures 11.6, 11.7), the label intensity was about the same as in the cortex.

The visual pathway displayed high concentrations of radioactivity in the lateral geniculate body (Figure 11.7), in the superior collicle (Figure 11.8), and in the central molecular layer of the visual cortex (Figure 11.9). In the auditory pathway, heavy label was found in the cochlear nuclei (Figure 11.9), in the inferior collicle, in the nucleus of the lateral lemniscus (Figure 11.8), and in the medial geniculate body (Figure 11.7). Radioactivity was also elevated in the central layer of the frontal and temporal regions including the auditory cortex (Figure 11.6). However, this labeling was less pronounced than that of the visual cortex.

Figure 11.6. Distributions of radioactivity in the forebrain region of the marmoset 30 min after IV injection of ^{14}C-Δ^9-THC. Gray matter is more heavily labeled than white matter. Accumulations of radioactivity are found in the nucleus paraventricularis hypothalami (PH), pituitary gland (PG), fiber bundles (*arrows*), and at clear-cut borders of white matter (*arrows*). Am—amygdala, CC—corpus callosum, Cd—nucleus caudatus, CI—capsula interna, GP—globus pallidus, Put—putamen, TO—tractus opticus, CF—cortex frontalis, CTp—cortex temporalis; × 3.8.

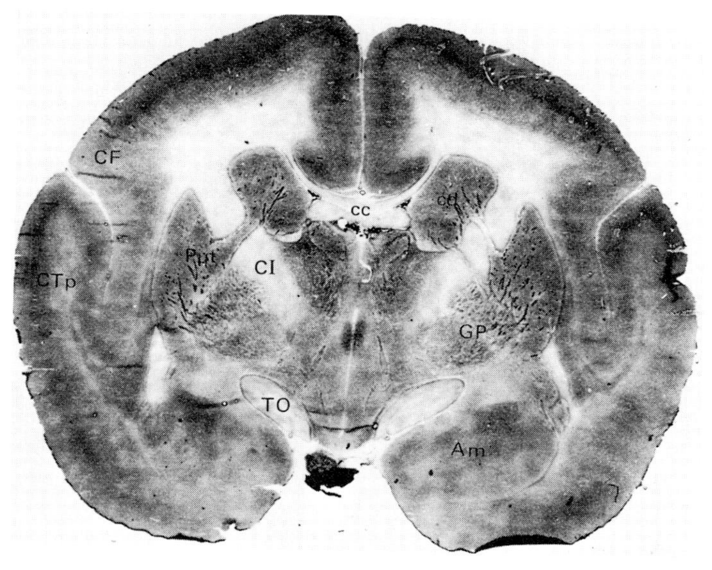

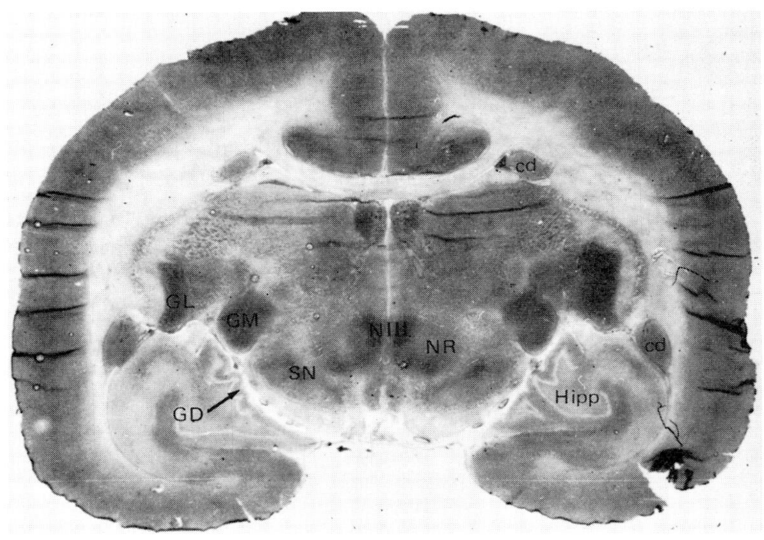

Figure 11.7. After $^{14}C-\Delta^9$-THC injection, the corpus geniculatum laterale (GL), the corpus geniculatum mediale (GM), and the nucleus nervi oculomotori (NIII) are the most heavily labeled structures in the thalamic region of the monkey's brain. Little radioactivity is observed in the hippocampus (Hipp), especially in the gyrus dentatus (GD). Cd—nucleus caudatus, NR—nucleus ruber, SN—substantia nigra; × 4.

Accumulations of radioactivity were also found in the supraoptic and the paraventricular nuclei and in the pituitary gland (Figure 11.6).

All white matter possessing a clear-cut border, such as the corpus callosum, the internal capsule, or the optic tract, was distinguished by a thin, distinct line of heavy label along the border of the white matter (Figure 11.6). Also, all bundles of myelinated fibers which pass through gray matter structures such as the striatum and the putamen were heavily labeled (Figure 11.6). In the cerebellum, a thin line of label next to the Purkinje cell layer (Figure 11.9) seemed also to be associated with myelinated fibers. This labeling has a striking resemblance to that seen in Fink-Heimer preparations demonstrating myelin distribution [3].

After 6 hours of $^{14}C-\Delta^9$-THC incorporation in the live animal, the radioactivity in the organs was strongly reduced, and in some organs—especially in the brain—the label distribution had changed completely. Little radioactivity remained in the gray matter, and

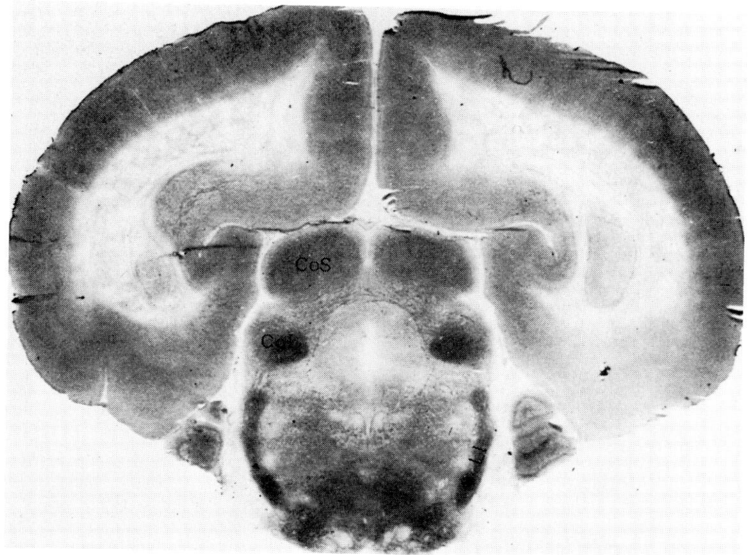

Figure 11.8. Cross section through the midbrain of the marmoset. 30 min after ^{14}C-Δ^9-THC administration, labeling is heavy in the colliculus superior (CoS), the colliculus inferior (CoI), and the nucleus lemnicus lateralis (LI); × 4.

the white matter—particularly the blood vessels (Figure 11.10)—was the most heavily labeled area. The midbrain and the medulla oblongata, however, maintained rather high levels of radioactivity with relatively little difference in the label intensities between white and gray matter (Figure 11.10). None of the nuclei containing accumulations of radioactivity after 30 min were conspicuously labeled after 6 hr.

Discussion

Several suitable methods of detecting Δ^9-THC in biological fluids have been recently reported. The most promising for routine analysis seem to be combined gas chromatography–mass spectroscopy [1] and radioimmunoassay techniques [7,24]. The latter method exhibits no absolute specificity for THC. Cross-reactions with other cannabinoids that may be pharmacologically inactive may occur. On the other hand, mass spectroscopic identification of

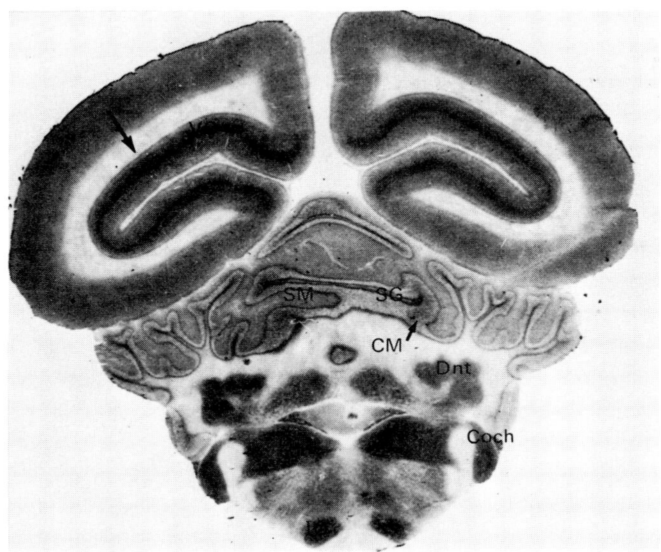

Figure 11.9. 30 min after IV injection of ^{14}C-Δ^9-THC, labeling is heavy in the visual cortex (VC); the dentate (Dnt), vestibular (Ves), and cochlear (Coch) nuclei; and in the inferior olive (IO). Arrows indicate labeling of white matter borders. Another thin line of label is located in the stratum moleculare (SM) next to the layer of Purkinje cells. CM—corpus medullare, SG—stratum granulosum; × 3.9.

DNS–THC has been accomplished following Silica Gel procedures and polyamide TLC, although after more than 2–3 hours after cannabis intake, only the fluorometric detection of DNS- Δ^9-THC was possible [5,10,12]. The use of high-pressure liquid chromatography for the nanogram scale identification of DNS–cannabinoids was recently reported by Loeffler *et al.* [20].

Hollister and Gillespie [9] and Karniol and Carlini [15] reported that the Δ^8-isomer had only minor psychopharmacological potency, whereas the 11-hydroxylated metabolites of Δ^8- and Δ^9-THC seemed to be equipotent in mice after both intravenous and intracerebral administration [25]. Furthermore, the monohydroxylated metabolites have been suggested to be responsible for most of the psychopharmacological effects [18,22]. Considering the various values of ratio 1 in all organs investigated 30 min after the injection of Δ^8- and Δ^9-THC, the initial metabolic rate of Δ^8-THC is markedly reduced, suggesting that the minor psycho-

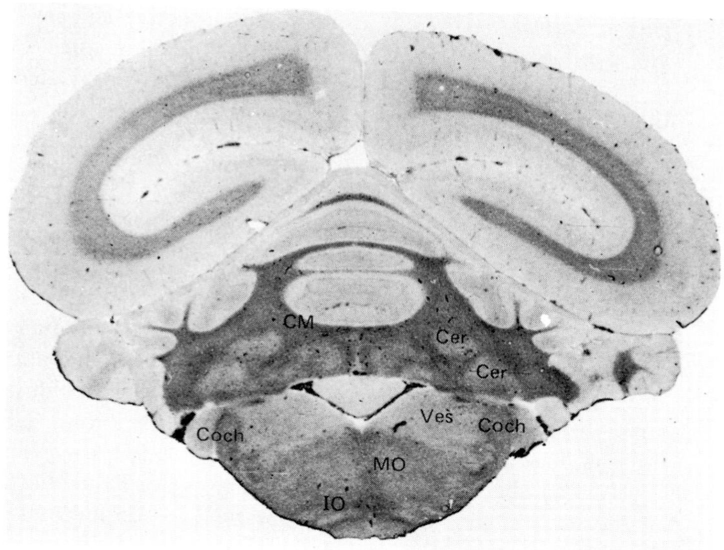

Figure 11.10. Six hr after IV injection of ^{14}C-Δ^9-THC, most label has been removed from the heavily labeled structures shown in Figure 11.9 and from the gray matter in general. The highest concentrations of radioactivity are now in the white matter. Labeling is relatively strong in the medulla oblongata (MO). Other abbreviations same as in Figure 11.9; × 4.2.

pharmacological activity of Δ^8-THC may be due to its slower rate of biotransformation to 11-OH- Δ^8-THC. Ho *et al.* [8] also reported slightly higher values of ratio 1 in the brain of rats 15 and 30 min after administration of a 5 mg/kg dose of Δ^8-THC as compared with the Δ^9-congener.

The heavy labeling of the cells lining the duct walls of the salivary glands as well as the presence of ^{14}C-Δ^9-THC in the monkey's saliva after the intravenous administration of the drug may indicate that also in man Δ^9-THC is secreted with saliva in spite of the lipophilicity of the drug. However, this must be reinvestigated.

The high label concentration in the adrenal gland may be governed by the high lipid content of this organ. Histological staining of the adrenal cortex with Sudan black correlates exactly with the labeling in the autoradiogram. In spite of the high drug accumulation in the adrenal gland, the results of Kubena *et al.* [16] suggest a centrally mediated pituitary-adrenal activation, rather than a direct influence of Δ^9-THC on hormone-producing cortical cells.

In the brain, Δ^8- and Δ^9-THC and their 11-hydroxylated metabolites comprise more than 90 percent of the total radioactivity. Therefore, the autoradiograms represent the distribution of a mixture of the parent compounds and their 11-hydroxylated metabolites. Yet, this hardly diminishes the value of the autoradiograms since the two substances seem to produce the same neuropharmacological effects although they are of different potencies [6,25].

The label distribution demonstrated in the marmoset's brain generally correlates well with that in the squirrel monkey reported by McIsaac *et al.* [21]. However, these authors did not mention drug accumulation in the cochlear, vestibular, oculomotor, and some other nuclei. On the other hand, the strong label these authors found in the cerebellar cortex (except the thin line of myelinated fibers next to the Purkinje cells) or in the hippocampus of the squirrel monkey was not observed in the marmoset's brain. The hippocampus appeared to be even less radioactive than gray matter in general, which agrees with the findings of Layman and Milton [17] in the rat hippocampus.

The labeling of extrapyramidal and other nuclei concerned with motor function may be related to the motor incoordination attributed to THC influence. Numerous further symptoms, such as impairment of visual and acoustic perceptions or hallucinations, may originate in changes in physiological functions in heavily labeled structures of the visual and acoustic pathway. This assumption is confirmed by the neurophysiological studies of Bieger and Hockman [2] on the effects of Δ^9-THC on lateral geniculate neurons of the rat.

REFERENCES

1. Agurell, S., B. Gustafsson, B. Holmstedt, K. Leander, J. Lindgren, I. Nilsson, F. Sandberg, and M. Asberg (1973) Quantitation of Δ^1-tetrahydrocannabinol in plasma from cannabis smokers. *J. Pharm. Pharmacol. 25:*554.
2. Bieger, D. and C. H. Hockman (1973) Differential effects produced by Δ^1-tetrahydrocannabinol on lateral geniculate neurons. *Neuropharmacology 12:*269.
3. Erdmann, G., W. W. Just, S. Thel, G. Werner, and M. Wiechmann (1975) Comparative autoradiographic and metabolic study of Δ^8- and Δ^9-tetrahydrocannabinol in the brain of the marmoset Callithrix jacchus. *Psychopharmacologia* (in press).
4. Forrest, I. S., D. E. Green, S. D. Rose, G. C. Skinner, and D. M.

Torres (1971) Fluorescent-labelled cannabinoids. *Res. Commun. Chem. Pathol. Pharmacol. 2*:787.
5. Friedrich-Fiechtl, J., G. Spiteller, W. W. Just, G. Werner, and M. Wiechmann (1973) Zu nachweis und identifizierung von tetrahydrocannabinol in biologischen flüssigkeiten. *Naturwissenschaften 60*:207.
6. Gill, E. W., G. Jones, and D. K. Lawrence (1973) Contribution of the metabolite 7-hydroxy-Δ^1-tetrahydrocannabinol towards the pharmacological activity of Δ^1-tetrahydrocannabinol in mice. *Biochem. Pharmacol. 22*:175.
7. Gross, S. J., R. J. Soares, S. R. Wong, and R. E. Schuster (1974) Marihuana metabolites measured by a radioimmune technique. *Nature 252*:581.
8. Ho, B. T., V. S. Estevez, and D. F. Englert (1973) The uptake and metabolic fate of cannabinoids in rat brains. *J. Pharm. Pharmacol. 25*:488.
9. Hollister, L. E., and H. K. Gillespie (1973) Δ^8- and Δ^9-tetrahydrocannabinol. *Clin. Pharmacol. Ther. 14*:353.
10. Just, W. W., G. Erdmann, S. Thel, G. Werner, and M. Wiechmann (1975) Metabolism and autoradiographic distribution of Δ^8- and Δ^9-tetrahydrocannabinol in some organs of the monkey Callithrix jacchus. *Naunyn Schmiedebergs Arch. Pharmacol. 287*:219.
11. Just, W. W., N. Filipovic, and G. Werner (1974) Detection of Δ^9-tetrahydrocannabinol in saliva of men by means of thin-layer chromatography and mass spectrometry. *J. Chromatogr. 96*:189.
12. Just, W. W., G. Werner, G. Erdmann, and M. Wiechmann (1975) Detection and identification of Δ^8- and Δ^9-tetrahydrocannabinol in saliva of man and autoradiographic investigation of their distribution in different organs of the monkey. *Strahlentherapie [Sonderb] 74*:90.
13. Just, W. W., G. Werner, and M. Wiechmann (1972) Bestimmung von Δ^1 and $\Delta^{1(6)}$-tetrahydrocannabinol in blut, urin und speichel von haschisch-rauchern. *Natruwissenschaften 59*:222.
14. Just, W. W., G. Werner, M. Wiechmann, and G. Erdmann (1973) Detection and identification of Δ^8- and Δ^9-tetrahydrocannabinol in the saliva of man and autoradiographic investigation of their distribution in the salivary glands of the monkey. *Jugoslav. Physiol. Pharmacol. Acta 9*:263.
15. Karniol, I. G. and E. A. Carlini (1973) Comparative studies in man and in laboratory animals on Δ^8- and Δ^9-*trans*-tetrahydrocannabinol. *Pharmacology 9*:115.
16. Kubena, R. K., J. L. Perhach, Jr., and H. Barry (1971) Corticosterone elevation mediated centrally by Δ^1-tetrahydrocannabinol in rats. *Eur. J. Pharmacol. 14*:89.
17. Layman, J. M. and A. S. Milton (1971) Distribution of tritium labelled Δ^1-tetrahydrocannabinol in the rat brain following intarperitoneal administration. *Br. J. Pharmacol. 42*:308.
18. Lemberger, L., R. Martz, B. Rodda, R. Forney, and H. Rowe (1973) Comparative pharmacology of Δ^9-tetrahydrocannabinol and its metabolite, 11-OH-Δ^9-tetrahydrocannabinol. *J. Clin. Invest. 52*:2411.
19. Liebman, A. A., D. H. Malarek, A. M. Dorsky, and H. H. Kaegi (1971) Synthesis of olivetol-4,6-$^{14}C_2$ and its conversion to (-)-Δ^9-6a,

10a-trans-tetrahydrocannabinol-2,4-$^{14}C_2$ via (-)-Δ^8-6a, 10a-trans-tetrahydrocannabinol-2,4-$^{14}C_2$. *J. Labelled Comp. 7:*241.

20. Loeffler, K. O., D. E. Green, F. C. Chao, and I. S. Forrest (1975) New approaches to assay of cannabinoids in biological extracts. *Proc. West. Pharmacol. Soc. 18:*363.
21. McIsaac, W. M., G. E. Fritchie, J. E. Idänpään-Heikkilä, B. T. Ho, and L. F. Englert (1971) Distribution of marihuana in monkey brain and concomitant behavioural effects. *Nature 230:*593.
22. Mechoulam, R. (1970) Marihuana chemistry. *Science 168:*1159.
23. Petrzilka, T., W. Haefliger, and C. Sikemeier (1969) 123. Synthese von haschisch-inhaltsstoffen. *Helv. Chim. Acta 52:*1102.
24. Teale, J. D., E. J. Forman, L. J. King, E. M. Piall, and V. Marks (1975) The development of a radioimmunoassay for cannabinoids in blood and urine. *J. Pharm. Pharmacol. 27:*465.
25. Wall, M. E. (1971) The in vitro and in vivo metabolism of tetrahydrocannabinol (THC). *Ann. N.Y. Acad. Sci. 191:*23.
26. Werner, G., H. Werner, P. G. Bosque, and J. Carreres-Quevedo (1966) Eine methode zur autoradiographischen darstellung hydrophiler substanzen in biologischem material. *Z. Naturforsch. [B] 21:*238.

I

Marihuana Chemistry

Kinetics and Biotransformation

12

Cannabinoids: Metabolites Hydroxylated in the Pentyl Side Chain

S. AGURELL, M. BINDER, K. FONSEKA, J.-E. LINDGREN, K. LEANDER, B. MARTIN, I. M. NILSSON, M. NORDQVIST, A. OHLSSON, AND M. WIDMAN

Introduction

This chapter—which also covers recent unpublished results from our laboratory—is mainly concerned with cannabinoid metabolites hydroxylated in the side chain. Other aspects of cannabinoid metabolism have recently been reviewed in other volumes [4,5,12].

Since the isolation of 7-hydroxy-Δ^1-tetrahydrocannabinol (*2*) as the first known metabolite of Δ^1-THC (*1*), it has been speculated that the CNS activity of Δ^1-THC is partly or solely due to the formation of active metabolites [4,5,9,12]. There is no general consensus as to the importance of the metabolites for the psychotomimetic effects of Δ^1-THC but recent clinical experiments (e.g., [4,2,9]) suggest that the marihuana "high" is at least partly induced by the formation of metabolites such as 7-OH-Δ^1-THC.

The metabolism of the cannabinoids has been found to be quite complex in both animals and man as discussed in recent reviews [4,5,12]. The metabolic patterns show marked species differences and vary also *in vitro* with the experimental conditions. However, the primary metabolic reactions, as shown for Δ^1-THC (Figure 12.3; *1*) and cannabidiol (CBD, Figure 12.5a; *11*), involve hydroxylation at C_7 to 7-OH-Δ^1-THC (*2*) and 7-OH-CBD (*12*) and at C_6 to the 6α- (*3, 13*) and 6β-hydroxylated (*4, 14*) compounds [4,8,10,13]. Further metabolism as exemplified by Δ^1-THC (Figure 12.3) leads to compounds such as *5, 6,* and *10.*

A potentially reactive intermediate, 1,2-epoxyhexahydrocannabinol (*7*), has been isolated, from *in vitro* preparations of squirrel monkey, dog, and rabbit tissues [cf. 12,18]. So far, no likely transformation product of 7 has been identified, which indicates

Marihuana: Chemistry, Biochemistry, and Cellular Effects, edited by Gabriel G. Nahas,

that the epoxide may react with macromolecular compounds. The metabolism of cannabinol (CBN; *28*) follows [4,5,12] a similar pattern (Figure 12.6) with C-7 hydroxylation as a major route (*29*).

Although in this chapter primarily the problems connected with side chain hydroxylated metabolites are emphasized, the presence of metabolites hydroxylated elsewhere in the molecule—usually the major route—obviously must also be considered (Figures 12.3, 12.5, and 12.6). McCallum and other [12] also have shown that Δ^1-THC to some extent will yield CBN; consequently, the formation of CBN metabolites from THC must not be overlooked. Moreover, before being eliminated, primary cannabinoid metabolites are often further oxidized or conjugated. Since these compounds are more polar and apparently lack psychotomimetic activity, we will not discuss them further.

Our earlier work indicated that side chain hydroxylation might be a metabolic route of importance at least in some species. A program was undertaken to synthesize side chain hydroxylated cannabinoids, develop methods of separating and identifying them, investigate their formation in some *in vitro* systems, and evaluate their psychotomimetic effects. The ultimate goal is to establish to what extent, if any, side chain hydroxylated Δ^1-THC metabolites contribute to the effects of Δ^1-THC and marihuana in man.

Some of these results reporting over a dozen not previously known side chain hydroxylated metabolites are also discussed in this chapter.

Synthesis of Side Chain Hydroxylated Cannabinoids

No available methods allow the synthesis of Δ^1-THC derivatives also carrying a hydroxyl group in the pentyl side chain. However, the syntheses of the corresponding compounds in the Δ^6 series—which may in many respects serve as useful reference compounds—have been described.

Fahrenholtz [6] has described the synthesis of 1″-OH-Δ^6-THC and 3″-OH-Δ^6-THC using dithioethylene as the protecting group in preparing the intermediate Δ^6-THC-3″-one. In connection with the synthesis of labeled cannabinoids, Pitt *et al.* [15] prepared 4″- and 5″-OH-Δ^6-THC. Both compounds were obtained from the common intermediate 5″-bromo-Δ^6-THC.

We have synthesized 1″-, 2″-, 3″-, and 5″-OH-Δ^6-THC as shortly outlined below and as described in detail elsewhere [1].

The side chain hydroxylated Δ^6-THCs were synthesized by condensation of (+)-*trans-p*-menthadien-(2,8)-ol-(1) with an appropriate olivetol derivative, followed by transformation to the hydroxy compound. Thus, 2″- and 5″-OH-Δ^6-THC were synthesized by reaction of the terpene with 1-(3,5-dihydroxyphenyl) pentan-2-one and methyl 5-(3,5-dihydroxyphenyl)pentanoate, respectively, followed by reduction. The 1″- and 3″-OH-Δ^6-THC were prepared according to Fahrenholtz [6] with the exception of minor differences in the preparation of 1-(3,5-dihydroxyphenyl) pentan-3-one, an intermediate in the synthesis of 3″-OH-Δ^6-THC. 1-(3,5-dihydroxyphenyl)pentan-2-one was prepared by reaction of 3,5-dimethoxyphenylacetyl chloride and dipropylcadmium, followed by demethylation with pyridinium chloride. The isomer 1-(3,5-dihydroxyphenyl)pentan-3-one, which could not be obtained by an analogous reaction with diethylcadmium, was synthesized as follows. Oxidation of 3,5-dibenzyloxybenzyl alcohol with aluminium isopropoxide in the presence of butanone gave a good yield of 1-(3,5-dibenzyloxyphenyl) pentan-3-one. Hydrogenation of the latter compound in ethanol with palladium as catalyst gave 1-(3,5-dihydroxyphenyl)pentan-3-one. The olivetol derivative used in the synthesis of 5″-OH-Δ^6-THC was prepared by a Wittig reaction from 3,5-dibenzyloxybenzaldehyde and methyl crotonyltriphenyl-phosophonium bromide. The resulting methyl 5-(3,5-dibenzyloxyphenyl)pentadienoate gave on catalytic reduction methyl 1-(3,5-dihydroxyphenyl)pentanoate.

The preparation of 2″- (*30*), 3″- (*31*), and 5″ OH-CBN (*33*) was recently described by our group [17]. In general, the compounds were obtained by sulfur dehydrogenation of a suitable Δ^6-THC intermediate, viz.Δ^6-THC-2″-one, Δ^6-THC-3″-one dithioethyleneacetal, and Δ^6-THC-5″-oic acid methyl ester with subsequent reduction to the alcohol.

The syntheses of 1″-OH-CBD (*15*) and the corresponding 2″- (*16*) and 3″-hydroxy (*17*) derivatives are discussed in a recent review [4, pp. 21–22] and along with some metabolic data in a previous paper [13]. The preparation of 5″-OH-CBD (*19*) will be reported later.

Separation and Identification

The metabolic patterns of the cannabinoids are complex on their own, and the products formed are difficult to separate from each other. As pointed out by other workers, thin-layer chromatography (TLC) techniques alone are usually not sufficient. To identify and quantify different metabolites, one must have reference compounds and a variety of separation techniques. We have found [7] that combinations of liquid chromatography on Sephadex LH-20, TLC, and gas-liquid chromatography (GLC) are suitable for separating mono- and dioxygenated cannabinoid metabolites before they are identified by spectral measurements.

Liquid chromatography

For column chromatography, Sephadex LH-20 (1 × 70 cm) is used [2] with a mixture of light petroleum, chloroform, and ethanol (10:10:1) as the eluent (flow rate 0.2 ml/min). The elution pattern for mixtures of cannabinoid metabolites as exemplified with Δ^6-THC, Δ^1-THC, and CBN is shown in Figure 12.1a. From these data and corresponding data with CBN the Sephadex LH-20 column appears to separate the side chain hydroxylated cannabinoids in the following order: 2″-, 1″-, 3″-, 4″-, and finally the 5″-hydroxylated compounds. The last of these compounds in turn have elution volumes similar to those of the 7-OH compounds. Certain compounds overlap, and this can probably be overcome by high-pressure liquid chromatography. However, the described Sephadex column has wide application and can be used for purifying a few nanograms as well as for separating a metabolite mixture containing several hundred milligrams of impurities.

Thin-layer and gas chromatography

As discussed by Mechoulam *et al.* [12], TLC has inherent limitations but also useful applications in the separation and purification of cannabinoids. For monohydroxylated cannabinoids, precoated Silica Gel F plates (10 × 5 cm) developed with diethyl ether and light petroleum (3:2) as the eluent gives a satisfactory separation as shown in Figure 12.1b for derivatives of Δ^1-THC, Δ^6-THC, and CBN. More polar compounds, such as 6,7-diOH-Δ^1-THC (*5*), must be chromatographed with a solvent like acetone-chloroform (7:13).

A 6-foot GLC column with 2 percent SE-30 ultraphase on Gas Chrom Q 125–150 mesh, at 250°C, was used for most separations both for ordinary GLC and GLC–MS. Some of the gas chromatographic results are presented in Table 12.1. Compounds such as 3″- (*8*) and 4″-OH-Δ^1-THC (*9*) are difficult to separate unless converted to their trimethylsilyl (TMS) derivatives [3]. Also, dihydroxylated compounds must be derivatized before GLC.

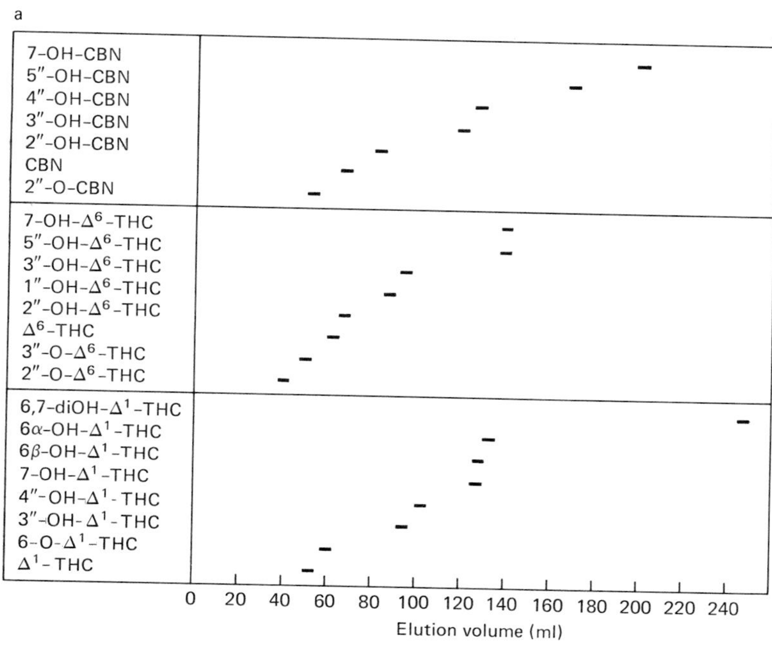

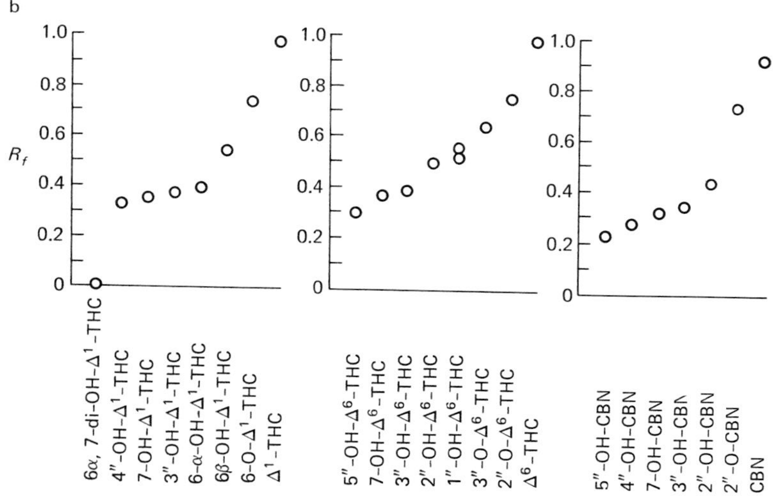

Figure 12.1(a). Elution pattern on Sephadex LH-20 of some cannabinoids and their oxygenated metabolites. 2″-O-CBN = CBN-2″-one, and so non. **(b)** TLC separation of some cannabinoids and their metabolites on Silica Gel F plates with diethyl ether and light petroleum (3:2) as solvent; CBN plate developed twice.

Table 12.1 Gas chromatographic separation of some cannabinoids and their metabolites

	Retention time (min)		*Retention time (min)*		*Retention time (min)*
Δ^1-THC	4.8	Δ^6-THC	4.4	CBN	6.0
6β-OH-Δ^1-THC	10.1	$2''$-O-Δ^6-THC	8.7	$2''$-O-CBN	11.8
6α-OH-Δ^1-THC	10.4	$2''$-OH-Δ^6-THC	8.9	$2''$-OH-CBN	12.2
$3''$-OH-Δ^1-THC	11.0	$1''$-OH-Δ^6-THC	9.3	$3''$-OH-CBN	14.1
$4''$-OH-Δ^1-THC	11.1	$3''$-OH-Δ^6-THC	10.1	$4''$-OH-CBN	14.3
7-OH-Δ^1-THC	14.2	7-OH-Δ^6-THC	14.1	7-OH-CBN	18.2
6,7-diOH-Δ^1-THC	—	$5''$-OH-Δ^6-THC	14.3	$5''$-OH-CBN	19.3
TMS ether		*TMS ether*			
$3''$-OH-Δ^1-THC	3.7	7-OH-Δ^6-THC	4.7		
$4''$-OH-Δ^1-THC	4.1	$5''$-OH-Δ^6-THC	5.1		
6,7-diOH-Δ^1-THC	4.5				

Spectroscopic identification

Nuclear magnetic resonance (NMR) spectra of cannabinoids have proven to be very helpful for structure elucidation [12], and the use of 100 MHz instruments with Fourier transforms has in numerous cases allowed us and others [4,10] to elucidate structures of metabolites using as little as 50–100 μg of compound. Still, the structural information obtained by GLC–MS requires only a few micrograms of metabolite, and mass fragmentography reveals partial information with only nanograms available, as shown by previous work [2] and papers published in the present volume.

The NMR and mass spectra (MS) of side chain hydroxylated cannabinoids have been studied in detail [3] and are discussed elsewhere in this volume by Binder. In short, using TMS ethers one can derive MS fragmentations specific for the site of hydroxylation. Thus, in the THC, CBD, and CBN series, a fragment M^+ -57 is typical for a silylated 1″-OH compound; the TMS ether of 2″-OH is characterized by an intense ion $m/e = 145$; 3″-OH by M^+ -29 and M^+ -144; 4″-OH by a major fragment $m/e = 117$; and the 5″-OH shows certain but not too characteristic features [3].

In summary, preliminary fractionation on Florisil columns [7,18] followed by combinations of liquid chromatography and TLC allow separation and preliminary identification (GLC) of primary side chain hydroxylated (and other) metabolites. A final structure determination is carried out by NMR and/or GLC–MS analysis of the silylated derivatives. Using these methods, we have isolated and determined the structures of some 20 side chain hydroxylated cannabinoid metabolites, only two of which were known previously.

Metabolites

Δ^1-THC—side chain hydroxylated metabolites

The liver is considered to be the main site for THC metabolism, but other tissues such as lung and spleen have been reported to be metabolically active [12,14,18].

Cannabis is usually inhaled as a smoke, and after smoking or IV administration THC accumulates in the lung. To minimize metabolic effects of other tissues, we have in collaboration with Dollery's group studied Δ^1-THC metabolism using the isolated perfused dog (greyhound) lung [18]. Tritiated Δ^1-THC was administered IV, and after a 2-hr perfusion, lung circuit plasma and lung tissue were extracted and found to contain similar metabolites. The elution pat-

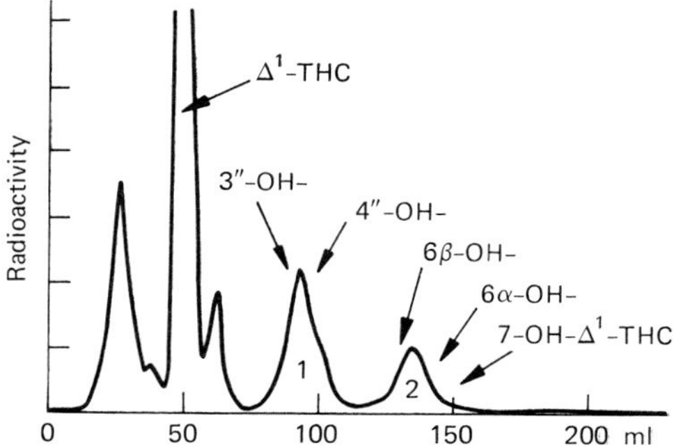

Figure 12.2. Elution pattern of Δ^1-THC derivatives from Sephadex LH-20 of metabolites extracted from the perfused dog lung plasma.

tern of metabolites isolated from lung plasma is shown in Figure 12.2. Further separation by Sephadex LH-20 and TLC followed by MS identification showed that the new metabolites 3″-OH-Δ^1-THC (*8*) and 4″-OH-Δ^1-THC (*9*) were major metabolites in the dog

Figure 12.3. Metabolic pathways for Δ^1-THC;* indicates metabolite not previously reported. Metabolic transformation established in (a) dog; (b) man; (c) monkey; (d) mouse; (e) rabbit; (f) rat.

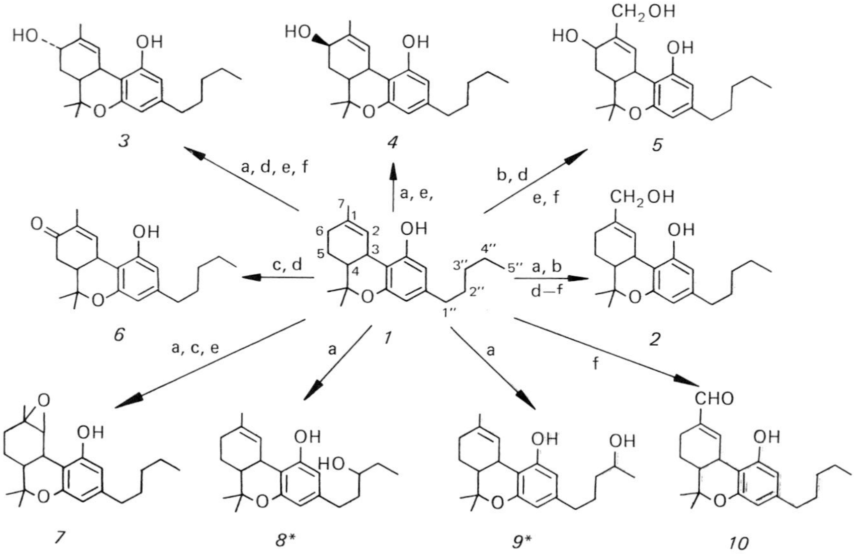

Table 12.2 Relative proportions of *in vitro* metabolites[a]

	Δ^1-THC		CBD	CBN	
	Dog lung	*Dog liver*	*Rat liver*	*Rabbit liver*	*Rat liver*
1″-OH	—	—	+	—	—
2″-OH	—	—	+	—	—
3″-OH	+++	+	+	—	tr
4″-OH	+++	+	++	+	tr
5″-OH	—	—	+	+++	+
				++	tr
7-OH	++	+	+++	+++	+++
6α-OH	+	+++	++		
6β-OH	+	+++	tr		

[a] Experimental conditions described in the text. +, ++, +++ indicate minor to major metabolite; tr indicates trace; — indicates "not found."

lung, whereas the previously known 6α- (*3*), 6β-OH-Δ^1-THC (*4*), and 7-OH-Δ^1-THC (*2*) were all minor compounds (Figure 12.3).

The same metabolites and in addition compound 7 were formed in the 10,000*g* liver supernatant from the same dog (Table 12.2). However, the proportions of the metabolites were reversed, with 6α- and 6β-OH-Δ^1-THC as the major compounds in the liver and *8* and *9* the minor compounds. Although the experimental conditions for lung (perfused) and liver (10,000*g* supernatant) tissues were not equivalent, a difference in the metabolism between the two organs is indicated.

The formation of 3″- and 4″-OH-Δ^1-THC by the lung is of special interest since these compounds probably both have higher psychotomimetic activity (Table 12.3) than Δ^1-THC itself.

Previously, only 1″-OH-Δ^6-THC and 3″-OH-Δ^6-THC have been isolated as Δ^6-THC metabolites from dog liver *in vitro* by Maynard *et al.* [11] and Δ^1-THC-7-oic acids carrying hydroxyl groups in the 1″- and 2″ positions from *in vivo* experiments by Burstein *et al.* [4].

CBD—side chain hydroxylated metabolites

CBD (*11*) has previously been found to be metabolized to 7-OH-, 6α-OH-, and 6β-OH-CBD by rat liver [8,13]. Also, the side chain hydroxylated metabolite 3″-OH-CBD (*17*) has been identified [13].

We have now further investigated the CBD metabolites produced by rat liver 10,000*g* supernatant [10]. After removing most

Table 12.3 Pharmacological effects[a] of Δ6-THC derivatives hydroxylated in the side chain [1]

Compound	*Dose (mg/kg)*	*Activity*
1″-OH-Δ6-THC	1	−
	5	+
	7	+
2″-OH-Δ6-THC	1	+
	2	++
	5	+++
3″-OH-Δ6-THC	0.05	−
	0.10	−
	0.20	++
	0.25	+++
	1	+++
5″-OH-Δ6-THC	0.25	−
	0.50	++
	1	+++
	2	+++

[a] Activity after IV injection into rhesus monkey was evaluated in comparison with Δ6-THC according to the following scale:

−	No behavioral changes
+	Behavioral changes equivalent to 0.1–0.3 mg/kg Δ6-THC
++	" " " " 0.4–0.9 " "
+++	" " " " 1.0–2.0 " "

The pharmacological tests in rhesus monkeys are described by Edery in *Psychopharmacologia 14:* 200, 1969, and *Arzneim. Forsch.* 22: 1995, 1972.

of the unchanged CBD with petroleum ether, investigators extracted metabolites with diethyl ether and fractionated them on a Florisil column; this was followed by chromatographic separation on Sephadex LH-20 (Figure 12.4) and TLC.

7-Hydroxy-CBD (*12*) was by far the major metabolite in the rat (Table 12.2) and was, together with 6α-OH-CBD (*13*) and 6β-OH-CBD (*14*), identified by comparison with authentic references and by spectral properties [8]. Hydroxylation was also found to occur in all possible positions of the pentyl side chain—from 1″ to 5″ (*15–19,* Figure 12.5 a). The identities of *15, 16,* and *19* were confirmed by chromatographic and spectroscopic comparison with synthetic references.

The structures of 3″- and 4″-OH-CBD were assigned according to ^{1}H–NMR and MS data. Apart from NMR data [3], the structure

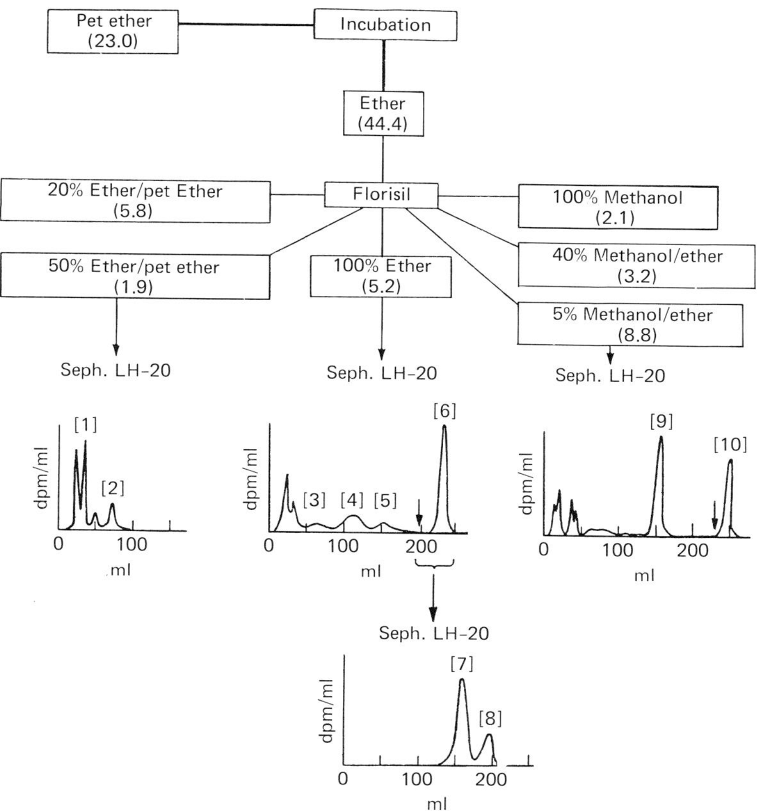

Figure 12.4. Extraction and separation of CBD and its metabolites on Florisil and Sephadex LH-20. Figures in parentheses show mg metabolites.

elucidation of 3″-OH-CBD (*17*) was based on the presence of $m/e = 301$ (loss of ethyl) in the nonsilylated derivative [10]. The TMS derivative showed the typical fragment M^+ -144 [3]. Fragment $m/e = 117$ [3] is typical for the identity of 4″-OH-CBD, and this structure was also verified by NMR (doublet at $\delta = 1.19$ instead of the usual triplet at $\delta = 0.87$; C 5″-protons). For a further discussion of spectral data, see the article of Martin *et al.* [10].

The fraction of more polar dihydroxylated metabolites (Florisil, 5 percent methanol/ether) was further separated by TLC as described earlier in this chapter. 3″, 7-Dihydroxy-CBD (*20,* Figure 12.5b) and 4″, 7-diOH-CBD (*21*) were isolated as major metabolites and their structures determined by spectroscopic methods.

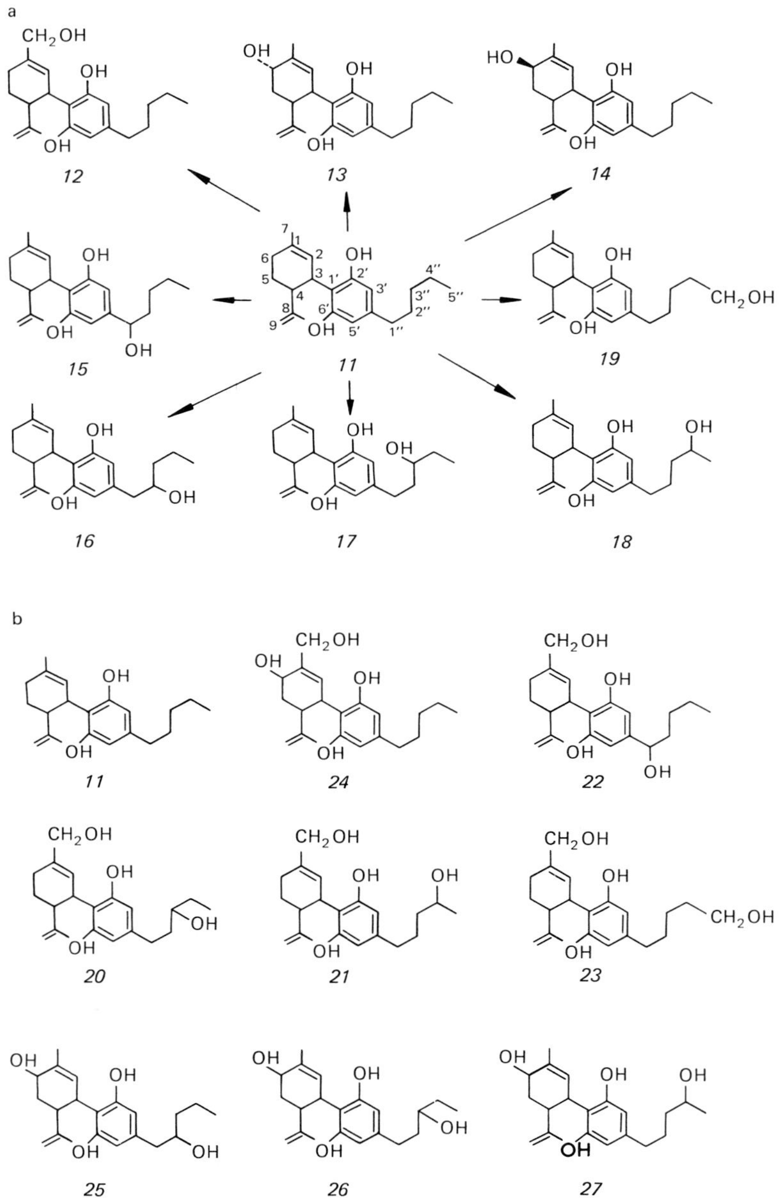

Figure 12.5. Metabolic products of CBD in rat liver. (a) Monohydroxylated metabolites; (b) dihydroxylated metabolites.

NMR showed the absence of the C_7 methyl groups and instead the presence of two proton singlets at $\delta = 4.12$ (-CH_2OH). The signals for the C_5''-methyl groups in *20* and *21* corresponded to the expected values for a C_4 and C_3-hydroxylated side chain. From spectral evidence, 1″, 7- (*22*) and 5″-, 7-diOH-CBD (*23*) were also identified although in smaller amounts. Four dihydroxylated minor metabolites (*24–27*), which apart from a hydroxyl group in the 6 or 7 position also contained a hydroxyl group in 2″, 3″, or 4″ position, were also identified.

In summary, the metabolism of CBD in rat liver is unusually diverse (Figure 12.5) and has yielded a variety of metabolites hydroxylated both in the monoterpene moitey and in all five positions in the side chain.

CBN—side chain hydroxylated metabolites

The biotransformation of CBN (*28*) to 7-OH-CBN (*29*) has been established *in vitro* with liver enzymes from rat (cf. [12,17]. Under similar conditions, Wall [16] tentatively identified 2″-OH-CBN—an interpretation which in the light of later information was correct.

We have now [17] investigated more extensively the metabolism

Figure 12.6. Metabolic products of CBN.

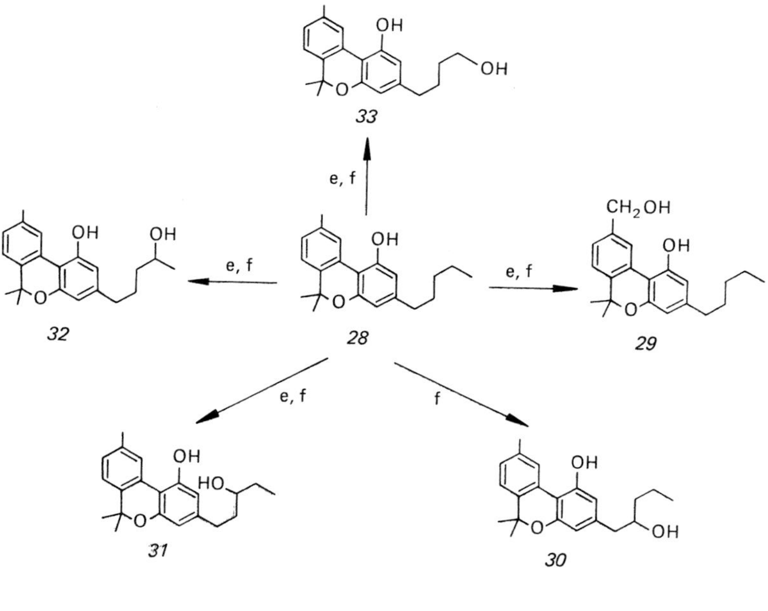

33

e, f

32 ← e, f — 28 — e, f → 29

28 — e, f → 31

28 — f → 30

of CBN in rat and rabbit liver 10,000*g* supernatant. Apart from the previously known 7-OH-CBN (*29,* Figure 12.6), rat liver produced small amounts of 2″- (*30*), 3″- (*31*), 4″- (*32*), and 5″-OH-CBN (*33*). The major biotransformation in the rabbit was to 7- and 4″-OH-CBN with minor amounts of 3″- and 5″-OH-CBN formed (Table 12.2).

Species Differences

Species differences in cannabinoid metabolism are indicated by available information [12]. However, it is difficult to make more meaningful comparisons also of *in vitro* work unless such factors as protein and substrate concentrations, cofactors, and induction of enzymes are compensated for. From the results presented in this chapter concerning the metabolism of Δ^1-THC in the dog, differences in metabolism between tissues also are indicated.

The relative proportions of metabolites of Δ^1-THC, CBD, and CBN formed *in vitro* under similar (except dog lung) conditions in our laboratory are shown in Table 12.2. But, as emphasized above, the results must be interpreted with caution because only a few experiments are available. However, the results suggest that in all the three tested species, if side chain hydroxylation occurs, hydroxylation in the 3″ and particularly the 4″ position is favored. This assumption is also supported by the isolation of 3″, 7- and 4″, 7-diOH-CBD as major dioxygenated metabolites from rat liver supernatant. Hydroxylation in 2″ and 5″ positions seems to be of less importance and occurs in the 1″ position to an even smaller extent.

Biological Activity

It is now well established (cf. [4,5,12,14]) both in man and animals that several metabolites of Δ^1-THC are potent pharmacological compounds. Thus, 7-OH-Δ^1-THC has been shown to be as potent as Δ^1-THC in man, whereas CBN is much less active than Δ^1-THC.

Several cannabinoids have been tested in the rhesus monkey for cannabis-type psychic effects—a model which seems to be reasonably correlated with activity in man [12]. Since the importance of side chain hydroxyl groups is related to the possible psychotomimetic effects in man of the corresponding metabolites, we have now in collaboration with the groups of Edery and Mechoulam tested the activities of 1″-, 2″-, 3″-, and 5″-OH-Δ^6-THC in the rhesus monkeys [1].

The results (Table 12.3) show that 3″-OH-Δ^6-THC is several times more potent than Δ^6-THC itself, whereas 5″-OH-Δ^6-THC is about equipotent than Δ^6-THC. 4″-OH-Δ^6-THC was not available, but an extrapolation of the results in Table 12.3 would suggest it to be at least as potent as Δ^6-THC. 2″-OH-Δ^6-THC is less potent than Δ^6-THC, and 1″-OH-Δ^6-THC shows only little activity. Thus, it would appear that those side chain hydroxylated metabolites which are the major metabolites are also the psychotomimetically most potent compounds.

Possible Human Significance of Side Chain Hydroxylated Metabolites

The possible human significance is, of course, related to the occurrence of side chain hydroxylated Δ^1-THC metabolites in man. 7-OH-Δ^1-THC has been identified by Wall *et al.* [16] as a Δ^1-THC metabolite in human plasma and tentative evidence suggest that also 6α- and 6β-OH-Δ^1-THC are present [12]. For example, in the present study we found in the rabbit that side chain hydroxylation is a major route for certain cannabinoids. Also, the lung (which in man usually is the tissue where Δ^1-THC is absorbed), as exemplified by the dog lung, has considerable metabolic capacity to form the presumably most active of the side chain hydroxylated metabolites, viz., 3″- and 4″-OH-THCs, as major metabolites. Our results suggest that they are generally present. Previously only three primary metabolites hydroxylated in the side chain were known (1″- and 3″-OH-Δ^6-THC, 3″-OH-CBD) and the occurrence of 19 new metabolites now reported may possibly be due to the development of new separation and identification techniques. Whether side chain hydroxylate metabolites are generally significant in man or in animals remains to be established.

The pharmacokinetics of each side chain hydroxylated compound is obviously important since these compounds have to be distributed to the CNS in high enough concentration relative to Δ^1-THC and 7-OH-Δ^1-THC to be able to contribute significantly to the effects. An extrapolation to man also necessitates that the potencies in the Δ^1-THC series be correlated with those measured in the Δ^6 series. Further work along these lines is in progress.

REFERENCES

1. Agurell, S., J. Dahmén, H. Edery, K. Leander, and R. Mechoulam (1975) Synthesis and biological activity of side chain hydroxylated tetrahydrocannabinols. (To be published.)
2. Agurell, S., S. Levander, M. Binder, A. Bader-Bartfai, B. Gustafsson, K. Leander, J.-E. Lindgren, A. Ohlsson, and B. Tobisson (1975) Pharmacokinetics of Δ^8-tetrahydrocannabinol in man after smoking—relations to physiological and psychological effects. *The Pharmacology of Cannabis* (M. Braude and S. Szara, eds.). Baltimore: University Park Press.
3. Binder, M., S. Agurell, K. Leander, and J.-E. Lindgren (1974) Zur identifikation potentieller metabolite von cannabis inhaltstoffen: kernresonanz und massenspektroskopische untersuchungen an seitenkettenhydrozylierten cannabinoiden. *Helv. Chim. Acta 57:*1626.
4. Burstein, S., J. Martinez, J. Rosenfeld, and T. Wittstruck (1972) The general pharmacology of cannabinoids. *Cannabis and Its Derivatives.* (W. D. M. Paton, and J. Crown, eds.). London: Oxford University Press, pp. 39–49.
5. Burstein, S. H. (1973) Labeling and metabolism of the tetrahydrocannabinols. *Marijuana* (R. Mechoulam, ed.). New York: Academic Press, pp. 167–190.
6. Fahrenholtz, K. E. (1972) The synthesis of two metabolites of (-)-Δ^8THC. *J. Org. Chem. 37:*2204.
7. Fonseka, K., M. Widman, and S. Agurell (1976) Chromatographic separation of cannabinoids and their monooxygenated derivatives. *J. Chromatogr.* (in press).
8. Lander, N., Z. Ben-Zvi, R. Mechoulam, B. Martin, M. Nordqvist, and S. Agurell (1976) Total synthesis of cannabidiol and Δ^1-tetrahydrocannabinol metabolites. *J. Chem. Soc.* (in press).
9. Lemberger, L., R. Martz, B. Rodda, R. Forney, and H. Rowe (1973) Comparative pharmacology of Δ^9-THC and its metabolite, 11-OH-Δ^9-THC. *J. Clin. Invest. 52:*2411.
10. Martin, B., M. Nordqvist, S. Agurell, J.-E. Lindgren, and K. Leander (1976) Identification of monohydroxylated metabolites of cannabidiol formed by rat liver. *J. Pharm. Pharmacol.* (in press).
11. Maynard, D. E., O. Gurny, R. G. Pitcher, and R. W. Kierstead (1971) (-)-Δ^8THC. Two novel *in vitro* metabolites. *Experientia 27:*1154.
12. Mechoulam, R., N. K. McCallum, and S. Burstein (1975) Recent advances in the chemistry and biochemistry of Cannabis. *Chem. Rev.* (in press).
13. Nilsson, I. M., S. Agurell, J. L. G. Nilsson, M. Widman, and K. Leander (1973) Two cannabidiol metabolites formed by rat liver. *J. Pharm. Pharmacol. 25:*486.
14. Paton, W. D. M. (1975) Pharmacology of marijuana. *Ann. Rev. Pharmacol. 15:*191.
15. Pitt, C. G., D. T. Hobbs, H. Schran, C. E. Twine, Jr., and D. L. Williams (1976) The synthesis of deuterium, carbon-14, and carrier-free tritium labelled cannabinoids. *J. Org. Chem.* (in press).
16. Wall, M. E. (1971) The *in vitro* and *in vivo* metabolism of tetrahydrocannabinol. *Ann. N. Y. Acad. Sci. 191:*23.

17. Widman, M., K. Dahmén, K. Leander, and K. Petersson (1975) *In vitro* metabolism of cannabinol in rat and rabbit liver. Synthesis of 2″-, 3″-, and 5″-hydroxycannabinol. *Acta Pharm. Suec. 12*:385.
18. Widman, M., M. Nordqvist, C. T. Dollery, and R. H. Briant (1975) Metabolism of Δ^1-tetrahydrocannabinol by the isolated perfused dog lung. *J. Pharm. Pharmacol. 27*:842.

13

Identification of Hydroxylated Cannabinoids by PMR and Mass Spectroscopy

MICHAEL BINDER

Introduction

The stereospecific synthesis of (-)-Δ^1-3,4-*trans*-tetrahydrocannabinol (Δ^1-THC = Δ^9-THC, IUPAC nomenclature) by Mechoulam and Gaoni [8] and by Petrzilka *et al.* [11,12] has initiated a number of studies concerning the metabolic fate of Δ^1-THC and other cannabinoids in different organisms. The first major metabolite of Δ^1-THC was isolated independently by Nilsson *et al.* [9] and by Wall *et al.* [15] in 1970, and its structure was shown to be 7-OH-Δ^1-THC (for the numbering of the cannabinoid skeleton, see Figure 13.1). In the meantime, the number of known metabolites has increased considerably. These include 6α,7-diOH-Δ^1-THC, 6α-OH-Δ^1-THC, 6β-OH-Δ^1-THC, 1,2α-epoxy-Δ^1-THC, and 6-oxo-Δ^1-THC. In addition to these metabolites, which are derived from Δ^1-THC by the introduction of an oxygen function around (or on) the isolated double bond of the isoprene moiety, another recently isolated group of metabolites contains hydroxyl groups in the aliphatic pentyl side chain of the molecule. Hydroxylation of the pentyl side chain seems to occur rather unspecificly, and compounds like 1″-OH-Δ^6-THC, 3″-OH-Δ^6-THC [7], 3″-OH-Δ^1-THC, and 4″-OH-Δ^1-THC have been isolated [17]. The two final compounds were identified unequivocally by the method we present here. Metabolic studies on other cannabinoids, e.g., cannabidiol (CBD) and cannabinol (CBN), showed in addition the occurrence of side chain hydroxylated metabolites. Thus, the tentative identification of 2″-OH-CBN and 2″,7-diOH-CBN and the identification of 3″-OH-CBN, 4″-OH-CBN, and 5″-OH-CBN [16] have been reported, as has the isolation of a side chain hydroxylated cannabidiol, 3″-OH-CBD [10].

Compared with metabolites bearing oxygen functions in the

Marihuana: Chemistry, Biochemistry, and Cellular Effects, edited by Gabriel G. Nahas, © 1976 by Springer-Verlag New York Inc.

isoprene moiety, side chain hydroxylated metabolites are obtained in small quantities from *in vitro* and *in vivo* experiments, thus posing rather tricky problems of isolation and identification. Therefore, we considered it desirable to develop a general method for identifying side chain hydroxylated cannabinoids that would depend only on the position of the hydroxyl group in the pentyl side chain, regardless of the basic type of cannabinoid. We have investigated the 100 MHz PMR spectra of a number of synthetic side chain hydroxylated cannabinoids, the mass spectra (MS) of these compounds, and the mass spectra of their trimethylsilyl (TMSO) ethers.

Materials and Methods

Materials

1″-OH-CBD (I), 1″-OH-Δ^6-THC (II), 2″-OH-CBD (III), 2″-OH-Δ^6-THC (IV), 2″-OH-CBN (V), 3″-OH-Δ^6-THC (VI), 3″-OH-CBN (VIII), 5″-OH-CBD (IX), 5″-OH-Δ^6-THC (X), and 5″-OH-CBN (XI) were prepared synthetically in varying amounts up to 50 mg. The details of these syntheses will be reported elsewhere [6]. 4″-OH-CBN (VIII) was obtained from an *in vitro* incubation of CBN with rat liver homogenate (300 μg) [10]; it contained about 20 percent of the 5″-OH isomer. The synthetic materials were purified by preparative thin-layer chromatography (TLC) and contained, according to TLC and gas-liquid chromatography (GLC), less than 5 percent impurities.

All compounds were silylated by reacting 250 μg of the synthetic material and 50 μg of 4″-OH-CBN (VIII) with an excess of *bis*-N,0-trimethylsilyl trifluoracetamide (BSTFA) at 50°C for 5 min in a closed vial. The reaction products were diluted with acetonitrile to give suitable concentrations of 2.5 μg/μl and 0.5 μg/μl, respectively, for GLC–MS analysis.

PMR spectra

One hundred MHz PMR spectra of all compounds were recorded in a $CDCl_3$ solution on a Varian XL-100 instrument with Fourier transform. The chemical shifts given in δ values were measured from the $CHCl_3$ signal as internal standard (δ7.26 ppm).

Mass spectra

All mass spectra were recorded on a GC–MS combination, type LKB 9000. GLC separation of the compounds was achieved on a 3 percent SE-30 / gaschrom Q column (1.8 m $\times$ 2 mm) between

180 and 240 °C. Ionization voltage ranged from 10 to 70 eV. If not otherwise stated, spectra were recorded at 20 eV. The given relative intensities (RI) of fragment ions were averaged from multiple runs, the spectra always being taken in the ascending slope of the GLC peak.

Results and Discussion

PMR spectra

The PMR spectra of the basic cannabinoids have been reported in detail [1,11]. Usually, the only distinguishable features of protons in the side chain are a 2-H triplet centered around δ2.5 ppm and a 3-H triplet around δ0.9 ppm, corresponding to the benzylic protons in the 1″ position and to the terminal methyl group (C-5″).

The δ values, the type of signal, and the coupling constants (in Hz) for side chain protons of the five varieties of side chain hydroxylated cannabinoids are listed in Table 13.1.

As a synopsis of the relevant details, parts of these PMR spectra have been compiled in Figure 13.1.

In the spectra of the 1″-OH-cannabinoids, the usual triplet of the benzylic protons has been replaced by a sharp 1-H triplet around δ4.5 ppm. On irradiation at δ1.7 ppm, the approximate place of the C-2″ protons, this triplet collapses to give a singlet.

Location of the hydroxyl group on C-2″ leads to a broad multiplet centered at δ3.8 ppm corresponding to H-2″. The protons on C-1″ have been shifted to a slightly lower field and appear as an AB system, which is further split by different couplings to H-2″. Irradiation of H-2″ destroys the additional splitting of the H-1″ AB system.

The spectra of 3″-OH-cannabinoids show a pentet centered at δ3.6 ppm that arises from equal couplings of H-3″ to the four protons on C-2″ and C-4″. The protons on C-1″ give rise to a complicated multiplet at δ2.6 ppm, while the 5″-methyl protons for the first time appear as a nicely resolved triplet.

The spectrum of 4″-OH-CBN (VIII) exhibits a broad multiplet at δ3.6 ppm, corresponding to the 4″-proton, while the triplet of the terminal methyl group has been replaced by a 3-H doublet centered at δ1.2 ppm. Irradiation at δ3.6 ppm leads to a singlet at δ1.2 ppm.

Location of the hydroxyl group on C-5″ results in the replacement of the 3-H triplet at δ0.9 ppm by a 2-H triplet at δ3.7 ppm.

Table 13.1 PMR data of protons located in the side chain of side chain hydroxylated cannabinoids

Cannabinoid		H—1″	H—2″	H—3″	H—4″	H—5″
1″-OH-CBD	(I)	4.50 t/6				0.87 t/5
1″-OH-Δ⁶-THC	(II)	4.50 t/8				0.97 t/7
2″-OH-CBD	(III)	2.7 2.39 AB/14/3/8	3.87 m			0.93 m
2″-OH-Δ⁶-THC	(IV)	2.7 2.42 AB/14/3/9	3.80 m			0.94 t
2″-OH-CBN	(V)	2.77 2.51 AB/14/4/8	3.88 m			0.94 t
3″-OH-Δ⁶-THC	(VI)	2.59 m		3.60 p/6		0.94 t/7
3″-OH-CBN	(VII)	2.67 m	1.81 m	3.62 p/6	1.4 m	0.95 t/7
4″-OH-CBN	(VIII)	2.56 t/7			3.66 m	1.21 d/6
5″-OH-CBD	(IX)	2.47 t/7				3.64 t/6
5″-OH-Δ⁶-THC	(X)	2.47 t/7				3.66 t/6
5″-OH-CBN	(XI)	2.53 t/7				3.66 t/6

Irradiation at the approximate place of the 4″-protons leads to the collapse of this triplet.

The PMR spectra exhibit typical signals for side chain protons in each of the five possible cases of hydroxylation. Chemical shifts, type of signal, and coupling constants are largely independent of the basic cannabinoid. The signals rarely overlap with signals due to protons located in other parts of the molecule. Even when, due to small quantities of compound, the signals obtained are not sharp, identification of metabolites by aimed decoupling experiments still seems possible.

Mass spectra

The mass spectra of the basic cannabinoids and the fragmentation mechanisms encountered have been discussed in detail [3,4]. Recently, Vree *et al.* [13,14] have described a method for identify-

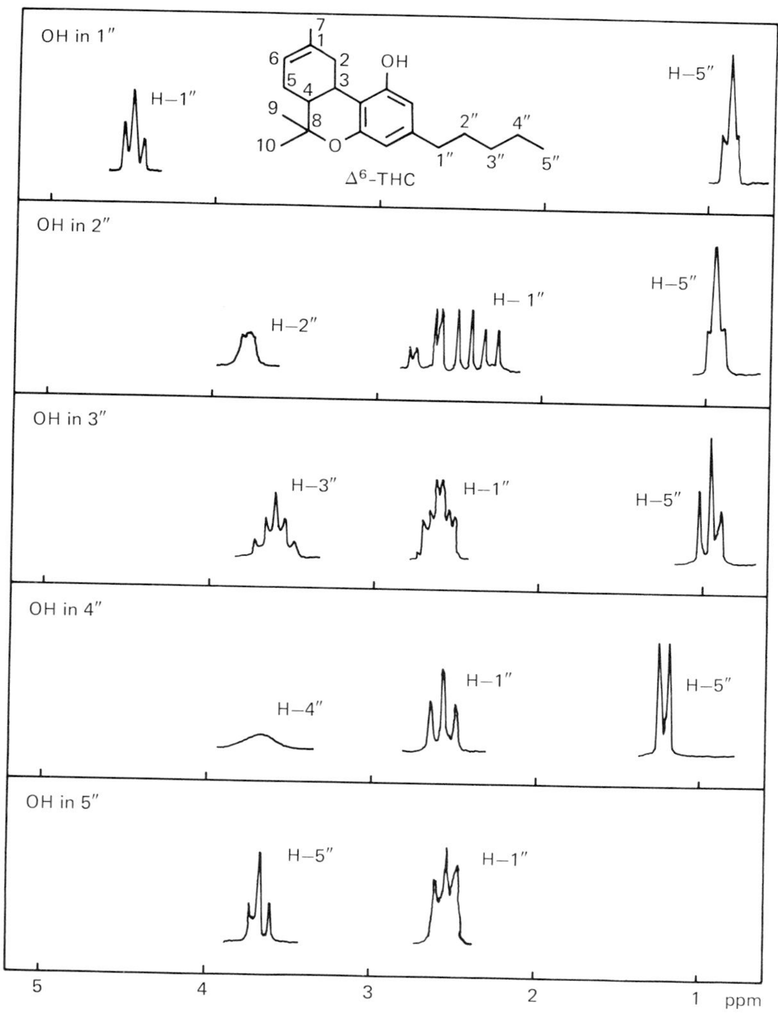

Figure 13.1. Details of the 100 mHz PMR spectra of side chain hydroxylated cannabinoids.

ing cannabinoids with varying side chains. By plotting the relative intensities of specific fragment ions against the ionization voltage, similar mass intensity graphs were obtained for fragment ions derived from THCs with pentyl, propyl, and methyl side chains.

We started looking for fragment ions common to cannabinoids of different basic types but possessing hydroxyl groups in the same position of the side chain. These mass spectra, however, were dominated by fragmentations of the isoprenoid moiety of the molecules, and even Vree's method was unsuccessful [2]. This was because ions resulting from α-cleavages in the side chain were of very low intensity, and were sometimes lacking completely, especially at ionization voltages below 20 eV.

Therefore, we investigated the mass spectra of the TMSO derivatives of these cannabinoids. The influence of the TMSO group on fragmentations of straight chain hydrocarbons has been discussed [5].

At 70 eV ionization voltage, the mass spectra were dominated by unspecific ions at $m/e = 73$, 75, and 147, which are common with mono- and poly-TMSO ethers. At 20 eV ionization voltage, the RI of these ions decreased and the spectra exhibited fragments of high RI resulting from cleavages influenced by the TMSO group in the side chain. Except for an increase in the RI of the molecular ion, there were no significant changes when the ionization voltage was lowered to 10 eV.

The typical fragmentation pattern for TMSO ethers of 1″-OH-cannabinoids is the loss of a butyl radical, leading either directly, as in the case of 1″-TMSO-Δ^6-THC (IIa), to the base peak M^+-57 (IIb), or in the case of 1″-TMSO-CBD (Ia) in combination with the well-known retro-Diels-Alder reaction to the base peak M^+-68-57 (Ib). There is no fragment corresponding to the loss of butene, indicating that the cleavage between C-1″ and C-2″ occurs without McLafferty rearrangement. Figure 13.2 summarizes the main fragment ions for both cases.

The mass of the fragment ions is given as difference to the molecular ion because we consider the similarities of fragmentations rather than absolute m/e values. The figures in parentheses give the RIs of the ions at 20 eV ionization voltage.

Location of the TMSO group on C-2″ leads in all cases to the fragment $[CH_3CH_2CH_2CH = OSi(CH_3)_3]^+$ at $m/e = 145$ (IIIb, IVb, Vb), which represents the base peak at all ionization voltages. The corresponding fragment M^+-145 does not occur, the charge always being retained on the TMSO fragment. α-Cleavage between C-1″ and C-2″ occurs to a small extent with McLafferty rearrangement and charge retention on the aromatic moiety, leading to the fragments IIId and Vc (cf. Figure 13.3).

Although loss of the side chain with McLafferty rearrangement plays no major role in the case of 1″- and 2″-TMSO-cannabinoids, it becomes important when the TMSO group is located in the 3″ position. The cleavage between C-1″ and C-2″ occurs exclusively with McLafferty rearrangement and charge retention on the aro-

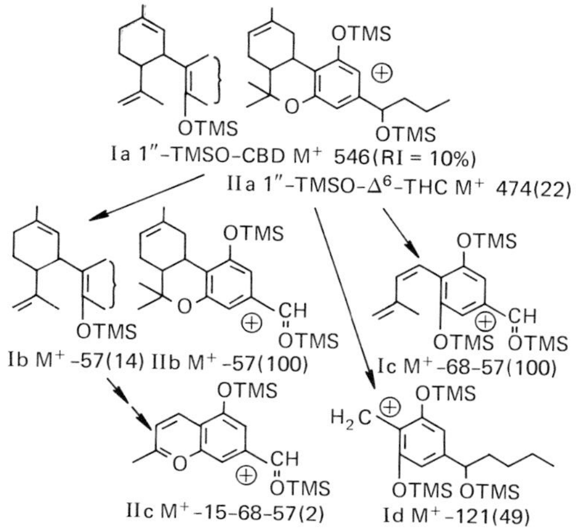

Figure 13.2. Typical fragment ions obtained from 1″-TMSO-cannabinoids.

matic moiety. Fragment ions at $m/e = 144$ or 145 do not occur. As shown in Figure 13.4, loss of 144 mass units leads in the case of 3″-TMSO-Δ[6]-THC (VIa) directly to the base peak M⁺-144 (VIc), or in the case of 3″-TMSO-CBN (VIIa) to the prominent ion M⁺-144 (RI 94 percent). Of the four possible ions that could

Figure 13.3. Typical fragment ions obtained from 2″-TMSO-cannabinoids.

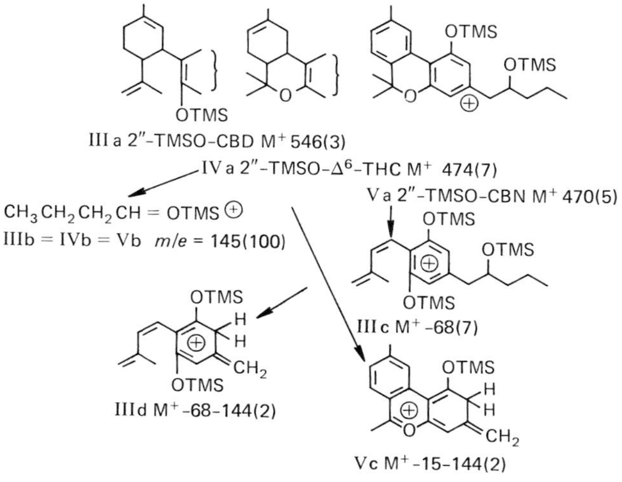

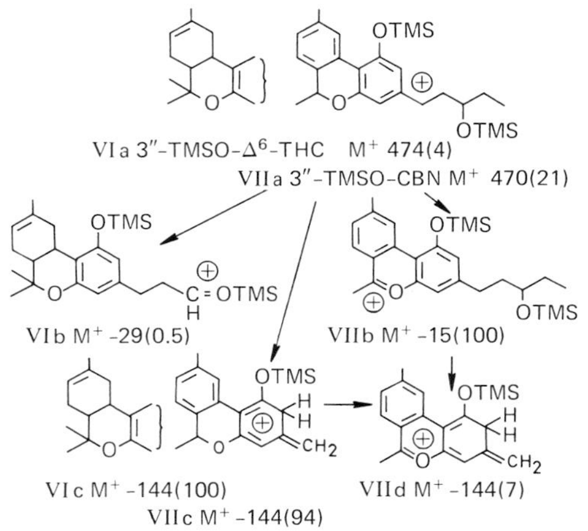

VIa 3″-TMSO-Δ⁶-THC M⁺ 474(4)
VIIa 3″-TMSO-CBN M⁺ 470(21)
VIb M⁺-29(0.5)
VIIb M⁺-15(100)
VIc M⁺-144(100)
VIIc M⁺-144(94)
VIId M⁺-144(7)

Figure 13.4. Typical fragment ions obtained from 3″-TMSO-cannabinoids.

result from α-cleavages in the side chain, only the weak fragment VIb derived from 3″-TMSO-Δ^6-THC (VIa) is found.

The mass spectrum of 4″-TMSO-CBN (VIIIa) exhibits a weak but characteristic fragment resulting from α-cleavage between C-3″ and C-4″ at $m/e = 117$ (RI 6 percent) $[CH_3CH=OSi(CH_3)_3]^+$. We would expect this ion to become more intense in other cannabinoids that are not dominated by the aromatization reaction of cannabinols.

According to our expectations, no typical fragmentation patterns were observable for the 5″-TMSO-cannabinoids. The presence of the TMSO group in the 5″ position can be deduced from weak fragment ions that arise from loss of the side chain, e.g., M^+-144 or M^+-145, alone or in combination with other major fragmentations. The 5″-TMSO-cannabinoids could be confused with the 3″-TMSO-cannabinoids, but a comparison of the relative intensities of the molecular ion and the fragment M^+-144 shows the latter to be of low intensity in 5″-TMSO-cannabinoids and of high intensity in 3″-TMSO-cannabinoids. The other cases of hydroxylation can be excluded by the negative evidence of the absence of fragments M^+-57, 145^+, or 117^+.

Conclusions

The sensitivity of the described method allows identification of metabolites by PMR spectroscopy in amounts of 100 μg. Mass spectroscopy requires quantities in the microgram range. We consider it possible to identify even smaller amounts by mass fragmentography, e.g., focusing on the predicted fragment ions. The presence of further metabolically introduced functions in the molecule will not disturb PMR identification but may complicate the mass spectra considerably. To extend our method to polyfunctional cannabinoid derivatives, we will have to perform further research.

ACKNOWLEDGMENT

We are greatly indebted to Dr. T. Drakenberg, Institute of Technology, Lund, Sweden, for recording the 100 MHz PMR spectra.

REFERENCES

1. Archer, R. A., D. B. Boyd, P. V. Demarco, I. J. Tyminski, and N. L. Allinger (1970) Structural studies of cannabinoids. A theoretical and proton magnetic resonance analysis. *J. Am. Chem. Soc. 92:*5200.
2. Binder, M., S. Agurell, K. Leander, and J.-E. Lindgren (1974) Zur identifikation potentieller metabolite von cannabis-inhaltstoffen. *Helv. Chim. Acta 57:*1626.
3. Budzikiewicz, H., R. T. Alpin, D. A. Lightner, C. Djerassi, R. Mechoulam, and Y. Gaoni (1965) Massenspektroskopie und ihre anwendung auf strukturelle und stereochemische probleme—LXVIII. *Tetrahedron 21:*1881.
4. Claussen, U., H.-W. Fehlhaber, and F. Korte (1966) Massenspektrometrische bestimmung von haschisch-inhaltstoffen—II. *Tetrahedron 22:*3535.
5. Diekman, J., J. B. Thomson, and C. Djerassi (1967) Mass spectrometry in structural and stereochemical problems. *J. Org. Chem. 32:*3904.
6. Leander, K., S. Agurell, K. Pettersson, and M. Binder Unpublished results.
7. Maynard, D. E., O. Gurney, R. G. Pitcher, and R. W. Kierstaed (1971) (-)-Δ^8-Tetrahydrocannabinol: two novel *in vitro* metabolites. *Experientia 27:*1154.
8. Mechoulam, R. and Y. Gaoni (1965) A total synthesis of dl-Δ^1-tetrahydrocannabinol, the active constituent of hashish. *J. Amer. Chem. Soc. 87:*3273.
9. Nilsson, I. M., S. Agurell, J. L. G. Nilsson, A. Ohlsson, F. Sandberg, and M. Wahlqvist (1970) Δ^1-Tetrahydrocannabinol: structure of a major metabolite. *Science 168:*1228.
10. Nilsson, I. M., S. Agurell, J. L. G. Nilsson, M. Widman, and K. Leander (1973) Two cannabidiol metabolites formed by rat liver. *J. Pharm. Pharmacol. 25:*486.

11. Petrzilka, T., W. Haefliger, and C. Sikemeier (1969) Synthese von haschisch-inhaltstoffen. *Helv. Chim. Acta 52:*1102.
12. Petrzilka, T., W. Haefliger, C. Sikemeier, G. Ohloff, and A. Eschenmoser (1967) Synthese und chiralität des cannabidiols. *Helv. Chim. Acta 50:*719.
13. Vree, T. B., D. D. Breimer, C. A. M. van Ginneken, and J. M. van Rossum (1972) Identification in hashish of tetrahydrocannabinol, cannabidiol and cannabinol analogues with methyl sidechain. *J. Pharm. Pharmacol. 24:*7.
14. Vree, T. B., D. D. Breimer, C. A. M. van Ginneken, J. M. van Rossum, R. A. de Zeeuw, and A. H. Witte (1971) Identification of cannabivarins in hashish by a new method of combined gaschromatography-mass-spectrometry. *Clin. Chim. Acta 34:*365.
15. Wall, M. E., D. R. Brine, A. Brine, C. G. Pitt, R. I. Freudenthal, and H. D. Christensen (1970) Isolation, structure and biological activity of several metabolites of Δ^9-tetrahydrocannabinol. *J. Am. Chem. Soc. 92:*3466.
16. Widman, M., J. Dahmén, K. Leander, and K. Pettersson (1975) In vitro metabolism of cannabinol in rat and rabbit liver. Synthesis of 2″-, 3″- and 5″-hydroxy-cannabinol. *Acta Pharm. Suec.* (in press).
17. Widman, M., M. Nordqvist, C. T. Dollery, and R. H. Briant (1975) Metabolism of Δ^1-tetrahydrocannabinol by the isolated perfused dog lung. *J. Pharm. Pharmacol. 27:*842.

14

Pharmacokinetics of Δ^9-Tetrahydrocannabinol and Its Metabolites: Importance and Relationship in Developing Methods for Detecting Cannabis in Biologic Fluids

LOUIS LEMBERGER

Although methods have been available for detecting *Cannabis sativa* and its component cannabinoids for many years, these methods could detect cannabinoids only in plant materials, such as the leaves and seeds. The methods used to date include colorimetry, spectrofluorimetry, gas-liquid chromatography, and thin-layer chromatography (TLC) [14,15,16]. Colorimetric tests such as the Duquenois–Negm [5] or the Beam [3] require the presence of the cannabinoid structure, that is, a C^{21} compound resembling cannabinol. Unfortunately, due to their lack of sensitivity, these methods require large concentrations of material and thus cannot be used for detecting cannabinoids in biologic fluids.

Problems Associated with Detecting Cannabinoids in Body Fluids

Several of the major problems associated with developing rational approaches for the detection of cannabis in biologic fluids are based on factors discussed below.

Identification of psychopharmacologically active component

First, marihuana is a mixture of cannabinoids (over 20 identified to date) and other chemicals. Just as we have learned that morphine was the active constituent of opium and ethanol the active component of beer, wine, and whiskey, one could have surmised that some distinct chemical or chemicals would be responsible for the pharmacologic effects of cannabis. Indeed, in 1965 Mechoulam and Gaoni [12,13] isolated Δ^9-tetrahydrocannabinol (Δ^9-THC) and subsequently demonstrated that it was responsible for the psycho-

Marihuana: Chemistry, Biochemistry, and Cellular Effects, edited by Gabriel G. Nahas,

pharmacologic effects of cannabis. Shortly thereafter, Isbell [7] and Hollister *et al.* [6] confirmed this effect in man. Although the active constituent of cannabis is Δ^9-THC, several genetic variants of cannabis exist, and thus the concentration of Δ^9-THC may vary considerably from lot to lot of marihuana.

Many of the other components of marihuana are relatively inactive. Thus, based upon this marked variation in the quantity of the active constituent in cannabis (ranging from 0.1 percent Δ^9-THC content for Indiana or Kansas marihuana to up to 4 percent of Δ^9-THC for Jamaican or Vietnamese marihuana), one must devise detection methods that are capable of measuring only the active constituent or one of its major metabolic products.

Physicochemical properties of cannabinoids

Second, several of the problems encountered in detecting cannabinoids in body fluids are due to their physicochemical properties. Δ^9-THC is very lipid soluble and is easily distributed to tissue, as demonstrated by Agurell *et al.* [1] and by Klausner and Dingell [8]. This is in contrast to drugs such as alcohol which distribute in total body water. The general properties involved in the physiologic

Figure 14.1. Schematic representation of the processes associated with the physiologic disposition of drugs.

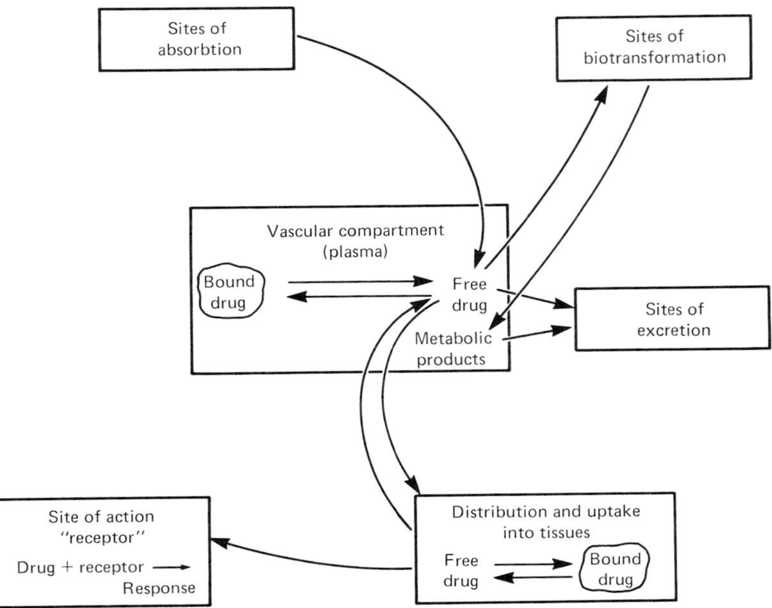

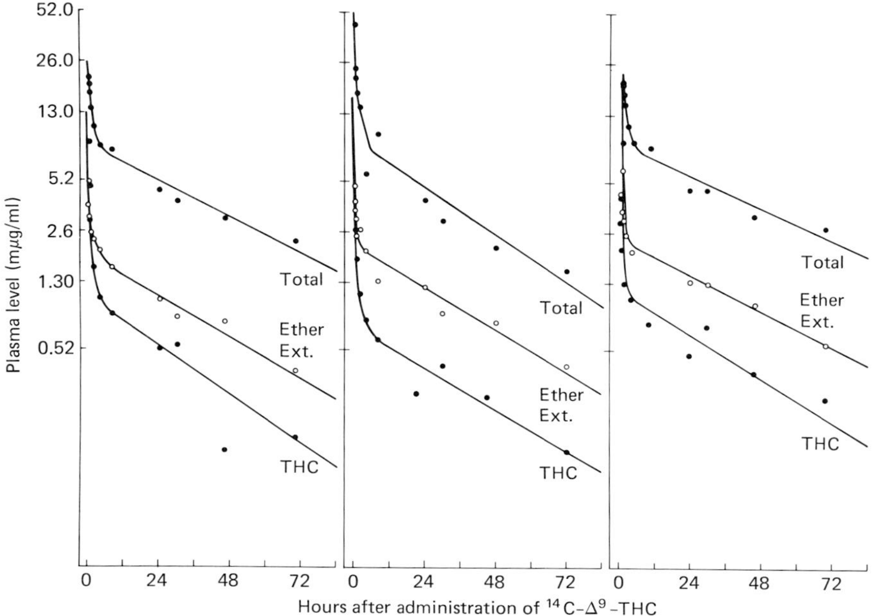

Figure 14.2. Plasma levels of Δ^{9}-THC, total radioactivity, and ether-extractable radioactivity after IV injection of ^{14}C-Δ^{9}-THC to chronic marihuana users.

disposition of drugs are illustrated in Figure 14.1. Thus, after its intravenous administration, Δ^{9}-THC is rapidly taken up from the central compartment and distributed to tissues where it is temporarily sequestered. This results in a marked drop in the plasma levels of ^{9}Δ-THC during a relatively short time [9]. This is illustrated in Figure 14.2. Similar effects are seen after the inhalation of Δ^{9}-THC [10] (Figure 14.3).

When Δ^{9}-THC is administered orally, the plasma concentration reaches a peak and then rapidly declines. The plasma levels of Δ^{9}-THC become quite low, relative to the levels of metabolites, probably secondary to a large first-pass phenomenon. As a result of its high tissue concentration and its inherent lipid solubility, Δ^{9}-THC exhibits a large apparent volume of distribution of about 500 liters (Table 14.1). However, when one estimates the apparent volume of distribution for total radioactivity, which is represented mainly by the metabolites of Δ^{9}-THC, it approaches that of the total body water compartment (about 50 liters), thus suggesting that the metabolites are more water soluble than the parent compound and are not sequestered in tissue to any great extent. The

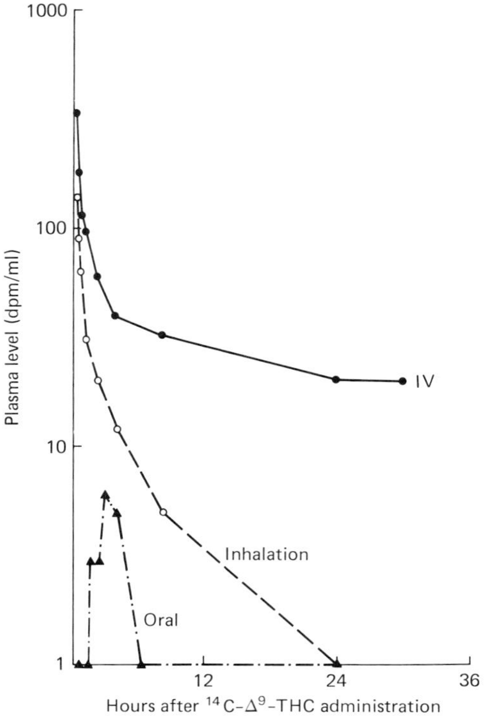

Figure 14.3. Plasma levels of unchanged ^{14}C-Δ^9-THC after oral or IV administration and inhalation of ^{14}C-Δ^9-THC. Each curve represents a typical subject.

combination of a considerable degree of uptake into tissues and the large volume of distribution, in effect, is responsible for the low plasma levels of Δ^9-THC and its metabolites, which make it difficult to develop a routine method for detecting cannabinoids in blood. Consequently, to determine the pharmacokinetics of these compounds, investigators have had to use radioactive compounds or develop sophisticated techniques such as gas chromatography–mass spectroscopy, the method developed by Agurell and his group [2]. Even though labeled Δ^9-THC has been shown to persist in plasma for as long as 72 hr, it is present in such low concentrations that even with the sensitive techniques of gas chromatography–mass spectroscopy, Δ^9-THC and its metabolites can be detected only for 4–6 hr after drug administration.

During the past 10 years, many investigators have tried to de-

Table 14.1 Apparent volumes of distribution of total radioactivity and Δ^9-THC[a]

Nonsmokers			Chronic smokers		
Subjects	*Total radioactivity (liters)*	*THC (liters)*	*Subjects*	*Total radioactivity (liters)*	*THC (liters)*
R. L.	34	497	W. D.	58	742
S. M.	60	516	F. B.	63	498
W. R.	50	439	C. R.	60	453
Mean	48 ± 7.5	484 ± 23.3		60 ± 1.5	564 ± 90

[a] Values represent mean ± standard error.

velop techniques for measuring Δ^9-THC and related cannabinoids in urine. Unfortunately, these approaches have been generally unsuccessful. The lack of success in these endeavors is now understandable and has a rational explanation. Before 1970, little was known of the pharmacokinetics of Δ^9-THC. However, once the active constituent of marihuana was identified, investigators could conduct studies to demonstrate the quantitative and qualitative nature of the metabolites of ^{9}Δ-THC and to determine to what extent they were excreted in urine. As a result of these pharmacokinetic studies using tritiated and ^{14}C-labeled Δ^9-THC, we now have a better understanding of the physiologic disposition of Δ^9-THC. Application of this basic knowledge has facilitated the development of better detection methods based on a more rational approach to the problem.

Excretion of Δ^9-THC and its metabolites

The third impediment to developing a method of detecting cannabinoids in body fluids is that the psychoactive constituent of marihuana is extensively metabolized, and virtually no Δ^9-THC is excreted in urine in its unchanged form. In addition, only a small percentage of the administered dose is excreted in urine as metabolites, the major portion being excreted in the feces.

Investigations with radiolabeled Δ^9-THC in man and animals revealed that this compound was excreted in urine and feces to variable degrees, depending on the species studied (Table 14.2). If, in humans, one examines the excretion of total radioactivity in urine and feces after the administration of Δ^9-THC by various routes, it is clear that only about 15–25 percent of the administered

Table 14.2 Excretion of radioactivity after administration of radiolabeled Δ^9-THC in several species

Species	*Route*	*Dose recovered (%)*	*Time period (days)*	*Radioactivity excreted (%)* In urine	*Radioactivity excreted (%)* In feces	*Reference*
Rat	IV	50	10	10	40	Agurell *et al.* (1969)
Rabbit	IV	60	3	45	15	Agurell *et al.* (1970)
Mouse	IP	90	5	10	80	Mantilla-Plata and Harbison (1971)
Man						
Nonuser	IV	67	7	22	45	Lemberger *et al.* (1971a)
Chronic user	IV	71	7	31	40	Lemberger *et al.* (1971a)

dose of radioactivity is excreted into the urine [10] (Table 14.3). The urinary excretion occurs predominantly within the first 12–24 hr. The remainder of the drug and its metabolites are excreted in the feces; thus, the detection of Δ^9-THC and its related cannabinoids in humans would be expected to be quite difficult to perform routinely since the routine collection of feces samples is difficult as well as lacking in aesthetic qualities.

Therefore, using the knowledge derived from metabolic studies with Δ^9-THC, one might attempt to develop a suitable method for its detection based on the urinary excretion of one of its metabolites. From animal studies and studies in man, it is known that Δ^9-THC is converted to a very polar acidic compound, the structure of which has been elucidated by Burstein and coworkers [4] (Figure 14.4). Because in man most of the urinary radioactivity is represented by this 11-carboxy compound [11], the measurement of unchanged Δ^9-THC in urine and the development of methods for detecting Δ^9-THC would be both foolish and fruitless since essentially no unchanged drug is excreted in urine. As an aside, in order to facilitate the development of a method for detecting cannabis usage, it would be advisable to subject the urine to extraction from an acidic pH in an attempt to concentrate the metabolites, thus ensuring a higher degree of accuracy with any potential method.

Table 14.3 Excretion of ^{14}C-Δ^9-THC and its metabolites after intravenous or oral administration and inhalation

Case number	Dose recovery (%)					
	Urine collection (hr)					
	0–24	24–48	48–72	0–72	Feces	Urine + feces
Intravenous administration:						
8	23.8	5.2	2.4	31.4	44.3	75.7
9	20.6	4.7	2.7	28.0	37.3	65.3
10	15.5	6.5	4.0	26.0	37.1	63.1
11	17.9	2.4	1.0	21.3	—	—
Oral administration:						
1	17.4	3.9	0.5	22.6	43.9	66.5
12	18.8	0.5	0.7	20.0	44.1	64.1
2	17.5	1.0	0.2	18.7	—	—
3	10.8	3.4	1.0	15.2	33.9	49.0
4	13.4	5.6	1.6	20.6	36.4	57.0
Inhalation:						
7[a]	7.6					
5[a]	5.7					
6[a]	15.4					

[a] Calculations based on assumption that 50% of administered dose was delivered to subject.

The effect of pH on the extraction of the urinary metabolites of Δ^9-THC is shown in Table 14.4.

From the preceding discussion of the pharmacokinetics relating to the urinary excretion pattern for Δ^9-THC metabolites, it becomes mandatory that urinary specimens be obtained shortly after drug administration, at times coinciding approximately with the duration of pharmacologic effects (about 2–3 hr). The major excretion

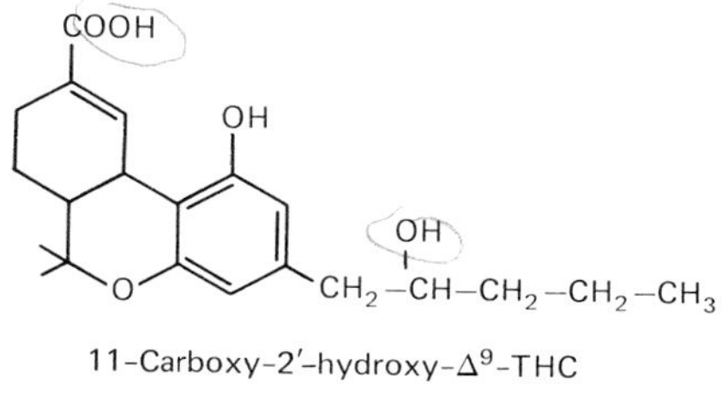

COOH, OH, O, OH, CH_2–CH–CH_2–CH_2–CH_3

11-Carboxy-2′-hydroxy-Δ^9-THC

Figure 14.4. Structure of an 11-carboxylic acid derivative of Δ^9-THC.

Table 14.4 Effect of pH on the extraction properties of radioactivity from urine and feces after the administration of ^{14}C-Δ^9-THC

	Radioactivity extracted (%)					
	Urine pH				*Feces pH*	
	6.5	*5.0*	*4.0*	*3.0*	*6.5*	*5.0*
Heptane	1	3	5	8	67	65
Ether	7	35	46	61	16	19
Ethyl acetate	13	16	21	18	5	4
Total extracted	21	54	71	87	88	88
Residual	79	46	29	13	12	12

of radioactivity in urine occurs during the first few hours after administration; after that time the urinary excretion of metabolites tapers off, making detection more difficult.

Methods

The pharmacokinetic data presented here for Δ^9-THC involved the use of methods such as radioactivity and/or gas chromatography–mass spectroscopy. Recent reports in the literature have suggested that methods using the principle of radioimmunoassay are available for detecting Δ^9-THC. However, at the present time, these methods lack specificity since several Δ^9-THC metabolites can also interact with the reagents. Furthermore, the methods are directed mainly toward detecting Δ^9-THC, a compound which is not present in sufficient quantities in any biologic fluid except plasma (and here it is present only in low concentrations). Thus, for a detection method based on radioimmunoassay to be of any value in positively identifying drug in the urine of cannabis smokers, it would have to be specific for the 11-carboxy metabolites. On the positive side, the radioimmunoassay does appear to have the most promise of the newer methods available or under consideration for detecting cannabinoids because it is simple to perform and can be used routinely.

Conclusion

In conclusion, I have stressed some of the pharmacokinetic reasons to explain the difficulties encountered in the past in developing methods for detecting Δ^9-THC (and, therefore, cannabis) in biologic fluids of humans. These difficulties include: (1) the low dose of drug necessary to produce its effects in man; (2) the low plasma levels present after the administration of this drug; (3) the drug's large apparent volume of distribution due to its high degree of tissue sequestration; (4) its predominant excretion via the feces, an excrement which is usually unaccessable for assay; and (5) the fact that an acidic metabolite rather than Δ^9-THC is present in urine, and its presence in high concentrations in urine occurs primarily during the first few hours after administration. Finally, and of utmost importance, is the fact that a marked variability in the chemical constituents from different genetic species of cannabis mandates that methods to be developed must possess specificity for Δ^9-THC and/or its *in vivo* metabolites.

REFERENCES

1. Agurell, S., I. M. Nilsson, A. Ohlsson, and F. Sandberg (1969) Elimination of tritium-labelled cannabinols in the rat with special reference to the development of tests for the identification of cannabis users. *Biochem. Pharmacol. 18:*1195.
2. Agurell, S., B. Gustafsson, B. Holmstedt, K. Leander, J-E. Lindgren, I. Nilsson, F. Sandberg, and M. Asberg (1973) Quantitation of Δ-^{9}-tetrahydrocannabinol in plasma from cannabis smokers. *J. Pharm. Pharmacol. 25:*554.
3. Beam, W. (1911) Fourth report of the Wellcome Tropical Research Laboratories, Vol. B. Khartoum: Gordon Memorial College, p. 25.
4. Burstein, S., J. Rosenfeld, and T. Wittstruck (1972) Isolation and characterization of two major urinary metabolites of Δ-1-tetrahydrocannabinol. *Science 176:*422.
5. Duquenois, P. and M. Mustapha (1938) Contribution á l'identification et au dosage du hachisch dans les zones sensorielles et les viscerés. *Ann. Med. Leg. 18:*485.
6. Hollister, L. E., R. K. Richards, and H. K. Gillespie (1968) Comparison of tetrahydrocannabinol and synhexyl in man. *Clin. Pharmacol. Ther. 9:*783.
7. Isbell, H. (1967) Effects of (-)Δ^9-trans-tetrahydrocannabinol in man. *Psychopharmacologia 11:*184.
8. Klausner, H. A. and J. V. Dingell (1971) The metabolism and excretion of Δ-9-tetrahydrocannabinol in the rat. *Life Sci. 10:*49.
9. Lemberger, L., N. R. Tamarkin, J. Axelrod, and I. J. Kopin (1971) Delta-9-tetrahydrocannabinol: metabolism and disposition in long-term marihuana smokers. *Science 173:*72.
10. Lemberger, L., J. L. Weiss, A. M. Watanabe, I. M. Galanter, R. J. Wyatt, and P. V. Cardon (1972) Delta-9-tetrahydrocannabinol. Temporal correlation of the psychologic effects and blood levels after various routes of administration. *N. Engl. J. Med. 286:*685.

11. Lemberger, L., R. Martz, B. Rodda, R. Forney, and H. Rowe (1973) Comparative pharmacology of Δ-9-tetrahydrocannabinol and its metabolite, 11-OH-Δ-9-tetrahydrocannabinol. *J. Clin. Invest. 52:*2411.
12. Mechoulam, R. and Y. Gaoni (1965) A total synthesis of dl-delta-1-tetrahydrocannabinol, the active constituent of hashish. *J. Am. Chem. Soc. 87:*3273.
13. Mechoulam, R. and Y. Gaoni (1967) The absolute configuration of delta-1-tetrahydrocannabinol, the major active constituent of hashish. *Tetrahedron 12:*1109.
14. Schou, J., A. Steenhoft, K. Worm, J. Morkholdt Andersen, and E. Nielsen (1971) A highly sensitive method for gas chromatographic measurement of tetrahydrocannabinol (THC) and cannabinol (CBN). *Acta Pharmacol. Toxicol. 30:*480.
15. Wall, M. E. (1971) The *in vitro* and *in vivo* metabolism of tetrahydrocannabinol (THC). *Ann. N.Y. Acad. Sci. 191:*23.
16. Willinsky, M. D. (1973) Analytical aspects of cannabis chemistry in marihuana. *Marihuana* (R. Mechoulam, ed.). New York: Academic Press, pp. 137–166.

15

Rate of Penetration of Δ^9-Tetrahydrocannabinol and 11-Hydroxy-Δ^9-Tetrahydrocannabinol to the Brain of Mice

MARIO PEREZ-REYES, JANE SIMMONS, DELORES BRINE, GARY L. KIMMEL, KENNETH H. DAVIS, AND MONROE E. WALL

During investigations designed to study the clinical pharmacology and metabolism of cannabinoids, tritium-labeled Δ^9-tetrahydrocannabinol (Δ^9-THC) and 11-OH-Δ^9-THC were intravenously infused to normal control volunteers.

Since it was found that the plasma concentrations of Δ^9-THC were significantly higher than those of 11-OH-Δ^9-THC during infusion, the question arose as to whether the 11-OH metabolite was passing more readily from the intravascular compartment to other tissues, particularly the brain. Consequently, mice were injected intravenously with radiolabeled Δ^9-THC or 11-OH-Δ^9-THC and sacrificed at different time intervals. Their brains were excised and chemically analyzed.

We wish to report in this communication the results of our human and animal studies.

Human Experiments

Twenty normal, paid, male volunteers, fully informed about the nature, risks, and benefits of the study and familiar with the effects of marihuana, participated in the experiment. Their average age was 24.7 ± 2.92 yr (range 20–31), and their average weight was 80.4 ± 8.52 kg (range 65–92). Fifteen were intravenously infused with ^{3}H-Δ^9-THC (33.4μCi/mg) and five with ^{3}H-11-OH-Δ^9-THC (38 μCi/mg). The drugs were suspended in 25 percent salt-free human serum albumin by the technique described elsewhere

Marihuana: Chemistry, Biochemistry, and Cellular Effects, edited by Gabriel G. Nahas,

Table 15.1 Percentage of the total radioactivity administered present in the total plasma volume at the specified times[a]

Time	*Δ⁹-THC*	*11-OH-Δ⁹-THC*	*p*
5′	23.09 ± 5.92	13.86 ± 2.92	0.01
10′	16.53 ± 3.70	10.29 ± 1.93	0.005
15′	13.48 ± 2.95	10.23 ± 1.31	0.05
20′	12.18 ± 1.97	9.36 ± 0.88	0.01
25′	10.49 ± 2.18	9.34 ± 1.03	N.S.
30′	8.79 ± 1.88	8.61 ± 0.73	N.S.

Figures represent the mean of the groups ± the standard deviation.

[4]. The rate of administration was 0.2 mg/min, and the drugs were infused to the maximal amount tolerated by each subject. The mean total dose of Δ^9-THC administered was 4.73 ± 1.23 mg (58.35 ± 15.81 μg/kg), and that of 11-OH-Δ^9-THC was 5.0 ± 1.28 mg (65.26 ± 18.42 μg/kg), which were statistically indistinguishable.

During the experiments, the heart rate was continuously recorded on a polygraph, and the subjective feelings of marihuanalike "high" were determined at frequent intervals in the manner previously described [2]. Blood samples were drawn at 5-min intervals during placebo and drug infusion and at longer intervals during the next 2 days. Total radioactivity present in duplicate aliquots of plasma was estimated by liquid scintillation spectrometry.

Table 15.1 summarizes the results obtained in human subjects. It can be seen that during the first 20 min of intravenous infusion of ^{3}H-Δ^9-THC, the total radioactive plasma levels were higher than those of ^{3}H-11-OH-Δ^9-THC. The difference between the means at these time periods was statistically significant. After 25 min at the end of the infusion, the plasma levels of the two cannabinoids became and remained similar throughout the 48 hr of observation.

These findings indicate that during intravenous infusion, Δ^9-THC remained in the intravascular compartment at significantly higher levels than its 11-hydroxylated metabolite. This result might be because 11-OH-Δ^9-THC penetrates to other tissues and possibly the brain more rapidly than Δ^9-THC. To investigate this possibility, we performed two experiments in mice by the techniques described below.

Animal Experiments

First experiment in mice

One hundred micrograms of either ^3H-Δ^9-THC (108 μCi/mg) or ^3H-11-OHΔ^9-THC (339 μCi/mg) were dissolved in a mixture of 5 percent Tween 80 and 5 percent ethanol and injected into the tail veins of two groups of 40 CF-1 male mice, 6 weeks old with an average weight of 25 gm. The injection volume was 0.2 ml. The mice were sacrificed by cervical fracture in groups of 10 at 30 sec and 2, 5, and 15 min. Their brains were quickly excised and divided at the midline. Half of each brain of the mice in the groups was pooled, homogenized, extracted with ether, and analyzed by thin-layer chromatography; the other half was individually oxidized in a Packard Tri-Carb Tissue Oxidizer to determine the total radioactivity present.

The results of the individual half-brain oxidations are shown in Table 15.2. The data indicate that four times more 11-OH-Δ^9-THC than Δ^9-THC penetrated to the brain ($p > 0.001$). Similar results were found in the chemical analysis of the pooled half brains. The maximal brain concentration of 11-OH-Δ^9-THC occurred 2 min after its intravenous injection and declined slightly at 15 min, whereas the brain concentration of Δ^9-THC steadily increased and reached its maximum at 5 min. However, the brain levels of cannabinoids did not decline appreciably during the short time elected for observation. For this reason, a second experiment was performed in which longer time intervals of sacrifice were selected.

Second experiment in mice

One hundred micrograms of either ^3H-Δ^9-THC (0.1 μCi/mg) or ^3H-11-OH-Δ^9-THC (0.1 μCi/mg) dissolved in a mixture of 5 percent Tween 80 and 5 percent ethanol were injected into the tail veins of two groups of 70 CF-1 male mice, 6 weeks old with an average weight of 29.2 gm (range 24.5–34.8 gm). The injection volume was 0.2 ml. The mice were sacrificed by cervical fracture in groups of 10 at 30 sec, at 5, 15, and 30 min and at 2, 4, and 24 hr. Their brains were quickly excised and divided at the midline. Half of each brain of the mice in the groups was pooled, homogenized, extracted with ether, and analyzed by thin-layer chromatography, and the other half was individually oxidized in a Packard Tri-Carb Tissue Oxidizer and counted in a liquid scintillation spectrometer to determine the total radioactivity present.

The results in Table 15.3 replicate those of the first experiment

Table 15.2 Percentage of the total dose of cannabinoids injected present in half of the brain at the specified time intervals

Individual half-brain oxidations

Time	*Δ⁹-THC*	*11-OH-Δ⁹-THC*	*p*
30″	0.16 ± 0.03	0.68 ± 0.22	>0.001
2′	0.17 ± 0.02	0.94 ± 0.07	>0.001
5′	0.22 ± 0.03	0.93 ± 0.07	>0.001
15′	0.24 ± 0.06	0.79 ± 0.14	>0.001

Chemical analysis of half-pooled brains

	30″	*2′*	*5′*	*15′*
Δ⁹-THC injected				
Δ⁹-THC	0.07	0.04	0.055	0.07
11-OH-Δ⁹-THC	0.007	0.009	0.013	0.020
8β-OH-Δ⁹-THC	0.009	0.009	0.011	0.015
Other metabolites[a]	0.025	0.035	0.045	0.055
Total	0.111	0.093	0.124	0.16
11-OH-Δ⁹-THC injected				
11-OH-Δ⁹-THC	0.24	0.345	0.295	0.27
Other metabolites[a]	0.175	0.215	0.24	0.215
Total	0.415	0.56	0.535	0.485

[a] Polar acids, polar neutral material, 11-COOH-Δ⁹-THC, and 8,11,diOH-Δ⁹-THC.

and again show that the 11-hydroxy metabolite penetrates to the brain in significantly larger amounts than its parent compound ($p > 0.001$). The data indicate that the maximal brain concentration of both compounds is reached at 30 sec after their intravenous injection, and that it does not appreciably decline until 30 min after injection. Unfortunately, we did not select intermediate times between 30 and 120 min. Therefore, it is not known at what precise moment the brain concentration of the drugs actually begins to decline.

The differences in the brain levels of Δ⁹-THC and its 11-hydroxylated metabolite are corroborated further in the results obtained by the chemical analysis of the pooled half brains. Thus, the lower portion of Table 15.3 shows that the levels of the pure cannabinoids and their total with their metabolites are very different at all intervals observed.

Table 15.3 Percentage of the total dose of cannabinoids injected present in half of the brain at the specified time intervals

Individual half-brain oxidations[a]

Time	*Δ⁹-THC*	*11-OH-Δ⁹-THC*	*p*
30″	0.1318 ± 0.0124	0.3197 ± 0.0564	>0.001
5′	0.1213 ± 0.0283	0.3342 ± 0.0445	>0.001
15′	0.1413 ± 0.0186	0.3120 ± 0.0360	>0.001
30′	0.1411 ± 0.0248	0.2903 ± 0.0650	>0.001
120′	0.0584 ± 0.0182	0.1365 ± 0.0231	>0.001
240′	0.0256 ± 0.0036	0.0731 ± 0.0094	>0.001
1440′	0.0130 ± 0.0024	0.0546 ± 0.0096	>0.001

Chemical analysis of half-pooled brains

	30″	*5″*	*15″*	*30′*	*120′*	*240′*	*1440′*
Δ⁹-THC injected							
Δ⁹-THC	0.0551	0.0552	0.0435	0.0802	0.0282	0.0107	0.0014
Metabolites[b]	0.0169	0.0365	0.0485	0.0604	0.0224	0.0116	0.0036
Total	0.0720	0.0917	0.0920	0.1406	0.0506	0.0223	0.0050
11-OH-Δ⁹-THC injected							
11-OH-Δ⁹-THC	0.2494	0.2158	0.1951	0.1926	0.0372	0.0061	0.0015
Metabolites[b]	0.0445	0.0866	0.1173	0.0794	0.0486	0.0213	0.0078
Total	0.2939	0.3024	0.3124	0.2720	0.0858	0.0274	0.0093

[a] Figures represent the means of the groups ± the standard deviation.

[b] Polar acids, polar neutral material, 11-COOH-Δ⁹-THC, and 8,11,diOH-Δ⁹-THC.

Commentary

The results of these experiments are surprising from a physicochemical point of view because Δ⁹-THC, which is less ionized and less polar, should have penetrated more readily to the brain than 11-OH-Δ⁹-THC. However, our results replicated by two different experiments indicate the contrary. Marked differences in protein binding between the two compounds might explain the results.

If our findings are correct, 11-OH-Δ⁹-THC, which penetrates to the brain more rapidly, should produce noticeable pharmacological effects faster than Δ⁹-THC. We have found this to be the case in both mice and man. Thus, behavioral effects in mice occurred 5 min after the injection of 11-OH-Δ^9-THC and 10 min after the injection of Δ^9-THC, whereas in 12 normal control volunteers rapidly injected intravenously with 400 μg of either compound in a double-blind, cross-over design, the average time of perception of drug effects was 5.9 $\pm$ 2.9 min for 11-OH-Δ^9-THC and 11.1 $\pm$ 3.9 for Δ^9-THC ($p > 0.005$).

The pharmacological potency of a drug is defined as its effectiveness per unit of weight administered. In man, equal doses of Δ^9-THC and 11-OH-Δ^9-THC produced similar effects; therefore, we concluded that the two drugs were equipotent. However, we have found in these experiments that 11-OH-Δ^9-THC leaves the intravascular compartment of humans more rapidly and penetrates to the brain of mice four times faster than Δ^9-THC. This difference in the rate of brain penetration explains the results of Christensen *et al.* [1], which showed that 11-OH-Δ^9-THC had twice the potency of Δ^9-THC when intravenously injected to mice.

We recognize that comparisons between human findings and those obtained in animals constitute a hazardous extrapolation. However, the results obtained in man and mice are so much in agreement that they suggest that the 11-hydroxylated metabolite penetrates to the brain of humans at a faster rate than its parent compound. It is not known whether the difference in brain penetration or plasma disappearance of the two compounds is because Δ^9-THC is more strongly bound to the plasma proteins, or 11-OH-Δ^9-THC diffuses more readily through the blood-brain barrier, or other factors.

Since the response to a drug is proportional to the concentration of the drug-receptor complex and Δ^9-THC produces maximal effects similar to those of 11-OH-Δ^9-THC at lower brain concentrations, Δ^9-THC must have a greater affinity for the specific receptor sites. Therefore, Δ^9-THC is more potent in eliciting marihuanalike effects than its 11-hydroxylated metabolite.

ACKNOWLEDGMENTS

These studies were conducted under Contract No. HSM-42-71-95 between the Center for Studies of Narcotic and Drug Abuse, NIMH, and the Research Triangle Institute. In addition, this investigation was supported by Public Health Service Research Grant No. RR-46 from the General Clinical Research Centers Branch of the Division of Research Resources.

REFERENCES

1. Christensen, H. D., R. I. Freudenthal, J. T. Gidley, R. Rosenfeld, G. Boegli, L. Testino, D. R. Brine, C. G. Pitt, and M. E. Wall (1971) Activity of Δ^8- and Δ^9-tetrahydrocannabinol and related compounds in the mouse. *Science 172:*165.
2. Perez-Reyes, M., M. C. Timmons, K. H. Davis, and M. E. Wall (1973) A comparison of the pharmacological activity in man of intravenously administered Δ^9-tetrahydrocannabinol, cannabinol and cannabidiol. *Experientia 29:*1368.
3. Perez-Reyes, M., M. C. Timmons, M. A. Lipton, H. D. Christensen, K. H. Davis, and M. E. Wall (1973) A comparison of the pharmacological activity of Δ^9-tetrahydrocannabinol and its monohydroxylated metabolites in man. *Experientia 29:*1009.
4. Perez-Reyes, M., M. C. Timmons, M. A. Lipton, K. H. Davis, and M. E. Wall (1972) Intravenous injection in man of Δ^9-tetrahydrocannabinol. *Science 177:*633.

16

Changes in the Metabolism of Δ^9-Tetrahydrocannabinol Caused by Other Cannabis Constituents

GUNNAR TOPP, JAN DALLMER, AND
JENS SCHOU

Although the psychological effects of cannabis preparations in general parallel their content of Δ^9-tetrahydrocannabinol (Δ^9-THC), several authors have claimed that the primary biotransformation product, 11-OH-Δ^9-THC, should be even more active than the parent compound. Lemberger *et al.* [3] reported results from investigations in man indicating that the rate of biotransformation is accelerated in chronic marihuana users compared to drug-naive individuals. They suggested that an increased formation rate of 11-OH-Δ^9-THC in chronic cannabis users should lead to a relatively higher brain concentration of the metabolite. As the metabolite is believed to have higher psychological activity than the parent compound, this could explain the "reversed tolerance" to cannabis, meaning the increased effect of the same dose in chronically exposed individuals.

In animal experiments, however, it has not been possible to provoke an increase in the rate of Δ^9-THC metabolism by pretreatment with cannabis products. There seems to be no change in drug hydroxylation capacity of liver microsomes from pretreated rats [2], and in swine we have been unable to stimulate Δ^9-THC metabolism by pretreatment with cannabis extract or Δ^9-THC [4].

This apparent discrepancy between the metabolic reactivity in man and conventional laboratory animals could be attributable to a species difference in microsomal reactivity to Δ^9-THC or to the fact that a component in cannabis other than Δ^9-THC caused the metabolic induction of microsomal enzymes in man, leading to accelerated THC metabolism. The purpose of our investigation was to determine whether fractions of cannabis other than Δ^9-THC could increase the metabolism of this compound. The only con-

Marihuana: Chemistry, Biochemistry, and Cellular Effects, edited by Gabriel G. Nahas,

stituent in cannabis which has been shown to affect the metabolism of Δ^9-THC is cannabinol, which is acting as an inhibitor of THC hydroxylation. This has been demonstrated in *in vitro* experiments and *in vivo* after a single dose of cannabinol was given to rats [1], but the effect of prolonged pretreatment has not been investigated. We intended to demonstrate the effects of acute and prolonged cannabidiol treatment on Δ^9-THC metabolism and the distribution of metabolites in the rat. Biotransformation seems to occur mainly in liver and lung, whereas the brain is unable to hydroxylate drugs and Δ^9-THC. Therefore, metabolites found in the brain had to gain access through the blood-brain barrier.

Figure 16.1. Schematic presentation of the 2 thin-layer chromatographic systems used for separating Δ^9-THC, 11-OH-Δ^9-THC, and 8,11-OH-Δ^9-THC. Dotted lines—separations between the zones a, b, c, and d, which are scraped off for liquid scintillation counting of radioactivity.

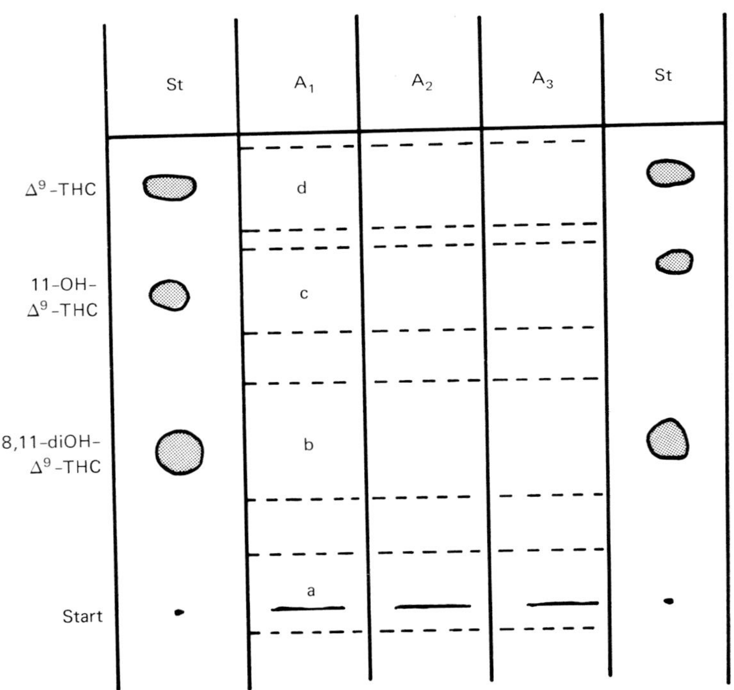

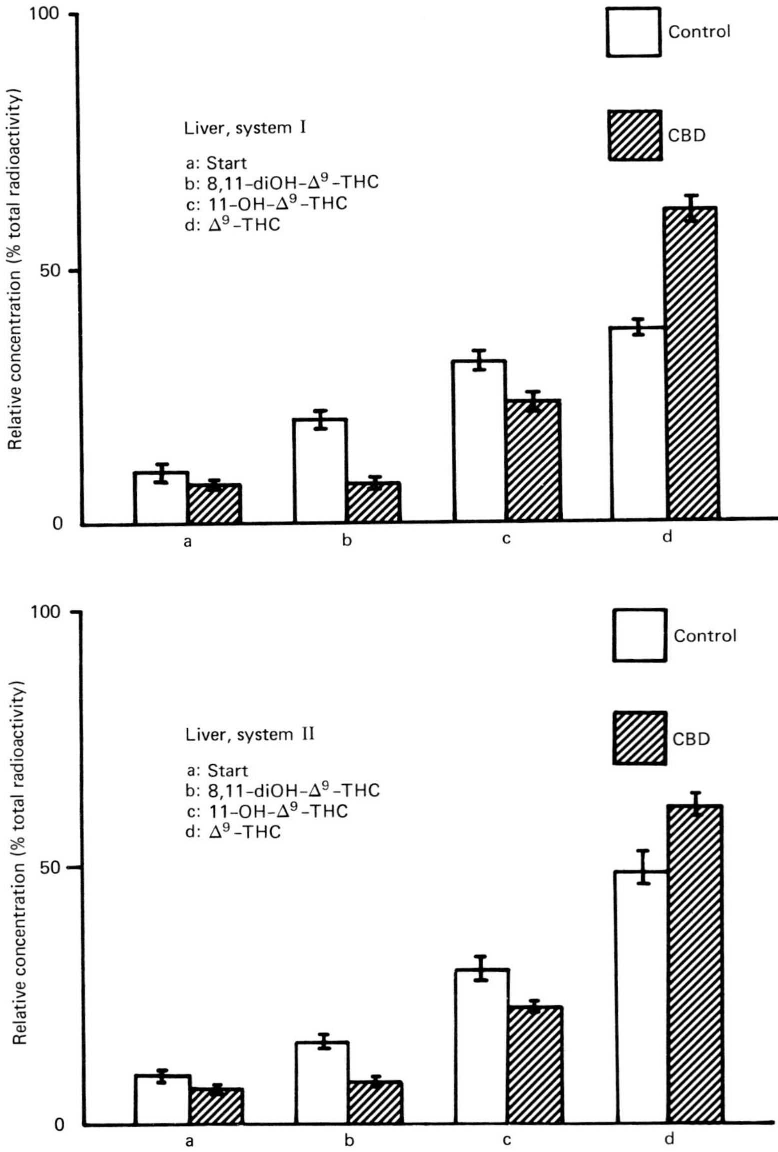

Figure 16.2. The relative concentrations (% of total radioactivity) of Δ^9-THC and the 11-OH and 8,11-OH metabolites in liver after pretreatment of rats with 50 mg/kg cannabidiol IP followed by ^{3}H-Δ^9-THC IV 40 min later and sacrifice after 30 min (*hatched bars*); control animals given vehicle for CBD (*open bars*). Nearly identical results were found with two different chromatographic systems (I and II).

Methods

The experiments were performed on male Wistar rats weighing approximately 150 gm. They were injected intraperitoneally with 50 mg/kg cannabidiol in 10 percent propylene glycol and 1 percent Tween 80 in saline (acute experiments), or every second day up to 20 days with 25 mg/kg daily. Forty minutes after the last injection of cold cannabidiol, 6 μCi/kg ^{3}H-Δ^9-THC in 10 percent Tween 80 in saline was injected into a tail vein, and after 30 min the animals were decapitated. Immediately the liver, lung, and brain were removed into ice-cold saline and homogenized with water (1:1).

One gram homogenate was extracted with 3 times 5 ml ethylacetate and subjected to thin-layer chromatography with labeled standards (Figure 16.1). The radioactivity of the fractions shown was determined by liquid scintillation counting, and the results for the liver, lung, and brain were expressed as percentage radioactivity

Figure 16.3. The relative concentrations (% of total radioactivity) of Δ^9-THC and the 11-OH and 8,11-OH metabolites in lung after pretreatment with 50 mg/kg cannabidiol IP followed by ^{3}H-Δ^9-THC IV 40 min later and sacrifice after 30 min (*hatched bars*); control animals given vehicle for CBD (*open bars*).

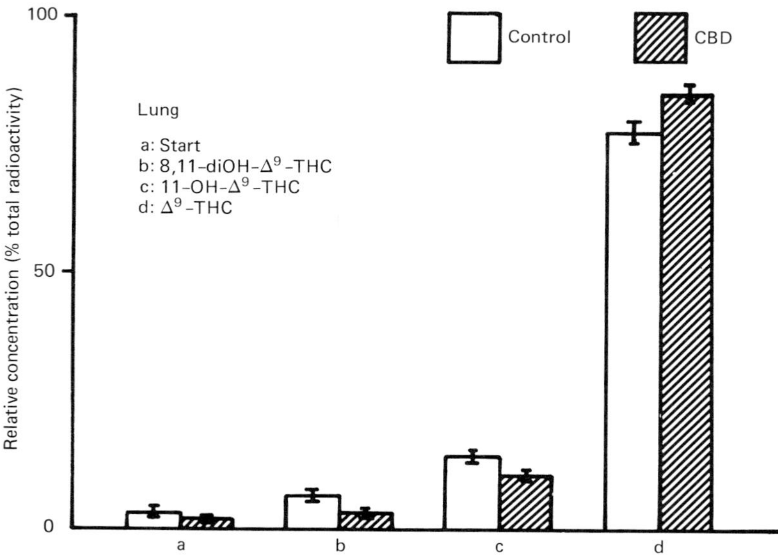

of total radioactivity of the samples found in the fractions of Δ^9-THC, and the 11-OH and 8,11-OH metabolites, respectively.

Results

The results are shown in Figures 16.2 to 16.4. Due to limitations of space, only results from the acute experiments are shown, but nearly identical results were found after prolonged pretreatment.

There is a marked inhibition of the biotransformation of Δ^9-THC into 11-OH and 8,11-OH-Δ^9-THC in cannabinol-pretreated animals compared to controls. The same pattern is found for all the organs investigated. That means that although the brain is not itself metabolizing THC, the metabolites penetrate into the brain and they are found in high concentrations in control animals, whereas the concentrations are significantly lower after cannabidiol pre-

Figure 16.4. The relative concentrations (% of total radioactivity) of Δ^9-THC and the 11-OH and 8,11-OH metabolites in brain after pretreatment with 50 mg/kg cannabidiol IP followed by ^{3}H-Δ^9-THC IV 40 min later and sacrifice after 30 min (*hatched bars*); control animals given vehicle for CBD (*open bars*).

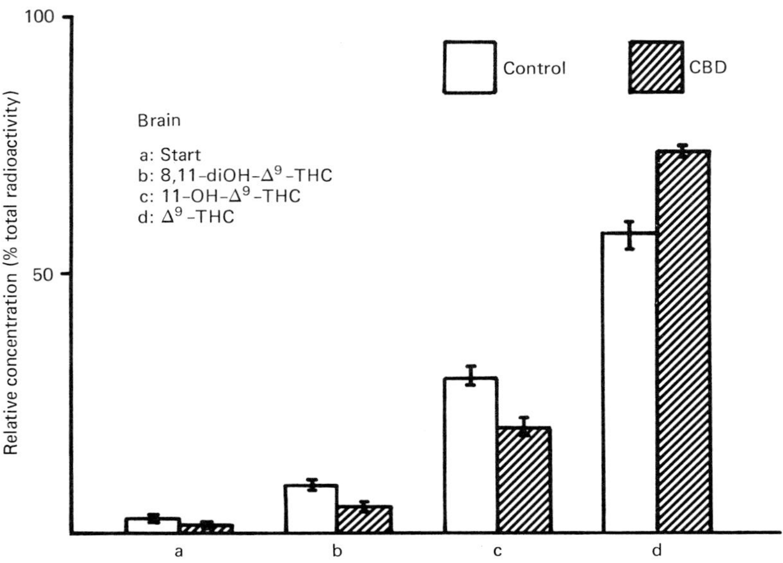

treatment. Exactly the same pattern was found after prolonged pretreatment with cannabidiol 25 mg/kg every second day for 20 days.

Our results seem to rule out the possibility of a metabolic induction of Δ^9-THC metabolism elicited by chronic cannabidiol stimulation in the rat. Other cannabis fractions do not influence the rate of Δ^9-THC hydroxylation by our method. This seems to rule out the possibility of an induction of THC metabolism by any cannabis components in the rat. Still, a species difference may explain the metabolic induction in man, but more likely the metabolic induction could be due to products formed from cannabis components by pyrolysis during smoking. Now that high amounts of pyrolytic products are being sampled and purified, this possibility should be investigated.

ACKNOWLEDGMENTS

Radiolabeled Δ^9-THC and the 11-OH and 8,11-OH metabolite were generously supplied by the National Institute of Drug Abuse, U.S.A., by courtesy of Monique C. Braude, Ph.D.

Supported by a grant from the Danish National Research Council (512–2541).

REFERENCES

1. Jones, G. and R. G. Pertwee (1972) A metabolic interaction in vivo between cannabidiol and Δ^1-tetrahydrocannabinol. *Br. J. Pharmacol. 45:*375.
2. Kupfer, D., E. Levin, and S. H. Burstein (1973) Studies on the effects of Δ^1-tetrahydrocannabinol (Δ^1-THC) and DDT on the hepatic microsomal metabolism of Δ^1-THC and other compounds in the rat. *Chem. Biol. Interact. 6:*59.
3. Lemberger, L., N. R. Tamarkin, J. Axelrod, and I. J. Kopin (1971) Delta-9-tetrahydrocannabinol: metabolism, and disposition in long-term marihuana smokers. *Science 173:*72.
4. Worm, K., J. M. Andersen, E. Nielsen, J. Schou, and A. Steentoft (1971) Studies on the metabolism and disposition of Δ^9-THC in Danish pigs before and after prolonged intravenous administration of Δ^9-THC. *Acta Pharm. Suec. 8:*690.

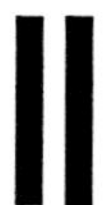

Marihuana: Biochemical and Cellular Effects

Effects on Isolated Cell Systems

17

The Influence of Marihuana on Eukaryote Cell Growth and Development

ARTHUR M. ZIMMERMAN AND
SELMA B. ZIMMERMAN

Introduction

Δ^9-Tetrahydrocannabinol (THC) is the major psychomimetically active compound in marihuana. An understanding of the action of THC on isolated cellular systems should prove helpful in evaluating the action of marihuana in animals and humans. Cell systems offer many advantages for studying the action of chemical agents. Among these is the ability to study specific cell parts and their related molecular mechanisms. Although considerable emphasis is placed on the importance of elucidating the action of marihuana on organismic and systemic levels, comprehension of the more overt psychological and physiological results of marihuana can come about only when there is sufficient information relating to its biochemical effects in the cell. The effect of THC on cell growth and cellular biosynthesis is currently being investigated in several laboratories around the world.

We chose the protozoan *Tetrahymena pyriformis* as a model cellular system for studying the action of THC. This eukaryote cell has been useful for investigating the action of several pharmacological agents [4,12,13], and a great deal of biochemical, physiological, and cytological information is available for this cell (cf. [1]). A unique characteristic of this model system is that it can be division synchronized, permitting one to obtain large numbers of cells before and after cell division. This makes it possible to investigate the cellular sensitivity to specific chemical agents at various stages throughout the cell cycle.

Marihuana: Chemistry, Biochemistry, and Cellular Effects, edited by Gabriel G. Nahas, © 1976 by Springer-Verlag New York Inc.

Action of THC on Tetrahymena

Influence of THC on log-growth cultures

The influence of THC on growth represents a sensitive parameter by which the action of this drug can be studied. The growth kinetics of log growth phase cultures of tetrahymena were determined in systematically varied concentrations of THC. The exponential growth rates were determined by establishing the increases in cell number over 24 hr. The cells were treated with THC (3.2–24 μM) and maintained in a growth medium. Samples were removed for analysis at specified times, and cell density was determined. At 16 hr the cell density was depressed 11 percent with 9.6 μM THC and 18 percent with 24 μM THC as compared with controls (Figure 17.1).

In general, 1–2 hr after immersion in THC at 3.2 or 9.6 μM, the cells, which are normally pyriform in shape, became ovoid, motility was sluggish, and the swimming pattern was irregular. These characteristics became more apparent as the concentration of THC was increased. Despite these changes, the cells continued to remain active throughout the log and stationary growth phases. There was a gradual reversal of the observed alterations of cell shape, motility, and swimming behavior, and after 8–12 hr the control cells were indistinguishable from the drug-treated cells.

Influence of THC on division-synchronized cells

As stated previously, one of the advantages of working with this model system is the ability to induce the cells to divide synchronously. Log growth phase tetrahymena that are induced to divide synchronously by thermal treatment proceed through a division maximum of 80–90 percent at approximately 70 min after the last thermal treatment. The synchronization procedure consisted of treating the cells with a series of eight 30-min heat shocks (34°C), each followed by a 30 min interval of growth at optimal temperature (28°C). The end of the last heat shock (designated EH) was the reference point for all experiments. The cells were transferred to inorganic media approximately 25 min before the last heat shock, at which time cell numbers could be adjusted for culture experiments. The experiments were divided into two phases. In one, the influence of THC throughout a division schedule was investigated, and in the other, the influence of a short pulse of THC on a division schedule was studied. In both these studies, division delay was related to the dose of THC, the duration

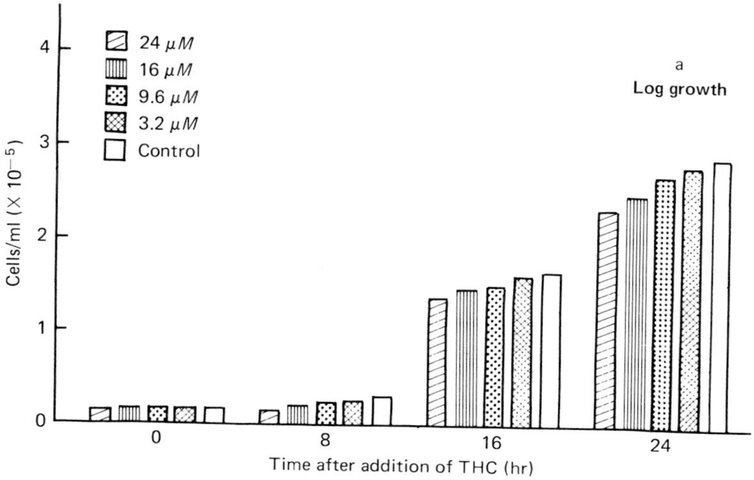

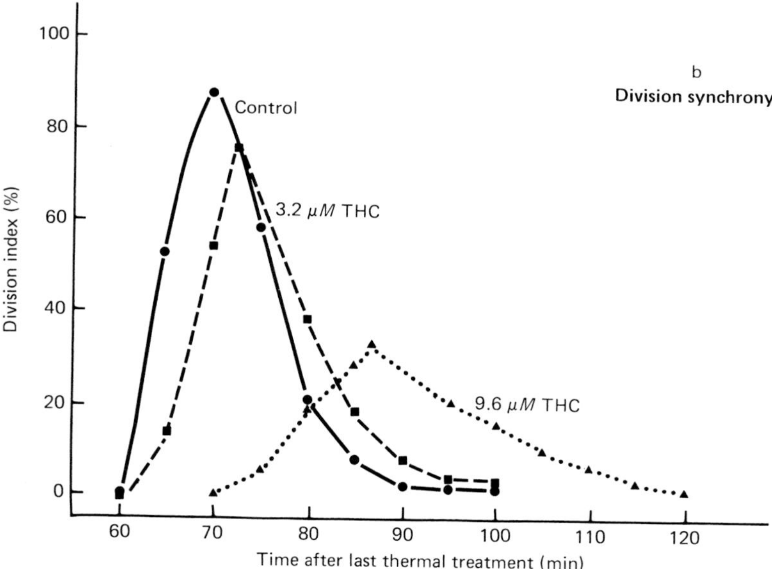

Figure 17.1. (a) The influence of THC on exponentially growing cultures of *Tetrahymena pyriformis*. THC was added to cells maintained in nutrient media. (b) Division-synchronized tetrahymena were exposed to THC immediately after the last thermal treatment. The cells were transferred to inorganic media before the final heat shock. The development of division maxima and the determination of division delays are illustrated.

(After Zimmerman and McClean [13].)

of exposure to THC, and the specific cellular stage at which THC treatment was initiated.

In the first series, the division-synchronized tetrahymena were continuously exposed to various concentrations of THC beginning immediately after the last thermal treatment. The effect of specific concentrations of THC on the first division profile is shown in Figure 17.1. In these studies, the division maxima for control cells was 88 percent at 70 min after the last thermal treatment. The cells incubated with 3.2 and 9.6 μM THC displayed a division maxima of 75 and 35 percent, respectively. The cells incubated with 3.2 μM THC were delayed 2.5 min and the cells treated with 9.6 μM THC were delayed 15 min as compared with control cells.

In the second series of experiments, it was demonstrated that the cells are differentially sensitive to THC throughout the division cycle. The synchronized cells were exposed to 9.6 and 3.2 μM THC for 10 min (treatment was initiated at 0, 10, 20, 30, 40, and 50 minutes EH). The cells were found to be most sensitive to THC approximately 30–40 min after the last thermal treatment (midway between the last heat shock and the first synchronous division). This period of greatest sensitivity was the same for both THC concentrations (Figure 17.2).

Figure 17.2. Effect of THC on the division schedule of tetrahymena. Hatched bars depict division delays induced in synchronized cells exposed to 9.6 μM and 32 μM THC. A 10-min drug exposure was initiated at various times after the last thermal treatment.

(After McClean [3].)

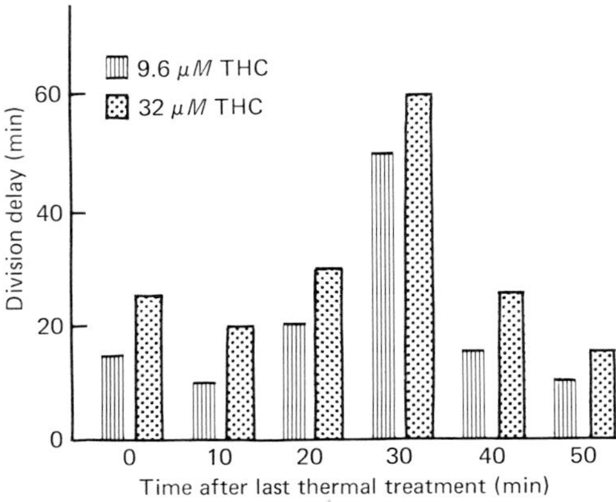

Influence of THC on macromolecular synthesis

The specific molecular mechanism through which THC acts has not been unequivocably established; however, there is sufficient information to suggest that macromolecular events are affected in cells treated with THC. The incorporation of radioactive precursors into the acid-insoluble fractions was used to study macromolecular synthesis. The uptake of ^{14}C-thymidine, ^{3}H-uridine, ^{14}C-phenylalanine, and ^{14}C-sodium acetate was monitored as an index of DNA, RNA, protein, and lipid synthesis, respectively. These radioactive precursors were added to the cells (which were suspended in an inorganic medium) immediately after the last thermal treatment, and incorporation into the acid-insoluble fraction was measured at specific stages throughout the first division schedule. Exposure to THC at 3.2 and 9.6 μM resulted in a reduced incorporation of labeled thymidine, uridine, and phenylalanine, although there was a slight stimulation of sodium acetate into the acid-insoluble fractions. The results of these studies are illustrated in Figure 17.3.

The effect of THC on the cellular precursor pool was also investigated since the incorporation of radioactive precursors into acid-insoluble fractions is related to the amount of radioactive material that enters into the cellular precursor pool. To investigate

Figure 17.3. Effects of THC on incorporation of radioactive thymidine, uridine, and phenylalanine into DNA, RNA, and protein. Division-synchronized tetrahymena were added to the appropriate radioactive precursor immediately after the last thermal treatment (0 EH). The incorporation of radioactivity into the TCA-insoluble material was determined at various times before synchronous division.

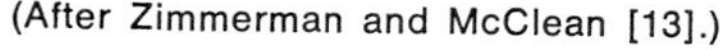
(After Zimmerman and McClean [13].)

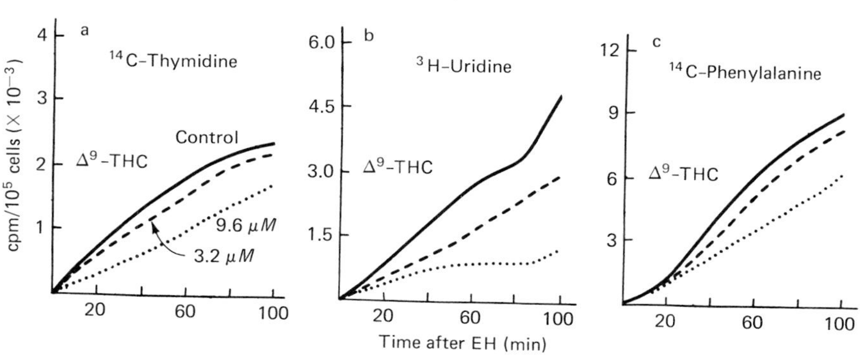

this problem, we pulsed division-synchronized tetrahymena (at 35 min EH) with ^{3}H-uridine for 10 min in the presence of 9.6 μM THC. The cells were then washed 3 times with 10 volumes of cold inorganic medium (fortified with nonlabeled uridine) and cold trichloracetic acid was added to the cells. The incorporation of radioactive uridine into the acid-insoluble and acid-soluble fractions was compared for control and drug-treated cells. The THC-treated cells showed a reduction of radioactivity in the acid-insoluble fraction (53–66 percent), which was comparable to the reduction of radioactivity in the acid-soluble fraction (50–64 percent).

The reduction of precursor incorporation into cellular macromolecules could reflect an inhibition of the uptake of exogenous precursor material. The studies with the precursor pool indicate that the THC interferes with the incorporation of precursors into the pool, and the observed reduction in the acid-insoluble fraction could be related to the availability of exogenous precursors in the cell pool. Thus, THC may alter the cell membrane, reducing the permeability of the precursors. This could result in a depression of metabolic synthesis.

Polyribosome studies

A reduction in the content of polyribosomes after treatment with narcotic agents has been reported for both prokaryotic and eukaryotic cells. In order to establish the effect of THC on total polyribosome content in tetrahymena, we incubated division-synchronized cells with 9.6 μM THC beginning 5 min after the last thermal treatment and ending just before division 60 min after EH. The cells were lysed and the polyribosomes were evaluated using sucrose density gradient analysis. Optical density profiles showed a reduction of polyribosomal material in the heavier cellular fractions after exposure to 9.6 μM THC. There was little difference between the amounts of recoverable monosomes in the THC and control preparations, but the amount of polysomes recovered was greatly reduced in the cellular fraction obtained from THC-treated cells.

Further studies were performed on the incorporation of precursor material by the newly synthesized polyribosomes. The association of messenger RNA with ribosomes and the synthesis of nascent proteins was investigated. Cells were labeled during the midterm of division I (35–50 min EH) with both radioactive uridine and 32 μM THC. During this period, the specific activities of ^{3}H-uridine- and ^{14}C-amino acid–labeled macromolecules were markedly reduced. The reduced specific activity of messenger RNA (^{3}H-uridine labeled) was evident throughout the polyribosomal region. The spe-

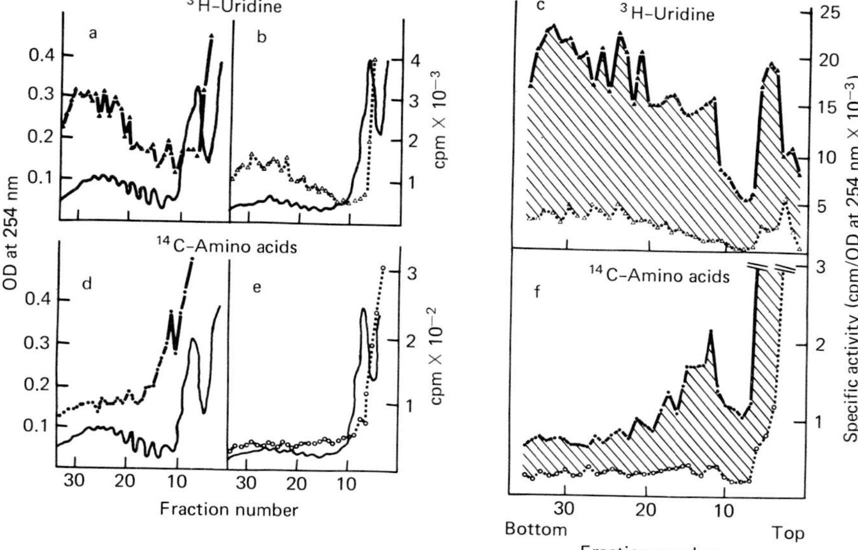

Figure 17.4. Sucrose density gradient sedimentation profiles of polyribosomes extracted from THC-treated tetrahymena. The hatched areas in (c) and (f) represent the reduction in specific activity of newly synthesized RNA and nascent proteins which result from THC treatment. THC (32 μM) was added to division-synchronized cells 35 min after EH; 5 min later, ^{3}H-uridine (20 μCi/ml) and ^{14}C-labeled amino acids (4 μCi/ml) were added to the culture. The cells were lysed at 50 min EH. The controls were not exposed to THC. The 12,000*g* supernatant was layered on a 15–30% sucrose density gradient and centrifuged for 2.5 hr at 27,000 rpm in an SW 27 rotor. Fractions of 1 ml were collected and analyzed spectrophotometrically, and the radioactivity was determined. (a) control (—); (▲) ^{3}H-uridine. (b) 32 μM THC (—); (△) ^{3}H-uridine. (c) Control (▲); 32 μM THC (△). (d) Control (—); (●) ^{14}C-amino acids. (e) 32 μM THC (—); (○) ^{14}C-amino acids. (f) control (●); 32 μM THC (○).
(After McClean [3].)

cific activity of the nascent polypeptides (^{14}C-amino acid) was also decreased by this short pulse of THC (Figure 17.4).

The RNA species affected by THC were evaluated further by analyzing phenol-extracted nucleic acids on a methylated albumin Kieselguhr column (MAK). The nucleic acids were monitored during the first synchronous division with a double labeling technique. The elution profiles showed that the drug caused a drastic reduction in the synthesis of all species of RNA; the ribosomal

RNA (5S, 17S, and 25S) as well as 4S RNA showed significant depressions. There were also depressions in the 35S ribosomal precursor RNA species (Q_1 RNA) and in the heterogeneous high molecular weight RNA species (Q_2 RNA and TD RNA) (Figure 17.5).

Studies with ^{14}C-THC

For further insight into the action of THC on tetrahymena, we incubated division-synchronized cells with labeled ^{14}C–THC beginning immediately after the last thermal treatment. The incorporation of radioactive material was monitored at 10 min intervals over a total duration of 60 min. Radioactivity was rapidly ac-

Figure 17.5. Characterization of nucleic acids in THC-treated cells. Methylated albumin Kieselguhr (MAK) column chromatographic profiles from division-synchronized cells treated with 32 μM THC and pulse labeled with ^{3}H-uridine (20 μCi/ml) from 35–50 min after the last thermal treatment. Simultaneously, control cells were pulse labeled with ^{14}C-uridine (2 μCi/ml). After the 15-min pulse, both groups were pooled and the cellular nucleic acids were extracted by the cold phenol–SDS procedure and separated on the MAK column. Fractions were analyzed for radioactivity and absorbance at 260 nm. ^{3}H and ^{14}C heights were adjusted from ratios obtained from identical experiments excluding the THC treatment.

(After McClean [3].)

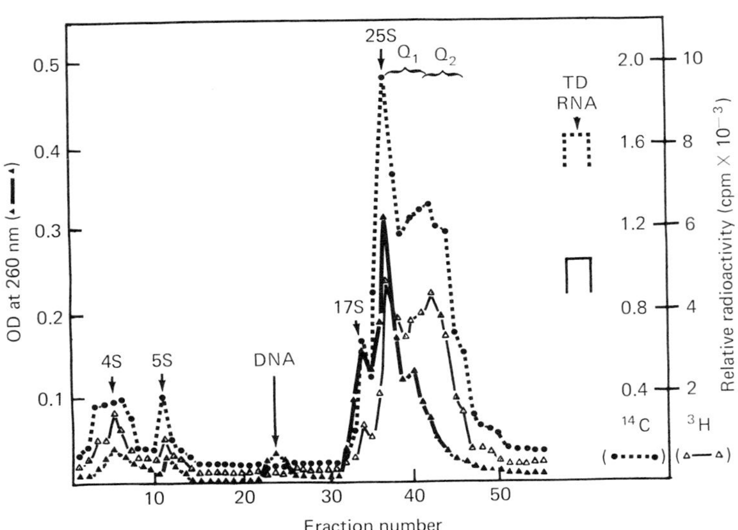

cumulated during the first 10 min of incubation; a plateau was reached which was maintained throughout the remainder of the study (50 min).

The accumulation of radioactive THC was also investigated by analysis of the cells at 30 and 60 min after initiation of THC using perchloric acid. Comparison of the acid-soluble and acid-insoluble fractions revealed that 60 percent of the total recoverable radioactivity was localized in the acid-insoluble fraction.

Discussion

In general, these studies show that THC depresses the exponential growth of tetrahymena, delays the onset of the first synchronous division in heat-synchronized cultures, and causes a reduction of DNA, RNA, and protein synthesis.

The reduction in macromolecular synthesis following exposure to THC was determined by: the incorporation of radioactively labeled precursors into the acid-insoluble fraction; the incorporation of labeled precursors into polyribosomes; and the incorporation of precursors into specific species of RNA. The depressed incorporation of specific radioactive precursors into DNA, RNA, and protein macromolecules might reflect the reduction of exogenous precursors found in the acid-soluble pool. A reduction of precursors in the cellular pool could influence the synthesis of macromolecules. Studies on the precursor pool suggest that the effects of THC on incorporation of precursors into macromolecules is related to the availability of exogenous precursors. The action of THC on cell membranes may be responsible for the reduction of macromolecular synthesis. In connection with this, Seeman [8] has proposed that anesthetics and tranquilizers disrupt molecules within the cell membrane resulting in subsequent metabolic alterations.

The binding of ^{14}C-labeled THC to tetrahymena was rapid and reached a plateau 10 min after exposure to THC. These studies also suggest that the cell surface is one of the main sites of THC accumulation. A major problem in evaluating the action of THC concerns its pronounced lipophilic character. Thus, many of the cellular changes induced by THC may result from its affinity for lipoprotein bonding sites on the cell membrane.

Disruption of the protein-synthesizing system is not unique to THC. Other drugs such as levallorphan [12] and levorphanol and morphine [4] have been shown to depress protein synthesis in tetrahymena. In different cellular systems such as *Escherichia coli*

[9] and HeLa cells [7], morphinans also affect RNA and protein synthesis.

The action of THC on DNA synthesis and cell replication has also been reported in other systems. THC caused a reduction in macromolecular synthesis in isolated rat brain slices [2] and in rat testis (see Chapter 20). Nahas and coworkers [5] demonstrated that THC alters the cellular-mediated immune responsiveness in rodents. They proposed that the reduction in cellular-mediated immunity might be related to an impairment of DNA synthesis [6]. Stenchever *et al.* [11] showed an increase in the incidence of chromosomal breakage in marihuana smokers, although no increase in chromosomal breakage was determined in *in vitro* studies with THC [10]. An important factor to consider in these studies is the possible synergistic action of THC with other drugs as well as with metabolites of cannabis.

ACKNOWLEDGMENTS

The research reported in this manuscript was conducted by Dr. Daniel K. McClean while a graduate student in the laboratory of A.M.Z.

Financial support from the National Research Council of Canada and the Non-Medical Use of Drug Directorate, Medical Research Council, is gratefully acknowledged.

REFERENCES

1. Hill, D. L. (1972) *The Biochemistry and Physiology of Tetrahymena.* New York: Academic Press.
2. Jakubovic, A. and P. L. McGeer (1972) Inhibition of rat brain protein and nucleic acid synthesis by cannabinoids *in vitro. Can. J. Biochem. 50:*654.
3. McClean, D. K. (1972) Cell division and macromolecular synthesis in *Tetrahymena pyriformis:* the action of tetrahydrocannabinol, morphine, levorphanol and levallorphan. Ph.D. Thesis, University of Toronto, Toronto.
4. McClean, D. K. and A. M. Zimmerman (1975) Response of division-synchronized protozoa to morphine and levorphanol. *Comp. Gen. Pharmac. 6:*171–179.
5. Nahas, G. G., D. Zagury, and I. W. Schwartz (1973) Evidence for the possible immunogenicity of Δ^9-tetrahydrocannabinol (THC) in rodents. *Nature 243:*407.
6. Nahas, G. G., N. Suciu-Foca, J. P. Armand, and A. Morishima (1974) Inhibition of cellular mediated immunity in marihuana smokers. *Science 183:*419.
7. Noteboom, W. D. and G. Mueller (1969) Inhibition of cell growth

and the synthesis of ribonucleic acid and protein in HeLa cells by morphinans and related compounds. *Mol. Pharmacol. 5:*38.

8. Seeman, P. (1972) The membrane actions of anesthetics and tranquilizers. *Pharmacol. Rev. 24:*583.
9. Simon, E. J. (1971) Single cells. *Narcotic Drugs: Biochemical Pharmacology* (D. H. Clouet, ed.). New York: Plenum Press, pp. 310–341.
10. Stenchever, M. A. and M. Allen (1972) The effect of delta-9-tetrahydrocannabinol on the chromosomes of human lymphocytes *in vitro. Am. J. Obstet. Gynecol. 114:*819.
11. Stenchever, M. A., T. J. Kunysz, and M. Allen (1974) Chromosome breakage in users of marihuana. *Am. J. Obstet. Gynecol. 118:*106.
12. Stephens, R. and A. M. Zimmerman (1973) Action of levallorphan: macromolecular synthesis and cell division. *Mol. Pharmacol. 9:*163.
13. Zimmerman, A. M. and D. K. McClean (1973) Action of narcotic and hallucinogenic agents on the cell cycle. *Drugs and the Cell Cycle.* (A. M. Zimmerman, G. M. Padilla, and I. L. Cameron, eds.). New York: Academic Press, pp. 67–94.

18

Inhibition of Proliferation and Differentiation of *Dictyostelium Discoideum* Amoebae by Tetrahydrocannabinol and Cannabinol

STANLEY BRAM AND PHILIPPE BRACHET

One of the major advantages of using the slime mold *Dictyostelium discoideum* for studying marihuana cytotoxicity is that cell proliferation and differentiation are separable in this mold. This unicellular amoeba proliferates in rich media. Under starvation conditions, proliferation is arrested and the cells undergo a differentiation cycle which begins with the aggregation of individual amoebae and results in the formation of a multicellular organism.

In our laboratory, we studied previously [1] the effects of a large number of hormones on the proliferation and aggregation of *D. discoideum.* For example, pregnenolone inhibits only cell multiplication, whereas progesterone and testosterone block both growth and differentiation. The actions of various compounds may be grouped into several categories: those with no effect, those which inhibit only growth, and those which affect both growth and differentiation. In this present study, Δ^9-tetrahydrocannabinol (Δ^9-THC) and cannabinol above a critical concentration were found to affect both growth and differentiation.

Methods

The Δ^9-THC and cannabinol we used were samples provided by NIDA. Multiplication was followed with a Coulter counter on aliquots from spinner cultures with an axenic strain AX2 [4]. Aggregation was examined in starvation media containing known amounts of drug. Media containing the cannabinoid were sonicated before adding cells in order to assure dispersal of the compounds. Cells were kept in Petri dishes at 22°C and monitored by direct light microscopy.

Marihuana: Chemistry, Biochemistry, and Cellular Effects, edited by Gabriel G. Nahas,

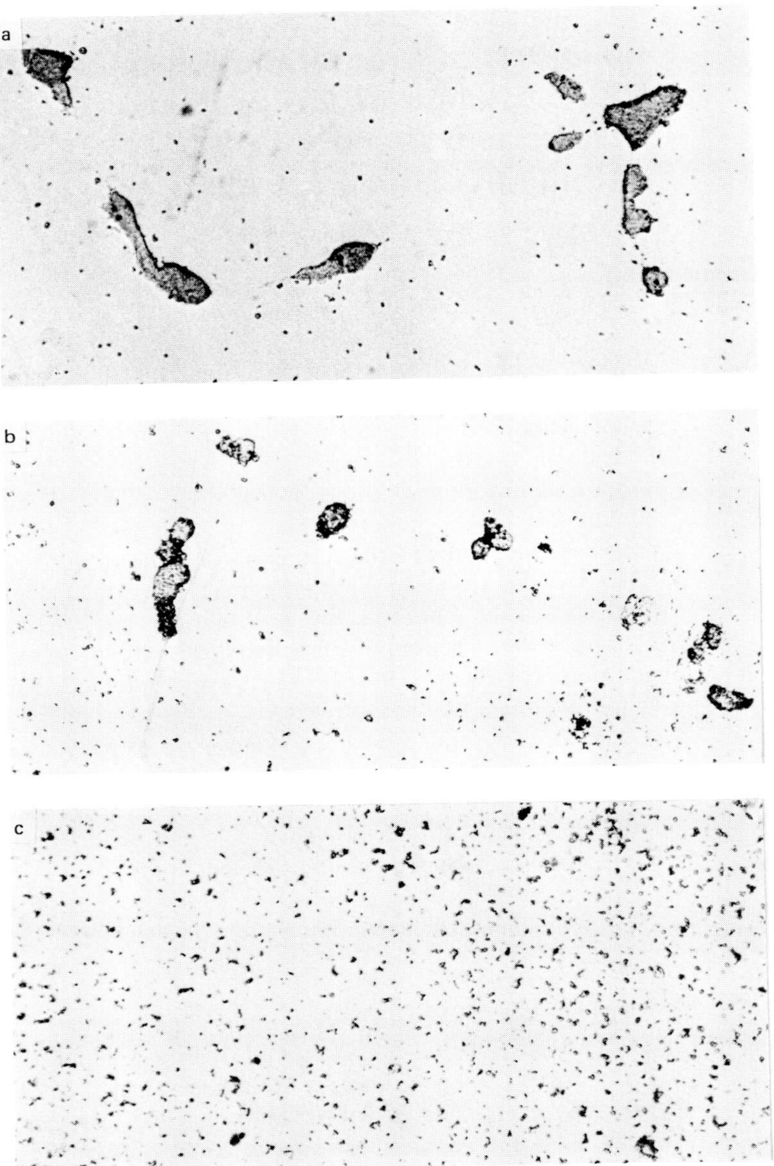

Figure 18.1. Direct photomicrographs (× 120) of *Dictyostelium discoideum* in a starvation medium after 24 hr in a Petri dish. (a) Control cells (no cannabinoid added): the majority of cells are found in large aggregates. (b) Amoebae incubated with 50 μM THC: like the control, most cells are aggregated. (c) Amoebae incubated in 50 μM cannabinol: few aggregates are seen; differentiation seems to have been blocked.

Results

Within a few minutes after being placed in media containing 60 μM THC, the cells became rounded. Their pseudopods retracted and the cells became immobilized. However, after a few hours, the cells generally recovered their normal form.

Figure 18.1a is a photomicrograph of a control population of *D. discoideum* after 24 hr in starvation media. Most cells are found in large aggregates. Smaller aggregates and individual cells were also observed. Essentially, all cells were fixed to the bottom of the Petri dish.

A photomicrograph of cells incubated for 24 hr with 60 μM THC is shown in Figure 18.1b. Most cells were found in aggregates that appeared slightly smaller than those of the control cell, but this may be due to the lag of the onset of aggregation caused by the rounding. As in the control group, individual cells were attached to the support.

When 50 μM of cannabinol was added, the cells became rounded but most never recovered their normal form. Figure 18.1c is a photomicrograph of cells after a 24-hr incubation in 50 μM can-

Figure 18.2. Growth of amoebae in the presence of various concentrations of cannabinol. Proliferation is significantly inhibited at concentrations above 60 μM.

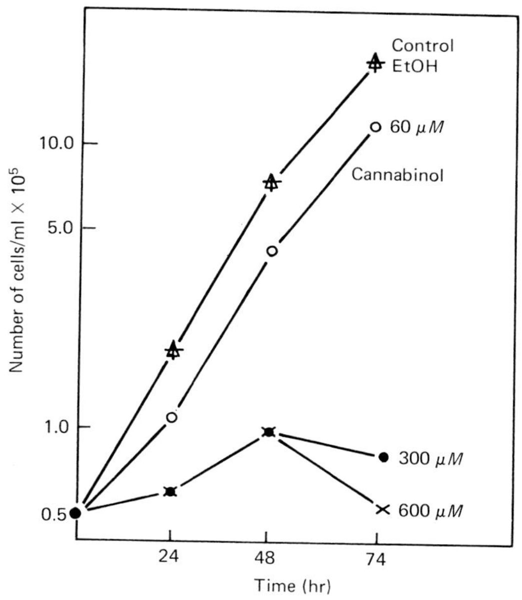

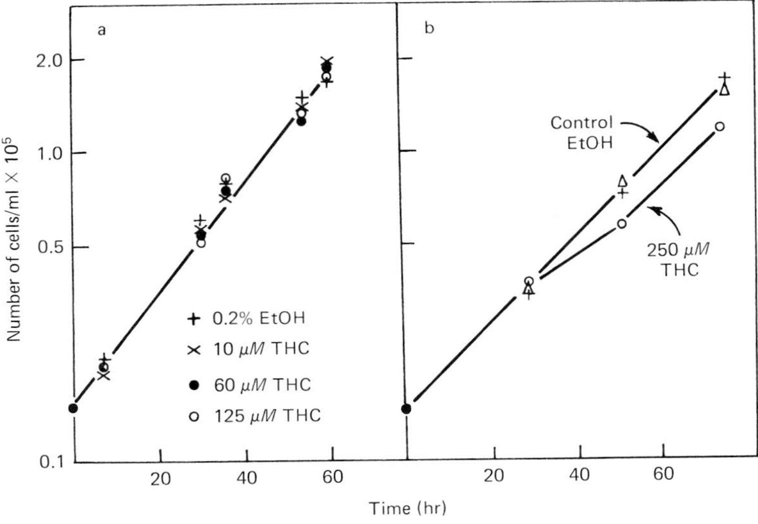

Figure 18.3. Growth of amoebae in the presence of THC. (a) An experiment with low concentrations; no appreciable effect is observed. (b) Another series at higher concentrations; proliferation begins to be inhibited at a concentration of about 200 *μM*.

nabinol. Few aggregates were seen, and those present were small. Most cells remained individual and not attached to the support. A dose-response curve for cannabinol on cells in a rapid multiplication medium is given in Figure 18.2. No effect on proliferation is observed below concentrations of about 50 *μM*.

Above this critical concentration, multiplication is inhibited progressively and at about 300 *μM* the cells begin to die.

Figure 18.3a,b shows the effect of THC on *D. discoideum* multiplication. We noticed no effect on proliferation until a concentration of about 200 *μM was* exceeded. A series of experiments at lower concentrations showed no difference from the controls.

Discussion

Cannabinol begins to inhibit *D. discoideum* proliferation and differentiation at concentrations of 30–50 *μM*, whereas THC is cytotoxic only at concentrations at least five times higher. An important facet of our studies is the comparison of cannabinol to steroid hormones. The inhibition of *D. discoideum* by cannabinol occurs at the same concentration as does inhibition by testosterone and estradiol [1]. Progesterone acts at a critical concentration of about 10 μM. Additional comparative studies may help us to determine the site of cytotoxic effects.

Nahas and coworkers have examined the influence of several cannabinoids on thymidine uptake in human leukocytes [3]. The critical concentrations for the onset of cytotoxic effects in human leukocytes are essentially the same as our values for *D. discoideum* with both THC and cannabinol. This similar effect of these two types of cells with different evolutionary patterns may be indicative of the mechanism of action. Furthermore, although Nahas and coworkers did not stress their relative fivefold difference in cytotoxicity between cannabinol and THC, we feel that the difference is significant.

REFERENCES

1. Brachet, P., and C. Klein (1975) Inhibition of growth and cellular aggregation of *Dictyostelium discoideum* by steroid compounds. *Exp. Cell. Res. 93:*159.
2. Isbell, H., G. Gorodetsky, D. Jasinski, U. Claussen, F. Spulak, and F. Korte (1967) Effects of (-)Δ^9-*trans*-tetrahydrocannabinol in man. *Psychopharmacologia 11:*184.
3. Nahas, G., B. Desoize, J. P. Armand, J. Hsu, and A. Morishima (1974) Inhibition in vitro de la transformation lymphocytaire par divers cannabinoides naturels. *C. R. Acad. Sci. (Paris) 279:*785.
4. Watts, D. J., and J. M. Ashworth (1970). Growth of myxamoebae of the cellular slime mould *Dictyostelium discoideum* in axenic culture. *Biochem. J. 119:*171.

19

Δ^9-Tetrahydrocannabinol: Effect on Macromolecular Synthesis in Human and Other Mammalian Cells

R. DEAN BLEVINS AND JAMES D. REGAN

Introduction

Some heavy marihuana smokers have a decreased blastogenesis of lymphocytes as measured following stimulation by mixed lymphocyte culture or phytohemagglutinin (PHA) [14]. This inhibition is believed to be due to interference with DNA synthesis by Δ^9-tetrahydrocannabinol (Δ^9-THC) and other cannabinoids. PHA-induced blastogenesis of human lymphocytes is completely inhibited with 20 μM Δ^9-THC [14]. Growth of mouse lung carcinoma cells *in vivo* is retarded significantly by Δ^9-THC [9]. The growth and DNA and RNA synthesis of Tetrahymena are inhibited by Δ^9-THC at 3–9 μM concentrations [24].

Evidence is accumulating for the action of THC at the membrane level, as shown by its effects on mitochondria [5,12], microsomes [6], and red blood cells [4,17]. Anesthetics can potentiate or alter many physiological responses. This may be particularly important with a lipophilic substance such as Δ^9-THC. Gill and Jones [8] suggested that the chemical structures of some cannabinoids and their metabolites resemble that of cholesterol. This analogy presents implications for the nature of the interaction between the cannabinoids and all membranes of and within the cell; and since some steroids have anesthetic and convulsant activities, investigators have considered the possibility of interactions between the cannabinoids and steroids in the body at various receptor and binding sites. Paton *et al.* [16] suggested that not only is the lipophilicity of THC at the center of its pharmacological action, but a limit to this action is set by its physiochemical properties in relation to those of the cell membrane.

This report shows that Δ^9-THC inhibits the incorporation of ^{3}H-thymidine, ^{3}H-uridine, and ^{14}C-leucine into DNA, RNA, and protein, respectively, in normal human fibroblasts, human neuroblastoma cells, and mouse neuroblastoma cells. This depression of macromolecular synthesis cannot be accounted for by reduced transport of radioactive precursors through the cell membrane, since the rate of transport of the precursors into the cell appeared to be essentially the same in the presence or absence of Δ^9-THC. Pool sizes of macromolecular precursors as measured radioisotopically (^{3}H-thymidine, ^{3}H-uridine, ^{14}C-leucine) appear to be reduced about 50 percent. This reduced pool size could account for the reduced macromolecular synthesis seen in the presence of Δ^9-THC. No inhibition of Δ^9-THC was observed in DNA repair synthesis after ultraviolet (UV) damage or τ-ray damage in human fibroblasts.

Materials and Methods

Cell culture and labeling of DNA, RNA, and protein

The cells used in these assays were: HSBP cells—normal human diploid fibroblasts cells derived from fetal foreskin [19], human neuroblastoma cells [15], and mouse neuroblastoma cells [11]. They were grown as monolayers—in 60×100 mm disposable Falcon Petri dishes with an original inoculum of 5×10^5 cells/ml —according to standard tissue culture procedures using Eagle's [7] minimal medium and 10 percent fetal calf serum. In this investigation, the concentrations of Δ^9-THC used were 3.2 times $10^{-7}M$ and $10^{-5}M$ (lethal to less than 5 percent of cells as determined at the end of the exposure). DNA, RNA, and protein syntheses were monitored by assaying the cell's incorporation of ^{3}H-thymidine, 5-^{3}H-uridine and ^{14}C-leucine into acid-insoluble material using slight modifications [13,18] of the filter disk method of Bollum [3]. Briefly, DNA synthesis was measured by incubating the cells in Eagle's medium with 10 percent calf serum and 1–5 μCi (1.9 Ci/mM) of ^{3}H-thymidine per milliliter for 18–24 hr with the culture medium containing (none in the untreated control) the desired concentrations of Δ^9-THC. The RNA synthesis was measured by incubating the cells in Eagle's medium with 10 percent calf serum and 1–5 μCi (5 Ci/mM) of 5-^{3}H-uridine per milliliter for 18–24 hr with the culture medium containing (none in the untreated control) the desired concentrations of Δ^9-THC. Protein synthesis was examined by incubating the cells in Eagle's medium with 10 percent calf serum and 3–5 μCi (130 μCi/mM) of ^{14}C-leucine per milliliter for 18–24 hr with the culture medium containing (none in the untreated control) the desired concentrations of Δ^9-THC. The labeled medium was removed, and the cells were thoroughly washed with phosphate-buffered solution (PBS). A nonradioactive medium was then placed on the cells for 4 hr to deplete the radioactive thymidine, uridine, or leucine pool. Total TCA-precipitable DNA, RNA, and protein were then collected. The acid-insoluble radioactivity of the precipitates was counted in a Packard Scintillation Counter.

Analysis of DNA repair

When the DNA of human cells is damaged by ionizing or UV radiation, a specific pattern of repair is initiated [23]. To measure DNA repair, we used an assay that involved the photolysis of bromodeoxyuridine (dBrUrd), an analog of deoxythymidine (dThd), incorporated into labeled parental DNA during repair [19,21]. Briefly, the DNA of the HSBP cells was labeled by incubation of the cells for 18 hr in a medium containing ^{3}H- or ^{14}C-deoxythymidine (1.9 Ci/mM) at 1–5 μCi/ml plus 10 percent fetal calf serum.

After the labeling period the radioactive medium was replaced with growth medium containing 10 percent fetal calf serum. After about 2 hr, hydroxyurea at 2 times 10^{-3} M and unlabeled dBrUrd at 10^{-4} M and Δ^9-THC (10^{-5} M) were added to the ^{3}H- and ^{14}C-labeled cultures. The radiation and/or Δ^9-THC (10^{-5} M) treatment was then delivered, and the cells were incubated for 20 hr. During this time, repair occurred with dBrUrd being inserted in place of the excised dThd residues. The labeled cells were then harvested, mixed together (2×10^5 cells/ml) in an ethylenediaminetetraacetate solution [22], and exposed to 313 nm light from a large quartz prism monochromator. This caused the dBrUrd-containing regions to become sensitive to alkali. Rejoining of DNA single-strand breaks induced by the γ-irradiation was studied by sedimentation of the cellular DNA in alkaline sucrose [2]. Briefly, 10,000 cells were lysed on top of, and their DNA was spun through (sedimented), an alkaline sucrose gradient (5–20 percent sucrose 2 M NaCl) at 30,000 rpm for 180 min in 4-ml tubes on an SW56 rotor of a Beckman model L centrifuge. Drops were collected from a hole punched in the bottom of each DNA sediment tube onto strips of filter paper, and the acid-insoluble ^{3}H or ^{14}C counts were measured in a toluene-based scintillation fluid in a Packard Scintillation Counter. The distributions of radioactivity were converted to weight-average molecular weights by a computer program based on the distances sedimented by phage DNAs of known molecular weights [19,21]:

T4 DNA, 55×10^6; λ DNA, 15×10^6; φχ174 DNA, 1.7×10^6. This assay is rapid and sensitive (one repair event in 10^8 daltons of DNA can be detected).

Ionizing radiation was delivered from a ^{60}Co source at about 3,500 R/min. The repair period for ionizing radiation was 90 min. UV radiation was delivered from a germicidal lamp at a fluence rate of ~ 7.4 ergs/mm²/sec. The repair period for UV radiation was 20 hr.

Uptake of radioactive precursors of RNA, DNA, and protein in the total intracellular pool

Rate of uptake of radioactive precursors was determined by exposing the cells that had been previously planted in Petri dishes at 5×10^5 per dish and incubated for 18 hr for 2 hr to 1×10^{-5} *M* Δ^9-THC. The medium containing the Δ^9-THC was then removed and replaced with phosphate-buffered saline (PBS), which contained the appropriate labeled precursor for DNA, RNA, or protein. Uptake of the radioactive precursor was monitored from zero to 60 min at intervals of 5 min. All of the above was done at 37°C. At the end of each time interval, the PBS was immediately removed from the cells and the cells were cold washed well and then lysed by exposing them to distilled water for a minimum of 30 min at room temperature. A Packard Tri-Carb Scintillation Counter was used to determine the disintegrations/min.

Results and Discussion

Table 19.1 shows the results of two concentrations of Δ^9-THC (both dosages were established to be lethal to less than 5 percent of the cells) on macromolecular synthesis of DNA, RNA, and protein, as measured by incorporation of radioactive precursors into acid-insoluble cell fractions, in normal human diploid fibroblasts, human neuroblastoma cells, and mouse neuroblastoma cells. At 3.2×10^{-7} *M* Δ^9-THC, the effect on nucleic acid synthesis was minimal, of the order of 11–17 percent inhibition in the three cell types used. There was no effect on protein synthesis at this concentration. At 10^{-5} *M* Δ^9-THC, there was 40–50 percent inhibition of nucleic acid synthesis and 30–40 percent inhibition of protein synthesis. The plasma concentration of Δ^9-THC in chronic users after smoking a marihuana cigarette containing 18.9 mg of Δ^9-THC is 250 ng/ml (7.95×10^{-7} *M*) [9]. Because of the manner in which successive dosages of Δ^9-THC lead to accumulation, consid-

Table 19.1 Effect of Δ⁹-THC on incorporation of radioactive precursors of DNA, RNA, and protein into acid-insoluble cell fractions in mammalian cells over an 18–24-hr period[a,b]

	Δ⁹-THC at 3.2 × 10⁻⁷ M			*Δ⁹-THC at 1 × 10⁻⁵ M*		
Cell type	*³H-thymidine*	*³H-uridine*	*¹⁴C-leucine*	*³H-thymidine*	*³H-uridine*	*¹⁴C-leucine*
Human diploid fibroblast	82.9	88.6	96.8	49.3	54.9	60.3
Human neuroblastoma	83.3	87.9	104.4	41.7	62.9	70.0
Mouse neuroblastoma	84.3	88.0	101.9	48.6	60.8	67.8

[a] Averages of three separate triplicate determinations. Variation among triplicates was always within ± 5 percent.

[b] Data show percent of controls.

eration of the effects of Δ⁹-THC concentrated in body tissues (and thus its effects on macromolecular synthesis and physiological action) is necessary.

As indicated above, although Δ⁹-THC inhibited (or greatly reduced) semiconservative DNA synthesis, tests for inhibition of DNA repair synthesis after UV or ionizing radiation were negative (Figure 19.1).

Figure 19.2 shows that when Δ⁹-THC at 10^{-5} *M* was in contact with the cells for 30 min, 1 hr, or 2 hr, there was no downward shift in the sedimentation constant of the DNA, and thus no induced lesions in the cell's DNA. Therefore, the DNA of the cells receiving Δ⁹-THC sedimented to positions corresponding to weight-average molecular weights of the DNA from cells receiving no treatment (control).

Studies of inhibitors of membrane transport [1,24] suggested that the nonspecificity of the inhibition of macromolecular synthesis by Δ⁹-THC may interfere with uptake of radioactive precursors. Thus, as discussed above, we examined the effect of Δ⁹-THC at 10^{-5} *M* on radioactive precursor uptake. Since no significant differences in the results were observed for the different cell types used in this study, Figures 19.3 (³H-thymidine), 19.4 (³H-uridine), and 19.5 (¹⁴C-leucine) are representative for all cell types observed. The rate of transport of the radioactive precursors (³H-thymidine, ³H-uridine, and ¹⁴C-leucine) into the cells is very rapid initially, continues in a

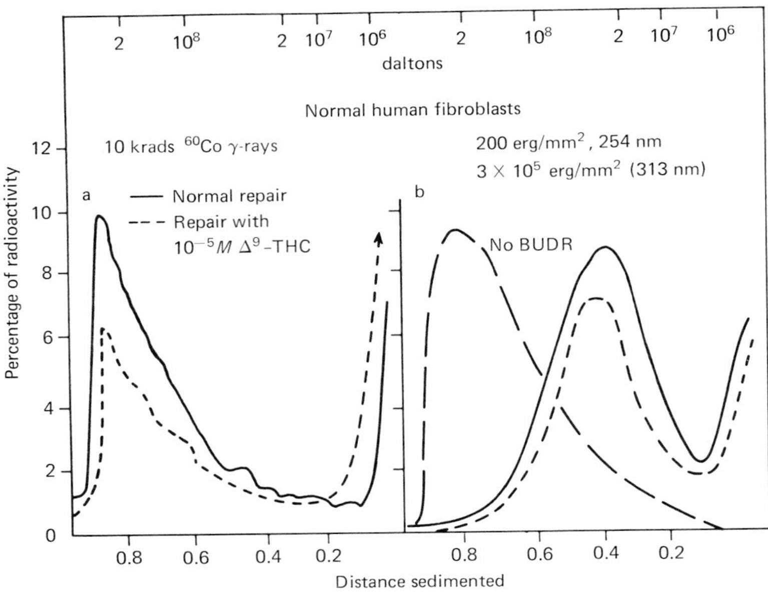

Figure 19.1. (a) Alkaline sucrose gradients of DNA from normal HSBP cells irradiated with 10 krad ^{60}Co γ-rays and then incubated for 90 min in dBrUrd and 10^{-5} *M* Δ^9-THC. A dosage of 313 nm radiation was 6×10^5 ergs/mm² before sedimentation in alkaline sucrose. (b) Alkaline sucrose gradients of DNA from normal HSBP cells irradiated with 200 ergs/mm², 254 nm UV radiation and then incubated for 20 hr in dBrUrd and 10^{-5} *M* Δ^9-THC. The dosage of 313 nm radiation was 3×10^5 ergs/mm² before sedimentation in alkaline sucrose. Each point of the curve represents the average of at least 6 determinations.

linear fashion, and then reaches a stable state. These experiments show that the depression of macromolecular synthesis cannot be accounted for by reduced transport of radioactive precursors into the cell since the rate of inward transport of these precursors is essentially the same in the presence or absence of Δ^9-THC in the three cell types used. A decreased pool size of macromolecular precursors as measured radioisotopically (^{3}H-thymidine for DNA, ^{3}H-uridine for RNA, and ^{14}C-leucine for protein) of about 50 percent was seen. Since Δ^9-THC inhibits the rate of incorporation of ^{3}H-thymidine into DNA, ^{3}H-uridine into RNA, and ^{14}C-leucine into protein, the decreased intracellular pool size of the precursors (all of which reach a steady state that is about 50 percent below that of the untreated cells) could contribute greatly to the reduced macromolecular synthesis of DNA, RNA, and protein seen in the pres-

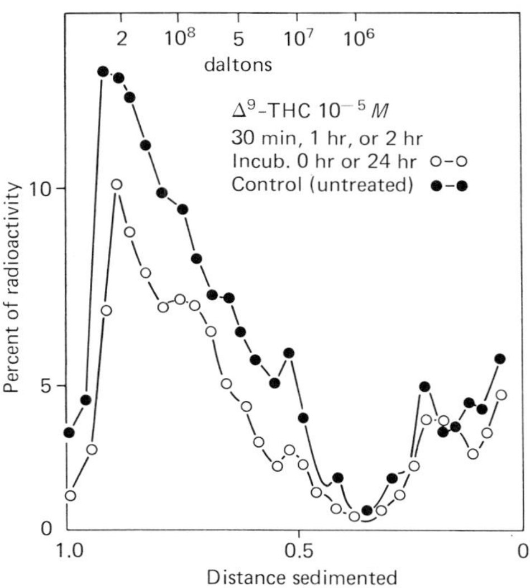

Figure 19.2. Type of effect observed after treatment with 10^{-5} *M* Δ^9-THC for 30 min, 1 hr, or 2 hr on the sedimentation profile of DNA from normal HSBP cells, human neuroblastoma, or mouse neuroblastoma cells in alkali both immediately after treatment and after 24 hr of post-treatment incubation. Each point of the curve represents the average of at least 6 determinations.

ence of Δ^9-THC. We do not know what causes this reduced stabilization of pool size. It is conceivable that the Δ^9-THC may, through solubilization in the lipid moiety of the cell membrane, cause the membrane to be "leaky." The cell may thus be unable to retain macromolecular precursor pools the same size as untreated cells.

Figure 19.3. Effect of 10^{-5} *M* Δ^9-THC on the total intracellular uptake of ^{3}H-thymidine (includes both the intracellular free ^{3}H-thymidine and the ^{3}H-thymidine incorporated into DNA) as a function of incubation time by normal HSBP cells. After the times indicated, the cells were cold washed well and lysed, and the thymidine radioactivity was then monitored. The medium (phosphate-buffered saline at 37°C) initially contained 1–5 μCi/ml of ^{3}H-thymidine. The ^{3}H-thymidine not found intracellularly was accounted for in the medium and in the discarded washings. Each point on the curve represents the average of at least 6 determinations.

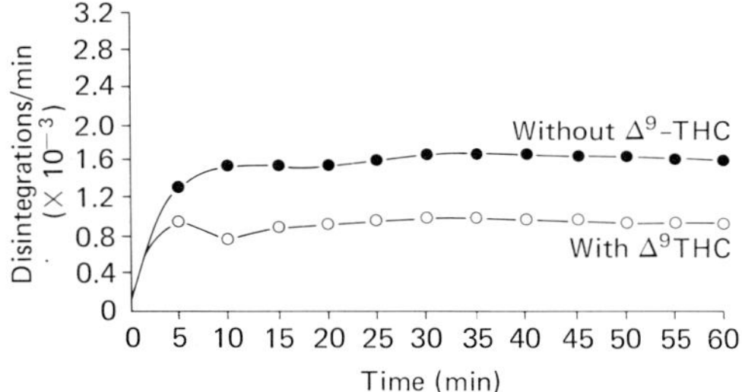

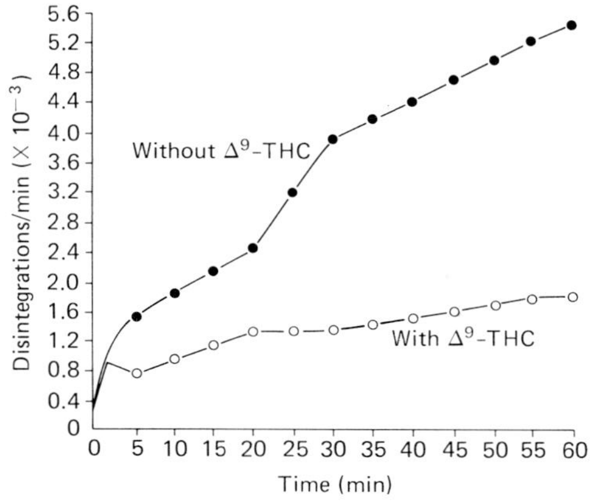

Figure 19.4. Effect of 10^{-5} *M* Δ^9-THC on the total intracellular uptake of ^{3}H-uridine (includes both the intracellular free ^{3}H-uridine and the ^{3}H-uridine incorporated into RNA) as a function of incubation time by normal HSBP cells. Procedure same as that described in Figure 9.3.

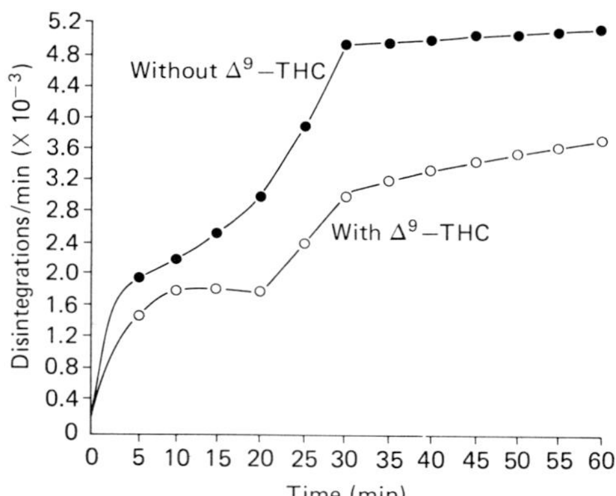

Figure 19.5. Effect of 10^{-5} *M* Δ^9-THC on the total intracellular uptake of ^{14}C-leucine (includes both the intracellular free ^{14}C-leucine and the ^{14}C-leucine incorporated into protein) as a function of incubation time by normal HSBP cells. Procedure same as that described in Figure 9.3.

REFERENCES

1. Adamson, L. F., A. C. Herington, and J. Borstein (1972) Evidence for the selection by the membrane transport system of intracellular and extracellular amino acids for protein synthesis. *Biochem. Biophys. Acta 282:*352.
2. Agurell, J. R. (1973) Quantitation of Δ^1-tetrahydrocannabinol in plasma from cannabis smokers. *J. Pharm. Pharmacol. 25*(7):554.
3. Bollum, F. J. (1959) Thermal conversion of non priming deoxyribonucleic acid to primer. *J. Biol. Chem. 234:*2733.

4. Chari-Bitron, A. (1971) Stabilization of rat erythrocyte membrane by Δ^1-tetrahydrocannabinol. *Life Sci. 10:*1273.
5. Chari-Bitron, A. and T. Bino (1971) Effect of Δ^1 (Δ^8)-tetrahydrocannabinol on ATPase activity of rat liver mitochondria. *Biochem. Pharmacol. 20:*473.
6. Cohen, G. M., D. W. Peterson, and G. J. Mannering (1971) Interactions of Δ^9-tetrahydrocannabinol with the hepatic microsomal drug metabolizing system. *Life Sci. 10:*1207.
7. Eagle, H. (1959) Amino acid metabolism in mammalian cell cultures. *Science 130:*432.
8. Gill, E. W. and G. Jones (1972) Brain levels of Δ^1-tetrahydrocannabinol and its metabolites in mice—correlation with behavior and the effect of the metabolic inhibitors SKF 525A and Piperonyl Butoxide. *Biochem. Pharmacol. 21:*2237.
9. Gross, S. J., J. R. Soares, S-L. R. Wong, and R. E. Schuster (1974) Marijuana metabolites measured by a radioimmune technique. *Nature 252:*581.
10. Harris, L. S., A. E. Munson, M. A. Friedman, and W. L. Dewey (1974) Retardation of tumor growth by Δ^9-tetrahydrocannabinol (Δ^9-THC). *Pharmacologist 16:*259.
11. Klebe, R. J. and F. H. Ruddle (1969) Clone neuro-2a. *J. Cell Biol. 43:*69A.
12. Mahoney, J. M. and R. A. Harris (1972) Effect of Δ^9-tetrahydrocannabinol on mitochondrial processes. *Biochem. Pharmacol. 21:*1217.
13. Mans, R. and G. D. Novelli (1961) Measurement of the incorporation of radioactive amino acids into protein by a filter-paper disk method. *Arch. Biochem. Biophys. 94:*48.
14. Nahas, G. G., N. Suciu-Foca, Jean-Pierre Armand, and A. Morishima (1974) Inhibition of cellular mediated immunity in marihuana smokers. *Science 183:*419.
15. Nichols, W. W., J. Lee, and S. Dwight (1970) The IMR-32 cell line. *Cancer Res. 30:*2110.
16. Paton, W. D. M., R. G. Pertwee, and D. M. Temple (1972) The general pharmacology of cannabinols. *Cannabis and Its Derivatives: Pharmacology and Experimental Psychology* (W. D. M. Paton and J. L. Crowns, eds.). London: Oxford University Press, pp. 50–75.
17. Raz, A., A. Schurr, and A. Livne (1972) The interaction of hashish components with human erythrocytes. *Biochem. Biophys. Acta 274:*269.
18. Regan, J. D. and E. H. Y. Chu (1966) A convenient method for assay of DNA synthesis in synchronized human cell cultures. *J. Cell Biol. 28:*139.
19. Regan, J. D., J. D. Setlow, and R. D. Ley (1971) Normal and defective repair of damaged DNA in human cells: A sensitive assay utilizing the photolysis of bromodeoxyuridine. *Proc. Natl. Acad. Sci. U.S.A. 68:*708.
20. Regan, J. D., R. B. Setlow, M. M. Kaback, R. R. Howell, E. Klein, and G. Burgess (1971) Xeroderma pigmentosum: a rapid, sensitive method for prenatal diagnosis. *Science 174:*147.
21. Setlow, R. B., J. D. Regan, J. German, and W. L. Carrier (1969) Evidence that xeroderma pigmentosum cells do not perform the first

step in the repair of ultraviolet damage to their DNA. *Proc. Natl. Acad. Sci. U.S.A. 64*:1035.
22. Setlow, R. B., and J. D. Setlow (1972) Effects of radiation on polynucleotides. *Annu. Rev. Biophys. Bioengineer. 1*:293.
23. Tscherne, J. S., I. B. Weinstein, K. W. Lanks, N. B. Gersten, and C. R. Canton (1973) Phenylalanyl transfer ribonucleic acid synthetase activity associated with rat liver ribosomes and microsomes. *Biochemistry 12*:3859.
24. Zimmerman, A. M. and D. N. McClean (1973) Action of narcotic and hallucinogenic agents on the cell cycle. *Drugs and the Cell cycle* (A. M. Zimmerman, G. M. Padilla, and I. L. Cameron, eds.). New York: Academic Press, pp. 67–94.

20

In Vitro Inhibition of Protein and Nucleic Acid Synthesis in Rat Testicular Tissue by Cannabinoids

A. JAKUBOVIC AND P. L. MCGEER

Several reports which describe the distribution, metabolism, and excretion of administered Δ^9-tetrahydrocannabinol (THC) in humans [19] and various mammalian species [1,12,16] indicate that THC and/or its metabolites are retained in different tissues, including the testes [11], for long periods of time. High doses of marihuana bring about a deterioration in sexual performance in male rats [4,22]. Reduced sperm counts, reduced sexual potency [17], and gynecomastia have been reported in human heavy cannabis users [8].

The reason for this apparent interference with gonadal function is unknown, but one possibility is a direct interference with protein and nucleic acid synthesis. We have reported this as one of the important effects of THC and other cannabinoids, distinct from their pharmacological action at receptor sites in brain tissue [13,14]. We have also reported that a possible structural correlate is the reduction of nuclear membrane-bound ribosomes found in brain tissue shortly after the administration of THC *in vivo* to neonatal rats [9,10]. A similar effect was obtained in brain tissue of suckling rats after THC was administered to the lactating mother [15]. This result showed that THC and/or its metabolites could be transferred from mother to suckling infant in amounts capable of bringing about structural and biochemical changes in the infant brain cells.

Several more recent reports [20] involving such diverse cellular systems as tetrahymena [27] and cultured human lymphocytes [23] also suggest that a widespread effect of cannabis derivatives may be interference with protein and nucleic acid synthesis.

The testis was chosen as a suitable organ for testing the generality of the inhibition since nucleic acids, proteins, and lipids are synthesized rapidly during spermatogenesis. Furthermore, the demonstration of such an inhibitory effect might help explain the observed decline in gonadal function in cannabis users. Metabolism

Marihuana: Chemistry, Biochemistry, and Cellular Effects, edited by Gabriel G. Nahas,

in vitro was measured so that direct effects could be observed in the absence of complicating *in vivo* hormonal relationships [5].

In this study different cannabinoids and a variety of radioactive precursors were used to evaluate protein and lipid synthesis as well as the salvage and *de novo* pathways of nucleic acid synthesis.

Methods

Testicular tissue was obtained from adult male Wistar rats (250–300 gm). Each testis was stripped of its tunica and sectioned into six parts of approximately 200–300 mg wet weight. The tissue sections were incubated in separate Warburg flasks containing a final volume of 3 ml of Krebs–Ringer phosphate buffer, pH 7.4, at 33 °C, for 90 min. In experiments in which 10 m*M* glucose was included, the incubation was at 37 °C. The addition of cannabinoids and work up of the slices were essentially as previously described for slices of brain tissue [13]. Except for SP-111A (1-[4-(morpholino) butyryloxy]-3-*n*-pentyl-6,6,9-trimethyl-10a,6a,7,8-tetrahydrodibenzo[b,d]pyran hydrobromide), the soluble derivative of THC [28] which was added in aqueous solution, all cannabinoids were introduced into the medium in 5 μl of 95 percent ethanol. An equal amount of ethanol was then added to the control incubations. The water-insoluble cannabinoids formed a fine suspension in the incubation medium. The solution containing radioactive substrate was placed in the side arm of the Warburg flask and tipped into the main vessel after 7 min equilibration. Respiration was measured by the conventional Warburg technique. Tissue fractionation was carried out as previously described [13]. In order to separate the RNA and DNA fractions, we performed digestions in 0.2 *M* KOH for 18 hr at 37° [25]. The nucleic acid precursors in the TCA-soluble, low molecular weight fraction were chromatographed on Whatman No. 3 paper with added cold carrier. The solvent systems were butanol: acetic acid: water (2:1:1 v/v) when labeled uridine, orotic acid, or adenine were substrates; and ethyl acetate: formic acid: water (7:2:1 v/v) when thymidine was the substrate. The metabolites were identified by their UV absorbance. The appropriate areas of the paper were cut out, and the radioactivity on the paper counted in a liquid scintillation counter. The di- and triphosphonucleotides were not separated by the solvent systems and thus were counted together. The ATP level in the tissue was determined by fluorometry [7].

The values reported for insoluble cannabinoids were always in comparison with alcohol controls. The values for SP-111A were in comparison with alcohol-omitted controls. The significance of the data was analyzed by Student's t test.

Results

L-Leucine-U-^{14}C and -1-^{14}C as substrates

The effect of different cannabinoids on the rate of incorporation of L-leucine-U-^{14}C into various fractions is shown in Table 20.1. The tested cannabinoids did not appear to affect seriously the respiration of the slices, as evidenced by only slight decreases of oxygen consumption and $^{14}CO_2$ evolution (Figure 20.1). Similarly, uptake of the leucine, indicated by total radioactivity in the soluble fraction, was virtually unaffected by the cannabinoids (Table 20.1, Figure 20.1), except in the case of 8-β-OH-Δ^9-THC, in which up-

Table 20.1 Effect of cannabinoids on the metabolism of L-leucine-U-^{14}C in rat testis slices[a]

Cannabinoids (0.1 m*M*)	*Percentage of control dpm/100 mg wet weight tissue*			
	Soluble fraction	*Nucleic acid*	*Lipid*	*Protein*
Δ^9-THC	96 ± 2	66 ± 15[d]	69 ± 11[d]	66 ± 10[e]
Δ^8-THC	94 ± 4	62 ± 10[e]	67 ± 6[d]	65 ± 6[e]
11-OH-Δ^9-THC[b]	98 ± 2	73 ± 11	65 ± 8[c]	76 ± 3[e]
8-β-OH-Δ^9-THC[b]	122 ± 14	55 ± 2[e]	47 ± 3[e]	57 ± 4[e]
Cannabidiol	108 ± 7	71 ± 10[d]	100 ± 25	70 ± 5[e]
Cannabinol	99 ± 4	68 ± 4[e]	79 ± 20	71 ± 11[e]
Cannabigerol	112 ± 3	68 ± 20[d]	80 ± 20	71 ± 10[e]
Alcohol omitted	96 ± 9	97 ± 5	125 ± 20	102 ± 9

[a] Slices were incubated for 90 min at 33°C in 3 ml Krebs-Ringer phosphate buffer containing 1 μCi of L-leucine-U-^{14}C (10 μCi/μM).

[b] Indicates addition of 10 m*M* glucose and incubation at 37°C for 90 min. Values for all cannabinoids were expressed as percentage of standard alcohol (28 m*M*) control. Each value represents mean ± SD, $n = 3$. Control values in dpm/100 mg tissue wet weight were (without glucose): soluble 106,124 ± 5,075; nucleic acid 3,694 ± 793; lipid 2,062 ± 469; protein 105,863 ± 13,389; $n = 9$; (with glucose): 87,665 ± 2,443; 7,051 ± 885; 14,237 ± 2,168; 204,452 ± 9,000, respectively; $n = 6$.

[c] Significance of experimental values compared with matched controls: $p < 0.05$.

[d] $p < 0.02$.

[e] $p < 0.01$.

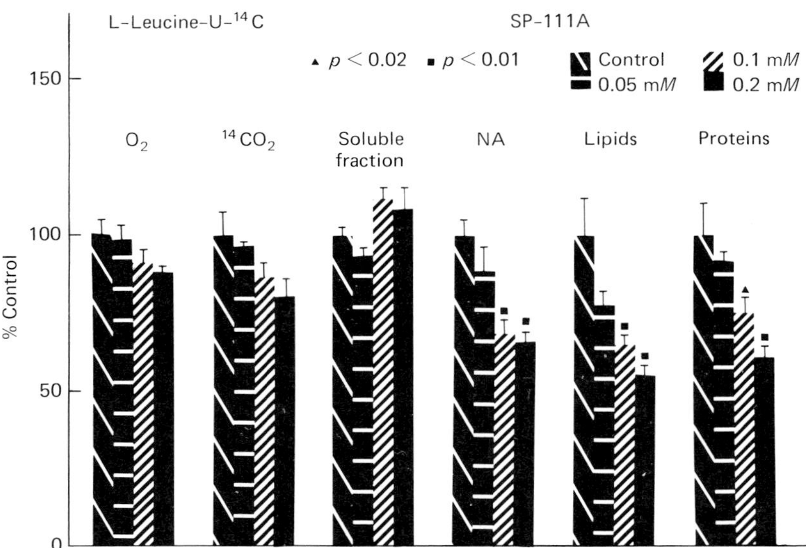

Figure 20.1. Effect of different concentrations of SP-111A on the metabolism of L-leucine-U-^{14}C in rat testis *in vitro*. Experimental conditions as described in Table 20.1 with 10 m*M* glucose. Control values in dpm/100 mg wet tissue weight were: soluble fraction 75,052 ± 1,565; NA 7,202 ± 315; lipids 16,616 ± 1,884; proteins 193,094 ± 18,930. Values are means ± SD; $n = 3$.

take appeared to be increased. In spite of this, the incorporation of radioactive carbon into nucleic acid and lipid fractions was significantly less in the presence of most of the tested cannabinoids. In the proteins, in which the whole molecule of leucine was presumably incorporated unchanged, all cannabinoids brought about a highly significant reduction of radioactivity. 8-β-OH-Δ^9-THC had the greatest effect (43 percent inhibition). Alcohol-omitted controls were not significantly different from the standard controls (i.e., 28 m*M* alcohol) (Table 20.1). The inhibitory effect of SP-111A was tested at three concentrations, and a dose-related inhibition of incorporation of ^{14}C into the macromolecular fractions was observed. Thus, at 0.2 m*M*, 0.1 m*M*, and 0.05 m*M* SP-111A, the incorporation of radioactivity was 60, 77, and 90 percent of control, respectively (Figure 20.1). A similar dose-response effect was obtained with Δ^9-THC.

In order to test the level of unmetabolized leucine in the acid-soluble low molecular weight fraction, L-leucine-1-^{14}C was used as

Table 20.2 Effects of cannabinoids on L-leucine-1-^{14}C metabolism in rat testis slices[a]

Cannabinoids (mM)		*Percentage of dpm/100 mg wet weight tissue*	
		Soluble fraction	*Protein*
Δ^9-THC	0.1	108 ± 6	76 ± 8[b]
Δ^8-THC	0.1	100 ± 2	70 ± 6[b]
11-OH-Δ^9-THC	0.1	133 ± 12[b]	68 ± 2[c]
8-β-OH-Δ^9-THC	0.1	183 ± 6[c]	42 ± 2[c]
	0.05	134 ± 14[b]	66 ± 2[c]
	0.025	114 ± 14	90 ± 4
Alcohol omitted		93 ± 3	100 ± 2
SP-111A	0.2	135 ± 9[b]	74 ± 2[c]

[a] Incubations were as described in Table 20.1 with 10 m*M* glucose except that 1 μCi L-leucine-1-^{14}C (20 μCi/μM) was the substrate. Each value represents mean ± SD, $n = 3$. Control values in dpm/100 mg tissue wet weight were: soluble 27,728 ± 609; protein 153,288 ± 17,257; $n = 9$. SP-111A values were compared with alcohol omitted controls.

[b] Significance of experimental values compared with matched controls: $p < 0.02$.

[c] $p < 0.01$.

the substrate instead of L-leucine-U-^{14}C (Table 20.2). Metabolism of L-leucine-l-^{14}C results in loss of the label as $^{14}CO_2$. With L-leucine-l-^{14}C, radioactivity was increased significantly in the soluble fraction by 11-OH-Δ^9-THC, 8-β-OH-Δ^9-THC, and SP-111A, in contrast to the apparent lack of change with these cannabinoids using L-leucine-U-^{14}C (Table 20.1). This increase clearly indicates that the inhibitory effects of the cannabinoids were not due to lack of labeled leucine as substrate and suggests that the observed inhibition with cannabinoids might have been even greater had labeled substrate concentration been taken into account.

L-Lysine-U-^{14}C as substrate

The effects of various cannabinoids on the metabolism and rate of incorporation of L-lysine-U-^{14}C are shown in Table 20.3. The results are similar to those of L-leucine-U-^{14}C (Table 20.1). There was an overall decrease of radioactive carbon incorporation into the nucleic acid and lipid fractions and of lysine-^{14}C incorporation into the protein fraction. Radioactivity in the acid-soluble fraction was

Table 20.3 Effect of cannabinoids on L-lysine-U-^{14}C metabolism in rat testis slices[a]

Cannabinoids (0.1mM)	Percentage of dpm/100 mg wet weight tissue			
	Soluble fraction	*Nucleic acid*	*Lipid*	*Protein*
Δ^9-THC	91 ± 8	69 ± 6[e]	78 ± 6[e]	73 ± 8[e]
11-OH-Δ^9-THC	95 ± 8	62 ± 7[e]	60 ± 6[e]	59 ± 1[e]
8-β-OH-Δ^9-THC	81 ± 5[c]	38 ± 20[e]	37 ± 12[e]	35 ± 10[e]
Cannabidiol	95 ± 7	66 ± 11[e]	64 ± 12[e]	69 ± 4[e]
Cannabinol	84 ± 3[c]	64 ± 2[e]	57 ± 2[e]	59 ± 11[e]
Cannabigerol	80 ± 5[c]	54 ± 10[e]	58 ± 10[e]	62 ± 6[e]
Δ^9-THC[b]	97 ± 5	63 ± 14[d]	66 ± 5[e]	67 ± 12[e]
8-β-OH-Δ^9-THC[b]	86 ± 4[c]	61 ± 6[d]	66 ± 6[d]	65 ± 5[e]
SP-111A[b]	86 ± 2[c]	70 ± 2[e]	67 ± 3[e]	77 ± 2[e]
Alcohol omitted[b]	105 ± 8	96 ± 14	110 ± 4	103 ± 5

[a] Incubations as described in Table 20.1 except 1 μCi L-lysine-U-^{14}C (10 μCi/μM) was the substrate.

[b] Indicates addition of 10 m*M* glucose. Each value represents mean ± SD, $n = 3$. Control values in dpm/100 mg tissue wet weight were (without glucose): soluble 130,522 ± 6,435; nucleic acid 2,392 ± 85; lipid 1,128 ± 16; protein 32,401 ± 435; (with glucose): 126,262 ± 10,323; 8,412 ± 1,225; 5,632 ± 200; 20,009 ± 1,033, respectively. SP-111A values were compared with alcohol-omitted controls.

[c] Significance of experimental values compared with matched controls: $p < 0.05$.

[d] $p < 0.02$.

[e] $p < 0.01$.

significantly decreased by 8-β-OH-Δ^9-THC, cannabinol, cannabigerol, 8-β-OH-Δ^9-THC, and SP-111A. The inhibition of metabolism and incorporation of labeled lysine into the tissue was apparent with or without glucose in the incubation medium. Alcohol, at 28 m*M*, had no effect on these biosynthetic processes (Table 20.3).

Glycine-U-^{14}C as substrate

As a further test of possible effects of cannabinoids, the incorporation and metabolism of glycine-U-^{14}C in rat testis tissue slices in the presence of SP-111A, 11-OH-Δ^9-THC, and 8-β-OH-Δ^9-THC were determined. The distribution of label among the various subcellular fractions is shown in Table 20.4. There was once again a significant inhibition of the incorporation of ^{14}C into nucleic acid and protein fractions with all these derivatives. Three concentrations of SP-111A were tested, and a dose-related effect was obtained (Table 20.4).

Table 20.4 Effect of cannabinoids on the metabolism of glycine-U-^{14}C in rat testis slices[a]

Cannabinoids (*m*M)		*Percentage of dpm/100 mg wet weight tissue*			
		Soluble fraction	*Nucleic acid*	*Lipid*	*Protein*
SP-111A	0.1	77 ± 4[d]	59 ± 9[c]	55 ± 1[d]	52 ± 5[d]
	0.05	78 ± 5[c]	68 ± 5[c]	72 ± 8[c]	67 ± 4[d]
	0.025	88 ± 4	75 ± 6[b]	76 ± 7[c]	82 ± 8
11-OH-Δ^9-THC	0.1	83 ± 2[d]	63 ± 9[d]	71 ± 9[b]	69 ± 10[c]
8-β-OH-Δ^9-THC	0.1	86 ± 6	57 ± 9[d]	78 ± 14	58 ± 7[d]
Alcohol omitted		102 ± 5	94 ± 4	111 ± 10	103 ± 2

[a] Incubations as described in Table 20.1 with 10 m*M* glucose except 1 μCi glycine-U-^{14}C (10 μCi/μM) was the substrate. Each value represents mean ± SD, $n = 3$. Control values in dpm/100 mg tissue wet weight were: soluble 121,228 ± 6,965; nucleic acid 2,907 ± 350; lipid 621 ± 52; protein 18,513 ± 1,750. SP-111A values were compared with alcohol-omitted controls.

[b] Significance of experimental values compared with matched controls: $p < 0.05$.

[c] $p < 0.02$.

[d] $p < 0.01$.

Uridine-2-^{14}C as substrate

The addition of different cannabinoids was found to produce a marked decrease in the radioactivity in the RNA fraction of rat testis tissue (Table 20.5). The incorporation of labeled uridine into RNA was progressively reduced with increasing concentrations of SP-111A (Figure 20.2).

The distribution of the radioactivity among the various components of the low molecular weight fraction showed that although radioactivity in the nucleoside was increased or unchanged by cannabinoids, there was a dramatic inhibition of synthesis of the nucleotides UMP and UDP + UTP (Table 20.5, Figure 20.2). Thus, the decline in incorporation of radioactivity into RNA correlated with the decline of formation of phosphorylated uridine derivatives.

There was also a slight effect of 28 m*M* alcohol (Table 20.5) since alcohol-omitted controls gave significantly higher values in the soluble and RNA fractions, as well as in the nucleotides.

Orotic acid-6-^{14}C as substrate

Orotic acid, as an intermediary product of pyrimidine biosynthesis, was used to test the effects of cannabinoids on the *de novo* pathways. The uptake and incorporation of orotic acid (Table

Table 20.5 Effect of cannabinoids on uridine-2-^{14}C metabolism in rat testis slices[a]

	Percentage of dpm/100 mg wet weight tissue					
Cannabinoids (0.1 mM)	*Soluble fraction*	*RNA*	*U*	*UR*	*UMP*	*UDP + UTP*
Δ^9-THC	81 ± 5[c]	59 ± 12[d]	74[d]	122[c]	71[d]	54[d]
11-OH-Δ^9-THC	92 ± 5	70 ± 3[d]	78[d]	145[d]	69[c]	66[d]
8-β-OH-Δ^9-THC	70 ± 10[c]	40 ± 14[d]	63[d]	130[c]	45[d]	27[d]
Cannabinol	80 ± 2[d]	66 ± 4[d]	78[d]	106	62[d]	65[d]
Cannabigerol	77 ± 11	58 ± 20[d]	81[c]	99	51[d]	52[d]
Cannabidiol	95 ± 4	76 ± 10[d]	83[d]	149[d]	74[c]	68[d]
Alcohol omitted	120 ± 5[c]	119 ± 10[b]	114	110	132[b]	137[b]

[a] Incubations as described in Table 20.1 except 1 μCi uridine-2-^{14}C (62 μCi/μM) was the substrate. Each value represents mean ± SD, $n = 3$. Control values in dpm/100 mg tissue wet weight were: soluble 60,444 ± 4,281; nucleic acid 16,202 ± 791. The percent distribution of labeled nucleic acid metabolites by chromatography was: U = 43 ± 2; UR = 27 ± 1; UMP = 7 ± 0.3; UDP + UTP = 23 ± 1.

[b] Significance of experimental values compared with matched controls: $p < 0.05$.

[c] $p < 0.02$.

[d] $p < 0.01$.

20.6) were much lower than those of uridine (Table 20.5, Figure 20.2). Nevertheless, all the tested cannabinoids brought about significant decreases in the radioactivity in the nucleic acids, even though the label in the acid-soluble fraction was not affected (Table 20.6). The distribution of various labeled derivatives obtained by chromatography from the soluble fraction of the slices showed that the cells contained not only labeled orotic acid but also labeled uracil metabolites (Table 20.6). Even though the relative amount of labeled orotic acid was slightly increased, there was a marked depletion of the phosphorylated metabolites of uridine, especially UDP + UTP. Thus, the transport system for orotic acid was apparently not affected by the cannabinoids. Alcohol, 28 m*M*, had no effect (Table 20.6).

Thymidine-$^{14}CH_3$ as substrate

The effect of cannabinoids on the metabolism and incorporation of labeled thymidine into DNA is shown in Table 20.7 and Figure 20.3. Unlike the situation with uridine-^{14}C (Table 20.5, Figure 20.2), the cannabinoids caused an increase in the amount of label

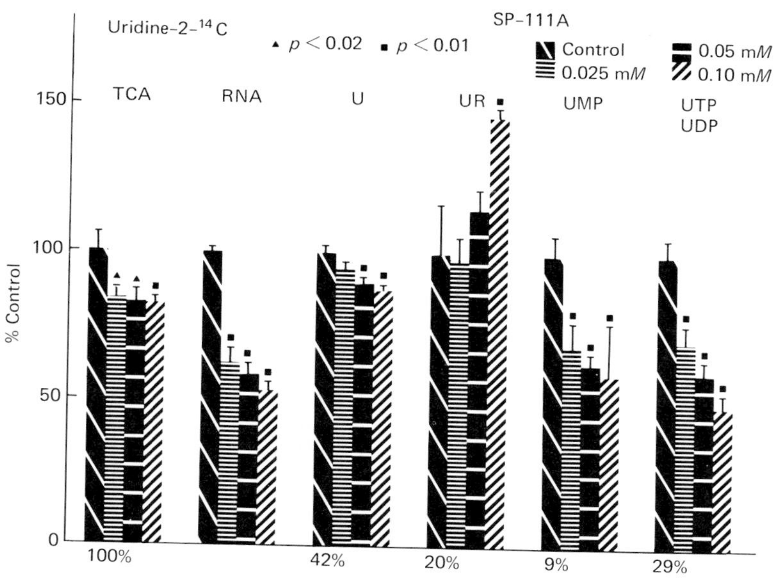

Figure 20.2. Effect of different concentrations of SP-111A on the metabolism and incorporation of uridine-2-^{14}C in rat testis *in vitro*. Experimental conditions as described in Table 20.1 with 10 m*M* glucose, except 1 μCi uridine-2-^{14}C (62 μCi/μM) was the substrate. Control values in dpm/100 mg wet tissue weight were: soluble fraction 76,788 ± 4,311; RNA 26,231 ± 293. The % on the X axis indicates the mean % distribution of labeled compounds compared with the control soluble fraction as 100%. Values are means ± SD, $n = 3$.

in the low molecular weight fraction. However, the rate of incorporation of radioactivity into DNA was decreased significantly. The distribution of label among the metabolites showed only a slight increase, or no change, in the hydrolytic pathway leading to thymine. Even with a marked increase in labeled nucleoside and no change in TMP, the synthesis of TDP + TTP was severely inhibited by all cannabinoids at 0.1 m*M* concentration (Table 20.7). 8-β-OH-Δ^9-THC (Table 20.7) and SP-111A (Figure 20.3) both exhibited a dose-related inhibition of TDP + TTP and the subsequent incorporation into DNA. These results indicate that the decreased synthesis of TDP + TTP might be responsible for the decreased incorporation of thymidine into DNA. Here again, 28 m*M* concentration of alcohol was without effect (Table 20.7).

Table 20.6 Effect of cannabinoids on orotic acid-6-^{14}C metabolism in rat testis slices[a]

	Percentage dpm/100 mg wet weight tissue					
Cannabinoids (*0.1 m*M)	*Soluble fraction*	*Nucleic acid*	*U + UR*	*OA*	*UMP*	*UDP + UTP*
Δ^9-THC	112 ± 4	74 ± 8[b]	106	115	100	73[d]
11-OH-Δ^9-THC	108 ± 9	61 ± 5[d]	91	122	69[c]	62[d]
Cannabidiol	98 ± 10	68 ± 4[d]	114	100	73[b]	64[d]
Cannabigerol	112 ± 7	74 ± 3[d]	100	122	73[b]	74[d]
Alcohol omitted	96 ± 3	100 ± 10	100	83	110	123[b]

[a] Incubations as described in Table 20.1 except 1 μCi orotic acid-6-^{14}C (61 μCi/μM) was the substrate. Each value represents mean ± SD, $n = 3$. Control values in dpm/100 mg tissue wet weight were: soluble 8,600 ± 230; nucleic acid 747 ± 76. The percent distribution of labeled nucleic acid metabolites in the soluble fraction by chromatography was: U + UR = 15 ± 1; orotic acid = 64 ± 1; UMP = 7 ± 1; UDP + UTP 13 ± 1.

[b] Significance of experimental values compared with matched controls: $p < 0.05$.

[c] $p < 0.02$.

[d] $p < 0.01$.

Table 20.7 Effect of cannabinoids on thymidine-$^{14}CH_3$ metabolism in rat testis slices[a]

		Percentage of dpm/100 mg wet weight tissue					
Cannabinoids (*m*M)		*Soluble fraction*	*DNA*	*T*	*TR*	*TMP*	*TDP + TTP*
11-OH-Δ^9-THC	0.1	129 ± 1[d]	71 ± 5[d]	135[c]	140[d]	118	60[d]
8-β-OH-Δ^9-THC	0.2	117 ± 8[b]	50 ± 8[d]	90	133[d]	103	44[d]
	0.1	115 ± 5[c]	54 ± 8[d]	97	128[d]	89	55[d]
	0.05	121 ± 10[b]	90 ± 11	98	131[b]	114	79[c]
Cannabidiol	0.1	121 ± 5[b]	70 ± 3[d]	130	135[d]	82	52[d]
Cannabinol	0.1	105 ± 6	88 ± 9	105	110	100	74[b]
Cannabigerol	0.1	105 ± 3	74 ± 6[c]	102	114	86	63[d]
Alcohol omitted		109 ± 8	105 ± 8	95	113	108	122

[a] Incubations as described in Table 20.1 except 1 μCi thymidine-$^{14}CH_3$ (59 μCi/μM) was the substrate. Each value represents mean ± SD, $n = 3$. Control values in dpm/100 mg wet tissue weight were: soluble 64,182 ± 4,281; DNA 10,421 ± 791. The percent distribution of labeled nucleic acid metabolites in the soluble fraction by chromatography was T = 20 ± 1, TR = 69 ± 1, TMP = 4 ± 0.5; TDP + TTP = 7 ± 1.

[b] Significance of experimental values compared with matched controls: $p < 0.05$.

[c] $p < 0.02$.

[d] $p < 0.01$.

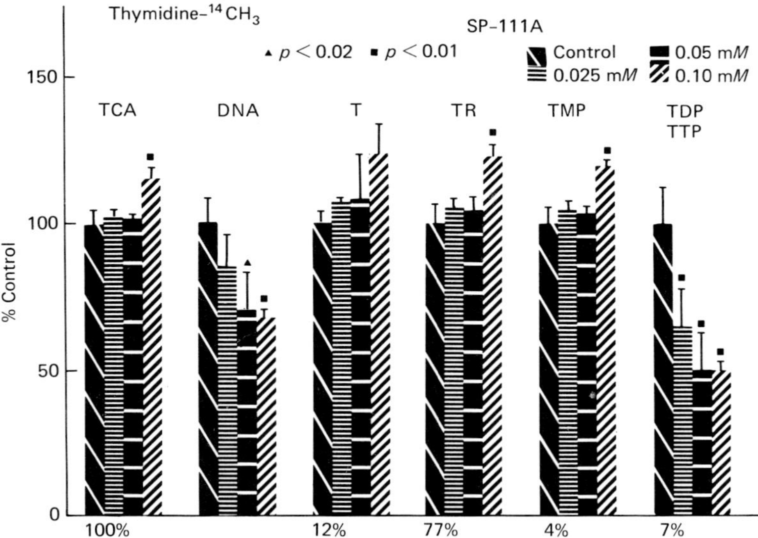

Figure 20.3. Effect of different concentrations of SP-111A on the metabolism and incorporation of thymidine-^{14}CH$_3$ in rat testis *in vitro*. Incubations were done as described in Table 20.1 with 10 m*M* glucose, except 1 μCi thymidine-^{14}CH$_3$ (59 μCi/μM) was the substrate. Control values in dpm/100 mg wet tissue weight were: soluble fraction 60,232 ± 3,089; DNA 11,662 ± 990. The % on the X axis indicates the mean % distribution of labeled compounds compared with the control soluble fraction as 100%. Values are means ± SD, $n = 3$.

Adenine-8-^{14}C as substrate

The effect of cannabinoids on the salvage pathway of nucleic acid synthesis was further ascertained by studying the metabolism and incorporation of labeled adenine into nucleic acid (Table 20.8). With all cannabinoids tested at a concentration of 0.1 m*M*, a significant decrease in the radioactivity in both the acid-soluble and nucleic acid fractions was found. The soluble fraction was explored further by chromatography. The results (Table 20.8) demonstrated a significant increase of the intracellular labeled adenine with only minor changes in adenosine and in AMP, although there was a marked decrease in the biosynthesis of the main soluble compounds, ADP + ATP. It is evident that the diminished radioactivity in the soluble as well as the nucleic acid fractions correlates with a decreased synthesis of labeled ADP + ATP (Table 20.8). Even

Table 20.8 Effect of cannabinoids on adenine-8-^{14}C metabolism in rat testis slices[a]

Cannabinoids (0.1 mM)	Percentage of dpm/100 mg wet weight tissue					
	Soluble fraction	Nucleic acid	A	AR	AMP	ADP + ATP
Δ^9-THC	68 ± 4[c]	75 ± 3[d]	111	97	90	59[d]
Δ^8-THC	82 ± 6[b]	78 ± 6[c]	117	101	102	72[d]
11-OH-Δ^9-THC	67 ± 6[d]	63 ± 7[d]	114	103	91	53[d]
8-β-OH-Δ^9-THC	73 ± 3[d]	65 ± 5[d]	92	123[c]	87	62[d]
Cannabidiol	74 ± 3[d]	71 ± 4[d]	119	113	95	61[d]
Cannabinol	72 ± 5[b]	82 ± 3[d]	117	107	97	61[d]
Cannabigerol	59 ± 5[d]	68 ± 8[d]	101	76	77	51[d]
SP-111A	77 ± 2[d]	78 ± 8[c]	185[d]	106	122[c]	60[d]
Alcohol omitted	110 ± 3	111 ± 3	51[d]	83[b]	86	124

[a] Incubations as described in Table 20.1 with 10 mM glucose except 1 μCi adenine-8-^{14}C (52.4 μCi/μM) was the substrate. Each value represents mean ± SD, n = 3. Control values in dpm/100 mg tissue wet weight were: soluble 497,763 ± 12,347; nucleic acid 43,403 ± 181. The percent distribution of labeled nucleic acid metabolites in the soluble fraction by chromatography was A = 2.5 ± 0.5; AR = 4.5 ± 0.5; AMP = 18 ± 2; ADP + ATP = 75 ± 3. SP-111A values were compared with alcohol-omitted controls.

[b] Significance of experimental values compared with matched controls: $p < 0.05$.

[c] $p < 0.02$.

[d] $p < 0.01$.

though it increased the amount of labeled adenine as well as adenosine, alcohol did not affect the nucleotides AMP and ADP + ATP (Table 20.8).

Glucose-U-^{14}C as substrate

To test the effects of cannabinoids on general metabolism, we tested the rate of incorporation of glucose-U-^{14}C into various fractions (Table 20.9). As noted in previous experiments, there was a mild reduction in O_2 consumption and $^{14}CO_2$ evolution, particularly at the higher (0.1–0.2 mM) concentrations of SP-111A. There was also a mild reduction in the amount of label in the soluble fraction. However, these dose-related effects were not as great as those noted in the nucleic acid and protein fractions, suggesting once more a particular interference of the cannabinoids with nucleic acid and protein metabolism. Again there was no effect of alcohol.

Table 20.9 Effect of cannabinoids on glucose-U-^{14}C metabolism in rat testis slices[a]

Cannabinoids (*0.1 m*M)	*% O_2* (*µl/100 mg*)	*Percentage of dpm/100 mg wet weight tissue*				
		$^{14}CO_2$	*Soluble fraction*	*Nucleic acid*	*Lipid*	*Protein*
Δ^9-THC	92 ± 9	90 ± 11	89 ± 3[b]	87 ± 6	94 ± 12	79 ± 6[c]
Δ^8-THC	92 ± 10	98 ± 5	91 ± 6	97 ± 6	81 ± 4	89 ± 4
11-OH-Δ^9-THC	86 ± 4	87 ± 12	94 ± 3	78 ± 7	81 ± 6	68 ± 5[c]
8-β-OH-Δ^9-THC	87 ± 4	84 ± 5	96 ± 4	78 ± 10	77 ± 7	72 ± 5[c]
Cannabidiol	94 ± 3	89 ± 5	84 ± 1[d]	89 ± 5	100 ± 15	91 ± 4
Cannabigerol	92 ± 5	86 ± 1[d]	86 ± 1[d]	75 ± 10[d]	104 ± 10	88 ± 10
Cannabinol	101 ± 2	96 ± 2	96 ± 2	90 ± 4	130 ± 5[d]	97 ± 6
Alcohol omitted	100 ± 2	100 ± 3	97 ± 6	104 ± 1	102 ± 6	112 ± 5
SP-111A 0.05 m*M*	86 ± 4[d]	71 ± 5[d]	87 ± 1[c]	70 ± 7[d]	76 ± 6[d]	72 ± 4[d]
0.1 m*M*	80 ± 2[d]	70 ± 5[d]	89 ± 2[c]	62 ± 6[d]	72 ± 7[d]	70 ± 8[c]
0.2 m*M*	78 ± 4[d]	66 ± 2[d]	86 ± 2[c]	53 ± 5[d]	70 ± 3[d]	49 ± 3[d]

[a] Incubations were as described in Table 20.1 with 10 m*M* glucose-U-^{14}C (0.014 µCi/µM). Each value represents mean ± SD, $n = 33$. Standard control values in dpm/100 mg tissue wet weight were: $^{14}CO_2$ evolution 7,576 ± 107; soluble 14,687 ± 790; nucleic acid 382 ± 6; lipids 606 ± 17; protein 1,219 ± 103. Standard control O_2 consumption 109 ± 2 µl/100 mg/90 min incubation. SP-111A values were compared with alcohol-omitted control.

[b] Significance of experimental values compared with matched controls: $p < 0.05$.

[c] $p < 0.02$.

[d] $p < 0.01$.

Table 20.10 Effects of cannabinoids on ATP content in the rat testis slices[a]

Cannabinoids (*m*M)		*% O_2 uptake* (*μl/100 mg wet weight*)	*% ATP*
Δ⁹-THC	0.1	85 ± 2[b]	62 ± 11[c]
Δ⁸-THC	0.1	85 ± 7	70 ± 3[c]
11-OH-Δ⁹-THC	0.1	89 ± 2	61 ± 4[c]
8-β-OH-Δ⁹-THC	0.1	95 ± 1	55 ± 4[c]
	0.05	100 ± 3	84 ± 1[c]
SP-111A	0.2	87 ± 3[b]	69 ± 2[c]
	0.1	96 ± 3	73 ± 5[b]
	0.05	103 ± 6	84 ± 7
Alcohol omitted		99 ± 2	95 ± 10

[a] Incubation as described in Table 20.1 with 10 m*M* glucose. Each value represents mean ± SD, $n = 3$. Control values per 100 mg tissue wet weight were: ATP = 158 ± 15 mμM; O_2 uptake 101 ± 6 μl/90 min.

[b] Significance of experimental values compared with matched controls: $p < 0.02$.

[c] $p < 0.01$.

Tissue concentration of ATP

ATP is one of the substrates for purine biosynthesis *de novo* and is also required for the synthesis of many other substrates. Furthermore, the syntheses of both nucleotides and nucleic acids are ATP dependent. Therefore, we studied the effect of cannabinoids on ATP content in the testis. Table 20.10 shows a dose-related depletion of ATP by SP-111A. Cellular concentrations of ATP were reduced even more by 8-β-OH-Δ⁹-THC. Other cannabinoids—e.g., 11-OH-Δ⁹-THC, Δ⁹-THC, and Δ⁸-THC—at concentrations of 0.1 m*M* also significantly decreased ATP levels when compared with the controls, even though the respiration was not usually affected by these cannabinoids. Alcohol had no effect on ATP levels under these experimental conditions (Table 20.10).

Discussion

In the present study, psychogenically active (e.g., Δ⁹-THC, Δ⁸-THC, 11-OH-Δ⁹-THC, and SP-111A, the water-soluble derivative of Δ⁹-THC) as well as the psychogenically less active or inactive (e.g., cannabidiol, cannabigerol, cannabinol, and 8-β-OH-Δ⁹-THC) cannabinoids [2,3,6,21,24,28] were tested for their possible effects on macromolecular synthesis in rat testis slices.

The results show that all tested cannabinoids, in incubation with or without exogenous glucose and with various labeled metabolites, significantly changed the biosynthesis of proteins, nucleic acids, and lipids in the rat testis. On the other hand, in most experiments the oxygen consumption, CO_2 evolution, and appearance of radioactivity in the soluble, low molecular weight fraction were only mildly or not significantly altered. These results compare with those previously obtained with Δ^9-THC in brain tissue slices [13].

Several aspects of metabolism were examined, and different radioactive precursors were used to illustrate these effects. Decreased protein synthesis was shown with leucine-U-^{14}C, leucine-1-^{14}C, lysine-U-^{14}C, glycine-U-^{14}C, and glucose-U-^{14}C. The inhibitions were generally comparable even though the precursors are not used to an equivalent extent in protein synthesis during spermatogenesis [5, 18]. The use of leucine-1-^{14}C illustrated that lack of substrate was not the principal reason for the inhibition of incorporation in the macromolecular fractions. Indeed, the counts in the soluble fraction in the presence of some cannabinoids (Table 20.2) increased with leucine-1-^{14}C, indicating less metabolism of the amino acid and therefore higher activity in the soluble fraction. The fact that even glucose-U-^{14}C was utilized less for protein synthesis suggests that some general inhibition was involved, and that this inhibition was not related to transport of the substrate into the cell or to oxygen consumption. Experiments, particularly with SP-111A, indicated that the effect was related to drug concentration (Tables 20.2, 20.4, 20.7, 20.9, 20.10 and Figures 20.1–20.3). In general, the psychogenically more active cannabinoids had the greatest influence.

Decreased lipid synthesis was also demonstrated with leucine-U-^{14}C, lysine-U-^{14}C, glycine-U-^{14}C, and glucose-U-^{14}C. Conversion into lipids was much less than into proteins, being roughly 0.5–4 percent as great.

The effects on nucleic acid metabolism were evaluated in a number of ways. The *de novo* synthesis of nucleic acids was tested generally by the incorporation of label from leucine-U-^{14}C, lysine-U-^{14}C, glycine-U-^{14}C, and glucose-U-^{14}C. All showed an inhibition, although the overall conversion was only 6–8 percent of that for protein. The *de novo* pathway for RNA synthesis was also tested using orotic acid-6-^{14}C. A similar result was obtained although once more the overall conversion was low.

Similar inhibition by the cannabinoids was also noted when the salvage pathway of nucleic acid synthesis was tested, even though higher incorporations into nucleic acid were always observed. The salvage pathway for RNA was tested using uridine-2-^{14}C and adenine-8-^{14}C, and for DNA, thymidine-$^{14}CH_3$. In each case, labeled RNA and DNA formation was substantially inhibited in the presence of the various cannabinoids.

The two basic pathways for the synthesis of phosphorylated nucleotides needed for nucleic acid synthesis are: (1) *de novo* synthesis, using small molecules and (2) the salvage pathway, using preformed purine and pyrimidine bases. The higher the proliferation of mammalian cells, the more important the latter pathway becomes.

Chromatographic analysis of the low molecular weight fractions indicated one possible mechanism for the overall observed results. When the distribution of uridine metabolites was examined, there was an increased uridine concentration with the cannabinoids, but decreased UMP and UDP + UTP, as well as uracil (Table 20.5, Figure 20.2). This result confirms our earlier work with brain slices in which Δ^9-THC had a similar effect [13]. When orotic acid-^{14}C was used to test the *de novo* pathway of uridine nucleotides and RNA, the phosphorylation to UMP and to UDP + UTP was also similarly inhibited even though the transport of orotic acid was not affected (Table 20.6). Thus, the decreased biosynthesis of labeled RNA appears to be directly related to the inhibition of phosphorylation of the precursors of RNA.

A somewhat comparable situation was observed when thymidine-$^{14}CH_3$ was the DNA salvage pathway precursor, with some differences in detail (Table 20.7, Figure 3). Unlike the situation with uridine, all the cannabinoids except cannabinol and cannabigerol caused a significant increase in the radioactivity of the soluble fraction. In this case there was also an increase in the activity of the TR fraction, with minor changes in the hydrolytic pathway to T, except for the case of 11-OH-Δ^9-THC. Even though there was no change in labeled TMP, there was a severe reduction in TDP + TTP. Despite these differences, the principal effect clearly was inhibition of the phosphorylation of TMP to TDP + TTP.

Further results of a similar nature were obtained with adenine-8-^{14}C as a precursor of the salvage pathway of nucleic acid synthesis (Table 20.8). Whereas AMP labeling was unchanged, there was a marked decrease in the labeling of ADP + ATP, which formed about 75 percent of the total soluble fraction. Total ATP levels in the testis slices also declined in comparison with the controls when incubation was carried out with cannabinoids (Table 20.10). Such a decrease of ATP content was also reported in bull sperm *in vitro* after incubation with Δ^9-THC [26].

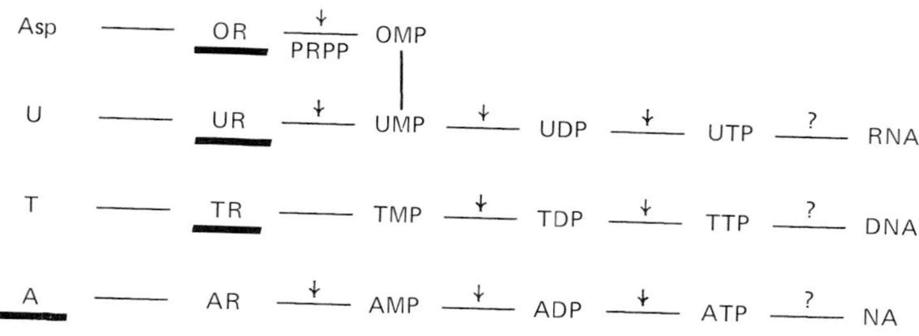

Figure 20.4. Schematic representation of the mechanism by which cannabinoids affect the *de novo* and salvage pathways of nucleic acid synthesis.

Since all biosynthetic processes in the testes—especially nucleic acid, protein, and lipid synthesis—are very active during spermatogenesis, the present *in vitro* results may help to explain the decreased spermatogenesis observed in cannabis users [17]. The reduced ATP levels in the cell and/or the phosphorylation, or perhaps even direct inhibition of nucleic acid polymerases may be the principal steps at which cannabis derivatives act on nucleic acid synthesis (Figure 20.4). The inhibition of protein synthesis, in turn, may be a result of decreased nucleic acid levels and/or decreased energy levels. The complete mode of action of cannabinoids at the subcellular level is still unknown and could be extremely complicated. However, the general action of the cannabis derivatives in inhibiting nucleic acid and protein synthesis may be applicable to other cellular systems [23,27]. In such circumstances, a cautious attitude should be taken regarding the potential effects of cannabis derivatives, and the particular contribution of the psychogenically inactive cannabinoids to the overall effects of such preparations as marihuana and hashish should be carefully scrutinized.

ACKNOWLEDGMENTS

We thank Elizabeth Sutherland for excellent technical assistance and the Canada NMUD and Providence of B.C. for financial support.

REFERENCES

1. Agurell, S., I. M. Nilsson, A. Ohlsson, and F. Sandberg (1969) Elimination of tritium-labelled cannabinols in the rat with special reference to the development of tests for the identification of cannabis users. *Biochem. Pharmacol. 18:*1195.
2. Ben-Zvi, Z. and R. Mechoulam (1971) 6β-hydroxy-Δ^1-tetrahydrocannabinol synthesis and biological activity. *Science 174:*951.

3. Christensen, H. D., R. I. Freudenthal, J. T. Gidley, R. Rosenfeld, G. Boegli, L. Testino, D. R. Brine, C. G. Pitt, and M. E. Wall (1971) Activity of Δ^8- and Δ^9-tetrahydrocannabinol and related compounds in the mouse. *Science 172:*165.
4. Corcoran, M. E., Z. Amit, C. W. Malsbury, and S. Daykin (1974) Reduction in copulatory behavior of male rats following hashish injections. *Res. Commun. Chem. Pathol. Pharmacol.* 7:779.
5. Davis, J. R. and G. A. Langford (1970) Testicular proteins. *The Testis* (A. D. Johnson, W. R. Gomes, and N. L. Vandemark, eds.) Vol. 2. New York: Academic Press, pp. 259–306.
6. Edery, H., Y. Grunfeld, Z. Ben-Zvi, and R. Mechoulam (1971) Structural requirements for cannabinoid activity. *Ann. N. Y. Acad. Sci. 191:*40.
7. Greengard, P. (1965) Determination by fluorometry. *Enzymatic Analysis* (H.-U. Bergmeyer, ed.). New York: Academic Press, pp. 551–555.
8. Harmon, J. and M. A. Aliapoulis (1972) Gynecomastia in marihuana users. *N. Engl. J. Med. 287:*936.
9. Hattori, T., A. Jakubovic, and P. L. McGeer (1972) Reduction in number of nuclear membrane-attached ribosomes in infant rat brain following acute Δ^9-tetrahydrocannabinol administration. *Exp. Neurol. 36:*207.
10. Hattori, T., A. Jakubovic, and P. L. McGeer (1973) The effect of cannabinoids on the number of nuclear membrane-attached ribosomes in the infant rat brain. *Neuropharmacology 12:*995.
11. Ho, B. T., G. E. Fritchie, P. M. Kralik, L. F. Englert, W. M. McIsaac, and J. Idänpään-Heikkilä (1970) Distribution of tritiated-1-Δ^9-tetrahydrocannabinol in rat tissues after inhalation. *J. Pharm. Pharmacol. 22:*538.
12. Jakubovic, A., R. M. Tait, and P. L. McGeer (1974) Excretion of THC and its metabolites in ewes' milk. *Toxicol. Appl. Pharmacol. 28:*38.
13. Jakubovic, A. and P. L. McGeer (1972) Inhibition of rat brain protein and nucleic acid synthesis by cannabinoids *in vitro. Can. J. Biochem. 50:*654.
14. Jakubovic, A. and P. L. McGeer (1972) The effect of Δ^9-tetrahydrocannabinol on infant rat brain nucleic acid and protein synthesis *in vivo.* Abstracts 2nd Annual Meeting Society for Neuroscience, Houston, Texas, p. 115.
15. Jakubovic, A., T. Hattori, and P. L. McGeer (1973) Radioactivity in suckled rats after giving ^{14}C-tetrahydrocannabinol to the mother. *Eur. J. Pharmacol. 22:*221.
16. Klausner, H. A. and J. V. Dingell (1971) The metabolism and excretion of Δ^9-tetrahydrocannabinol in the rat. *Life Sci. 10:*49.
17. Kolodny, R. C., W. H. Masters, R. M. Kolodner, and G. Toro (1974) Depression of plasma testosterone levels after chronic intensive marijuana use. *N. Engl. J. Med. 290:*872.
18. Lee, I. P. and R. L. Dixon (1972) Antineoplastic drug effects on spermatogenesis studied by velocity sedimentation cell separation. *Toxicol. Appl. Pharmacol. 23:*20.
19. Lemberger, L., N. R. Tamarkin, J. Axelrod, and I. J. Kopin (1971)

Delta-9-tetrahydrocannabinol: metabolism and disposition in long-term marihuana smokers. *Science 173:*72.

20. Luthra, V. K. and H. Rosenkrantz (1974) Cannabinoids: neurochemical aspects after oral chronic administration to rats. *Toxicol. Appl. Pharmacol. 27:*158.
21. Mechoulam, R., A. Shani, H. Edery, and Y. Grunfeld (1970) Chemical basis of hashish activity. *Science 169:*611.
22. Merari, A., A. Barak, and M. Plaves (1973) Effects of $\Delta^{1(2)}$-tetrahydrocannabinol on copulation in the male rat. *Psychopharmacologia 28:*243.
23. Nahas, G. G., N. Suciu-Foca, J.-P. Armand, and A. Morishima (1974) Inhibition of cellular mediated immunity in marihuana smokers. *Science 183:*419.
24. Perez-Reyes, M., M. C. Timmons, M. A. Lipton, H. D. Christensen, K. H. Davis, and M. E. Wall (1973) A comparison of the pharmacological activity of Δ^9-tetrahydrocannabinol and its monohydroxylated metabolites in man. *Experientia 29:*1009.
25. Schmidt, G. and J. J. Thannhauser (1945) A method for determination of desoxyribonucleic acid, ribonucleic acid, and phosphoproteins in animal tissues. *J. Biol. Chem. 161:*83.
26. Shahar, A. and T. Bino (1974) *In vitro* effects of Δ^9-tetrahydrocannabinol (THC) on bull sperm. *Biochem. Pharmacol. 23:*1341.
27. Zimmerman, A. M. and D. K. McClean (1973) Action of narcotics and hallucinogenic agents on the cell cycle. *Drugs and the Cell Cycle* (A. M. Zimmerman, G. M. Padilla, and I. L. Cameron, eds.). New York: Academic Press, pp. 67–94.
28. Zitko, B. A., J. F. Howes, R. K. Razdan, B. C. Dalzell, H. C. Dalzell, J. C. Sheehan, and H. G. Pars (1972) Water-soluble derivatives of Δ^1-tetrahydrocannabinol. *Science 177:*442.

21

Cytological and Cytochemical Effects of Whole Smoke and of the Gas Vapor Phase from Marihuana Cigarettes on Growth and DNA Metabolism of Cultured Mammalian Cells

CECILE LEUCHTENBERGER,
RUDOLF LEUCHTENBERGER, J. ZBINDEN,
AND E. SCHLEH

Introduction

Even though during the last decade smoking marihuana cigarettes has become widespread, with the exception of its hallucinogenic effects relatively little information is available regarding biological effects of the marihuana smoke on tissues, cells, and their metabolism. We considered an experimental investigation necessary especially to examine the following questions: 1. Does marihuana smoke alter the respiratory system; in particular, does long-term exposure contribute to or evoke pulmonary carcinogenesis? 2. Does marihuana smoke disturb DNA metabolism in somatic and germ cells; that is, does marihuana smoke interfere with the genetic material? 3. If alterations are demonstrable, are the responsible chemical constituents in the particulate or in the gas vapor phase of the marihuana smoke?

Our interest in exploring experimentally the biological effects of smoke from marihuana cigarettes was stimulated by our long-standing experimental studies started in 1956 on the effects of smoke from tobacco cigarettes on the respiratory system [10]. In our work on marihuana, we compared the biological effects of smoke from marihuana cigarettes with those of smoke from tobacco cigarettes. Such a comparison is necessary to obtain a standard of reference for assessing the alterations observed after marihuana smoke and also to avoid the pitfalls of interpreting results being

Marihuana: Chemistry, Biochemistry, and Cellular Effects, edited by Gabriel G. Nahas, © 1976 by Springer-Verlag New York Inc.

specific to marihuana smoke only. We also considered it essential to use exclusively fresh smoke, instead of individual components or condensates. The latter material has quite different physicochemical properties from those of fresh smoke. Fresh smoke—tobacco or marihuana—contains many components in the form of particles (particulate phase) and as gases and vapors (gas vapor phase) [20]. Thus, fresh smoke composed of particles, gases, and vapors, rather than condensates or extracts, comes into contact with the tissues and cells of the human who inhales cigarette smoke.

We report here comparative studies on animal and human lung cultures and on animal testis cultures after exposure to smoke from marihuana or tobacco cigarettes. In the model system we developed, cultures are exposed to puffs of fresh smoke under standardized conditions, proved to be a suitable bioassay to assess simultaneously time-sequential alterations in morphology, growth, and DNA metabolism of the various cells and chromosomes after short- and long-term exposure to fresh smoke from tobacco and/or marihuana cigarettes [1,3–6,8–12].

Material and Methods

For these studies cultures were prepared from (1) lungs (nontrypsinized, trypsinized) from mice, hamsters, and humans; and (2) testis from mice (nontrypsinized).

The cultures were exposed under standardized conditions in a Filtrona CSM_{12} smoking machine to puffs of fresh cigarette smoke. Cigarettes, all made with the same paper, were prepared with tobacco alone (Kentucky standard), with the same tobacco mixed with marihuana (0.5–1gm), and with marihuana alone (1.8 gm). The marihuana (UNC 303, 0.04 percent, 0.6 percent, and 4 percent THC) was obtained, after permission of the Health Department of the Swiss government, from Dr. Olav J. Braenden, Director, United Nations Narcotics Laboratory, Geneva, Switzerland. Detailed methods of preparation of cigarettes and of lung cultures, as well as the techniques of exposure to smoke, have been described in previous publications [8,9,11]. For these studies, 12 different experiments including over 5000 lung cultures have been employed.

Mouse testis explants were prepared from 3–5-month-old male mice (C57B1, C3H) by cutting 1-mm pieces and growing them on cover slips in Falcon dishes in Dulbecco-Eagle medium + 20 percent calf serum. Although no cell division was observed, there was a gradual outgrowth of interstitial and spermatogenic cells, especially of spermatids, which was most marked when testis explants were 12–18 days old. Twelve consecutive experiments were carried out on over 500 cultures. For each experiment, cover slips with matched testis explants were used. Besides unexposed controls, each set included cultures exposed to 2–6 puffs per day (25 ml at intervals of 58 sec) of fresh smoke from marihuana cigarettes for 2–6 days, and cultures exposed in the same manner to 2–4 puffs from Kentucky standard cigarettes. The lower number of puffs from Kentucky standard cigarettes was given because of the relatively high cytotoxic effects of this type of smoke on the cultures. The gas vapor phase of tobacco or marihuana smoke was obtained by passing the smoke through a Cambridge Filter, as previously described [6,7,9].

To assess time sequential changes, we examined regularly live cultures under a phase contrast microscope and original unsquashed stained cultures from 6 hr to over 1 yr after exposure. Cytological and cytochemical alterations were assessed simultaneously, focusing in the cytochemical studies special attention on the behavior of DNA. DNA metabolism was examined by autoradiography and by special quantitative cytochemical methods, such as Feulgen microspectrography and Feulgen microfluorometry [6]. These latter methods are unique for two reasons. First, the DNA content can be determined in a single cell or in part of a cell, such as the nucleus or the chromosomes; and second, the DNA can be analyzed *in situ* in the original cultures without destroying cell or tissue architecture. Thus, it is possible to compare morphology and DNA behavior directly on the same cell and from cell to cell and to detect changes in DNA before morphological alterations are apparent under the microscope. To determine whether the transformation obtained in the lung cultures was of malignant character, we injected the cultures subcutaneously into nude mice [3,5]. Malignancy of tumors observed in nude mice was established by histological diagnosis.

Results

We have performed four different types of experimental studies on mammalian cells with the following results.

Type 1

The first type of study consisted of comparing the effects on mouse lung cultures of short-term exposure to small doses of smoke from tobacco cigarettes and from cigarettes made of the same tobacco but to which marihuana was added.

We used a relatively small puff volume (8 ml) and a short exposure time so that the effects of tobacco cigarette smoke on lung cultures were minor.

We found that adding marihuana to tobacco cigarettes produced a smoke which evoked morphological and cytochemical alterations in cells of these lung explants to a significantly higher degree than did smoke from cigarettes without marihuana. Whereas after receiving small doses of cigarette smoke without marihuana the cells of the cultures resembled closely those of the monolayers in unexposed controls, after receiving the same small dose of cigarette smoke with marihuana, the cells assumed abnormal shapes, the size of nuclei and nucleoli increased markedly, and lagging of chromosomes and criss-cross formation were seen. These indications of abnormal proliferation were accompanied by a significant increase in the mitotic index and by stimulation of DNA synthesis. These features were statistically significant not only in comparison with the values of nonexposed controls, but also when compared with the frequencies of cultures exposed to tobacco cigarette smoke without marihuana. There were also striking differences in the DNA content. In control cultures and in cultures exposed to cigarette smoke without marihuana, cells with 2 DNA content were 8–10 times more common than cells with 4 DNA content; yet in cultures exposed to cigarette smoke with marihuana, the number of cells with 2 DNA content decreased, whereas those with 4 DNA content increased significantly, displaying 2 DNA: 4 DNA ratios of 2:1 instead of 10:1 or 8:1 in controls or after exposure to cigarette smoke, respectively.

Results mentioned here were published in detail previously [9].

Type 2

The second type of study consisted of comparing the effects on human lung cultures of longer term exposure to larger doses of smoke from cigarettes made of Kentucky standard tobacco and of smoke from cigarettes made of marihuana only.

For this study on human lung cultures, we used longer exposure times and larger puff volumes (25 ml) of smoke from Kentucky tobacco and marihuana cigarettes than in the study on mouse lung cultures (8 ml). This larger puff volume was chosen because it resembles more closely the standard puff volume of 35 ml inhaled by human smokers.

We found that the sequential alterations in human lung cultures (adult or fetal lung) were similar after exposure to smoke from marihuana cigarettes and after exposure to smoke from Kentucky

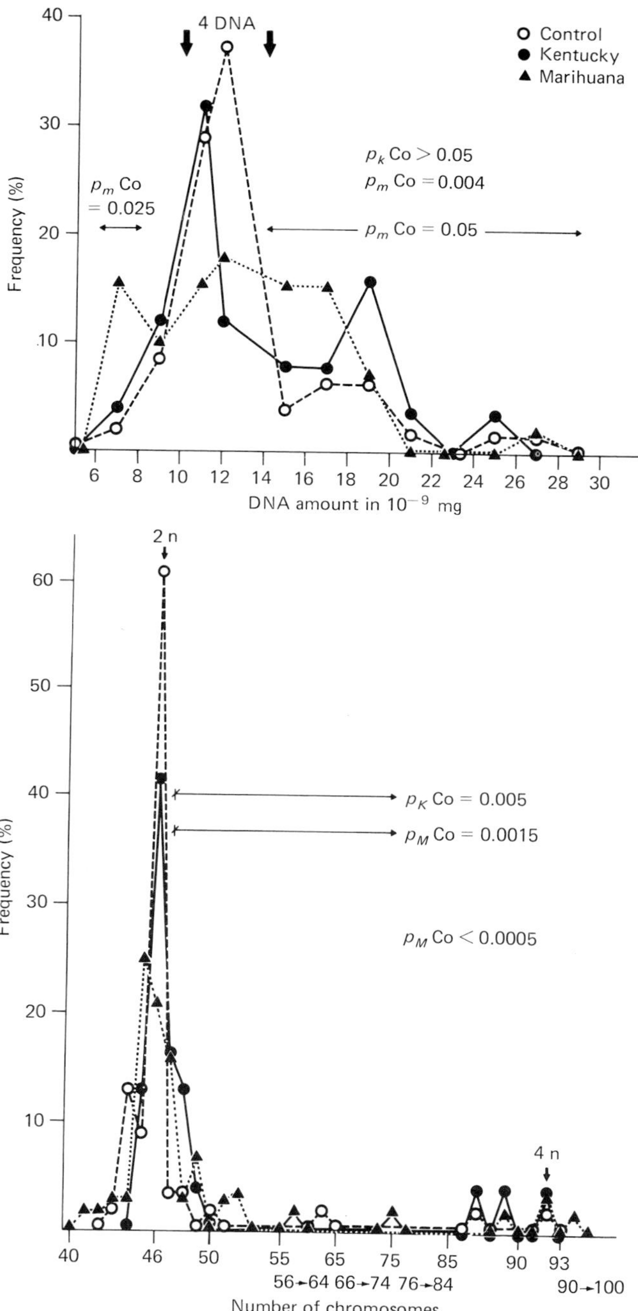

Figure 21.1. Comparison between the DNA content (Feulgen microfluorometry) in telophases ($n_1 = 224$) and number of chromosomes ($n_2 = 633$) from control adult human lung explants, and after exposure to fresh smoke from marihuana (M) and Kentucky (K) cigarettes. n_1 = number of cells measured; n_2 = number of metaphases counted.

standard cigarettes. Each type of smoke evoked first inhibition of DNA synthesis and mitosis, followed by abnormalities in cell morphology and mitosis and irregular, abnormal growth. Furthermore, after exposure to each type of smoke, the human lung cultures had an increased number of dividing cells characterized by a marked variability in number and DNA content of chromosomes; in other words, there was a disturbance of the genetic equilibrium of the cell population (Figure 21.1). This derangement was especially pronounced after exposure to smoke from marihuana cigarettes. After marihuana smoke, there was greater variability in the DNA content of chromosomes, and there appeared to be a more notable tendency toward lower DNA content and lower numbers of chromosomes than after tobacco (Kentucky) cigarette smoke (Figure 21.1).

Therefore, fresh smoke from marihuana cigarettes appears to produce atypical growth in human lung cultures as does smoke from tobacco cigarettes, and marihuana also seems to evoke even more marked changes in the genetic material and chromosomes than does tobacco. The similarity of atypical growth of human lung cultures after marihuana and tobacco smoke gains special significance when the role of tobacco cigarette smoke in pulmonary carcinogenesis is considered. Unfortunately, neither the human adult nor the human fetal lung cultures survived long enough to examine the effects of continued long-term exposure to tobacco or marihuana cigarette smoke. Therefore, these studies on human lung cultures do not provide conclusive evidence as to whether the atypical changes observed were precancerous changes that would progress to cancer when exposure to smoke was continued for a long period. For this reason, the following study on hamster lung cultures, which have a longer survival time, was carried out. The results reported here were published in detail previously [8,11].

Type 3

In the third type of study, we compared the effects on hamster lung cultures of short- and long-term exposure to larger doses of smoke from cigarettes made of Kentucky standard tobacco and of smoke from cigarettes made of marihuana only (whole smoke, gas vapor phase). Attention was focused on the following questions:

1. Does continued and long-term exposure to fresh smoke from tobacco or from marihuana cigarettes evoke sequential alterations that progress to malignant cell transformation?
2. Are the changes produced only by whole smoke—that is, by smoke which contains particulate phase and gas vapor phase—

or by the gas vapor phase alone (smoke which does not contain particulate matter)?

In order to answer these questions, we exposed the hamster lung cultures to fresh puffs of whole tobacco smoke, the gas vapor phase of tobacco smoke, whole marihuana smoke, or the gas vapor phase of marihuana smoke. Puff volumes were 25 ml. The cultures were exposed daily to 4–6 puffs for 3 consecutive days per week for periods up to 35 weeks. The time-sequential changes in control and exposed cultures were assessed regularly in live and fixed cultures from 1 day to 35 weeks or longer.

The salient features of the sequential changes observed in hamster lung cultures after exposure and in nonexposed control cultures are presented in the Figure 21.2. The three stages were observed in all exposed cultures, regardless of whether whole tobacco or whole marihuana smoke or their gas vapor phases alone were used. However, the cytotoxic effect after marihuana smoke was less than that after tobacco smoke in stage I, which occurred from 1–7 days after exposure. This decreased cytotoxicity may be due to the fact that smoke from marihuana cigarettes has a larger side stream than smoke from tobacco cigarettes; that is, less marihuana smoke reached the cultures than tobacco smoke. In spite of this lesser cytotoxicity, proliferative alterations in stage II occurring within 3–10 weeks of exposure to whole smoke or the gas vapor phase were especially striking after marihuana smoke. This was particularly the case after exposure to the gas vapor phase of marihuana, when the size of nucleoli, nuclei, and cytoplasm increased enormously. Furthermore, mitotic abnormalities—such as lagging of chromosomes, presence of pieces of chromosomes in the cytoplasm, enlarged spindles, variability of DNA content, and rapid abnormal growth—were more marked after the gas vapor phase or whole smoke from marihuana than after smoke from tobacco cigarettes.

On continued exposure to either type of smoke, the cells gradually lost their epithelial appearance, and the cultures displayed more and more irregular growth of abnormal fibroblasts with criss-cross formation and piling up. Stage III, the malignant transformation of the cells, occurred in these cultures within 6 months of exposure. When 1×10^6 cells of such exposed cultures were injected into nude mice, fibrosarcomas were observed at the injection site within 10–20 days. At this period the nonexposed control cultures rarely displayed alterations, and even when more than 1×10^6 cells of the control cultures were injected into nude mice, no fibro-

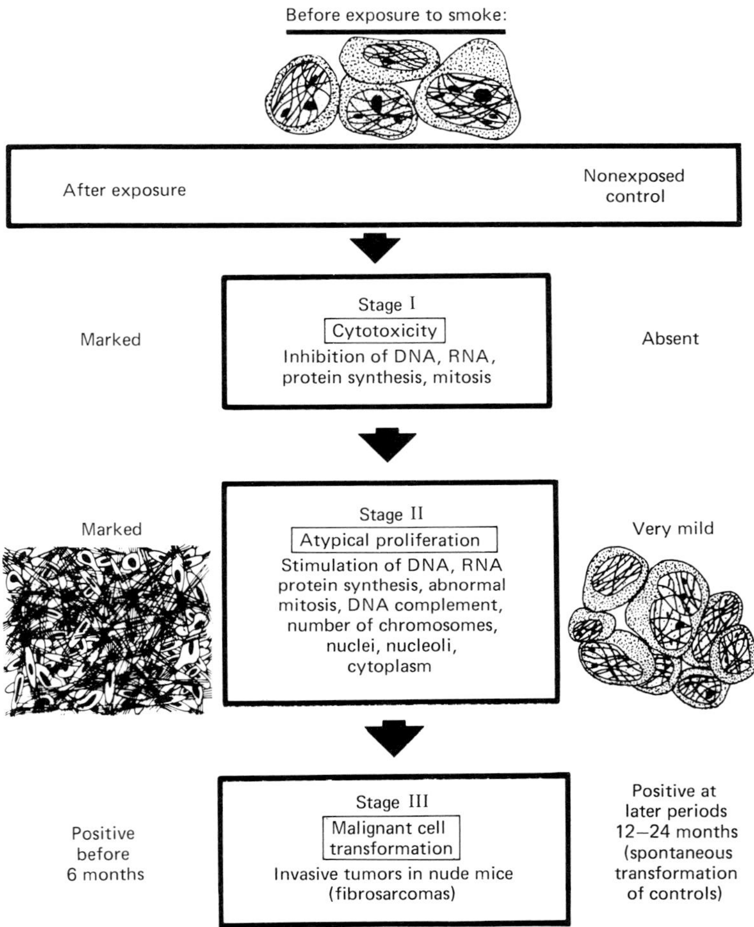

Figure 21.2. Time sequential effects of fresh tobacco and marihuana cigarette smoke on hamster lung cells.

sarcomas were produced. The growth rate of the control cultures at 6 months was only about 10–30 percent of that of the exposed cultures. However, on continued aging, the control cultures underwent alterations similar to those seen in stages II and III of the exposed cultures. Between the ages of 12 and 24 months, a considerable number of the control cultures displayed malignant transformation, producing on injection the same fibrosarcomas in nude mice [5]. The spontaneous malignant transformation of aged hamster lung cultures has also been reported by Okumura [15].

Therefore, smoke from marihuana cigarettes appears to accelerate malignant transformation of cultured lung cells as does smoke from tobacco cigarettes. The finding that this effect was obtained not only with whole smoke, but also with the gas vapor phase alone of marihuana or of tobacco smoke, indicates that mainly gas vapor phase constituents were responsible for enhancing malignant transformation.

Type 4

In the fourth type of experiment, we compared the effects on mouse testis cultures of short-term exposure to smoke from cigarettes made of Kentucky standard tobacco and from cigarettes made of marihuana only (whole smoke, gas vapor phase). We studied primarily the behavior of the spermatids regarding alterations in morphology and DNA content.

In living as well as in fixed and stained cultures, there were no significant differences in morphology of spermatids between control cultures and those exposed to whole smoke from Kentucky standard cigarettes. However, after exposure to whole smoke from marihuana cigarettes, a considerable number of spermatids had smaller nuclei and showed less staining with basic dyes when compared with spermatids of control cultures and those after exposure to Kentucky smoke. There were also no significant differences in the DNA complement of spermatids between control cultures and those exposed to Kentucky tobacco smoke. However, after whole marihuana smoke there was a statistically significant increased frequency of spermatids carrying a DNA complement lower than 1 DNA (Figure 21.3). Results were reproducible in all 12 experiments except in one set in which marihuana smoke had no effect on the DNA complement.

The observation that whole smoke from marihuana cigarettes evokes abnormalities in DNA complement of spermatids in cultured mouse testis is in good agreement with results obtained in living mice. Male mice inhaling whole smoke from marihuana cigarettes had a disturbance in spermatogenesis and an increased frequency of spermatids with reduced DNA content [5]. Furthermore, degenerating forms of spermatids and fragmented sperms were seen in mice after tetrahydrocannabinol (THC) administration (2).

To determine whether the responsible factors in the marihuana smoke are in the particulate or in the gas vapor phase, we also exposed testis cultures to the gas vapor phase of marihuana smoke.

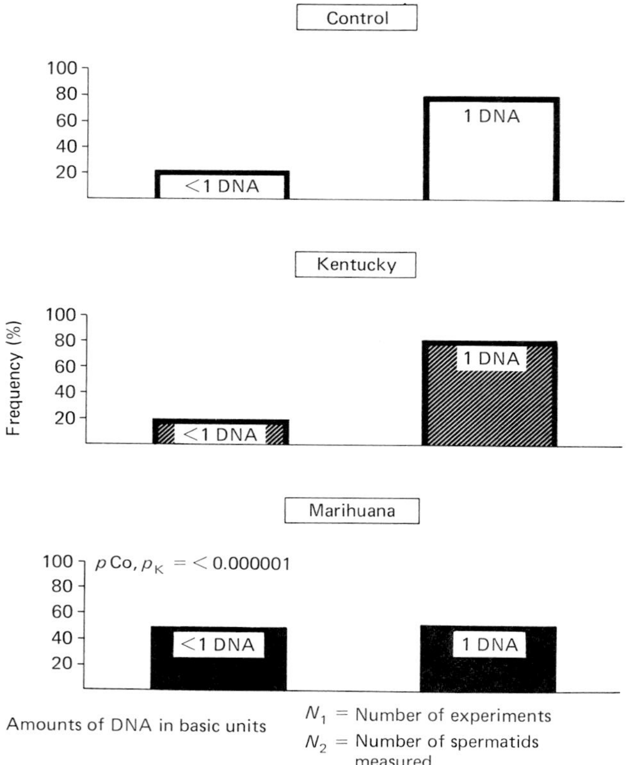

Figure 21.3. Comparison between DNA content (microfluorometry) in spermatids ($n_1 = 12$; $n_2 = 1750$) from mouse testis explants in control cultures and after exposure to 2–6 puffs daily for 2–6 days of fresh smoke from standard Kentucky and marihuana cigarettes.

No significant alterations in morphology or in the DNA content of the spermatids were observed after exposure to the gas vapor phase of marihuana smoke.

Discussion

The essential findings in each study were:

1. Adding marihuana to tobacco produced smoke that evoked more abnormalities in mouse lung cells than did smoke from tobacco cigarettes alone.

2. Smoke from marihuana cigarettes evoked in human lung cultures atypical growth similar to that of smoke from tobacco cigarettes. However, smoke from marihuana cigarettes produced more severe alterations in DNA content and number of chromosomes in these cultures than smoke from tobacco cigarettes.
3. Malignant cell transformation of hamster lung cultures was enhanced after whole smoke or the gas vapor phase of tobacco cigarettes.
4. After exposure of mouse testis cultures to whole smoke from marihuana cigarettes, the frequency of spermatids with reduced DNA complement was increased. Such a deviation was not observed after whole smoke from tobacco or after the gas vapor phase of marihuana cigarettes.

It thus appears that fresh smoke from marihuana cigarettes has a harmful effect not only on cultured cells of the respiratory system, but also on cultured spermatids of the male reproductive system. We found that smoke from marihuana cigarettes contributes to pulmonary carcinogenesis, and marihuana smoke interferes with the genetic material in somatic and germ cells. Furthermore, the data also indicate that the factors responsible for the abnormal alterations in the respiratory system are in the gas vapor phase of marihuana smoke, whereas the alterations in the DNA complement in the germ cells are probably mainly due to constituents in the particulate phase of marihuana smoke.

The finding that sequential changes of atypical growth and malignant transformation were similar between lung cultures after exposure to smoke from marihuana and from tobacco cigarettes indicates that the effects on the lungs are not specific for the marihuana smoke and also strongly suggests that chronic inhalation of marihuana smoke may play a similar role in human pulmonary carcinogenesis as does chronic inhalation of tobacco smoke. This concept gains support from the studies of Tennant on human marihuana smokers [19]. However, no definite conclusions can be drawn until extensive epidemiological data on human marihuana smokers become available.

That the gas vapor phase of marihuana smoke led to the same abnormal growth and enhancement of malignant transformation in lung cultures as did whole smoke of marihuana is noteworthy. It also indicates the similarity between effects on lungs of marihuana and tobacco smoke, the gas vapor phase of which is as effective as the whole smoke [7,10,12], but it also points to the necessity to search for carcinogenic or cocarcinogenic constituents in the gas vapor phase of marihuana smoke and their effects on other tissues and organs.

The striking abnormalities in mitosis and number of chromosomes demonstrable after exposure of animal and human lung cultures to marihuana smoke resembled those found in cultured white blood cells derived from human marihuana smokers. Morishima observed disturbance in chromosomal numbers [13], Stenchever *et al.* reported increased chromosome breakage [18], and Nahas and coworkers demonstrated inhibition of mitosis [14].

Although the enhancement of malignant cell transformation in the cultured lungs after marihuana smoke cannot be considered to be specific for marihauna smoke per se, the greater disturbance of the genetic equilibrium in chromosomes of the lung cell population after marihuana than after tobacco smoke would suggest that smoke from marihuana has special constituents that may affect DNA. The observation that a significant increase in frequency of spermatids with reduced DNA complement was noted only after exposure to whole marihuana smoke and not after exposure to tobacco smoke supports this concept. Since the gas vapor phase of marihuana smoke had no significant effect on the DNA complement of the spermatids, it is not unreasonable to ascribe the difference in biological activity to a difference in chemical composition of the particulate phase of tobacco and marihuana smoke [16,17].

Whether cannabinoids, THC, or other particulate components of marihuana smoke are responsible, and whether they have a direct effect on the DNA or impair reduction division cannot be determined at present. Nevertheless, the low DNA complement in spermatids of cultured mouse testis after whole marihuana smoke is an alteration that may have serious consequences for the genetic information if a sperm derived from a spermatid with low DNA content fertilizes an egg. The finding of a reduced DNA complement in mouse spermatids after exposure to whole marihuana smoke demands not only similar studies on spermatids of cultured human testis, but also comparative DNA analysis in sperm cells of human tobacco and marihuana smokers.

ACKNOWLEDGMENT

We thank Dr. O. Braenden, Director, Division of Narcotic Drugs, U.N.O., Geneva, for the marihuana.

This work was supported by grants from WHO and ASFC, Switzerland.

REFERENCES

1. Davies, P., G. S. Kistler, C. Leuchtenberger, and R. Leuchtenberger (1975) Ultrastructural studies on cells of hamster lung cultures after chronic exposure to whole smoke or the gas vapour phase of cigarettes. *Beitr. Pathol. 155:*168.
2. Dixit, V. P., V. P. Sharma, and N. K. Lohiya (1974) The effect of chronically administered cannabis extracts on the testicular function of mice. *Eur. J. Pharmacol. 26:*111.
3. Leuchtenberger, C. (1974) Enhancement of malignant transformation in hamster lung cultures after exposures to fresh cigarette smoke (Kentucky standard). Abstract Florence, XIth International Cancer Congress, October.
4. Leuchtenberger, C. and R. Leuchtenberger (1972) Abnormalities of mitosis, DNA metabolism and growth in human lung cultures, exposed to smoke from marihuana cigarettes, and their similarity with alterations evoked by tobacco cigarette smoke. Scientific Research on Cannabis. United Nations Bulletin, ST/SOA/SER.S/37, November.
5. Leuchtenberger, C. and R. Leuchtenberger (1975) Correlated cytological and cytochemical studies of the effects of fresh smoke from marihuana cigarettes on growth and DNA metabolism of animal and human lung cultures. Proceedings of the International Conference on the Pharmacology of Cannabis, Savannah, Dec. 3–6, 1974 (in press).
6. Leuchtenberger, C. and R. Leuchtenberger (1970) Differential cytological and cytochemical responses of various cultures from mouse tissues to repeated exposures to puffs from the gas phase of charcoal-filtered cigarette smoke. *Exp. Cell Res. 62:*161.
7. Leuchtenberger, C. and R. Leuchtenberger (1970) Effects of chronic inhalation of whole fresh cigarette smoke and of its gas phase on pulmonary tumorigenesis in Snell's mice. *Morphology of Experimental Respiratory Carcinogenesis.* U.S. Atomic Energy Commission, division of technical information, 21st AEC Symposium Series, December, pp. 329–346.
8. Leuchtenberger, C. and R. Leuchtenberger (1973) Effects of marihuana and tobacco smoke on human lung physiology. *Nature 241:* 137.
9. Leuchtenberger, C. and R. Leuchtenberger (1971) Morphological and cytochemical effects of marihuana cigarette smoke on epitheloid cells of lung explants from mice. *Nature 234:*227.
10. Leuchtenberger, C. and R. Leuchtenberger (1974) The experimental exploration of health damaging factors in cigarette smoke. *Sozial Präventivmed. 19:*41.
11. Leuchtenberger, C., R. Leuchtenberger, U. Ritter, and N. Inui (1973) Effects of marihuana and tobacco smoke on DNA and chromosomal complement in human lung explants. *Nature 242:*403.
12. Leuchtenberger, C., R. Leuchtenberger, and I. Zbinden (1974) Gas vapour phase constituents and SH reactivity of cigarette smoke influence lung cultures. *Nature 247:*565.

13. Morishima, A. (1974) Marihuana-hashish epidemic and its impact on United States security. Ninety-Third Congress, Second Session, May 9,16,17,20,21 and June 13, 1974. U.S. Government Printing Office, Washington D.C. 20402, pp. 109–117.
14. Nahas, G. G., N. Suciu-Foca, J. P. Armaud, and A. Morishima (1974) Inhibition of cellular mediated immunity in marihuana smokers. *Science 183*(4123):419.
15. Okumura, H. (1968) Spontaneous malignant transformation of hamster lung cells in tissue culture. *Cancer Cells in Culture.* (Hajim Katsuta, ed.). Baltimore: University Park Press, pp. 229–274.
16. Paton, W. D. M. (1975) Pharmacology of marihuana. *Annu. Rev. Pharmacol. 15:*191.
17. Report of a working group on the chemistry of cannabis smoke. Athens, United Nations Document MNAR/6/1975.
18. Stenchever, M. A., T. J. Kunysz, and M. A. Allen (1974) Chromosome breakage in users of marihuana. *Am. J. Obstet. Gynecol. 118*(1):106.
19. Tennant, F. S. (1974) Marihuana-hashish epidemic and its impact on United States security. Ninety-Third Congress, Second Session, May 9,16,17,20,21 and June 13, 1974. U.S. Government Printing Office, Washington D.C., 20402, pp. 288–314.
20. Wynder, E. L. and D. Hoffman (1967) *Tobacco and Tobacco Smoke.* New York: Academic Press.

22

Effects of Δ^8-Tetrahydrocannabinol, Δ^9-Tetrahydrocannabinol, and Crude Marihuana on Human Cells in Tissue Culture

MORTON A. STENCHEVER, KATHRYN J. PARKS, AND MARC R. STENCHEVER

In recent years a moderate controversy has arisen with respect to the possible cytotoxic effects of marihuana and its related compounds. Neu *et al.* [6] studied Δ^9-tetrahydrocannabinol (Δ^9-THC) in *in vitro* experiments with human leukocytes and found no increase in chromosome abnormalities. Stenchever and Allen [9] demonstrated similar negative findings in an experiment in which the Δ^9-THC was placed in tissue culture media after phytohemagglutinin had been added to the leukocytes. In these experiments the Δ^9-THC was present throughout the entire 72 hr of culture, and a number of concentrations ranging from 0.1–100 μg/cc of culture medium were studied. At the higher concentrations, there was a noticeable increase in cell death and decreased mitotic activity. Pace *et al.* similarly could find no chromosome damage in rat cells after exposure to marihuana resins [8]. Martin and coworkers [4] exposed both embryonic rat fibroblasts and human leukocytes to cannabis resins *in vitro* in separate studies and demonstrated a dose-related decrease in mitotic rate but no increase in chromosome abnormalities.

Gilmour and coworkers [1] studied several psychoactive drugs and found no increase in chromosome aberrations in "slight" users of marihuana. However, they did find an increase in chromosome breakage in 11 "heavy" users. Most of these users were taking multiple drugs. Stenchever *et al.* [10] demonstrated a significant chromosome breakage rate in a group of 49 college students who were using marihuana when this group was compared with a group of control individuals. These investigators could not relate the degree of damage to the extent of use, association with other drug use, or sex of the individual. However, all users had been smoking marihuana for a minimum of 5 months. Morishima has presented

Marihuana: Chemistry, Biochemistry, and Cellular Effects, edited by Gabriel G. Nahas,

data which imply that aneuploidy may be increased in lymphocytes of marihuana users [5].

The purpose of the present group of experiments was to investigate possible chromosome damage and aneuploidy in human leukocytes pretreated in tissue culture for 4 hr with Δ^8-THC, Δ^9-THC, and crude marihuana extract in varying concentrations.

Materials and Methods

Appropriate amounts of Δ^8-THC, Δ^9-THC, and crude marihuana were dissolved in 0.1 ml dimethyl sulfoxide (DMSO) so that when the agent was added to 10 ml of whole blood, the desired concentration of the particular agent would be produced. For each agent, 60 ml of whole blood was drawn in a heparinized syringe from a male and a female donor. These were young, healthy, individuals who had never used marihuana and who had not been exposed knowingly to a chromosome-breaking agent for at least 1 yr. In addition, each donor had had no x-ray exposure for at least 6 months. For each study the blood was divided into six 10-ml aliquots. For Δ^9-THC, the study compound was added to each of four tubes to give final concentrations of 100.0 μg, 10.0 μg, 1.0 μg, and 0.1 μg/ml. Added to a fifth tube was 0.1 ml DMSO, and a sixth tube had nothing added and served as a pure control.

For the crude marihuana extract and Δ^8-THC experiments, four cultures were inoculated with aliquots of the agent to make final concentrations of 200.0 μg, 100.0 μg, 10.0 μg, and 1.0 μg/ml of blood. For each agent, a DMSO and pure control was established. All experiments were handled in a fashion similar to that stated above, and all were incubated at 37 °C for 4 hr. Phytohemagglutinin was then added, and the tubes were placed in ice for 30 min. The material was centrifuged at 500 rpm for 5 min, and the serum containing leukocytes was removed and split into three equal aliquots. Minimal Eagle's medium was added to make final volumes of 10 ml, and the cultures were incubated at 37 °C for 72 hr. Two hours before harvesting, 0.3 ml Colcemid was added to each culture. The cells were then harvested in a manner standard for the laboratory. Air-dried preparations were made, and slides were coded for blind scoring. Each concentration was evaluated by two individuals with each scoring 50 consecutive, intact-appearing, metaphase spreads for chromatid and isochromatid gaps and breaks and for abnormal forms such as tetraploids, rings, triradials, and quadriradials. In addition, the cells in the crude marihuana experiment were evaluated for chromosome number with each 100 spreads being counted. All spreads demonstrating either chromosome damage or aneuploidy were photographed for more complete evaluation.

Results

Table 22.1 summarizes the data found in the crude marihuana experiments with respect to breaks, gaps, and aneuploidy. Isochromatid and chromatid lesions are combined because of the small number involved in each case. No significant differences were noted between any of the study concentrations and either control culture in both the male and the female subject. No abnormal forms were noted. A statistically significant increase in cells with aneuploidy exists at the 200 and 100 μg concentrations in the male and at the 100 μg concentration in the female when compared to the control cultures ($p < 0.05$). No significant differences were noted at the lower concentrations, although in some cases a trend toward aneuploidy seemed to be present.

Table 22.2 summarizes the data with respect to gaps and breaks seen in the Δ^9-THC experiments. Table 22.3 demonstrates similar data for the Δ^8-THC experiments. In neither group of experiments

Table 22.1 Breaks, gaps, and aneuploidy seen in cells exposed to crude marihuana extract

	Concentration (μg/ml)	Cells scored (No.)	Cells with breaks No.	Cells with breaks %	Cells with gaps No.	Cells with gaps %	Aneuploid No.	Aneuploid %
Female	200	100	3	3	0	0	4	4
	100	100	2	2	0	0	12	12
	10	100	0	0	1	1	4	4
	1	100	1	1	0	0	2	2
	(DMSO) 0	100	2	2	0	0	2	2
	0	100	4	4	0	0	2	2
Male	200	100	3	3	2	2	10	10
	100	100	5	5	0	0	9	9
	10	100	0	0	0	0	7	7
	1	100	5	5	1	1	4	4
	(DMSO) 0	100	2	2	1	1	4	4
	0	100	0	0	1	1	1	1

Table 22.2 Breaks and gaps seen in cells exposed to Δ^9-THC

	Concentration (μg/ml)		Cells (no.)	Cells with breaks		Cells with gaps	
				No.	%	No.	%
Female		100.0	100	1	1	2	2
		10.0	100	3	3	3	3
		1.0	100	2	2	4	4
		0.1	100	1	1	2	2
	(DMSO)	0.0	100	1	1	1	1
		0.0	100	2	2	1	1
Male		100.0	100	0	0	3	3
		10.0	100	0	0	0	0
		1.0	100	1	1	2	2
		0.1	100	0	0	1	1
	(DMSO)	0.0	100	0	0	2	2
		0.0	100	0	0	0	0

were any significant differences noted for any of the concentrations when compared to the controls. Again no abnormal forms were seen. At the 200 μg concentration of Δ^8-THC, little mitotic activity was noted.

Table 22.3 Breaks and gaps seen in cells exposed to Δ^8-THC

	Concentration (μg/ml)		Cells (no.)	Cells with breaks		Cells with gaps	
				No.	%	No.	%
Female		200	0	—	—	—	—
		100	90	1	1.1	3	3.3
		10	100	1	1.0	3	3.0
		1	100	1	1.0	4	4.0
	(DMSO)	0	100	4	4.0	0	0.0
		0	100	2	2.0	0	0.0
Male		200	38	1	2.6	0	0.0
		100	100	1	1.0	2	2.0
		10	100	1	1.0	0	0.0
		1	100	1	1.0	0	0.0
	(DMSO)	0	100	2	2.0	0	0.0
		0	100	0	0.0	0	0.0

Discussion

All of the studies described in this report were carried out on cultures that had been incubated with the respective study substance for 4 hr before adding phytohemagglutinin. This is a short exposure time, and since no chromosome damage was noted, two possible conclusions may be reached. The first is that the substances studied did not cause chromosome damage; the second is that these substances are capable of causing chromosome damage but require a longer exposure time in order to induce possible abnormalities. The latter is very likely since lymphocytes are in all stages of the cell cycle until phytohemagglutinin is added, and it is possible that only a small number are susceptible at any particular point. It is also likely that the production of chromosome damage requires a critical period of time, perhaps to activate certain biological systems within the cells. Four hours may be far too short a time to accomplish this. Therefore, it seems reasonable to institute more chronic studies in tissue culture systems using a cell that may be transferred through several passages in order to ascertain the effect of chronic exposure. Such experiments are currently underway in our laboratory.

It is of interest that the 4-hr exposure to the stronger doses of the crude marihuana extract did lead to an increase in aneuploidy. This is in keeping with the observations made on chronic users by Morishima [5] and suggests that the spindle may be somewhat sensitive to the effects of something in the cannabis resin. These observations have definite clinical implications: if exposure to cannabis can increase the degree of aneuploidy, then the possible production of cells with aneuploidy within the human may lead to such problems as trisomy if the germ cells are affected or to aneuploid cells with tumor potential in somatic cell systems. Certainly more studies and observations are necessary in this respect to clarify precise mechanisms involved.

Chromatid and isochromatid breaks and abnormal forms are undoubtedly signs of cytotoxicity, but newer tools are now available to diagnose more subtle changes such as inversions, insertions, and sister chromatid exchanges. By using special staining and banding techniques, one can identify some of these problems. The *in vitro* chromosome breakage studies should probably be repeated using these techniques.

There are several reasons why various laboratories seem to be reporting different results in studies on cannabis users and on cannabis substances in tissue culture. First, it is rather useless to study the effects of cannabis given to individuals who are already using marihuana. If one assumes that lymphocytes have an average life span of 6 months *in vivo,* the stopping of cannabis use for a few weeks and then the reinstitution of exposure under laboratory control does not really establish the potential damaging effects of the laboratory-administered drug since the effects of chronic use are probably still present. Therefore, it does not seem reasonable to consider as "control" the individual's blood before starting the laboratory portion of the experiment. Although it is morally and philosophically unacceptable to use naive subjects to determine the effects of cannabis, it is possible through studies of large, youthful populations at varying times to detect the effects of cannabis use with the individual serving as his own control before beginning to use the drug. Perhaps other study systems can be designed to help answer this baffling question of whether cannabis use does lead to chromosome damage.

A second reason for variation may involve the route of ingestion. Stenchever *et al.* studied smokers [10], whereas Leuchtenberger and Leuchtenberger [2] and Leuchtenberger *et al.* [3] exposed fatal mouse lung cells to marihuana smoke and noted positive morphological and cytochemical effects. However, Nichols *et al.* [7] found no cytogenetic changes in users who ingested the marihuana. Again, the experimental designs must be standardized before the studies can be compared appropriately.

A third consideration concerns the exposure time in *in vitro* systems and, indeed, even on the *in vitro* system chosen for study. For data from different laboratories to be meaningful, the same systems, the same exposure time, and certainly the same scoring techniques are necessary. In addition, the exchange of material for scoring spot checks between laboratories would seem useful. Certainly, every effort must be made to eliminate observer bias. The use of coded slides, blind scoring techniques, and a clear understanding of criteria for scoring would seem to be minimum requirements for such collaborative efforts.

Unlike studies of other drugs, cannabis studies, especially when human subjects are concerned, pose so many social and philosophical problems that it is extremely common for qualified investigators to avoid them. However, because of the widespread use of cannabis, such research is extremely necessary and should be encouraged.

ACKNOWLEDGMENTS

This research was supported by a grant from the Brush Foundation of Cleveland. Cannabis substances supplied by the National Institute of Health.

REFERENCES

1. Gilmour, D. G., A. D. Bloom, K. P. Lele, E. S. Robbins, and C. Maximilian (1971) Chromosome aberrations in users of psychoactive drugs. *Arch. Gen. Psychiatry 24:*268.
2. Leuchtenberger, C. and R. Leuchtenberger (1971) Morphological and cytochemical effects of marijuana cigarette smoke on epitheloid cells of lung explants from mice. *Nature 234:*227.
3. Leuchtenberger, C., R. Leuchtenberger, and A. Schneider (1973) Effects of marijuana and tobacco smoke on human lung physiology. *Nature 241:*137.
4. Martin, P. A., M. J. Thorburn, and S. A. Bryant (1974) In vivo and in vitro studies of the cytogenetic effects of cannabis sativa in rats and men. *Teratology 9:*81.
5. Morishima, A. (1974) Statement before the subcommittee on internal security committee on the judiciary, United States Senate, May 16.
6. Neu, R. L., H. O. Powes, S. King, and L. I. Gardner (1969) Cannabis and chromosomes. *Lancet 1:*675.
7. Nichols, W. W., R. C. Miller, W. Heneen, C. Bradt, L. Hollister, and S. Kanter (1974) Cytogenetic studies on human subjects receiving marijuana and Δ-9-tetrahydrocannabinol. *Mutat. Res. 26:*413.
8. Pace, H. D., W. M. Davis, and L. A. Borgen (1971) Teratogenesia and marihuana. *Ann. N.Y. Acad. Sci. 191:*123.
9. Stenchever, M. A. and M. Allen (1972) The effect of delta-9-tetrahydrocannabinol on the chromosomes of human lymphocytes in culture. *Am. J. Obstet. Gynecol. 114:*819.
10. Stenchever, M. A., T. J. Kunysz, and M. A. Allen (1974) Chromosome breakage in users of marihuana. *Am. J. Obstet. Gynecol. 118:*106.

23

Errors of Chromosome Segregation Induced by Olivetol, a Compound with the Structure of C-Ring Common to Cannabinoids: Formation of Bridges and Multipolar Divisions

AKIRA MORISHIMA, RICHARD T. HENRICH,
SEN JOU, AND GABRIEL G. NAHAS

In a previous study, we observed an increased incidence of metaphase nuclei containing less than 30 chromosomes ("micronuclei") [6] in cultured human lymphocytes obtained from chronic marihuana smokers. In the same study, we reported that a similar increase in "micronuclei" could be induced in lymphocytes of nonsmokers by adding Δ^9-tetrahydrocannabinol (Δ^9-THC) in a concentration of 6.4×10^{-6} *M* or olivetol in a concentration of 1.5×10^{-4} *M* to the culture medium. Olivetol, or 5-*n*-amylresorcinol, has the C-ring structure common to all cannabinoids.

In separate studies we have shown that ^{3}H-thymidine incorporation by partially purified thymus-derived lymphocytes (T-cells) obtained from chronic marihuana smokers is inhibited [11] and that a similar inhibition can be induced in T-cells of nonsmokers by adding Δ^8-THC or Δ^9-THC, their hydroxylated derivatives, and four nonpsychoactive cannabinoids—cannabinol, cannabidiol, cannabichromene, and cannabicyclol—to the culture medium in concentrations between 10^{-4} *M* and 10^{-5} *M* [7–10]. A similar effect was observed after adding olivetol to the medium [7–10].

A rapid inhibition of RNA and protein synthesis by lymphocytes exposed to Δ^9-THC, other cannabinoids, or olivetol has also been observed [9,10].

The depressant effects of marihuana products on DNA, RNA, and protein synthesis by various cells have been corroborated by the studies of others, many of which are reported in this book.

In consideration of the experimental evidence cited above, we developed a tentative model of action of the cannabinoids and olivetol on cellular function [6]: cannabinoids and olivetol may

Marihuana: Chemistry, Biochemistry, and Cellular Effects, edited by Gabriel G. Nahas,

first inhibit the cellular synthesis of protein and RNA, which in turn may decrease DNA synthesis. The decreased protein synthesis may also lead to disturbance in the formation of microtubules and spindles, resulting in segregational errors of chromosomes. "Micronuclei" arising from this process will have decreased DNA templates per cell, and hence the total DNA synthesis will be diminished. The present study was designed to determine whether olivetol could induce segregational errors of chromosomes.

Materials and Methods

Six healthy adult males, 23–45 yr of age, were used for the study. None of these subjects had ever used marihuana products. One individual who smoked tobacco was included in the study, since a previous study revealed that no cytogenetic changes are attributable to tobacco smoking [4]. Women were excluded from the study in order to eliminate the possible effect of estrogen on mitosis [5].

Twenty milliliters of heparinized blood was obtained from each subject. Partially purified T-cells were obtained from these samples by density gradient centrifugation using Ficoll-Isopaque [1]. After three washings with RPMI 1640 medium, cells were counted and aliquots of the suspension sufficient to yield 10^6 cells/ml of culture medium were placed in the flasks. The medium consisted of 3.6 ml of RPMI 1640 to which 15 percent autologous plasma and 1 percent phytohemagglutinin (PHA) were added.

Four cultures were established from each blood specimen. Two cultures served as the control, and the other two as the experimental series. Olivetol solution in absolute ethanol was diluted with RPMI 1640 and was added to the experimental culture in a final concentration of 5×10^{-5} *M*. The final ethanol concentration in the culture was 0.01 percent. An identical amount of ethanol was added to the control series of cultures. The cells were incubated for 3 days at 37 °C in an incubator saturated with water vapor and containing 5 percent CO_2.

After 72 hr of incubation, the cells were centrifuged for 5 min at 800 rpm. The supernatant was removed. Freshly mixed fixative, consisting of three parts absolute ethanol and one part of glacial acetic acid, was added to the cells immediately after removal of the supernatant. The fixative was changed twice, and slides were prepared by the air-drying technique. Cells were stained with Giemsa solution. Three to ten slides were prepared from each culture. Slides were coded so that they could not be recognized by the observers.

Microscopic observation started from a point selected at random on each slide and was carried through edge-to-edge of the slide in a zigzag fashion. All cells under the field of observation that were in prophase, metaphase, anaphase, or telophase of nuclear division were subjected to photomicrography. Each photomicrograph was examined independently by three observers in a double-blind fashion. The cells were classified into three groups: normal, abnormal, and questionable nuclear divisions. The questionable cells included those that could not be classified as normal or abnormal with confidence and a few cells about which the three observers disagreed.

Results

One set of control cultures failed to grow and was eliminated from the study. Thus, the observations were made in six sets of experimental and five sets of control cultures. A total of 405 nuclear divisions in the cells exposed to olivetol and 315 cell divisions in the control group were analyzed. Of the cells exposed to olivetol, 69.1 percent were judged to be normal, 24.7 percent questionable, and 6.2 percent abnormal (Table 23.1). This contrasted to 81.6 percent, 17.5 percent, and 0.95 percent, respectively, for the controls. All abnormalities were of segregational errors of chromosomes. When the questionable nuclear divisions were omitted from tabulation, abnormal nuclear divisions were present in 8.2 percent of the olivetol-treated cells and in 1.2 percent of the control group.

The types of segregational errors of chromosomes in the experimental group included formation of a bridge or multiple bridges in anaphase and telophase nuclei, anaphase lagging,

Table 23.1 Frequency of normal, questionable, and abnormal nuclear divisions in olivetol-treated human T-cells compared with controls[a]

Olivetol-treated cells (5×10^{-5} M; 405 cells)			*Controls (315 cells)*		
Normal	*Questionable*	*Abnormal*	*Normal*	*Questionable*	*Abnormal*
69.1	24.7	6.2	81.6	17.5	0.95

[a] Values expressed in %.

Table 23.2 Number of nuclei with various types of abnormal chromosome segregation induced by olivetol in cultured human lymphocytes

Type of abnormalities	*Cells in olivetol-treated cultures*	*Cells in controls*
Anaphase or telophase chromosome bridges, including multiple bridge formation	7	2
Anaphase lag	6	0
Abnormal anaphase, including unequal chromosome segregation in bipolar nuclear division	10	0
Multipolar chromosome segregation in anaphase or telophase	5	1

anomalous chromosome behavior in anaphase cells including unequal distribution of chromosome material in bipolar anaphase nuclei, and tripolar or multipolar segregation of chromosomes in anaphase and telophase cells (Table 23.2 and Figure 23.1). In three cells, two types of abnormalities coexisted in the nucleus. In contrast, only three cells with abnormal chromosome segregation were observed in the control group. These consisted of two nuclei with a single anaphase bridge formation and one tripolar anaphase.

Discussion

Olivetol clearly appears to induce segregational errors of chromosomes *in vitro.* The observed bridge formations in anaphase and telophase cells are likely to result in chromosomal breakages observable during the metaphases of subsequent cell generation. Unequal segregation of chromosomes in bipolar and multipolar cell divisions can give rise to hypodiploid and/or hyperdiploid nuclei. Thus, the previously reported "micronuclei" induced by olivetol are likely to have arisen as a consequence of abnormal chromosome segregation during the preceding cell division. We did not attempt to detect hyperdiploid cells in our previous study.

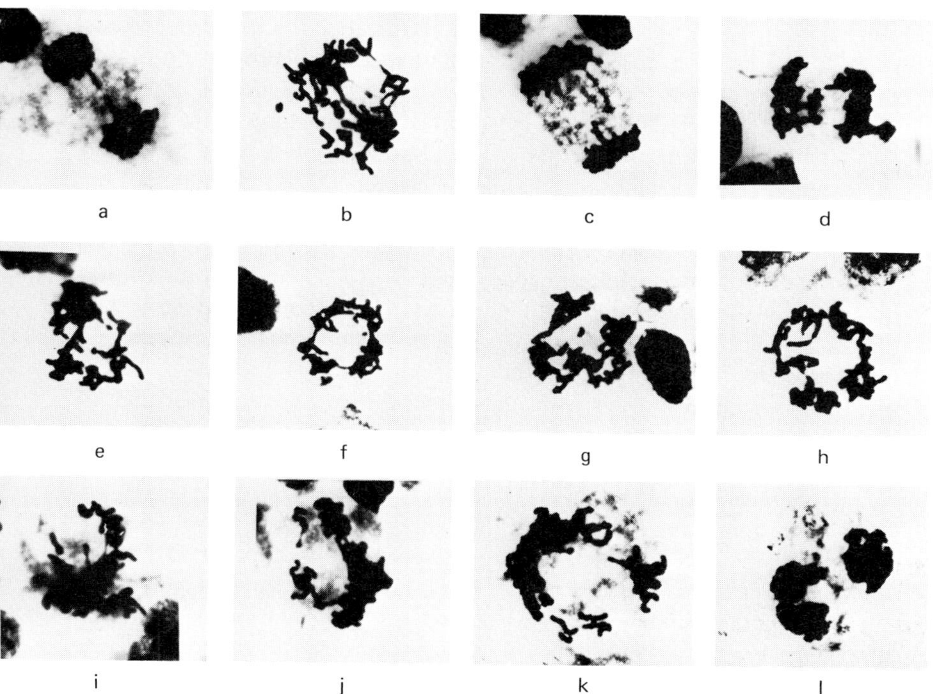

Figure 23.1. Various types of abnormal chromosome segregation induced by olivetol in cultured human lymphocytes. (a) A bridge formation in a telophase nucleus. (b) Formation of multiple anaphase bridges. (c) Anaphase lagging. (d) Anomalous chromosome behavior in an anaphase nucleus. (e, i) Unequal segregation of chromosomes in anaphase nuclei. (g, h) Multipolar anaphase. (j, k) Tripolar anaphase. (l) Tripolar telophase.

Whether cannabinoids and marihuana smoking can induce segregational errors of chromosomes is yet to be examined. However, in our pilot study, similar errors of chromosome segregation were induced in cultured human lymphocytes by exposing them to 3.2×10^{-6} M of Δ^9-THC.

Cannabinoids and olivetol appear to inhibit rapidly RNA and protein synthesis [9,10]. This inhibition seems to affect the intrachromosomal structure profoundly, resulting in the formation of anaphase and telophase bridges and to affect the formation of microtubules and spindles. Abnormal spindle formation gives rise to unequal segregation of chromosomes, including the formation of multipolar divisions. The resulting hypodiploid nuclei can readily explain the observed "micronuclei" [6]. Since the number of cells in cell division at any given moment is a small proportion of the cell population compared with those in the synthetic phase of DNA (S-period), it may be assumed that a comparatively large number of interphase cells in the S-period will have a decreased number of chromosomes and, therefore, DNA templates. This would explain the observed inhibition of ^{3}H-thymidine incorporation induced by cannabinoids and olivetol [7–10] as well as observed in chronic marihuana smokers [11], if one assumes that marihuana smoking has an effect similar to that of olivetol. The observation of increased "micronuclei" in marihuana smokers [6] supports this contention.

Stenchever and his colleagues detected an increased incidence of chromosomal breakage in chronic marihuana smokers [12]. The induction of chromosomal bridges by olivetol and Δ^9-THC corroborates their observation.

A significant decrease in the number of cells with euploid complements of chromosomes or with euploid amounts of DNA has been reported in cells derived from human lung explants exposed to marihuana smoke [2,3]. In these cells chromosomal breakage, anaphase lagging, tripolar metaphases, and the formation of large spindles were observed. The present study suggests that olivetol, a compound whose structure is that of the C-ring common to the cannabinoids, has the same effect as marihuana smoke.

The observation of uneven chromosome segregation, including the formation of multipolar cell divisions, is of particular interest since such a phenomenon has been reported rarely by students of human cytogenetics. Olivetol and cannabinoids may have a unique ability to disturb the formation of microtubules and spindles.

ACKNOWLEDGMENT

This study was supported by grants from the Health Research Council of the City of New York (U-2215), The National Foundation—March of Dimes, and the National Institute On Drug Abuse (1R01 DA 00894–01A1).

REFERENCES

1. Boyum, A. (1968) Isolation of leukocytes from human blood. *Scand. J. Clin. Lab. Invest. 21* (suppl. 97):31.
2. Leuchtenberger, C., R. Leuchtenberger, and U. Ritter (1973) Effects of marijuana and tobacco smoke on DNA and chromosomal complement in human lung explants. *Nature 242:*403.

3. Leuchtenberger, C., R. Leuchtenberger, and A. Schneider (1973) Effects of marijuana and tobacco smoke on human lung physiology. *Nature 241:*137.
4. Morishima, A. Unpublished data.
5. Morishima, A. and R. T. Henrich (1974) Blastogenesis of lymphocytes in patients receiving estrogens. *Lancet 2:*646.
6. Morishima, A., M. Milstein, R. T. Henrich, and G. G. Nahas (1976) Effects of marihuana smoking, cannabinoids and olivetol on replication of human lymphocytes: formation of micronuclei. *Pharmacology of Marihuana* (M. C. Braude and S. Szara, eds.). New York: Raven Press.
7. Nahas, G. G. and B. Desoize (1974) Effet inhibiteur du 5-n-amyl-resorcinol sur la transformation lymphoblastique. *C.R. Acad. Sci. (Paris) 279:*785.
8. Nahas, G. G., B. Desoize, J. P. Armand, J. Hsu, and A. Morishima (1974) Inhibition in vitro de la transformation lymphocytaire par divers cannabinoides naturels. *C.R. Acad. Sci. (Paris) 279:*785.
9. Nahas, G. G., B. Desoize, J. Hsu, A. Morishima, and P. R. Srinivasan (1976) Inhibition by natural cannabinoids and olivetol of lymphocyte transformation. *Pharmacology of Marihuana* (M. C. Braude and S. Szara, eds). New York: Raven Press.
10. Nahas, G. G., B. Desoize, A. Morishima, and P. R. Srinivasan (1976) Inhibitory effects of delta-9-tetrahydrocannabinol on nucleic acid synthesis and protein in cultured lymphocytes. *Marihuana: Chemistry, Biochemistry, and Cellular Effects* (G. G. Nahas, W. D. M. Paton, and I. Heikkila, eds.). New York: Springer-Verlag.
11. Nahas, C. G., N. Suciu-Foca, J. P. Armand, and A. Morishima (1974) Inhibition of cellular mediated immunity in marihuana smokers. *Science 183:*419.
12. Stenchever, M. A., T. J. Kunysz, and M. A. Allen (1974) Chromosome breakage in users of marihuana. *Am. J. Obstet. Gynecol. 118:* 106.

24

Effect of Δ^1-Tetrahydrocannabinol on Red Blood Cell Membranes and on Alveolar Macrophages

A. CHARI-BITRON

Introduction

Recent studies involving the major constituent of hashish, Δ^1-tetrahydrocannabinol (THC) [9,10], in its purified form [14] have provided important information on its pharmacological and biochemical effetcs in general, and at the membrane level in particular. THC is highly lipophilic (the expected partition coefficient, based on a corrected octanol/water partition, is 1200 [16]) and has great affinity for lipoproteins [20]. It does not demonstrate good anesthetic characteristics, and its mode of action on membranes is of a peculiar pattern.

This presentation includes two parts: first, a discussion of the dose-dependent action of THC on membranes, based on biochemical and morphological findings; second, a review of recent studies on the effect of THC on alveolar macrophages.

Dose-dependent Action of THC on Membranes

Up to a given concentration (about 20 μM for erythrocytes and 150 μM for liver mitochondria), THC appears to act on one type of membrane site and involve biochemical changes only, without causing observable configurational modifications. Beyond this "limiting concentration," additional sites are attacked, and structural changes occur concomitantly. A variety of supporting evidence for this concept is presented below.

Protection of erythrocytes and liposomes against hypotonic lysis

Adding THC *in vitro* to red blood cells of either rats [5] or humans [7] provides protection against hypotonic hemolysis. Figure 24.1, curve A, shows a monotonic increase in protection with rising

Marihuana: Chemistry, Biochemistry, and Cellular Effects, edited by Gabriel G. Nahas,

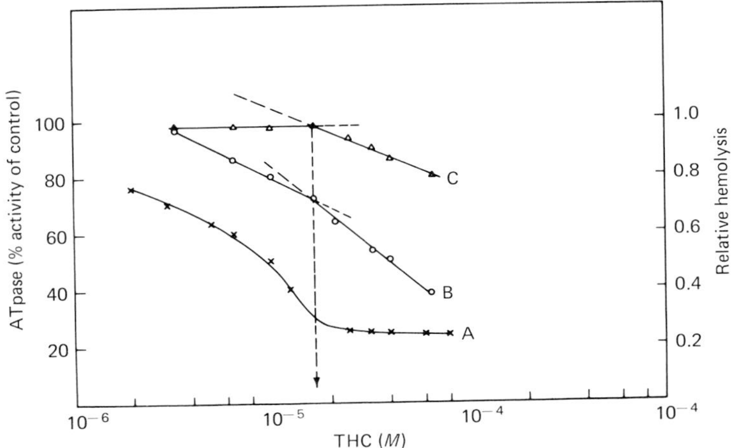

Figure 24.1. Dose response curves for the effect of THC on: A—hypotonic hemolysis; B—Na-K ATPase activity; C—Mg ATPase activity.

THC concentration, up to about 20 μM; beyond this value, protection remains unchanged, up to the highest concentration studied (100 μM). Obviously, this pattern is quite different from that observed with other surface-active substances such as tranquilizers, anesthetics, and hormones [18], vitamin A [8] and anti-inflammatory drugs [11]; at high concentrations, all these protecting agents produce hypotonic hemolysis.

In hypotonic solutions, the effect of THC on liposomes prepared from lipids of brain or erythrocytes is of a similar pattern [1]. For both these types of liposomes, there is a monotonic increase of protection with rising THC concentration to values approaching the "limiting concentration." At higher THC concentrations, no further increase of protection has been observed.

Partition coefficient (membrane/buffer) of THC

Measurements conducted by Seeman *et al.* [19] show that the membrane/buffer partition coefficient for THC, adsorbing to either erythrocyte ghost membranes or synaptosomes, decreases when the free concentration of THC is increased. At about 20 μM, a break in the curve for erythrocytes occurs, and the decrease of the partition coefficient with increasing THC concentration becomes much more pronounced. The curve for synaptosomes even demonstrates a marked anomaly in the vicinity of this concentration. (The inability of THC to produce anesthesia has been attributed by Paton and Pertwee [16] to its limited solubility in the membrane tissue; their estimates and the measurements of Seeman *et al.* [19] indicate a solubility for THC which is lower by 0.5–1 order of magnitude than that commonly found for other anesthetics obeying the Meyer–Overton rule.)

Precipitation and shape of red blood cells

When THC is added to red blood cells suspended in saline and the cells are allowed to precipitate, the pattern of the blood precipitate changes sharply at a concentration of around 20 μM THC (Figure 24.2). Neither the hematocrit measurements nor the sedimentation rate is affected by adding THC. However, microscopically, we have seen that at the limiting concentration, most of the red blood cells change their shape (Figure 24.3), usually from bioconcave discs to cups, and tend to form aggregates.

Figure 24.2. Effect of THC on erythrocyte precipitation. Numbers on test tubes represent concentrations in μg/ml. Note pattern of precipitate below (a) and beyond (b) the "limiting concentration."

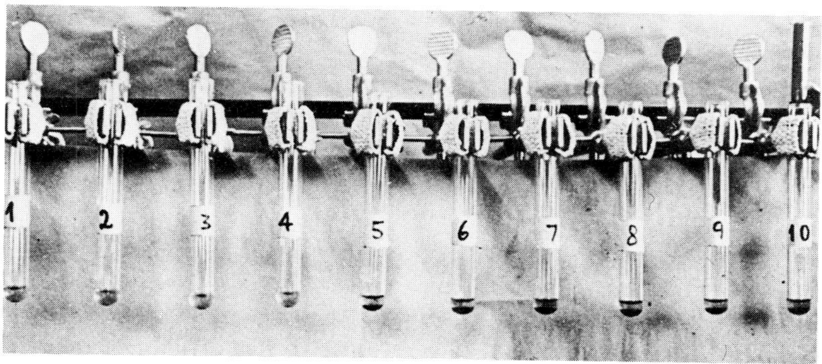

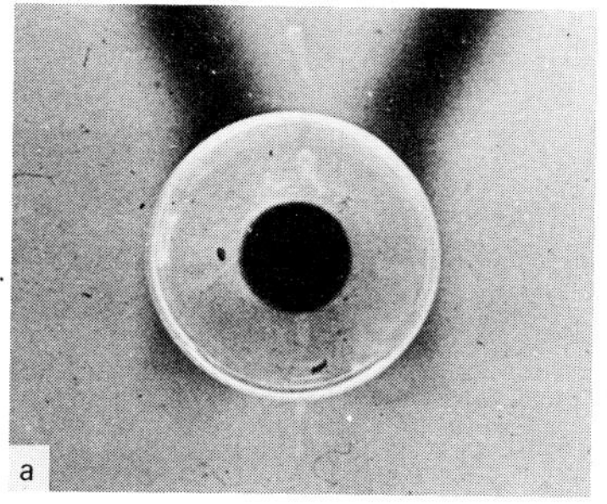

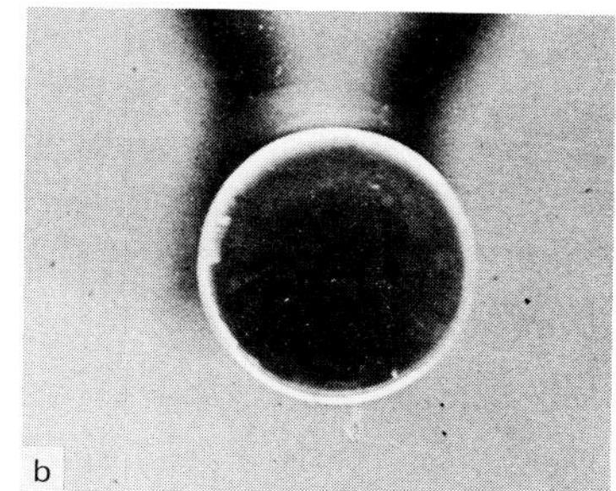

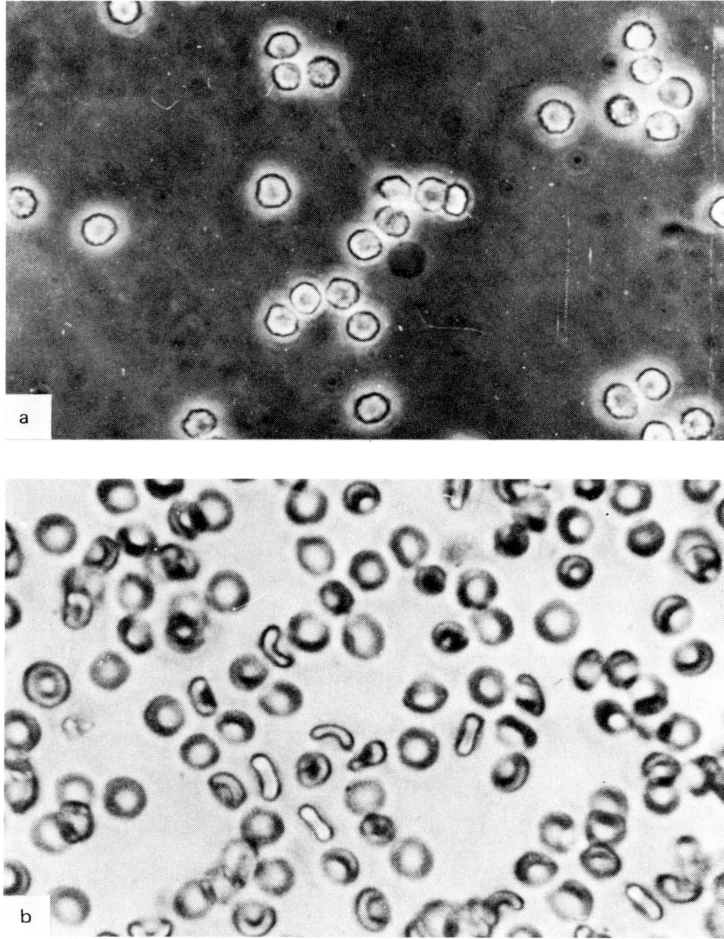

Figure 24.3. Shape of red blood cells. (a) Control containing alcohol 2.5 μl/ml. (b) Red blood cells in solution containing 20 μM THC.

Adenosine triphosphatase (ATPase) activity of red blood cell membrane

The action of THC on red blood cell membranes causes a pronounced decrease in Na-K ATPase activity (Figure 24.1, curve B) but does not affect Mg ATPase activity below the limiting concentration (Figure 24.1, curve C). At this concentration, a break in the Na-K ATPase activity curve appears, indicating an enhanced increase in inhibition, and, concomitantly, Mg ATPase activity also becomes inhibited notably. According to Laurent *et al.* [12], THC at a concentration of about 20 μM completely abolishes Na-K ATPase activity of a microsomal fraction from rat ileum.

Oxygen uptake, ATPase activity, and swelling of rat liver mitochondria

In our study [2] on the effects of THC on rat liver mitochondria, we suggested a biphasic dose dependence. The suggestion was based on comparing the biochemical and configurational changes, the latter being traced by ultrastructural examinations. The limiting concentration in this organelle was found to be about 150 μM. At this concentration oxygen uptake (after having passed through a maximum at about 50 μM) declines to zero, and swelling and ATPase activity reach a maximum, but no clear configurational changes are observed. At concentrations higher than 150 μM, the structural integrity of the mitochondria is no longer preserved. Mahoney and Harris [13] observed similar biochemical phenomena for liver mitochondria with the same limiting concentration.

Interpretation of experimental evidence

The mechanism of action of THC on membranes remains obscure. However, the experimental evidence presented suggests the existence of two different modes of action, each characterized by its respective range of concentration, above or below a membrane-dependent limiting concentration. In the low concentration range, THC presumably acts primarily on the membrane lipids—which are important in preserving its structure—and their amount therein constitutes one of the significant factors determining the magnitude of the limiting concentration. The higher the amount of lipids in the attacked cell membrane, the higher the limiting concentration. The specific types of lipids and lipoproteins probably also affect the value of this concentration (erythrocytes contain about 5 percent lipids, whereas the lipid content of liver mitochondria is approximately 30 percent). Beyond the limiting concentration, the contribution of the lipid–lipoprotein bond to safeguarding membrane integrity is no longer functioning properly, and the cell is destroyed.

Effect of THC on Alveolar Macrophages

The usual route of administration of hashish is via inhalation of its smoke. Therefore, we studied the effect of THC on alveolar macrophages, which are considered to be the first line of pulmonary defense and are exposed to the inhaled hashish before it enters the bloodstream or is metabolized.

As has been shown [3], THC has a marked disruptive effect on rat liver lysosomes *in vitro,* causing them to release hydrolytic enzymes. Since the macrophage contains an active complement of lysosomal enzymes, which can be released on treating the macrophages with surface-active substances, we studied the release of hydrolases after incubating macrophages with THC at various concentrations. Some of the results are presented below.

Selectivity of lysosomal enzyme release

Adding THC to alveolar macrophages *in vitro* causes the release of β-glucuronidase and (probably) β-galactosidase, but surprisingly not acid phosphatase (which is present in considerable amounts in the lysosomes of macrophages).

Figure 24.4 demonstrates that increasing concentrations of THC induce β-glucuronidase release progressively. Possibly the cause of this selective effect of THC is its attacking a nonlysosomal site. By using the trypan blue staining method, we ascertained that the release of β-glucuronidase by THC was not due to cell death.

Effect on macrophages in hypotonic solution

Alveolar macrophages, when transferred into 0.2 percent NaCl, have been shown to be relatively resistant to osmotic shock, with little loss of viability [15]. Our findings indicate that adding THC (35 μM) to the macrophages suspended in 0.2 percent NaCl causes

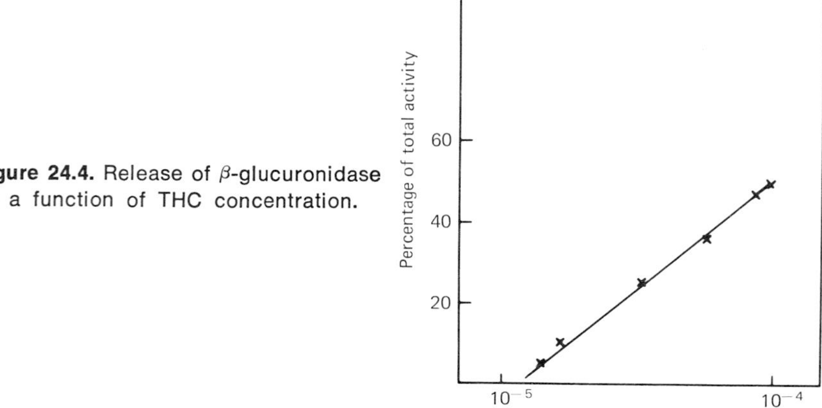

Figure 24.4. Release of β-glucuronidase as a function of THC concentration.

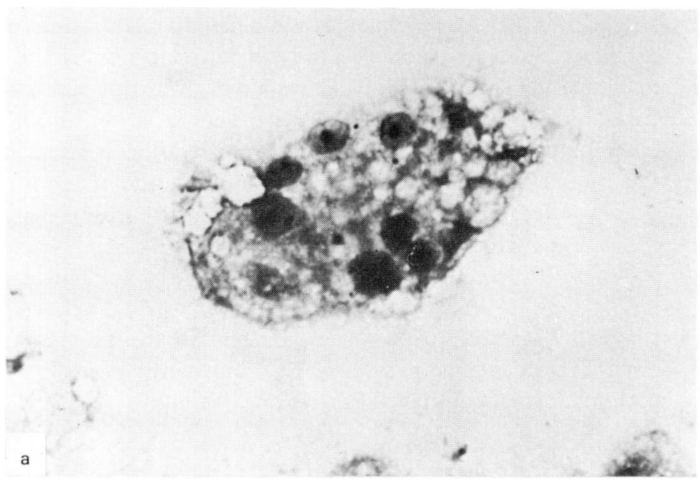

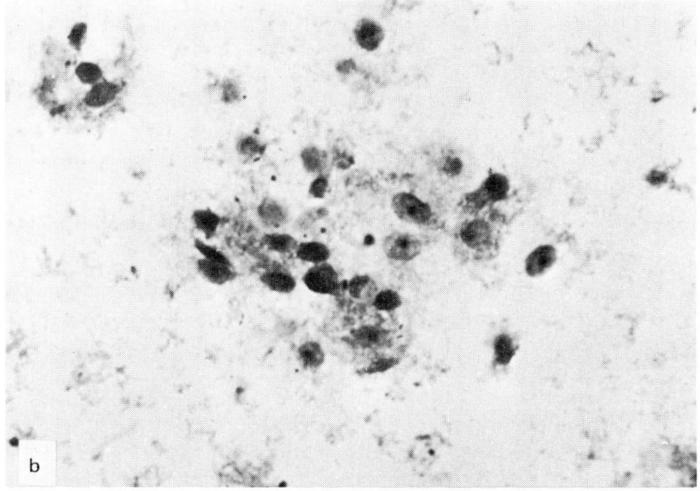

Figure 24.5. Cytolysis of macrophages by THC in hypotonic solutions. (a) Control; (b) after adding 20 μM THC.

complete cytolysis of the cells, accompanied by extrusion of lysosomal hydrolytic enzymes (Figure 24.5).

Inhibition of cell motility

Cinematography provides an excellent tool for studying the effect of THC on macrophage motion. Alcohol (2.5 μl/ml), which served as control, has no effect on the movement of the macrophage, but adding THC at 30 μM causes a spectacular inhibition of cell motility leading to actual paralysis without noticeably changing the macrophage's shape. We are now studying: the lowest concentration of THC that affects the organelle's motility, the reversibility of the effect, and the possible correlation between the selective release of β-glucuronidase and the inhibition of motility.

The effect of THC on macrophages resembles that of cytochalasin B, which inhibits cell movement [4] and selectively releases β-glucuronidase and β-galactosidase, but not acid phosphatase [6,7]. Davies *et al.* have postulated that these effects of cytochalasin B are due to its interference with the function of a contractile microfilament system that normally contributes to the maintenance of cellular organization.

ACKNOWLEDGMENTS

The skillful technical assistance of Miss Levana Motola is greatly appreciated. Thanks are due to Mr. M. Peled for his photographic work, to Dr. A. Shahar for the cinematography, and to Prof. R. Mechoulam for providing the THC.

REFERENCES

1. Alhanaty, E. and A. Livne (1974) Osmotic fragility of liposomes as affected by antihemolytic compounds. *Biochim. Biophys. Acta 339:* 146.
2. Bino, T., A. Chari-Bitron, and A. Shahar (1972) Biochemical effects and morphological changes in rat liver mitochondria exposed to Δ^1-tetrahydrocannabinol. *Biochim. Biophys. Acta 288:*195.
3. Britton, R. S. and A. Mellors (1974) Lysis of liver lysosomes in vitro by Δ^1-tetrahydrocannabinol. *Biochem. Pharmacol. 23:*1342.
4. Carter, S. B. (1967) Effects of cytochalasins on mammalian cells. *Nature 213:*261.
5. Chari-Bitron, A. (1971) Stabilization of rat erythrocyte membrane by Δ^1-tetrahydrocannabinol. *Life Sci. 10:*1273.
6. Davies, P., A. C. Allison, and A. D. Haswell (1973) Selective release of lysosomal hydrolases from phagocytic cells by cytochalasin B. *Biochem. J. 134:*33.
7. ——— R. Fox, M. Polyzonis, A. C. Allison, and D. Haswell (1973) The inhibition of phagocytosis and facilitation of exocytosis in rabbit polymorphonuclear leucocytes by cytochalasin B. *Lab. Invest. 28:*16.
8. Dingle, J. T. and J. A. Lucy (1962) Studies on the mode of action of excess of vitamin A. *Biochem. J. 84:*61.
9. Grunfeld, Y. and H. Edery (1969) Activity of the active constituents of hashish and some related cannabinoids. *Psychopharmacologia 14:* 200.
10. Hollister, L. E. (1970) Tetrahydrocannabinol isomers and homologues: contrasted effects of smoking. *Nature 227:*968.

11. Inglot, A. P. and E. Wolna (1968) Reaction of non-steroidal anti-inflammatory drugs with the erythrocyte membrane. *Biochem. Pharmacol. 17:*269.
12. Laurent, B., E. R. Roy, and L. Galis (1974) Inhibition by Δ^1-tetrahydrocannabinol of a Na^+K^+ transport adenosine triphosphatase from rat ileum. *Can. J. Physiol. Pharmacol. 52:*1110.
13. Mahoney, J. M. and R. A. Harris (1972) Effect of Δ^9-tetrahydrocannabinol on mitochondrial process. *Biochem. Pharmacol. 21:*1217.
14. Mechoulam, R. (1970) Marihuana chemistry. *Science 168:*1159.
15. Myrvik, Q. N., E. S. Leake, and B. Farris (1961) Lysozyme content of alveolar and peritoneal macrophages from the rabbit. *J. Immunol. 86:*128.
16. Paton, W. D. M. and R. G. Pertwee (1973) The pharmacology of cannabis in animals. *Marihuana Chemistry, Pharmacology, Metabolism and Clinical Effects* (R. Mechoulam, ed.). New York: Academic Press, pp. 280,81.
17. Raz, A., A. Schurr, and A. Livne (1972) The interaction of hashish components with human erythrocytes. *Biochim. Biophys. Acta 274:* 269.
18. Roth, S. and P. Seeman (1971) All lipid soluble anaesthetics protect red cells. *Nature 231:*284.
19. Seeman, P., M. Chan-Wong, and S. Moyyen (1972) The membrane binding of morphine, diphenylhydantoin and tetrahydrocannabinol. *Can. J. Physiol. Pharmacol. 50:*1181.
20. Wahlqvist, M., I. M. Nilsson, F. Sandberg, and S. Agurell (1970) Binding of Δ^1-tetrahydrocannabinol to human plasma protein. *Biochem. Pharmacol. 19:*2579.

25

Cannabinoids: Effects on Lysosomes and Lymphocytes

ALAN MELLORS

Introduction

A wealth of information has been accumulated in recent years to indicate that cannabinoids disrupt the structure and function of biological membranes. The major psychoactive constituent of cannabis, Δ^9-tetrahydrocannabinol (Δ^9-THC), resembles other isoprenoid alcohols such as sterols and vitamin A in that it has marked lipophilic properties and binds readily to hydrophobic regions of biological membranes. The lipophilic properties of cannabinoids aid the rapid passage of these molecules across lipoprotein membranes in the lung and in the vascular system. Excretion of these nonpolar molecules is slow; compared with water-soluble drugs, traces of cannabinoids persist in membranous structures for relatively long periods after administration. Tracer studies indicate that membranous organelles within the cell—especially mitochondria, lysosomes, plasma membranes, and synaptosomes—have an especially high affinity for cannabinoids and their metabolites. This chapter describes the interactions between cannabinoids and some of these membranous structures and proposes several mechanisms by which such interactions may impair normal cellular function.

Lysosomal Membranes

It has been shown in our laboratory [2] and in independent studies by Raz *et al.* [15] that Δ^9-THC has a marked lytic action on rat liver lysosomes *in vitro*. Figure 25.1 shows that these lysosomes are split *in vitro* by Δ^9-THC, Δ^8-THC, and the major liver metabolite of Δ^9-THC, 11-OH-Δ^9-THC. A partially purified hashish resin was also active in splitting lysosomes *in vitro*. The four substances have similar potencies in lysosomal lysis, with maximum

Marihuana: Chemistry, Biochemistry, and Cellular Effects, edited by Gabriel G. Nahas, © 1976 by Springer-Verlag New York Inc.

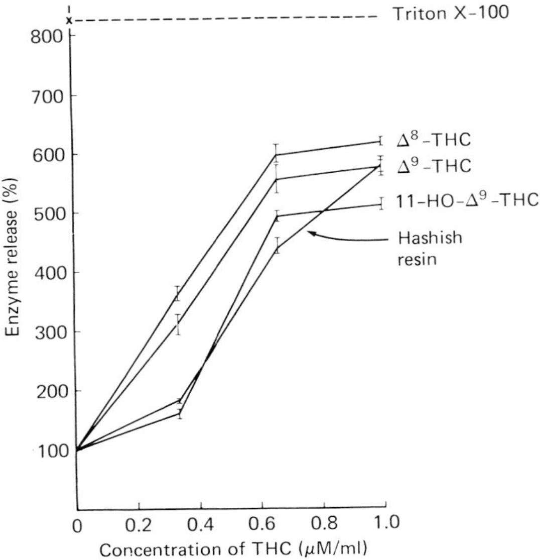

Figure 25.1. Lysis of rat liver lysosomes *in vitro* by cannabinoids.

effects seen for Δ^9-THC and Δ^8-THC. It is clear that the lytic effect of cannabinoids on lysosomal membranes is unspecific, as was shown previously using cannabidiol [15], and is unrelated to the psychoactive specificity of these compounds. The major difference between the data of Figure 25.1 and those reported earlier is that lysis was carried out here in an isotonic medium, without any osmotic stress exerted through the use of a hypotonic medium. This difference accounts for the somewhat lower proportion of total acid phosphatase released here compared with that reported in previous studies.

Do cannabinoids accumulate in lysosomes?

To determine whether the *in vivo* administration of cannabinoids results in the deposition of these potentially damaging agents in cell lysosomes, we performed a tracer study using ^{14}C-Δ^9-THC [10]. Rats were given ^{14}C-Δ^9-THC by intravenous injection, they were sacrificed at various times after the injection, and the distribution of ^{14}C-Δ^9-THC or its metabolites within subcellular fractions of rat liver homogenates was determined. In the first experiments, the lysosomes were obtained by the method of Trouet [21], which utilizes the detergent Triton WR 1339. Consequently, the lysosomes obtained contain this nonionic detergent.

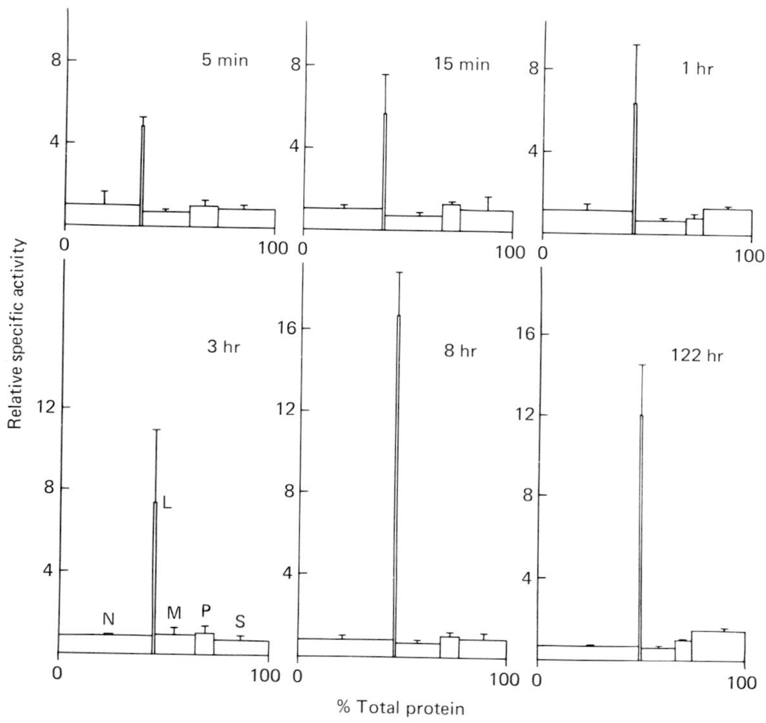

Figure 25.2. The distribution of ^{14}C-radioactivity within rat liver subcellular fractions at various times after the administration of ^{14}C-Δ^9-THC. The relative specific activity is the specific radioactivity of each fraction divided by that of the homogenate. Means are shown, with bars for SD, for 3 or 4 separate subcellular fractionations at each time period. N—nuclear and cell debris; L—Triton WR 1339-filled lysosomes; M—remaining protein from the sucrose density gradient consisting mainly of mitochondria; P—endoplasmic reticulum; S—soluble fraction.

The Δ^9-THC radioactivity is taken up rapidly by the liver so that the whole liver contains at 5 min 8.7 percent of the dose, at 15 min 15.5 percent, at 1 hr 7.5 percent, at 3 hr 7.8 percent, at 18 hr 3.9 percent, and at 122 hr 0.8 percent. Figure 25.2 shows that this radioactivity is concentrated in the lysosomes at all time periods studied. All other subcellular fractions show lower uptake of radioactivity, not greatly differing in specific activity (dpm per mg protein) from the homogenate. However, lysosomes have a specific activity five times that of the homogenate within 5 min of the injection of ^{14}C-Δ^9-THC. This specific activity of the isotope in lysosomes increases to a maximum of 17-fold compared to the homogenate at 18 hr after the injection, and thereafter the specific activity declines slowly.

In separate experiments, similar lysosomal fractions containing ^{14}C-Δ^9-THC prepared by the method of Trouet were subfractionated into lysosomal membrane fractions and lysosomal soluble enzyme fractions. This was done by lysing the organelles and centrifuging the lysate at 100,000*g* for 2 hr. The results (Table 25.1) show that radioactivity from ^{14}C-Δ^9-THC is distributed mainly in the lysosomal soluble fraction. To verify that this content of cannabinoid metabolites was not due to plasma membrane contamination of the lysosomal preparation, we established that rat liver plasma membranes were very low in ^{14}C activity 3 hr after the *in vivo* administration of ^{14}C-Δ^9-THC. We determined plasma membrane purity by measuring the marker enzymes 5′-nucleotidase and adenyl cyclase. Another control experiment that we undertook was to measure the uptake of ^{14}C-Δ^9-THC by rat liver lysosomes prepared by a method that did not use Triton WR 1339. The elevated levels of specific radioactivity in the lysosomal fractions in the above experiments could have been due to association between radioactive cannabinoids and Triton WR 1339. The radioactive complex could then accumulate within Triton WR 1339–filled lysosomes. To determine whether this had happened, we prepared lysosomes from rat livers of animals given ^{14}C-Δ^9-THC as before, but that were not given Triton WR 1339. Differential centrifugation by the method of Sawant *et al.* [18] was used to prepare lysosomes 3 hr after the administration of the labeled cannabinoid.

Table 25.1 The distribution of radioactivity between lysosomal soluble and membrane fractions of rat liver 18 hr after the administration of ^{14}C-Δ^9-THC[a]

	Acid phosphatase	*^{14}C-radioactivity*	
Lysosomal fraction	*Relative specific activity*	*Relative specific activity*	*Recovery (%)*
Soluble	22.1 ± 3.7	9.2 ± 0.8	5.8 ± 1.6
Membrane	15.2 ± 5.3	6.5 ± 4.7	0.6 ± 0.3

[a] All values mean ± SD for 4 fractionations.

The relative specific activity (fold purification over the homogenate) for cannabinoid-derived radioactivity in these rat liver lysosomes was 3.3 ± 0.4 ($n = 6$) at 3 hr after administration of the dose, compared to 7.4 ± 3.6 ($n = 4$) for lysosomes prepared by the Triton WR 1339 method. The higher figure for the latter lysosomes may indicate that the detergent carries some of the radioactive cannabinoid with it into the lysosomes, although it is more likely due to the increased lysosomal purification that is possible through the use of Triton WR 1339. Even in the absence of a detergent, the level of accumulation of radioactivity from ^{14}C-Δ^9-THC is substantially higher within lysosomes than within other cellular subfractions.

Effects on lysosomes *in vivo*

We have looked for biochemical evidence of damage to lysosomes *in vivo* during the development of subacute and acute Δ^9-THC toxicity in rats. This was done by monitoring lysosomal and other enzyme levels in serum and by measuring the fragility of rat liver lysosomes from some animals post mortem after 30 days of administration of subacute toxic levels of Δ^9-THC. Five groups of 9 male Wistar rats (150 gm) were given daily intraperitoneal injections of 0.3 ml propylene glycol containing Δ^9-THC. The doses were: group I, 30 mg/kg; group II, 15 mg/kg; group III, 7.5 mg/kg; group IV, 3.75 mg/kg; and group V, propylene glycol carrier only. Blood samples were taken from the tail veins on days 7, 13, 19, 25, and 31, and the sera obtained were assayed for several enzymes. Glutamate oxaloacetate transaminase (GOT), glutamate pyruvate transaminase (GPT), and lactic dehydrogenase (LDH) were all assayed by the methods of Henry *et al.* [7]; alkaline phosphatase [5], phosphodiesterase I [20], 5′-nucleotidase [14], and β-N-acetylglucosaminidase [1] were also assayed. No significant increases were seen in any group for the liver function marker enzymes LDH, GPT, GOT, the plasma membrane marker enzyme 5′-nucleotidase, or the lysosomal marker enzyme β-N-acetylglucosaminidase. From this biochemical evidence we conclude that there was no appreciable liver damage or any significant release of lysosomal enzymes from tissues into the serum. Toxicity caused by Δ^9-THC was apparent in the weight gain curves for groups I–IV, and by the acute toxicity at the highest dose (30 mg/kg) which resulted in the death of 5 of the 9 animals in this group in the 30-day period. Serum alkaline phosphatase levels were lowered in the higher dose groups, as shown in Table 25.2.

An enzyme which in rat liver is associated with plasma mem-

Table 25.2 Serum phosphodiesterase I and alkaline phosphatase levels in rats during the development of subacute Δ^9-THC toxicity

	Δ^9-*THC dose (mg/kg/day)*				
Day	*0*	*3.8*	*7.5*	*15.0*	*30.0*
Phosphodiesterase I[a]					
1	—	—	92 ± 16	131 ± 19	124 ± 20
7	118 ± 24	118 ± 36	105 ± 12	89 ± 12	76 ± 24
13	121 ± 22	133 ± 17	116 ± 11	108 ± 18	76 ± 25
19	126 ± 20	121 ± 12	116 ± 12	113 ± 9	37 ± 0
Alkaline phosphatase[a]					
1	98 ± 10	103 ± 7	114 ± 43	90 ± 21	85 ± 27
7	82 ± 20	67 ± 23	55 ± 18	33 ± 2	36 ± 1
13	86 ± 10	81 ± 28	75 ± 14	59 ± 11	39 ± 18
19	80 ± 31	65 ± 21	64 ± 17	57 ± 12	51 ± 7
25	91 ± 13	83 ± 14	57 ± 10	57 ± 19	31 ± 0

[a] Serum enzyme units are nmoles substrate hydrolyzed per ml serum per minute.

branes, phosphodiesterase I [20], was also significantly lowered in the higher dose groups. These changes would appear to be associated only with the acute toxicity seen in groups I and II receiving daily 30 and 15 mg/kg Δ^9-THC, respectively. Decreased levels of serum alkaline phosphatase are rarely encountered in pathological states, and clinical examples are restricted to the genetic syndrome known as "refractory rickets," or hypophosphatasia. Decreased levels of this enzyme due to acute Δ^9-THC toxicity may indicate impaired osteoblast function. The origin of the decreased phosphodiesterase I activity in serum is also uncertain. In rat liver cells the enzyme is associated with plasma membranes, and the decrease may reflect damage to cell membrane structure and function.

Fragility of rat liver lysosomes after *in vivo* administration of Δ^9-THC

Table 25.3 shows the fragility of lysosomes from the livers of rats from groups I–IV in the above experiment, sacrificed after receiving Δ^9-THC for 30 days. Lysosomal fragility was determined by incubating a lysosomal-mitochondrial pellet in hypotonic sucrose for 45 min at 37°C, and lysosomal acid phosphate release was measured as before [2]. Lysosomes from groups of rats given high

Table 25.5 Prevention of concanavalin A-induced MIF activity by *in vitro* treatment of lymphocytes with 40 μM Δ^9-THC

Supernatant[a]	*Macrophage migration cm²; mean* ± SD (n = 5)
Control-supernatant[b]	0.029 ± 0.005
THC-supernatant[c]	0.036 ± 0.003
Con A-supernatant[d]	0.011 ± 0.001
[THC-Con A] supernatant[e]	0.041 ± 0.004

[a] The various supernatants were dialyzed, lyophilized, and redissolved in one-tenth of the original volume. Aliquots (0.1 ml) of each were then included in the migration chamber.

[b] Supernatant of lymphocyte culture without addition of lectin.

[c] Supernatant of THC-treated lymphocyte culture without addition of lectin.

[d] Supernatant of Con A-stimulated lymphocyte culture.

[e] Supernatant of Con A-stimulated, THC-treated lymphocyte culture.

Lymphocytes were purified from lymph nodes of immunized guinea pigs [12], and after various treatments the supernatants from these lymphocytes were tested for MIF activity against untreated guinea pig peritoneal exudate macrophages. Table 25.5 shows that Con A–stimulated lymphocytes produced MIF, but that this stimulation was almost entirely abolished in the presence of 40 μM Δ^9-THC *in vitro.* Table 25.6 shows the effect of Δ^9-THC, given *in vivo* (0.8 mg/kg) to guinea pigs immunized with PPD, on the migration of peritoneal exudate cells from these animals. The cells were collected 19 hr after Δ^9-THC administration and

Table 25.6 Effect of *in vivo* treatment with Δ^9-THC on the cellular immune response in immunized guinea pigs

Δ^9-*THC dose (mg/kg)*	*Macrophage migration, cm²; Mean* ± SD (n = 3)	
	Without PPD	*With PPD*
0	0.037 ± 0.007	0.010 ± 0.002
0.79	0.033 ± 0.004	0.027 ± 0.003

were stimulated to produce MIF *in vitro* by the presence of PPD (10 μg/ml) in the culture medium. It can be seen from Table 25.6 that MIF production, stimulated by PPD, is greatly reduced by a single *in vivo* injection of Δ^9-THC.

Although the *in vivo* administration of Δ^9-THC in rats and in guinea pigs at levels of 0.3–1.25 mg/kg had no effect on the viability of peritoneal lymphocytes, Δ^9-THC strongly influences lymphocyte viability *in vitro.* Table 25.7 shows that there is dose-related killing of lymphocytes at concentrations of Δ^9-THC above 10 *μM*. The mitogen Con A (10 μg/ml) has a marked protective effect against loss of viability in the presence of Δ^9-THC concentrations up to 100 *μM*. Lineweaver-Burk kinetic plots indicate the "competitive" appearance of protection against Δ^9-THC–induced loss of viability by Con A. Thus, Con A and Δ^9-THC have mutually antagonistic effects on MIF production by lymphocytes, and loss of lymphocyte viability in the presence of Δ^9-THC can be prevented by Con A. Con A is known to stimulate blastogenesis through interaction at the lymphocyte cell membrane, and it appears that this triggering process can be overcome by Δ^9-THC, another membrane-active compound. Conversely, the membrane damage induced by Δ^9-THC can be minimized by the binding of Con A to the membrane. We have performed competitive binding experiments with radioactive ^{14}C-Δ^9-THC and ^{3}H-concanavalin A, in which we studied their binding to intact lymphocytes. We were unable to detect displacement of bound Con A by Δ^9-THC, or vice versa. Any

Table 25.7 Effect of Δ^9-THC on lymphocyte viability, showing protection by concanavalin A

Δ^9-THC concentration (μM)	*% viable cells*[a]	
	Without Con A	*With Con A*
0	91	100
10	74	93
25	64	89
50	63	72
100	56	69
500	53	52
1000	51	48

[a] Viability was determined by the trypan blue exclusion method. Preincubation with 10 μg/ml Con A for 30 min at 27°C was followed by 30-min incubation with Δ^9-THC.

competitive interaction apparently is not for binding at common binding sites but via antagonistic effects on membrane structure or function.

Biochemical events in lymphocyte transformation

Blastogenesis is a complex phenomenon, and many biochemical events can be used to characterize the process. The production of lymphokines such as MIF can, according to some reports [16], be induced in the absence of cell division and may be restricted to a special subpopulation of lymphocytes. We have studied other biochemical markers of lymphocyte transformation—namely, tritiated thymidine uptake, ^{14}C-choline uptake, calcium uptake, and membrane ATPase activities. Nahas' group [13] reported the inhibition of thymidine uptake by Δ^9-THC. We have studied the time course of the inhibition of ^{3}H-thymidine uptake in purified guinea pig lymph node lymphocytes. This was done to determine whether Δ^9-THC inhibited only certain stages in the Con A–induced transformation, or whether it would act at all stages. Nine duplicate aliquots of lymphocytes were exposed to Con A (10 μg/ml) for 7 hr, and Δ^9-THC(50 μM) was added to each set at 0, 3, 6, 9, 20, 24, 32, 48, and 56 hr, respectively. Tritiated thymidine was added at 56 hr, and its incorporation was measured at 70 hr.

The results showed that Δ^9-THC inhibited ^{3}H-thymidine uptake over 96 percent at all intervals of exposure to cannabinoid. This indicates that in spite of prolonged prior exposure to Con A alone, cells cannot incorporate thymidine in the presence of Δ^9-THC. Thymidine uptake appears to be blocked directly by Δ^9-THC rather than by subsequent events in DNA replication. Cells transformed by stimulation with Con A alone for many hours do not take up thymidine in the presence of Δ^9-THC to any greater extent than cells that have been exposed to Con A briefly.

Another biochemical marker of lymphocyte transformation, which is even more sensitive to Δ^9-THC than is thymidine uptake, is the synthesis of phospholipids by the lymphocyte membrane. In preliminary experiments we have pretreated purified mouse spleen lymphocytes with low concentrations of Δ^9-THC (5, 10, 15, and 25 μM) for only 10 min. Then after the lymphocytes had been stimulated with Con A (10 μg/ml) and incubated for 2 hr in the presence of ^{14}C-choline, we observed marked decreases in the incorporation of ^{14}C into lipids, measured as described by Fisher and Mueller [4]. As shown in Table 25.8, only 5 μM Δ^9-THC considerably inhibits Con A–stimulated lipid synthesis in these lymphocytes. The early acceleration of phospholipid synthesis by Con A

Table 25.8 The inhibition of concanavalin A-stimulated ^{14}C-choline incorporation into phospholipids of mouse spleen lymphocytes after *in vitro* treatment with low levels of Δ^9-THC

Δ^9-THC concentration (μM)	*^{14}C-choline incorporation* (*% of controls*)
0	100
5	66
10	46
25	24

or PHA is known to be independent of protein synthesis stimulation [4]. These studies suggest that the lectins (Con A or PHA) induce rapid and early changes in membrane metabolism, resulting in increased membrane growth and changes in the surface properties of the membrane. Inhibition of the increased phospholipid synthesis accompanying these changes by 5 μM Δ^9-THC indicates antagonism between Δ^9-THC and Con A at the membrane level at an early stage in lymphocyte transformation.

ACKNOWLEDGMENTS

The author wishes to acknowledge generous research support by Canada Health and Welfare and the Medical Research Council of Canada. He is indebted to Dr. H. N. Aithal, Dr. M. G. Anderson, Dr. A. B. Kamble, and C. C. Gaul for their help in conducting this research.

REFERENCES

1. Beck, C. and A. L. Tappel (1968) Rat-liver lysosomal β-glucosidase: a membrane enzyme. *Biochim. Biophys. Acta 151:*159.
2. Britton, R. S. and A. Mellors (1974) Lysis of rat liver lysosomes *in vitro* by Δ^9-tetrahydrocannabinol. *Biochem. Pharmacol. 23:*1342.
3. David, J. R. and R. David (1971) Assay for inhibition of macrophage migration. *In Vitro Methods in Cell-mediated Immunity* (B. R. Bloom and P. R. Glade, eds.). New York: Academic Press, p. 249.
4. Fisher, D. B. and G. C. Mueller (1969) The step-wise acceleration of phosphatidyl choline synthesis in phytohemagglutinin-treated lymphocytes. *Biochim. Biophys. Acta 176:*316.

5. Garen, A. and C. Levinthal (1960) A fine-structure genetic and chemical study of the enzyme alkaline phosphatase of E. coli. *Biochim. Biophys. Acta 38:*470.
6. Gaul, C. C. and A. Mellors (1975) Δ^9-Tetrahydrocannabinol and decreased macrophage migration inhibition. *Res. Commun. Chem. Pathol. Pharmacol. 10:*559.
7. Henry, R. J., N. Chiamori, O. J. Golub, and S. Berkman (1960) Revised spectrophotometric methods for the determination of glutamic-oxaloacetic transaminase, glutamic-pyruvic transaminase and lactic acid dehydrogenase. *Am. J. Clin. Pathol. 34:*381.
8. Hirschorn, R., J. M. Kaplan, A. F. Goldberg, K. Hirschorn, and G. Weissmann (1965) Acid phosphatase-rich granules in human lymphocytes induced by phytohemagglutinin. *Science 147:*55.
9. Ignarro, L. J. (1972) Lysosome membrane stabilisation *in vivo:* effect of steroidal and non-steroidal anti-inflammatory drugs on the integrity of rat liver lysosomes. *J. Pharmacol. Exp. Ther. 182:*179.
10. Irvin, J. E. and A. Mellors (1975) Δ^9-Tetrahydrocannabinol: uptake by rat liver lysosomes. *Biochem. Pharmacol. 24:*305.
11. Lau, R. J., C. B. Lerner, D. G. Tubergen, N. Benowitz, E. F. Domino, and R. T. Jones (1975) Non-inhibition of phytohemagglutinin (PHA) induced lymphocyte transformation in humans by Δ^9-THC. *Fed. Proc. 34:*783.
12. Manheimer, S. and E. Pick (1973) The mechanism of action of soluble lymphocytic mediators. *Immunology 24:*1027.
13. Nahas, G. G., N. Suciu-Foca, J.-P. Armand, and A. Morishima (1974) Inhibition of cellular mediated immunity in marihuana smokers. *Science 183:*419.
14. Neu, H. C. (1967) The 5′-nucleotidase of Escherichia coli: 1. Purification and properties. *J. Biol. Chem. 242:*3896.
15. Raz, A., A. Schurr, A. Livne, and R. Goldman (1973) Effect of hashish compounds on rat liver lysosomes *in vitro. Biochem. Pharmacol. 22:*3129.
16. Rocklin, R. E. (1973) Production of migration inhibitory factor by nondividing lymphocytes. *J. Immunol. 110:*674.
17. Roels, O. A. (1969) The influence of vitamins A and E on lysosomes. *Lysosomes in Biology and Pathology.* (J. T. Dingle and H. B. Fell, eds.), Vol. 1. Amsterdam: North Holland, pp. 254–275.
18. Sawant, P. L., S. Shibko, U. S. Kumta, and A. L. Tappel (1964) Isolation of rat liver lysosomes and their general properties. *Biochim. Biophys. Acta 85:*82.
19. Schwartzfarb, L., M. Needle, and M. Chayez-chase (1974) Dose-related inhibition of leucocyte migration by marijuana and delta-9-tetrahydrocannabinol *in vitro. J. Clin. Pharmacol. 14:*35.
20. Touster, O., N. N. Aronson, J. T. Dulaney, and H. Hendrickson (1970) Isolation of rat liver plasma membranes: use of nucleotide pyrophosphatase and phosphodiesterase I as marker enzymes. *J. Cell Biol. 471:*604.
21. Trouet, A. (1964) Immunisations de lapins par des lysosomes hépatiques de rat traités au Triton-WR 1339. *Arch. Int. Physiol. 72:*698.

22. Weissmann, G. and L. Thomas (1963) Studies on lysosomes. II. The effect of cortisone on the release of acid hydrolases from a large granule fraction of rabbit liver induced by an excess of vitamin A. *J. Clin. Invest. 42:*661.
23. Weissmann, G., J. W. Uhr, and L. Thomas (1963) Acute hypervitaminosis A in guinea pigs. I. Effect on acid hydrolases. *Proc. Soc. Exp. Biol. Med. 112:*284.
24. White, S. C., S. C. Brin, and B. W. Janicki (1975) Mitogen-induced blastogenic responses of lymphocytes from marijuana smokers. *Science 188:*71.
25. Zimmerman, A. M. and D. F. McLean (1973) Action of narcotic and hallucinogenic agents on the cell cycle. *Drugs and the Cell Cycle* (A. M. Zimmerman, G. M. Padilla, and I. L. Cameron, eds.). New York: Academic Press, p. 67.

26

Inhibitory Effects of Δ^9-Tetrahydrocannabinol on Nucleic Acid Synthesis and Proteins in Cultured Lymphocytes

GABRIEL G. NAHAS, BERNARD DESOIZE, JOY HSU, AND A. MORISHIMA

We have reported in other publications [16,17] that two natural psychoactive cannabinoids, Δ^8- and Δ^9-tetrahydrocannibinol, their hydroxylated derivatives, and four nonpsychoactive cannabinoids: cannabinol, cannabidiol, cannabichromene, and cannabicyclol, inhibit in similar concentrations (10^{-5} *M* to 10^{-4} *M*) blastogenesis of human lymphocytes. It was suggested that this inhibitory effect of the natural cannabinoids was induced in part by olivetol or 5*n*-amylresorcinol, which has the structure of the C ring of these compounds.

We investigated the inhibitory effect of Δ^9-tetrahydrocannabinol (Δ^9-THC) on the uptake and incorporation of thymidine, uridine, and leucine in cultured lymphocytes. Experiments were also performed to study the reversibility of this inhibition, its time course, and the interactions of THC with the culture medium, especially serum.

Methods

Culture preparation

The technique used is that of Hartzman *et al.* [7]. Venous blood is collected under heparin (50 IU/ml) from healthy male donors. Mononucleated cells are collected according to the technique of Boyum [3] by density gradient centrifugation with Ficoll Isopaque. After three washings, the cells are suspended in RPMI 1640 with streptomycin and glutamine added. Contamination with polymorphonuclear cells is less than 5 percent. Cell concentration is set at 10^6 cells per milliliter. Cell suspensions are transferred with an automatic Hamilton syringe into the wells of the disposable culture plate. Each well is filled with 0.2 ml of cell suspension (2×10^5 cells) and 0.5 ml of pooled human serum. Phytohemagglutinin

Marihuana: Chemistry, Biochemistry, and Cellular Effects, edited by Gabriel G. Nahas, © 1976 by Springer-Verlag New York Inc.

(PHA) is added to a final concentration of 4 mg/μ. The cells are incubated at 37°C for 3 days in an incubator saturated in water vapor and containing 5 percent CO_2. Macromolecular synthesis is evaluated by measuring the incorporation of ^{3}H-leucine (25 Ci/mM), ^{3}H-uridine (25 Ci/mM), and ^{3}H-thymidine (2 Ci/mM). ^{3}H-leucine and ^{3}H-uridine are added at the onset of culture. In the experiments in which ^{3}H-leucine incorporation is studied, RPMI leucine free and serum dialyzed against RPMI leucine free are used. ^{3}H-thymidine is added 2–6 hr before harvesting the cells.

Harvesting and measuring radioactivity

Cell death is determined by the cells' inability to exclude trypan blue. This micoscopic examination also allows for a morphological examination of lymphoblastic transformation. Cells are harvested with a Multiple Automatic Sample Harvester (MASH) described by Hartzman *et al.* [6]. Uptake of radioactivity in cells is measured after washing with saline; incorporation of radioactivity into DNA, RNA, and proteins is measured after washing twice with 5 percent trichloroacetic acid and methanol. Filters are dried and transferred into vials for scintillation counting. Radioactivity is measured in counts per minute (cpm). Each measurement represents the mean plus or minus standard error of three or four cultures.

Preparation of THC

THC is available in a 95 percent ethanol solution containing 20 mg/ml. This solution is mixed with serum. The final alcohol concentration in the culture medium is always less than 0.5 percent, which does not inhibit cell growth [10,16].

Incubation of cells with THC and reversibility of inhibition

In a group of experiments, cells are first incubated 24–48 hr with THC 2.5×10^{-4} *M*. Half the cultures contain PHA and half do not. After this first incubation, cells are washed three times by centrifugation with RPMI. After washing, the cells are cultured again and harvested at regular intervals. Results are compared with cultures free of THC.

Results

Inhibition of precursor uptake and incorporation

THC starts to inhibit ^{3}H-thymidine incorporation at a concentration of 10^{-4} *M* [17]. The same concentration of the drug inhibits ^{3}H-uridine and ^{3}H-leucine incorporation (Figure 26.1). Inhibition

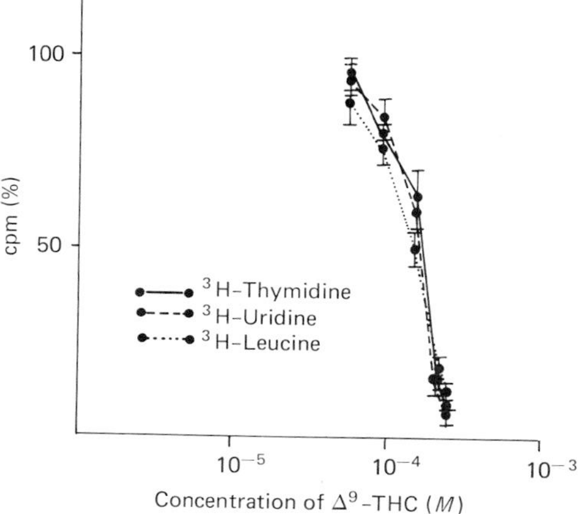

Figure 26.1. Dose response curve of the inhibition of incorporation of ^{3}H-thymidine, ^{3}H-uridine, and ^{3}H-leucine. Radioactivity is expressed in % cpm of parallel control cultures. Each point represents the mean of 2 experiments ± SE.

of cellular uptake of these precursors is similar to the inhibition of their incorporation into the macromolecules DNA, RNA, and proteins [5].

Interactions of THC with lymphocytes and serum

The inhibition of thymidine incorporation by THC is a function of serum concentration in the culture medium (Figure 26.2). With serum concentrations of less than 1 percent, thymidine incorporation is almost completely inhibited by 1.6×10^{-5} M THC, whereas it is marked in the control culture (cpm = 15,000–20,000). With the same dose of THC in the presence of 10 percent serum concentration, thymidine incorporation is only weakly inhibited. A Lineweaver–Burke plot of the data in Figure 26.2 indicates a competitive inhibition between serum and THC (Figure 26.3).

Furthermore, the degree of inhibition produced by the same dose of THC is the same when the cell concentration in the culture medium increases from 0.4 to 1.3×10^6/ml (Table 26.1).

Reversibility of inhibition

Lymphocytes are incubated for 24 or 48 hr without PHA and with 2.5×10^{-4} M THC, a dose which inhibits 85 percent of precursor incorporation. After the cells are washed and reset in culture

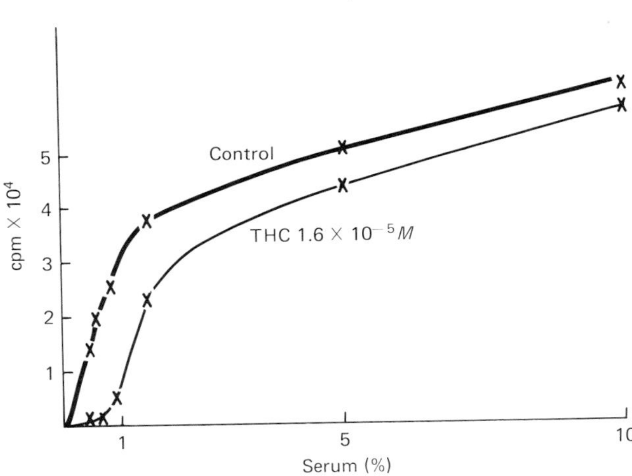

Figure 26.2. Effects of THC and serum on ^{3}H-thymidine uptake in cultured lymphocytes.

with PHA, thymidine incorporation at 3 days in experimental cultures is not significantly different from that observed in controls.

In another series of experiments, we incubated lymphocytes for 24 hr with THC (2.5×10^{-4} *M*) and PHA (Figure 26.4). After washing, the cells are reset in culture without PHA. There is a

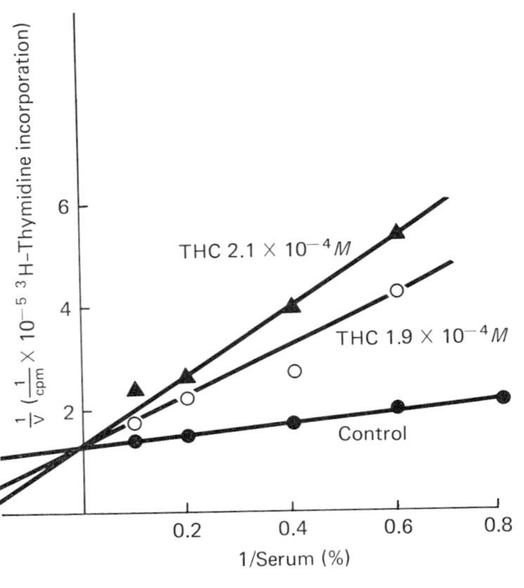

Figure 26.3. Lineweaver–Burke curve indicating the interactions of serum and THC in inhibiting ^{3}H-thymidine uptake. The inhibition is competitive.

Table 26.1 Inhibition of ^{3}H-thymidine incorporation by THC in a medium containing increasing amounts of cells[a]

	Cell concentration ($\times 10^5$/ml)			
THC concentration	4	5.3	8	13
1.5×10^{-4} M (2 exp.)	65.6% ±1.4	76.7% ±0.4	76.8% ±13.3	79.3% ±10.1
2.5×10^{-4} M (1 exp.)	24%	21%	19%	21%

[a] This inhibition was calculated in % incorporation of the precursor in a parallel control culture.

significant time lag in the incorporation of ^{3}H-thymidine by the cells preincubated with THC and stimulated with PHA, as compared with cells incubated with PHA alone (Figure 26.4). At 72 hr, incorporation in both sets of cultures is the same; microscopic

Figure 26.4. Reversibility of the inhibition of thymidine incorporation by THC in lymphocytes stimulated by PHA. Half the cultures are incubated for 24 hr with THC (2.5×10^{-4} *M*) and PHA; the other half is incubated during the same time with PHA alone. After 24 hr the cells are washed 3 times with RPMI and replaced in culture. Each point represents the mean of the radioactivity incorporated in the cells ± SE.

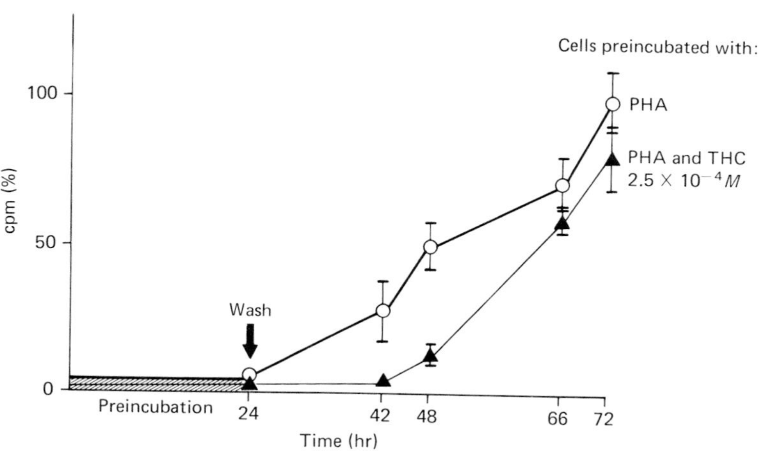

examinations show no significant difference between cells in both cultures.

Time course and nature of inhibition

It was reported previously [19] that THC inhibits leucine, uridine, and thymidine incorporation into cells after 16 hr, and that this inhibition remains constant throughout the culture period. Using different concentrations of precursors and different doses of THC, we observed that the rate of precursor incorporation was constant during 3 days of cultures. This is a necessary condition in order to use the Lineweaver–Burke plot.

In the present experiments, we studied leucine and uridine incorporation during the first 6 hr of culture (Figure 26.5a,b), and we observed that the presence of PHA did not interfere with the inhibitory effect of THC. In other experiments, we studied at the third day of culture the time required for THC to act on precursor incorporation (Figure 26.6). The inhibition is significant after 15 min and remains constant thereafter. In other experiments, different doses of THC were used with different concentrations of precursor in the culture medium. Results were plotted on a Lineweaver–Burke plot (Figure 26.7). The curves intersect on the abscissa, indicating a noncompetitive inhibition of precursor uptake by THC. Values of K_i and K_m for leucine, uridine, and thymidine are given in Table 26.2.

Discussion

Investigators reported previously that the degree of inhibition, by a given dose of THC, of ^{3}H-thymidine incorporation into lymphocytes was a function of serum concentration in the culture medium. With the same dose of THC, we observed ten times less inhibition when the serum concentration of the medium was increased from 10 to 20 percent [15,16].

Present results confirm these observations. As Klausner [9] and Wahlqvist [26] showed, 85 to 95 percent of THC is bound to serum lipoproteins. Widman also showed that the drug was bound to blood cells. Cellular binding of THC would take place by a displacement of its bond from the lipoproteins onto the cells. We have also observed that cellular toxicity of THC is reversed by washing, and the drug may therefore become "unbound" from the cell.

We suggest the following scheme to describe the interactions

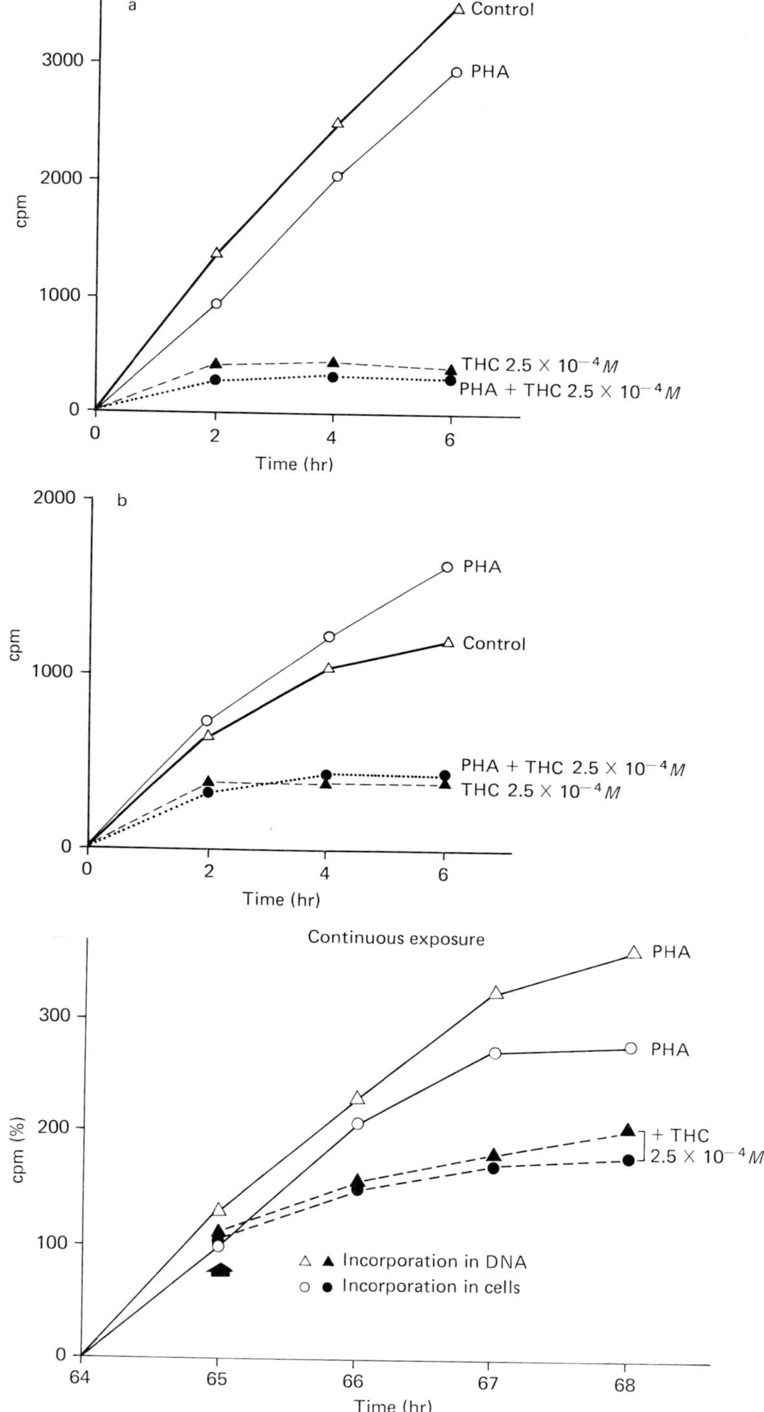

Figure 26.5. Inhibition by THC of the incorporation of (a) leucine or (b) uridine during the first 6 hr of incubation, with or without PHA. (c) Inhibition of thymidine uptake measured after 64 hr incubation.

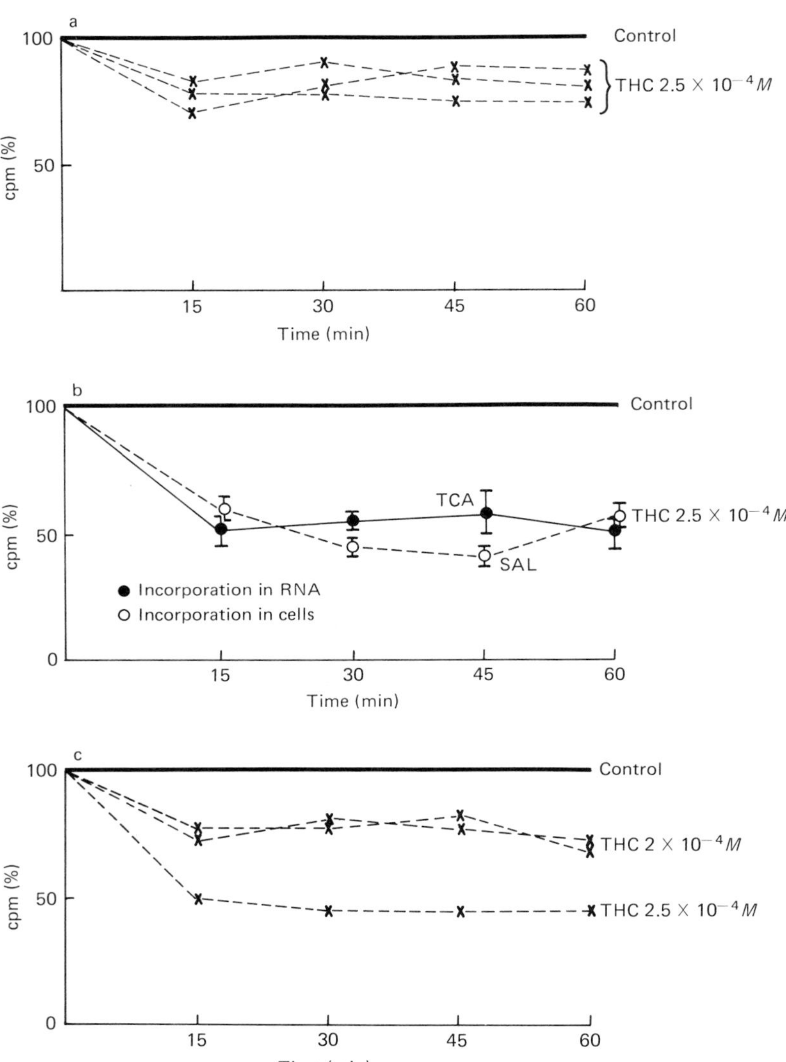

Figure 26.6. Time lag of the incorporation of (a) ^{3}H-leucine, (b) ^{3}H-uridine, and (c) ^{3}H-thymidine after adding THC. In (b), each point represents the mean of 2 experiments ± SD. THC and tritiated precursors were added in the middle of the 64th hr (timed). Thereafter, cells were harvested every 15 min. Results are expressed in % incorporation of precursors in a parallel control culture.

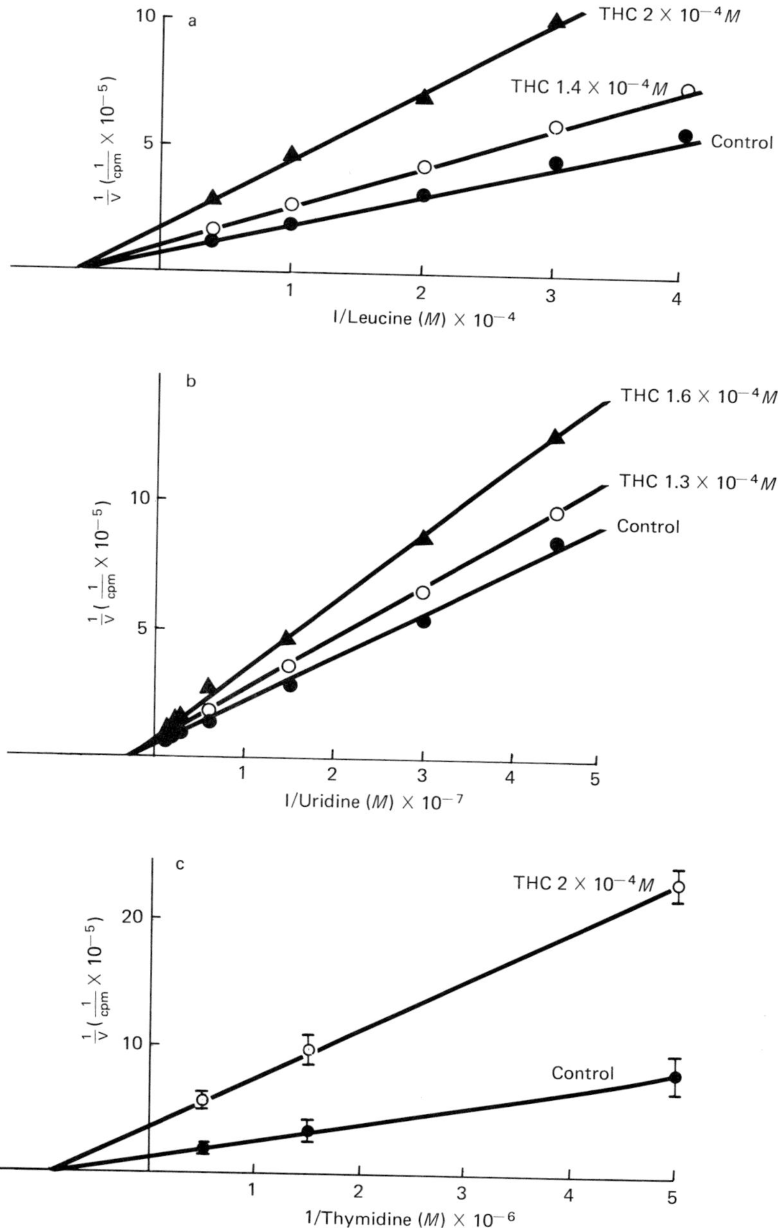

Figure 26.7. Lineweaver–Burke plot of the inhibition by THC of (a) leucine, (b) uridine, and (c) thymidine uptake. In (c), each point represents the mean of 2 experiments ± SE.

Table 26.2 Constants[a] of Michaelis-Menten (K_m) for the incorporation of the 3 precursors and constants of inhibition (K_i) for THC.

Precursors	K_m (*M*)	K_i (*M*)
Thymidine	9.5×10^{-7}	1.1×10^{-4}
Uridine	4.8×10^{-7}	3.0×10^{-4}
Leucine	1.9×10^{-4}	1.4×10^{-4}

[a] Constants are expressed in moles (M) and are calculated on the basis of the results of Figure 26.2.

between THC, cells, and the serum concentration of the culture medium:

$$(\text{cells}) + (\text{serum-THC}) \rightleftharpoons (\text{THC-cells}) + (\text{serum})$$

Therefore, if the serum concentration increases, cells are less inhibited by THC (Figure 26.2), and the equilibrium of the above reaction is displaced toward the left. If the cell concentration increases, there is a similar inhibition of lymphocyte transformation (Table 26.1), indicating that more molecules of THC are bound to cells, and the equilibrium of the reaction is displaced toward the left. These interactions between THC, serum, and cells explain why different authors report the same inhibitory effects of THC with concentrations varying from 10^{-5} *M* to 10^{-4} *M*, depending upon the serum concentration of the culture medium used.

Cellular toxicity with concentration of 10^{-5} *M* THC or less have been reported by Zimmerman [29] and by Blevin and Regan [2] in culture media containing 10 percent serum or less. These results are in agreement with ours [15].

The nature of the binding of THC to lymphocytes is not known. It can be reversed by washing the cells with RPMI even after they have been stimulated with a mitogen. In the latter case, however, the cells cannot be recovered (Figure 26.4) for at least 24 hr. The reversibility of the cytotoxicity of THC by washing of the cells might explain the discrepancies reported by different investigators who studied mitogen-induced blastogenesis of chronic marihuana smokers. In these subjects, Nahas *et al.* [15] reported an inhibition of lymphocyte transformation, but White *et al.* [28] did not. To isolate lymphocytes from the blood of marihuana smokers, one must wash the cells three times. During such a procedure THC might be washed away from the lymphocytes.

In cultured lymphocytes, a mitogen is required to induce blastogenesis; therefore, it is important to note that there is no interference between the inducer and the inhibitor of blastogenesis, between PHA and THC: THC does not prevent the induction of blastogenesis by PHA (Figure 26.2), and PHA does not alter the inhibition qualitatively or quantitatively (Figure 26.4a,b).

The mechanism of THC-induced inhibition is not clear. DNA, RNA, and protein syntheses are interrelated, and the inhibition of one impairs that of the other. The present data indicate that THC does not exert its inhibitory effect specifically on the synthesis of a single macromolecule: such a type of specific inhibition is characterized by a lag in the synthesis of the macromolecules that are not primarily affected by the inhibitor. For instance, Pogo [23] has shown that cells treated with cordycepin, which inhibits mRNA synthesis, display a lag of 2–6 hr before showing a decrease in protein synthesis. The present experiments indicate that all three precursors are inhibited within 15 min after adding THC and without any lag between them.

Inhibition of precursor uptake by THC is noncompetitive (Figure 26.7). This noncompetitive inhibition indicates that the enzymes regulating the transport of the precursors have the same affinity for their substrate (the same coefficient of Michaelis-Menten, or K_m) in the presence of increasing concentrations of inhibitor. However, their maximum rate (V_m) decreases with increasing amounts of THC. The coefficients of inhibition (K_i) calculated for leucine, uridine, and thymidine are similar (Table 26.2). Since the transport mechanisms of these three precursors are different [14], it would appear that THC would act through a similar mechanism. THC, which is very fat soluble [7], binds according to Chari-Bitron [4] to the double lipid layer of the plasma membrane. This binding alters the physical property of the membrane [6], as well as the function of its enzymes [11,22]. Because of its action on membranes, Seeman [24] classifies THC among the central nervous system depressants and anti-inflammatory agents.

Such an effect of THC on cell membranes could explain its mechanism of action on macromolecular synthesis. THC could inhibit the transport of precursors through the plasma membrane by a direct action on the enzymes specialized in this function. THC could also act indirectly by inhibiting nucleic acid, which is required in their transport across the membrane [25].

At the level of the mitochondrial membrane, THC could also exert an inhibitory effect. Martin *et al.* [13] have reported that 45 percent of ^{3}H-THC administered is recovered in mitochondria, where THC might inhibit energy production or transfer [1]. However, how such mechanisms inhibit cell anabolism must still be explained.

Whatever its mechanism, the depressant effect of marihuana products on protein and nucleic acid synthesis is now an established fact: the present studies corroborate those of Zimmerman, the Leuchtenbergers, Jakubovic and McGeer, Mellors, Blevin and Regan, Huot, and Carchman and Harris, which are included in this volume. This inhibitory effect could also explain the observations made by Rosenkranz and Hembree, in their studies using animals and human subjects exposed to heavy doses of marihuana. These observations suggest that the cannabinoids in doses reached in heavy human consumption might have an *in vivo* effect on macromolecular synthesis similar to the one described *in vitro.*

ACKNOWLEDGMENTS

This research was supported by grants from SAODAP (DA-4PG015) and NIDA (DA-00894-01A1). The Δ^9-THC used in this study was gracefully provided by NIDA (National Institute of Drug Abuse), Rockville, Maryland.

REFERENCES

1. Birmingham, M. K. and A. Bartova (1976) Effects of cannabinol derivatives on blood pressure, body weights, pituitary-adrenal function and mitochondrial respiration in the rat. *Marihuana: Biochemical and Cellular Effects* (G. G. Nahas, W. D. M. Paton, and J. Idanpään-Heikkelä, eds.). New York: Springer-Verlag.
2. Blevin, R. D. and R. D. Regan (1976) Delta-9-THC: Effect on macromolecular synthesis in human and other mammalian cells. *Marihuana: Biochemical and Cellular Effects* (G. G. Nahas, W. D. M. Paton, and J. Idanpään-Heikkelä, eds.). New York: Springer-Verlag.
3. Boyum, A. (1968) Isolation of leukocytes from human blood. *Scand. J. Clin. Lab. Invest. 21* (suppl. 97):31–50.
4. Chari-Bitron, A. (1971) Stabilisation of rat erythrocyte membrane by delta-9-THC. *Life Sci. 10:*1273–1279.
5. Desoize, B. and G. G. Nahas (1975) Effet inhibiteur du delta 9-tétrahydrocannabinol sur la synthése des protéines et des acides nucléiques. *C. R. Acad. Sci.* [*D*] (*Paris*) *280:*475–478.
6. Gill, E. W., G. Jones, and D. K. Lawrence (1972). Chemical mecha-

nisms of action of THC in cannabis and its derivatives (W. D. M. Paton and J. Crown, eds.). London: Oxford University Press pp. 76–87.

7. Hartzman, R. J., M. Segall, M. L. Bach, and F. M. Bach (1971) Miniaturization of the mixed leukocyte culture test. *Transplantation 11*(3):268–273.
8. Kreuz, D. S. and J. Axelrod (1973) Delta-9-THC: Localisation in body fat. *Science 179:*391–392.
9. Klausner, H. A. and J. V. Dingel (1971) The metabolism and excretion of delta-9-THC in the rat. *Life Sci 10:*49–59.
10. Koch, F. and Y. Koch (1974) Reversible inhibition of macromolecular synthesis in HeLa cells by ethanol. *Res. Commun. Chem. Pathol. Pharmacol.* 9(2):291–298.
11. Laurent, B. and P. E. Roy (1974) Alteration of membrane integrity by delta-9-THC. *Int. J. Clin. Pharmacol.* 10(2):154.
12. Leuchtenberger, C., R. Leuchtenberger, U. Ritter, and N. Inui (1973) Effects of marihuana and tobacco smoke on DNA and chromosomal complement in human lung explants. *Nature 242:*403–404.
13. Martin, B. R., W. L. Dewey, L. S. Harris, and J. S. Beckner (1974) Subcellular localization of ^{3}H-THC in dog brain after acute or chronic administration. *The Pharmacologist 16*(2):260.
14. Mizel, B. G. and L. Wilson (1972) Nucleoside transport in mammalian cells, inhibition by colchicine. *Biochemistry 11*(14):2573–2578.
15. Nahas, G., J. P. Armand, and J. Hsu (1974) Inhibition in vitro de la blastogénése des lymphocytes T par le delta-9-THC. *C. R. Acad. Sci.* [*D*] (*Paris*) *278:*679–680.
16. Nahas, G., B. Desoize, J. P. Armand, J. Hsu, and A. Morishima (1974) Inhibition in vitro de la transformation lymphocytaire par divers cannabinoides naturels. *C. R. Acad. Sci.* [*D*] (*Paris*) *279:* 785–787.
17. Nahas, G. and B. Desoize (1974) Effet inhibiteur du 5-n-amylresorcinol sur la transformation lymphoblastique. *C. R. Acad. Sci.* [*D*] (*Paris*) *279:*1607–1608.
18. Nahas, G. G., N. Suciu-Foca, J. P. Armand, and A. Morishima (1974) Inhibition of cellular mediated immunity in marihuana smokers. *Science 183:*419–420.
19. Nahas, G. G., B. Desoize, J. Hsu, A. Morishima, and P. R. Srinivasan (1975) Inhibition by natural cannabinoids and olivetol of lymphocyte transformation. *Pharmacology of Cannabis* (Szara, S. and M. Braude, eds.). New York: Raven Press.
20. Neu, R. L., M. O. Powers, S. King, and L. I. Garner (1970) Delta-8 and delta-9-THC: Effect on cultured lymphocytes. *J. Clin. Pharmacol. 10*(4):228–230.
21. Parker, J. R. and J. F. Mowbray (1971) Peripheral blood leukocyte changes during human renal allograft rejection. *Transplantation 11:*201–209.
22. Poddar, M. K. and J. J. Ghosh (1975) Neuronal membrane as the site of action of delta-9-THC. *Pharmacology of Cannabis* (Braude M. and S. Szara, eds.). New York: Raven Press.
23. Pogo, B. G. and L. Wilson (1974) Inhibition of RNA synthesis and transformation by cordycepin. *Cell. Immunol. 14:*134–138.

24. Seeman, P. (1972) The membrane actions of anesthetics and tranquilizers. *Pharmacol. Rev. 24:*583–615.
25. Scholtissek, C. (1968) Nucleotide metabolism in tissue culture cells at low temperatures. *Biochem. Biophys. Acta 155:*14–23.
26. Wahlqvist, M., I. M. Nilsson, F. Sandberg, and S. Agurell (1970) Binding of delta-9-THC to human plasma proteins. *Biochem. Pharmacol. 19:*2579–2584.
27. Widman, M., S. Agurell, M. Ehrnebo, and G. Jones (1974) Binding of delta-1-THC and 7-OH-delta-1-THC to blood cells and plasma proteins in man. *J. Pharm. Pharmacol. 26:*914–916.
28. White, J. C., J. C. Brin, and B. W. Janicki (1975) Mitogen induced blastogenetic responses of lymphocytes in marihuana smokers. *Science 188:*71–72.
29. Zimmerman, A. M. and D. K. MacClean (1973) Action of narcotic and hallucinogenic agents on the cell cycle. *Drugs and the Cell Cycle* (A. M. Zimmerman, G. M. Padilla, and I. L. Cameron, eds.). New York: Academic Press, pp. 67–94.

27

Cellular and Biochemical Alterations Induced *in Vitro* by Δ^1-Tetrahydrocannabinol: Effects on Cell Proliferation, Nucleic Acids, Plasma Cell Membrane ATPase, and Adenylate Cyclase

JACQUES HUOT

Introduction

The psychodysleptic effect produced by Δ^1-tetrahydrocannabinol (Δ^1-THC) is well known and was described in detail by Moreau [20] in 1845. However, the basic cellular mechanisms which underlie the development of the psychodysleptic syndrome still are not very clear. This present work describes some cellular and biochemical alterations induced by THC in cells cultivated *in vitro,* an experimental model which offers many advantages in the investigation of the mechanism of action of a drug on the cell. However, the results of such *in vitro* studies should not be extrapolated hastily to interpret the action of these drugs in man.

Material and Methods

Cell cultures

The experiments were carried out on three types of cells cultivated as monolayers: human epidermoid neoplastic KB cells, African green monkey kidney fibroblastic (AGMK) cells, and mouse cholinergic neuroblastoma cells NS-20. KB cells and AGMK cells were maintained in Eagle's minimal essential medium (MEM) containing 10 percent of calf serum and the following antibiotics: penicillin G 50 IU, streptomycin sulfate 50 μg/ml, and neomycin 50 μg/ml. Neuroblastoma cells were cultivated in MEM supplemented with 10 percent fetal calf serum and with 100 IU/ml of penicillin G, and 100 μg/ml of streptomycin sulfate. The cultures were incubated at 37°C and at pH 7.0 to 7.3 in a humidified

Marihuana: Chemistry, Biochemistry, and Cellular Effects, edited by Gabriel G. Nahas,

atmosphere of 10 percent CO_2: 90 percent air. The experiments reported below were performed on cultures of cells that were in the exponential phase of proliferation.

Determination of cell proliferation

Cell proliferation was measured by counting the isolated cell nuclei with a hemocytometer.

Determination of nucleic acid content

The effects of Δ^1-THC on nucleic acids were studied in fluorescence microscopy on cells stained with a solution of acridine-orange (1:10,000) in McIlwain buffer (pH 3.8). Details of the technique were described previously [14]. Under the experimental conditions used, nuclear DNA exhibits a greenish fluorescence, whereas the RNA-containing structures emit a yellowish-orange (nucleolus) or a reddish-orange fluorescence (cytoplasm). The characteristic and the intensity of the reaction are related to the cellular content of DNA and RNA as well as to their molecular conformation.

Determination of the plasma cell membrane ATPase activity

The plasma cell membrane ATPase activity was demonstrated histochemically by a technique adapted from that originally described by Padykula and Herman [25]. After the cells were treated by the various agents investigated, they were fixed for 15 min in 10 percent neutral formaldehyde (4°C). They were then incubated for 90 min at 37°C in a medium containing sodium barbital 100 m*M* (pH 9.4), calcium 2 m*M*, magnesium 2 m*M*, sodium 5 m*M*, potassium 1 m*M*, and ATP 5m*M*. The cells were then treated successively with a solution of cobalt chloride and one of ammonium sulfide. Under the light microscope, the enzyme activity was shown by black deposits of cobalt sulfide located mainly at the level of the plasma cell membrane. The specificity and the characteristic of the reaction were controlled by incubating some cultures in ATP-free media and others in ouabain (1 m*M*) containing media.

Determination of adenylate cyclase activity

The assay of the adenylate cyclase activity was performed on permeabilized preparations of NS-20 neuroblastoma cells. The techniques used to prepare the cells and to perform the enzyme assay were detailed in a recent paper [27]. The adenylate cyclase activity was measured by the conversion of α-^{32}P-ATP into cyclic ^{32}P-AMP. The enzymic reaction was initiated by adding the cellular preparation (100–125 μg of proteins under 25 μl) to the following incubation mixture (final volume 50 μl): Tris-HCl (pH 8.0) 100 m*M;* ATP 0.1 m*M;* $MgCl_2$ 0.25 m*M;* cyclic GMP 1.0 m*M;* papaverine hydrochloride 0.1 m*M;* creatine phosphate 20 m*M;* creatine kinase 50 μg; α-^{32}P-ATP 0.7 μCi; and the appropriate concentrations of the agents investigated. The mixture was incubated for 10 min at 37°C. The reaction was stopped by cooling and diluting α-^{32}P-ATP with an excess of unlabeled ATP. The cyclic AMP was separated from other nucleotides, nucleosides, or other eventually labeled metabolites by chromatography on Dowex columns. The chromatographic yield was controlled by adding cyclic ^{3}H-AMP to the final medium before filtration. Radioactivity was measured by liquid scintillation spectrometry.

Pharmacological agents and other chemicals

The effects of various concentrations of the following agents given alone or in simultaneous combination were studied: Δ^1-THC, ouabain, diphenylhydantoin (DPH), $CaCl_2$, and prostaglandin E_1 (PGE_1). Most of these drugs (concentrations indicated in the text) were added directly in the culture medium or in the incubation medium used for the adenylate cyclase assay. However, the original solution of THC (32 m*M*) was in a 1:1 mixture of propylene glycol: ethanol 95 percent. The solution was further diluted serially in the appropriate medium specified in the text. The final concentrations of PGE_1 in the incubation medium for the adenylate cyclase assay were obtained after the serial dilution of the initial ethanolic solution of PGE_1 (28 m*M* in 70 percent ethanol). In any case, two series of controls were employed when studying the effect of THC: one containing the same amount of vehicle brought about by the drug, and the other containing only the culture medium. Both controls and treated media were sterilized through passage on Millipore sweenex filters (0.22 μ) before being added for various times to the cultures.[1]

[1] THC was a gift from Dr. S. Radouco-Thomas, Laval University; and PGE_1 was furnished by Upjohn. Diphenylhydantoin (Dilantin) was purchased from Parke-Davis, and ouabaïn from NBC. α-^{32}P-ATP (1 Ci/mM) was from NEN, and cyclic ^{3}H-AMP (29 Ci/mM) from the Commissariat à l'Energie Atomique (Saclay). Creatine phosphate and creatine kinase were purchased from Boehringer. All other reagents were A grade.

Results

Effects on cell proliferation

The concentration-dependent effects of THC on the proliferation of KB and AGMK cells treated for 48 hr are given in Figure 27.1. Concentrations lower than 10 μM did not induce any significant alterations in both cell types. Nevertheless, a weak but reproducible stimulatory effect was observed in AGMK cells treated with 0.1 μM and 1.0 μM of THC. Conversely, cell proliferation was impaired by concentrations of THC greater than 10 μM. This is shown by the decreased number of cells in the treated cultures. Concentrations from 10–100 μM only retarded cell proliferation, whereas concentrations equal to or greater than 1 mM were cytotoxic since after the exposure period (48 hr) the number of cells in the treated cultures was less (by 40 percent) than at the beginning. The inhibitory action of THC was more pronounced in neo-

Figure 27.1. Concentration-dependent alterations induced by THC on the proliferation of KB and AGMK cells. The effects were evaluated after a 48-hr exposure period. The results are expressed as the percentage of cells found after 48 hr in comparison to the number of cells present at time 0.

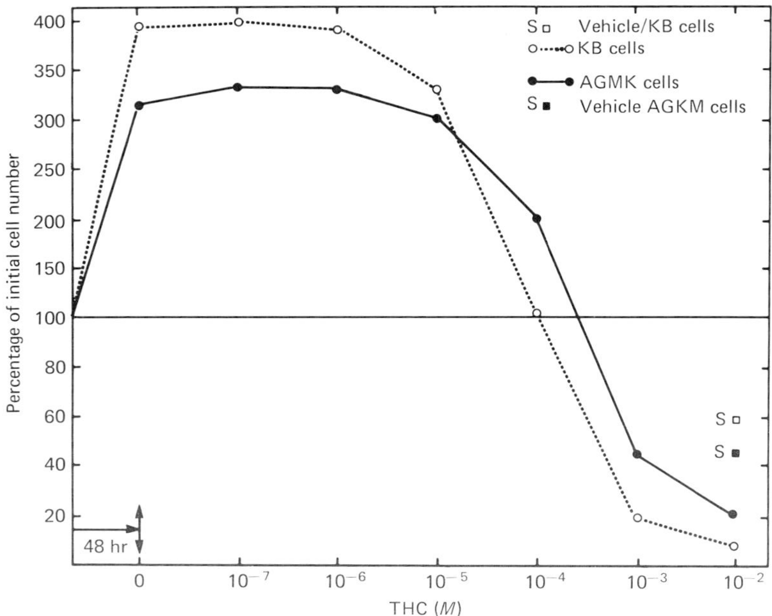

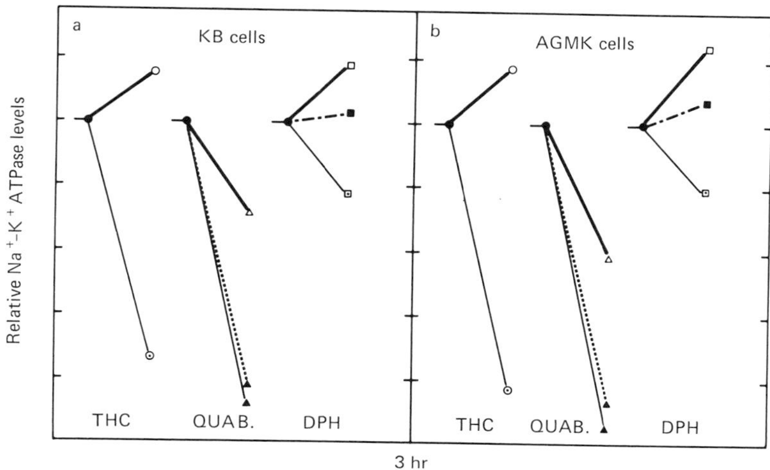

Figure 27.4. Effects of THC, ouabain, and DPH alone or in combination on the activity of the plasma cell membrane ATPase. The enzyme activity was determined by a histochemical technique described in the section on methods. The results are expressed in terms of relative levels of the ATPase activity, which were established from microscopic examination (by 2 investigators) of the histochemical reaction. (a) Effects on KB cells; (b) effects on AGMK cells.
Basal activity (——●); THC 10 μM (○); THC 0.5 mM (⊙); ouabain 1 mM (△- - -△); ouabain 1 mM/THC 0.5 mM (◬——◬); ouabain 1 mM/THC 10 μM (△——△); DPH 10 μM (■); DPH 10 μM/THC (□); DPH 10 μM/THC (0.5 mM (⊡).

markedly inhibited by ouabain 1 m*M*, whereas it was to some extent stimulated by DPH 10 μM. These latter two observations suggest that the measured activity corresponds mainly to that of the Na^+-K^+ ATPase. The inhibitory effect of ouabain was partially antagonized by THC 10 μM. This was more marked in KB cells. Conversely, there was a weak inhibitory synergy between ouabain 1 m*M* and THC 0.5 m*M*. A combination of DPH 10 μM and THC 10 μM seemed to have an additive stimulatory effect, at least in AGMK cells. On the other hand, DPH 10 μM partially antagonized the inhibition induced in both types of cells by THC 0.5 m*M*.

Effects on neuroblastoma cells' adenylate cyclase activity

In concentrations between 5 μM and 1 m*M*, THC progressively stimulated the adenylate cyclase activity of NS-20 neuroblastoma cells. Lower dosages ($< 5\ \mu M$) were inactive, whereas concentra-

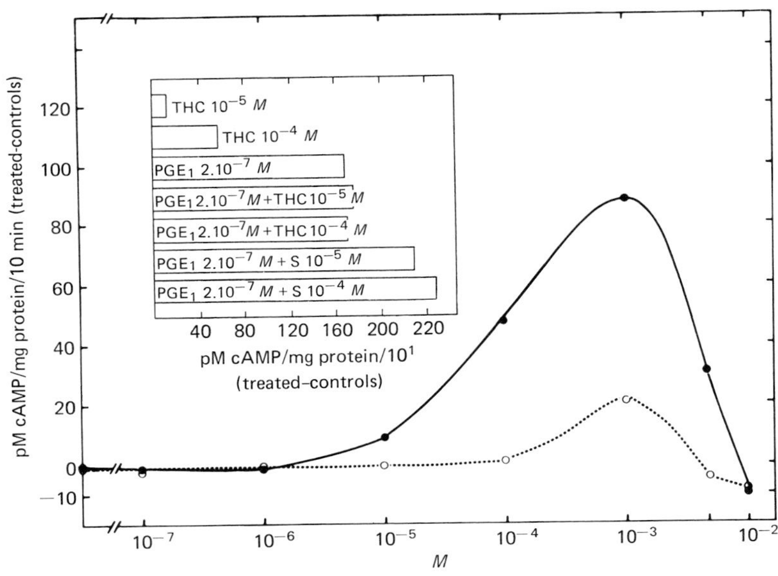

Figure 27.5. Concentration-dependent effects of THC on the adenylate cyclase from permeabilized neuroblastoma cells. (The assay of the adenylate cyclase is described in the section on methods.) Adenylate cyclase activity is expressed as the difference between the basal activity and that of the treated samples. Basal activity was 45–50 pM cAMP formed/10 min/mg of protein. The cellular preparations used contained 100 μg protein under 25 μl.
THC (●—●); vehicle (○. . . . .○).
The insert shows the effects resulting from the interaction between THC (10 μM–0.1 mM) and PGE_1 (0.2 μM) and between PGE_1 and the vehicle accompanying THC.

tions greater than 1 m*M* were inhibitory (Figure 27.5). The results are expressed by values (pmoles cAMP/mg protein/10 min) obtained after subtracting the basal activity from those of the treated samples. The vehicle brought by THC 1 m*M* stimulated the enzyme activity weakly. Conversely, when given in amounts accompanying THC 10 m*M*, the vehicle inhibited the basal activity the same amount as did the 10 m*M* solution of THC. The insert of Figure 27.5 shows that neither THC 10 μ*M* nor 0.1 m*M* could modify the stimulation induced by PGE_1 given in a concentration corresponding to its apparent K_m (0.2 μ*M*). On the other hand, the stimulating action of PGE_1 was increased by the presence of the vehicle in the amount used to solubilize THC 10 μ*M* and 1 m*M*.

Discussion

Our results, which indicate that THC impaired cell proliferation in concentrations greater than 10 μM, are in agreement with those obtained by other authors [5,22,34,35]. It is difficult to evaluate the *in vivo* significance of this effect. The range of concentrations which were effective appears to be greater than the blood level which could be reached in casual users. However, the concentrations of cannabinoids might be reached in heavy chronic users and induce deleterious effects during some particularly critical period of embryogenesis or during the development of the immune process [33].

The type of chromatin alterations induced by THC does not suggest that the DNA content was decreased. The reduction of the greenish fluorescence observed in some regions of the nucleus reflects probably only a local loss of chromatin material which had aggregated and formed clumps without any significant alterations of the net DNA content of the nucleus. Our observations would rather indicate a redistribution of chromatin or a molecular rearrangement which could result from the binding of THC with DNA or even with some nuclear proteins. These cytochemical alterations could be the reflection of some biochemical data previously reported [13]. It was demonstrated in the rat that THC might impair the template activity of chromatin, as a result of their mutual binding.

The reduced synthesis of RNA observed in the latter study was interpreted as being due to interference with the DNA template activity [13]. The THC-induced decrease in the fluorescence of the RNA-containing structures may be a manifestation of such a reduced synthesis of RNA through impairment occurring at the transcriptional level. The inhibition of RNA synthesis by THC has also been reported by others, as has the interference of the drug with other types of macromolecular synthesis [2,12,16,17,19,24,34,35]. It is also possible that the decrease of the RNA content reflects an accelerated breakdown. Nucleic acids play a vital role in the normal function of the cell, and their alterations by THC might be involved in the inhibitory effect of this drug on cell proliferation. Both inhibition of cell proliferation and alterations of nucleic acids were observed for the same range of THC concentrations. Similar alterations were also observed *in vivo* [11,12] with large dosages of THC that seem beyond those reached in human consumption. However, THC and its metabolites accumulate in the brain [9] where they may reach elevated concentrations in heavy users. The loss of memory sometimes reported by chronic users of cannabis could somehow be related to an action of THC on RNA or protein synthesis. The toxic reactions which may possibly result from the action of THC on nucleic acids *in vivo* should not necessarily be restricted to the brain and may affect those from other cells as shown by Stefanis and Issidorides [32]. Chromatin alterations observed in neutrophils and lymphocytes of chronic marihuana smokers indicate that our *in vitro* observations might have more than a test tube significance.

The following gross morphological alterations of the cells incubated with THC were observed: nucleus with irregular contours, general cellular enlargement, and loss of the elongated aspect of fibroblasts. Comparable effects were observed in nerve cells of dogs treated chronically with cannabis resin [11] and in explants of lung cells exposed to marijuana smoke [18]. These alterations may be the manifestation of an action at the plasma membrane level. Cellular enlargement could result partially from membrane expansion in a manner similar to that allegedly produced by anesthetics [30,31]. This membrane expansion would be caused by the hydrophobic binding of THC with the cell membrane. According to Paton *et al.* [26], THC should act like a "partial" anesthetic because its solubility in relation to that of the membrane lipids does not allow it to achieve the volume fraction needed for complete anesthesia. The antagonistic effect of 5.0 m*M* $CaCl_2$ on the THC-induced changes of the AGMK morphology may indicate that THC, like other drugs such as chlorpromazine [10] and reserpine [15], acts at membrane sites normally occupied by calcium. Therefore, addition of calcium would competitively dislodge or antagonize THC and neutralize its effect on cell morphology. The antagonism of THC by $CaCl_2$ also may result from the membrane-stabilizing properties of this ion. This functional antagonism is likely to occur since THC 1 m*M* may induce its effect through membrane lysis.

The biphasic action of THC on membrane ATPase is possibly related to changes in the structural conformation of the enzyme due to the high hydrophobicity of THC, which may give this drug detergent-like properties. Various detergents are known to induce a biphasic pattern of ATPase activity [29]. In low concentrations, THC would stimulate the enzyme by increasing the number of exposed enzymatic sites. At high concentrations (1m*M*), the interactions of THC with the membrane alter the state of the lipids which are required for the catalytic activity of the enzyme and which are involved in the modulation of the enzyme conformation

[29]. This will lead to inhibition of the enzyme activity. The inhibition of ATPase activity by THC has been reported previously [8]. The sensitivity of the enzyme to ouabain and DPH strongly suggests that the measured activity corresponds to that of Na^+-K^+-ATPase [29].

THC was used separately or in combination with DPH and ouabain in cell culture in order to investigate the possible relationship between alterations of the Na^+-K^+-ATPase and cell proliferation produced by the drug. The results obtained do not suggest that the effects of THC on cell proliferation are mediated through membrane ATPase.

THC also alters the adenylate cyclase activity of NS-20 neuroblastoma cells. Only the stimulation of the enzyme is clearly related to THC. The inhibitory effects are unspecific since the vehicle has the same action. The vehicle also weakly stimulates the enzyme activity when given in an amount equal to that brought by THC 1 m*M*. Consequently, this should be taken into account when evaluating the stimulation of THC 1 m*M*. The stimulation of adenylate cyclase is compatible with the inhibition of cell proliferation if it is accompanied by an elevation of the intracellular level of cAMP. This nucleotide is generally considered to impair cell proliferation in most types of cells, whereas cGMP would promote proliferation [4]. Phosphodiesterase activity should be assayed and the intracellular level of cAMP measured before a correlation between the inhibition of cell proliferation and the stimulation of the adenylate cyclase can be established. Nahas [23] has reported that comparable concentrations of THC (0.5 m*M*) stimulated the activity of the adenyl cyclase from uterine muscle preparation. However, the phosphodiesterase activity was not affected. In our study, THC maximally stimulated the adenylate cyclase in concentrations (0.1 m*M* to 1 m*M*) which otherwise inhibited the ATPase activity. This is consistent with the postulated antagonistic relationship between the adenyl cyclase activity and the ATPase activity [21].

The stimulatory action of THC on adenylate cyclase activity may be involved in the development of the psychodysleptic effect of this drug. It would be important to clarify whether THC alters the cyclase activity through a direct action on the molecule or through some unspecific detergent-like action related to its high hydrophobicity. It is difficult to imagine that a specific receptor to THC exists at the regulatory site of a given adenylate cyclase. However, THC may interact with a receptor site that is specific for a given agonist; THC would then act like a partial agonist and would be able to induce some degree of enzyme activation. If THC stimulates adenylate cyclase activity in such a way, a systematic investigation should be undertaken to characterize the nature of the adenylate cyclase system that responds to it. However, it is also possible that THC causes some conformational changes of the enzyme molecule leading to an increased accessibility of the agonist to the regulatory site or of ATP to the catalytic site.

The characterization of the eventual THC-sensitive adenylate cyclase is complicated by the fact that the drug shows no clear structural relationship with the various known agonists of the adenylate cyclase system. However, THC has structural similarity with LSD-25, psylocibin, and mescaline, and it has been reported that LSD-25 stimulates the activity of the dopamine-sensitive adenylate cyclase from rat caudate nucleus [3]. This effect is antagonized by neuroleptics.

Preliminary results with PGE_1 showed that THC does not alter the stimulating action of PGE_1. This suggests that the eventual involvement of PGE_1 in the effects induced by THC does not occur on the regulatory site of the PGE_1 sensitive adenylate cyclase, at least of neuroblastoma cells. However, experimental evidence indicates that THC inhibits the synthesis of PGE_1 [6,7]. On the other hand, it is unclear why the vehicle enhanced the effect of PGE_1, yet had no effect when given alone in the same amount. This paradoxical effect could be interpreted tentatively on the basis that the vehicle may facilitate the access of PGE_1 to its receptor site.

Summary and Conclusions

In concentrations greater than 10 μM, THC impairs cell proliferation, may interact with DNA, and decreases template activity. THC reduces the cellular content of RNA, probably through inhibition of synthesis occurring at the transcriptional level; THC induces various morphological alterations which may reflect its hydrophobic binding with membranes; in concentration of 10 μM, THC stimulates Na^+-K-ATPase while inhibiting this enzyme in concentration of 1mM. These effects might result from a conformational change, caused by the drug, in the state of the membrane lipids of the enzyme. In 0.5 μM–1 mM, THC stimulates the adenylate cyclase activity of NS-20 neuroblastoma cells. The range of concentrations used *in vitro* are higher than those which could be reached in man following casual use of marihuana, but they could be reached in long-term heavy users because of the cumulative properties of THC and of its metabolites.

ACKNOWLEDGMENTS

The author greatly appreciates the collaboration and advice of Drs. J. Penit, B. Canteau, and S. Jard from the Laboratoire de Physiologie Cellulaire of the Collège de France. Thanks are also addressed to Miss L. Lemire who participated in this study. Finally, he is indebted to Miss D. Huot for her secretarial assistance.

This work was supported by the Canadian Department of Health and Welfare (Grant No. 605/23/8) and by Le Conseil de la recherche médicale du Québec (Grant No. 730099).

The study concerning the effects of THC on adenylate cyclase activity was performed while the author was studying under a fellowship from the Medical Research Council of Canada. This investigation was done in collaboration with Drs. J. Penit, B. Canteau, and S. Jard from the Collège de France, Paris.

REFERENCES

1. Barnett, R. E. and J. Palazzoto (1974) Mechanism of the effects of lipid phase transitions on the Na^+-K^+-ATPase and the role of protein conformational changes. *Ann. N.Y. Acad. Sci. 242:*69.
2. Blevins, D. and J. D. Regan (1976) Δ^9-THC: Effect on macromolecular synthesis in human and other mammalian cells. *Marihuana: Chemistry, Biochemistry, and Cellular Effects* (G. G. Nahas *et al.,* eds.). New York: Springer-Verlag.
3. Bockaert, J. Personnal communication.
4. Bourne, H., P. Coffino, P. Insel, P. Jones, K. L. Melmon, G. M. Tomkins, and S. Wilbert (1975) Cyclic nucleotides and control of cell proliferation. Abstracts VI Int. Congress of Pharmacology, Helsinki, p. 536.
5. Bram, S. and P. Brachet (1976) Inhibition of proliferation and differentiation of D. discoideum amoebae by THC and cannabinol. *Marihuana: Chemistry, Biochemistry, and Cellular Effects* (G. G. Nahas *et al.,* eds.). New York: Springer-Verlag.
6. Burnstein, S. and A. Raz (1972) Inhibition of prostaglandin E_2 biosynthesis by delta 1-tetrahydrocannabinol. *Prostaglandins 2:*369.
7. Burnstein, S., L. Levin, and C. Varanelli (1973) Prostaglandins and cannabis-11. Inhibition of biosynthesis by the naturally occurring cannabinoids. *Biochem. Pharmacol. 22:*2905.
8. Chari-Bitron, A. and T. E. Bino (1970) Effects of Δ^1-tetrahydrocannabinol on ATPase activity of rat liver mitochondria. *Biochem. Pharmacol. 20:*473.
9. Colburn, R. W., N. G. Kylorenz, L. Lemberger, and I. J. Kopin (1974) Subcellular distribution of Δ^9-tetrahydrocannabinol in rat brain. *Biochem. Pharmacol. 23:*873.
10. Despopoulos, A. (1970) Antihemolytic actions of tricyclic tranquilizers. Structural correlations. *Biochem. Pharmacol. 19:*2907.
11. Durandina, A. I. and V. A. Romazenko (1972) Troubles fonctionnels et morphologiques observées dans l'intoxication chronique par des

substances résineuses tirées du cannabis de Yujnochuisk. *Bull. Stupéfiants 24:*31.

12. Hattori, T., A. Jakubovic, and P. L. McGeer (1972) Reduction in number of nuclear membrane-attached ribosomes in infant rat brain following acute Δ^9-tetrahydrocannabinol administration. *Exp. Neurol. 36:*207.
13. Hodgson, J. R., E. I. Woodhouse, and T. R. Castles (1972) Brain chromatin template activity of rats treated with Δ^9-tetrahydrocannabinol. *Can. J. Physiol. Pharmacol. 51:*401.
14. Huot, J. (1971) Effects des flavonoides sur des systèmes cellulaires cultivés in vitro. Ph.D. Thesis, Québec, Université Laval, pp. 45–55.
15. Hunt, J. and Simone Radouco-Thomas (1975) Alterations of Hela calcium by reserpine. Effects on cell proliferation. *Biochem. Pharmacol.* (submitted for publication).
16. Jakubovic, A. and R. L. McGeer (1976) *In vitro* inhibition of protein and nucleic acid synthesis in rat testicular tissue by cannabis. *Marihuana: Chemistry, Biochemistry, and Cellular Effects* (G. G. Nahas, *et al.,* eds.). New York: Springer-Verlag.
17. Jakubovic, A. and P. L. McGeer (1972) Inhibition of rat brain protein by cannabinoids *in vitro. Can. J. Biochem. 50:*654.
18. Leuchtenberger, C. and R. Leuchtenberger (1971) Morphological and cytochemical effects of marijuana cigarette smoke on epithelioid cells of lung explants of mice. *Nature 234:*227.
19. McClean, D. K. and A. M. Zimmerman (1972) The influence of morphinans and tetrahydrocannabinol on cellular biosynthesis. *Proc. Can. Fed. Biol. Soc. 15:*436.
20. Moreau, J. J. (1845) *Du Hashish et de l'Aliénation Mentale. Etudes Psychologiques.* Paris: Masson.
21. Moszik, G. (1969) Some feedback mechanisms by drugs in the interrelationship between the active transport system and adenyl cyclase system localized in the cell membrane. *Eur. J. Pharmacol. 7:*319.
22. Nahas, G. G. (1974) Effects of cannabis and cannabinoids on cell replication and replication and DNA synthesis in man. *J. Pharmacol. 5:*71.
23. Nahas, G. G. (1971) Results cited in the discussion of the following paper. Forney, R. B. and G. F. Kiplinger: Toxicology and pharmacology of marijuana. *Ann. N.Y. Acad. Sci. 391:*80.
24. Nahas, G. G., B. Desoize, J. Hso, A. Morishima, and P. R. Srinivesan (1975) Inhibition of nucleic acid and proteins synthesis by natural cannabinoids and olivelol. Abstract VI. Int. Congress of Pharmacol., Helsinki, p. 495.
25. Padykula, K. and E. Herman (1966) Calcium method for adenosine triphosphatase. *Selected Histochemical and Histopathological Methods* (S. V. Thomson, ed.). Springfield, Ill.: Charles C. Thomas.
26. Paton, W. D., R. G. Putwee, and D. Temple (1972) The general pharmacology of cannabinoids. *Cannabis and Its Derivatives* (W. D. M. Paton and J. Crown, eds.). London: Oxford University Press, pp. 50–75.
27. Penit, J., J. Huot, and S. Jard (1975) Neuroblastoma cell adenylate

cyclase: direct activation by adenosine and prostaglandins. *J. Neurochem.* (in press).

28. Petrzilka, T. (1970) Synthesis of (-) tetrahydrocannabinol and analogous compound. *The Botany and Chemistry of Cannabis* (C. R. B. Joyce and S. H. Curry, eds.). London: J. A. Churchill, pp. 79–92.
29. Schwartz, A., E. Lindenmayer, and J. C. Allen (1975) The sodium-potassium adenosine triphosphatase: pharmacological, physiological and biochemical aspects. *Pharmacol. Rev. 27:*3.
30. Seeman, P. (1972) The membrane actions of anesthetics and tranquilizers. *Pharmacol. Rev. 24:*583.
31. Seeman, P., M. Chau-Wong, and S. Moyyen (1972) The membrane binding of morphine, diphenylhydantoin and tetrahydrocannabinol. *Can. J. Physiol. Pharmacol. 50:*1193.
32. Stefanis, C. N. and M. Issidorides (1976) Cellular effects of chronic cannabis use in man. *Marihuana: Chemistry, Biochemistry, and Cellular Effects* (G. G. Nahas *et al.*, eds.). New York: Springer-Verlag.
33. Tinklenberg, J. R. (1975) What a physician should know about marijuana. *Rational Drug Therapy* 9(7):1.
34. Zimmerman, A. M. and S. B. Zimmerman (1976) The influence of marihuana on eukaryote cell growth and development. *Marihuana: Chemistry, Biochemistry, and Cellular Effects* (G. G. Nahas *et al.*, eds.). New York: Springer-Verlag.
35. Zimmerman, A. M. and D. K. McClean (1973) Action of narcotic and hallucinogenic agents on the cell cycle. *Drugs and the Cell Cycle* (A. Zimmerman, G. M. Padilla, and I. L. Cameron, eds.). New York: Academic Press, pp. 67–74.

28

Cannabinoids and Neoplastic Growth

R. A. CARCHMAN, W. WARNER, A. C. WHITE, AND L. S. HARRIS

Introduction

Marihuana is the botanical source of a variety of compounds termed cannabinoids. The cannabinoids represent a group of compounds that are scientifically important primarily because of the psychoactive properties of several members of this chemical family [22,27]. The major psychoactive ingredient in marihuana is Δ^9-tetrahydrocannabinol (Δ^9-THC). This compound has recently been shown to have effects in various systems that may not be directly related to its CNS actions. Our interest in the cannabinoids involves this latter aspect of their interactions with biological systems. We have reported [9,18] that certain of the cannabinoids inhibit the growth of the Lewis lung adenocarcinoma *in vivo* and significantly prolong the survival time of mice bearing these tumors. Some of these compounds also inhibit the splenomegaly induced by the Friend leukemia virus. Preliminary *in vitro* data corroborate the *in vivo* results obtained with the Lewis lung adenocarcinoma [4,9]. Others have shown that human lung cells grown in tissue culture exhibit alterations in DNA synthesis after exposure to marihuana smoke [15]. Complicated effects involving the impairment of different parts of the immune system in both man [20] and animals [11] have been reported. Δ^9-THC at micromolar concentrations inhibits macromolecular synthesis (RNA, DNA, protein) in tetrahymena and can also produce cytolysis [31]. Other reports have indicated that Δ^9-THC lowers testosterone levels [12], causes chromosomal abnormalities [28], and inhibits spermatogenesis [14].

The mechanisms by which Δ^9-THC and other cannabinoids alter cellular function are exceedingly complex and at present poorly understood. Our approach has been to examine the effects of several of the cannabinoids on cells *in vitro* and in tissue culture. These systems then afford us the ability to study the actions of the cannabinoids at different levels of cellular organization (e.g., transport, macromolecular synthesis). This ability to isolate and re-

Marihuana: Chemistry, Biochemistry, and Cellular Effects, edited by Gabriel G. Nahas,

integrate cellular function in the presence of a drug may shed further light on its mechanism of action.

In addition to the use of Lewis lung cells *in vitro* and in culture, we have evaluated the effects of Δ^9-THC on steroid-secreting cells (normal and malignant) *in vitro*. These systems enable us to study the effects of Δ^9-THC on a specialized cellular function (steroidogenesis) and relate its *in vitro* effects to responses seen *in vivo* [12,17,21].

Materials and Methods

Isolated Lewis lung cells

Tumors (Lewis lung) were aseptically removed from C57BL/6 mice 2 weeks after tumor transplant. Following debridement, the tumor was washed and carefully minced (1-mm^3 fragments) in a solution of Dulbecco's modified Eagles medium (Earle's salts) supplemented with 50 IU/ml penicillin and 50 μg/ml streptomycin. Trypsinization (0.25 percent) with constant stirring for 90 min effected a unicellular suspension. Pelleted cells were resuspended in minimal essential medium (MEM) (with Earle's salts) containing 20 percent heat-inactivated fetal calf serum. Cell viability was determined using trypan blue dye exclusion (0.5 percent), and cell number was ascertained on a Coulter counter (model ZB1). Cells were centrifuged (600 *g*, 10 min) and brought up in MEM (containing Earle's salts) supplemented with (for every 500 ml MEM) 5 ml penicillin/streptomycin (5000 IU/ml:5000 μg/ml). (Reagents were obtained from Flow Labs, Rockville, Maryland 20852; or Grand Island Biologicals, Grand Island, New York 14072.) The cell number was diluted to a final concentration of 10^7 cells/ml and aliquoted into 20-ml disposable glass scintillation vials (3–5 ml/flask) containing 10 μl of drug or drug vehicle (ethanol). Vials were equilibrated for 15 min at 37°C under 5 percent CO_2–95 percent O_2 with moderate shaking in a Dubnoff metabolic bath. Tritiated thymidine was then added, and 1-ml aliquots were removed at various times.

Isolated bone marrow cells

The tibias and fibulas were removed from mice (BDF_1). After removing the distal portions of these bones, we injected 1 ml MEM (with heparin, 1 unit/ml) through the bone using a 1-ml syringe with a needle (26 gauge). The cells were centrifuged (600*g*, 10 min) and resuspended (three times) in MEM. Cell viability was ascertained using trypan blue dye exclusion, and the cell number was adjusted to 10^7 cells/ml; the cells were then incubated as described above for isolated Lewis lung cells.

"In vitro" DNA and RNA synthesis

Methyl-^{3}H-thymidine (6.7 Ci/mM) and /or uridine-2-^{14}C (57 mCi/mM) was added (10 μCi/vial) after 15 min of equilibration of cells with drug or drug vehicle. One-milliliter aliquots were removed at various times and placed in test tubes containing 2 ml of 10 percent trichloroacetic acid (TCA; 4°C). The samples were mixed and allowed to stand for several minutes before filtration. Filters were placed into scintillation vials containing 10 ml of toluene-liquiflor cocktail and counted in a Beckman liquid scintillation spectrometer. The incorporation of radioactive precursors into acid (TCA)-insoluble material (DNA, RNA) was linear during the 45-min incubation period for Lewis lung and bone marrow cells.

Lewis lung cells in tissue culture

Cells for use in culture were prepared as for isolated Lewis lung cells with the following modifications. After centrifugation and resuspension (after trypsination), the cells were dispersed in Dulbecco's medium containing 20 percent heat-inactivated fetal calf serum and placed in culture. Falcon 250-ml T-flasks were inoculated with 10^7 viable (trypan blue dye exclusion) cells. Cultures were grown in a humidified 5 percent CO_2 Wedco incubator at 37°C. Growth medium consisted of Eagles MEM with Earle's salts, 10 percent glutamine supplemented with 20 percent heat-inactivated fetal calf serum, 10 percent vitamins, 10 percent amino acids, 50 IU/ml penicillin, and 50 μg/ml streptomycin. The medium was buffered with 3.5 percent $NaHCO_3$.

Maintenance of Lewis lung cells in culture

Lewis lung cells were maintained in logarithmic growth by multiple subculturing (e.g., dispersing one flask of cells into three flasks) every other day. Cells selected for rapid growth could be stored frozen (−70°C) in a medium containing dimethyl sulfoxide (DMSO; 10 percent) or glycerol (10 percent). Cells from culture are routinely inoculated (10^5–10^6 cells) into isogenic mice to assure continued tumorigenicity. Tumors produced by such techniques are indistinguishable from tumors continuously passed in animals, and the former are readily reestablished in culture.

Population growth in culture

The population doubling time of Lewis lung cells in culture was obtained by determining cell number over several days. Cultured cells were harvested, triturated to achieve a unicellular suspension, and diluted to contain between 10^4 and 10^5 cells/ml. The suspension was then aliquoted into 60-mm diameter plastic Petri dishes. At irregular intervals, triplicate cultures were harvested and the number of cells counted either microscopically or on a ZB1 Coulter counter. Viability was determined by trypan blue dye exclusion.

The effect of drugs on population growth was similarly quantitated. Populations were inoculated at low density into Petri dishes. Drugs and drug vehicle (for control) were added in 10 μl volumes 24 hr after plating and at 24 hr intervals thereafter. The medium (5 ml/dish) was changed daily. As with untreated populations, triplicate cultures were harvested and counted at various intervals.

Incorporation of ^{3}H-thymidine into Lewis lung DNA in culture

Tritiated thymidine (10 μCi/plate) was added to plates 15 min after adding the drug or drug vehicle (10 μl/3 ml). At the appropriate times, triplicate plates were removed from the incubator and the medium discarded. The plates were then washed three times in phosphate-buffered saline (PBS; 4°C), 3 ml of 10 percent TCA (4°C) was added to each plate, and the cells were removed with a Teflon scrapper and transferred to chilled Sorvall tubes. The broken cell suspension was then centrifuged at 15,000*g* for 20 min, and the supernatant was saved for measurements of acid-soluble radioactivity. The remaining pellet was resuspended in 3 ml TCA (4°C) and centrifuged at 15,000*g* for 15 min, and the supernatant was discarded. A solubilizer (NCS, 0.5 ml) was added to each pellet and transferred to a 55°C water bath (15 min). After dissolution and cooling of the pellet, 10 ml of toluene-liquiflor was added for scintillation spectrometry. Then 1 ml of the acid-soluble fraction was added to 1 ml of Aquasol and counted as above.

Adrenal steroid secretion

Functional mouse adrenal tumor cells (Y-1) were obtained from the American Type Culture Collection. The growth medium was Ham's F-10 nutrient mixture supplemented with horse serum (12.5 percent), fetal calf serum (2.5 percent), glutamine, penicillin, and streptomycin. (All tissue culture reagents were obtained from Grand Island Biological Co.) Cells were grown at 37°C in Falcon flasks (75 cm^2) in a Wedco CO_2 incubator. The medium was changed every 72 hr. Experiments were performed in Falcon Petri dishes (60-mm diameter) containing 3 ml incubation medium and a cell population of approximately 1.2×10^6 cells per plate. To remove residual steroids before incubation, we washed the cells twice and performed the experiments in unsupplemented Ham's F-10 medium. Inhibitors were added to cells first, then after 15 min steroidogenic stimulants were added, and the incubation was continued for 2 hr. Cannabidiol (CBD) and Δ^9-THC were dissolved in ethanol (0.01 ml added to each plate); all other solutions were aqueous. After the incubation was completed, the Petri dishes were drained, washed, and assayed by the sulfuric acid fluorescence method of Kowal and Fiedler [13]. Cells were scraped off the dishes and counted on a Coulter counter.

Experiments measuring incorporation of radioactivity into protein were performed as described above. Tritiated mixed amino acids were added 15 min after ACTH. After completing the incubation (at 1 and 2 hr), we drained the supernatant and washed the cells three times in phosphate-buffered saline (PBS) and denatured them with 10 percent TCA. After centrifugating the scraped cells, we counted an aliquot of the supernatant in a Unilux III scintillation counter. The pellet was dissolved in NCS and counted.

The normal cat adrenal cortical cell suspension was prepared by the procedure of Rubin and Warner [26]. Hydrocortisone was assayed by the competitive protein binding method of Murphy [19].

Results

Structure activity relationship of cannabinoids

Isolated Lewis lung and bone marrow cells incorporate radioactive precursors (^{3}H-thymidine, ^{14}C-uridine, and ^{3}H-amino acids) into DNA, RNA, and protein, respectively, at a linear rate for at least 45 min. Table 28.1 represents the concentration of cannabinoid required to produce a 50-percent inhibition of DNA synthesis (calculated by the method of Litchfield and Wilcoxin) during a 15-min incubation. Δ^9- and Δ^8-THC, abnormal Δ^8-THC (abn Δ^8-THC), and cannabinol (CBN) all have ED50's in the micromolar range, whereas CBD, abnormal cannabinol (abn CBD), cannabichromene, 8β,11-diOH-Δ^9-THC, and cannabicyclol are all much less active in the isolated Lewis lung system. Several experiments with Lewis lung cells using CBD (data not shown)

Table 28.1 Inhibition of DNA synthesis by cannabinoids

Drug	σED50[a] Lewis lung	Bone marrow
Δ^9-THC	4×10^{-6} *M*	2×10^{-4} *M*
Δ^8-THC	3×10^{-6} *M*	1.3×10^{-6} *M*
Abn Δ^8-THC	1.5×10^{-6} *M*	3.6×10^{-6} *M*
Cannabinol	2×10^{-6} *M*	3.1×10^{-7} *M*
Cannabidiol	3.4×10^{-5} *M*	5×10^{-4} *M*
Abn cannabidiol	9.3×10^{-5} *M*	5.5×10^{-6} *M*
Cannabichromene	$>10^{-4}$ *M*	—
8β, 11-diOH-Δ^9-THC	$>10^{-4}$ *M*	—
Cannabicyclol	$>10^{-4}$ *M*	—

[a] Cells were prepared as described in methods. The ED50 (50% inhibition) was calculated by the method of Litchfield and Wilcoxin [16]. Slopes from which the ED50 was calculated were not significantly different. Drugs were made fresh daily in ethanol (10 μl/flask) and preincubated for 15 min with cells before adding ^{3}H-thymidine (10 μCi/flask). Incorporation of ^{3}H-thymidine was linear for at least 45 min.

indicated a stimulation of thymidine uptake into acid-precipitable material by this cannabinoid.

Isolated bone marrow cells incubated *in vitro* were used for their possible value in predicting *in vivo* toxicity (bone marrow suppression). Of those cannabinoids that had an ED50 at micromolar levels, only Δ^9-THC was less inhibitory when compared to isolated Lewis lung cells. Cannabinol, which is slightly more active against the Lewis lung than Δ^9-THC, was approximately ten times more potent than Δ^9-THC against bone marrow cells. This *in vitro* observation correlates very well with *in vivo* measurements which showed that the greatest weight loss (toxicity) occurred in those animals treated with cannabinol [18].

Δ^9-THC: Lewis lung versus bone marrow cells (*"in vitro"*)

When the dose responsiveness of isolated Lewis lung and bone marrow cells in the presence of Δ^9-THC are compared, a clearer picture of the apparent selectivity of Δ^9-THC is easily seen. Figures 28.1 and 28.2 show the effect of various concentrations of Δ^9-THC on ^{3}H-thymidine and ^{14}C-uridine uptake (acid-precipitable radioactivity) in Lewis lung and bone marrow cells. The maximal separation of inhibition between Lewis lung and bone marrow cells

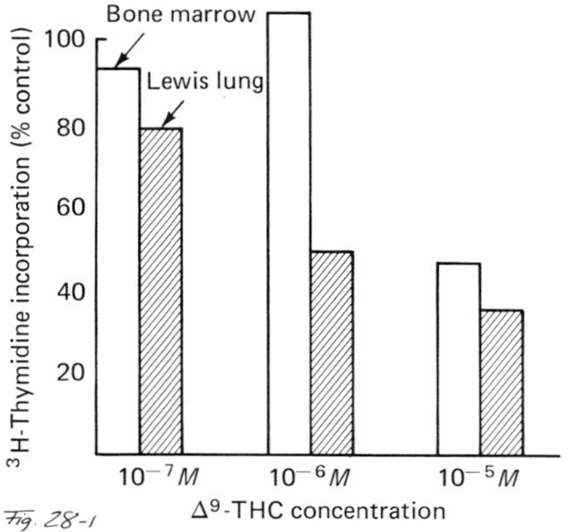

Figure 28.1. ^{3}H-Thymidine incorporation with increasing $^{9}\Delta$-THC concentration in bone marrow and Lewis lung cells. Results expressed as a percentage of control parallel culture.

is seen at micromolar concentrations of Δ^9-THC, which is comparable to the drug's ED50 (Table 28.1).

Lewis lung cells in tissue culture

Growing cells in tissue culture affords a milieu that demonstrates clear how certain cannabinoids inhibit tumor growth *in vivo.* Lewis lung cells grown in tissue culture exhibit many characteristics of transformed cells (e.g., lack of contact or density-dependent in-

Figure 28.2. ^{14}C-Uridine incorporation with increasing $^{9}\Delta$-THC concentration in bone marrow and Lewis lung cells. Results expressed as a percentage of control parallel culture.

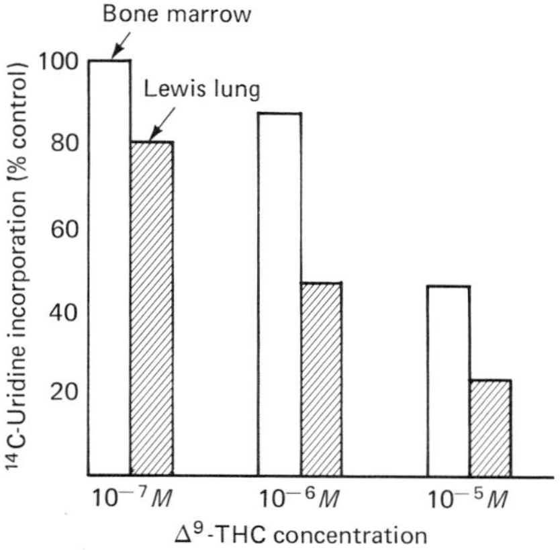

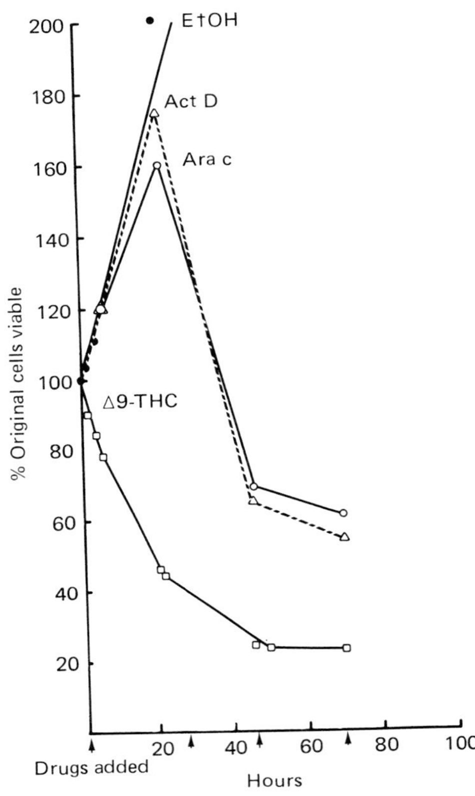

Figure 28.3. Inhibition of growth by Δ^9-THC, ARA-C, and Act D in Lewis lung cells grown in culture as described in text. At zero time, drugs or drug vehicle, ethanol, was added to a series of identical cultures. At various times cultures were harvested and cells counted. Every 24 hr after introduction of drugs, medium and drug were replenished in all cultures remaining. Cell number was determined on a Coulter counter (model ZB1).

hibition of growth, tumorigenicity); therefore, we have used this system to evaluate the effects of Δ^9-THC on these cells. If Δ^9-THC (10^{-4} *M*) is added to a culture of logarithmically growing Lewis lung cells, the number of viable cells decreases rapidly (within a few hours; Figure 28.3). After nutrient and drug replenishment, the Δ^9-THC–treated cells continue to die. When treated with potent inhibitors of macromolecular synthesis, such as cytosine arabinoside (10^{-6} *M*) [8] or actinomycin D (10^{-7} *M*) [24], these tumor cells show no observable changes in cell growth. Only after nutrient and drug replenishment (24–48 hr) is a decrease in cell number detectable.

DNA synthesis

Effect of Δ^9-THC

When ^{3}H-thymidine is added to logarithmically growing Lewis lung cells, a rapid increase in incorporation into acid-insoluble material (DNA) over 3–4 hr is observed (Table 28.2). The

Table 28.2 Time course of ^{3}H-thymidine uptake in culture[a]

	cpm (acid insoluble)			*cpm (acid soluble)*		
Hours	*Control*	*Δ⁹-THC*	*Inhibition (%)*	*Control*	*Δ⁹-THC*	*Inhibition (%)*
0.5	1.6×10^{5}	0.8×10^{5}	50	1.1×10^{4}	1.15×10^{4}	—
1.0	4.5×10^{5}	2.7×10^{5}	40	1.3×10^{4}	1.1×10^{4}	16
2.0	1.4×10^{6}	0.76×10^{6}	46	0.64×10^{4}	0.64×10^{4}	—
4.0	1.9×10^{6}	1.3×10^{6}	32	0.56×10^{4}	0.54×10^{4}	4

[a] Cells were prepared as described in methods. Δ^{9}-THC was prepared at a final concentration of 4×10^{-5} *M*. Values represent the mean of duplicate plates with less than 10% variability.

addition of $4 \times 10^{-5} M$ Δ^{9}-THC produces a 50-percent inhibition of DNA synthesis, which is seen as early as 30 min after adding the drug and is maintained over the next 3–4 hr (Table 28.2). The possibility that this inhibition of DNA synthesis was due to inhibition of radioactive precursor uptake by this lipophilic substance (Δ^{9}-THC) was tested by measuring the radioactivity in the acid-soluble pool (e.g., ^{3}H-thymidine, TMP, TDP, TTP). As can be seen in Table 28.2, $4 \times 10^{-5} M$ Δ^{9}-THC had no significant effect on the radioactive acid-soluble pool during the experiment.

In any analysis of complex drug interactions, concentrations of the agent should be tested over a wide range. When exposed to concentrations of Δ^{9}-THC (10^{-5}, 5×10^{-5}, $10^{-4} M$), rapidly growing Lewis lung cells exhibit an inhibition of DNA synthesis (12.5,

Table 28.3 Dose response of Δ^{9}-THC in Lewis lung cells in tissue culture: DNA synthesis[a]

	Percentage of control	
Final drug concentration	*Acid-insoluble radioactivity*	*Acid-soluble radioactivity*
10^{-5} *M*	87.5 ± 2.5	102.5 ± 5
5×10^{-5} *M*	52.5 ± 2	110 ± 4
10^{-4} *M*	17.5 ± 1.2	75 ± 2.5

[a] Cells were maintained and ^{3}H-thymidine uptake was measured as described in methods. Values represent the mean ± SE of triplicate Petri dishes. Drug was incubated with cells for 2 hr.

Table 28.4 Effect of cytosine arabinoside on ^{3}H-thymidine uptake[a]

	Percentage of control	
Final drug concentration	*Acid-insoluble radioactivity*	*Acid-soluble radioactivity*
10^{-9} *M*	99 ± 2.5	100 ± 7.5
10^{-8} *M*	97.5 ± 4	112 ± 3
10^{-7} *M*	75 ± 5	116 ± 3
10^{-6} *M*	21 ± 1.2	153 ± 5
10^{-5} *M*	10 ± 1.2	135 ± 2.5

[a] Cells were prepared as described in the methods. Cytosine arabinoside was incubated with the cells and radiolabel for 2 hr. Values represent the mean ± SE.

47.5, and 82.5 percent, respectively; Table 28.3). An analysis of the radioactivity in the acid-soluble fraction reveals that only at $10^{-4}M$ Δ^9-THC is there a measurable decrease in radioactivity (Table 28.3). This 25-percent decrease in acid-soluble radioactivity should be viewed in light of the large 82.5-percent inhibition of DNA synthesis at this same drug concentration.

Table 28.5 Effect of Δ^9-THC on ACTH-induced steroidogenesis in Y-1 cells[a]

	Steroid released per 10^6 cells (mcg)			
	Experiments			
Treatment	*5/6*	*5/12*	*6/30*	*Inhibition (%)*
None	3.9	4.9	2.5	
ACTH + vehicle	10	10	5.5	
+ 1 × 10^{-6} Δ^9-THC	9.3	9.4	5.3	5.3 ± 1.2 ($p < 0.05$)
+ 1 × 10^{-5} Δ^9-THC	6.7	6.5	3.9	26 ± 5.1 ($p < 0.01$)
+ 1 × 10^{-4} Δ^9-THC	4.8	4.7	4.1	43 ± 9.2 ($p < 0.05$)

[a] Cells were preincubated with the indicated concentrations of Δ^9-THC for 15 min, then ACTH was added (final concentration 125 μIU/ml). One set of cells received no drugs, another received ACTH and 0.01 ml ethanol (vehicle for Δ^9-THC). After 2 additional hours, the incubation medium was decanted, extracted, and assayed as described in the methods section. Cells were scraped and counted. Data were normalized for 10^6 cells. Each data point represents duplicate incubations. Statistical significance was determined by paired *t* test.

Cytosine arabinoside

In view of the paucity of information on Δ^9-THC and the present use of the heretofore uncultured Lewis lung cells, we evaluated cytosine arabinoside, a known inhibitor of DNA synthesis [8]. This agent (10^{-9}, 10^{-8}, 10^{-7}, 10^{-6}, 10^{-5} *M*) produces a dose-dependent inhibition of DNA synthesis (1, 2.5, 25, 79, and 90 percent, respectively; Table 28.4). Unlike Δ^9-THC, this drug causes a large increase in the radioactivity (~ 50 percent in the acid-soluble pool; Table 28.4). Cytosine arabinoside is much more active *in vitro* against the Lewis lung than Δ^9-THC [4], although its efficacy against this tumor *in vivo* has not been demonstrated.

ACTH-induced steroidogenesis

Inhibition by Δ^9-THC

The use of steroid-secreting cells in tissue culture allows the investigator to study the effects of agents on a differentiated cellular function. Y-1 cells respond to various stimulants by synthesizing and secreting steroids. Table 28.5 is a compilation of three experiments (5/6, 5/12, 6/30). ACTH (125 μIU/ml) caused approximately a twofold increase in steroid output in the presence of a drug vehicle (ethanol). Δ^9-THC (10^{-6}, 10^{-5}, 10^{-4} *M*) produces a dose-dependent inhibition of steroid synthesis (5, 26, and 43 percent, respectively). Measurement of the cellular steroid content indicates that the inhibition seen with Δ^9-THC was not due to

Table 28.6 Effect of cannabidiol on ACTH-induced steroidogenesis in Y-1 cells[a]

Treatment	Steroid released per 10^6 cells (mcg) — Experiments 6/30	7/7	Inhibition (%)
None	2.5	0.9	
ACTH + vehicle	5.5	1.6	
+ 1 × 10^{-6} CBD	3.9	0.8	33.8
+ 1 × 10^{-5} CBD	1.8	0.5	68.6
+ 1 × 10^{-4} CBD	1.7	0.3	77.5

[a] Cells were preincubated 15 min with indicated concentrations of CBD followed by additional 2 hr with 125 μIU/ml ACTH. One set of cells received no drugs, and one received only ACTH and CBD vehicle (0.01 ml ethanol). Each data point represents the mean of duplicate incubations.

inhibition of steroid release (unpublished observation). Similar data were obtained using normal trypsin-dispersed cat adrenal cells, although these cells appear to be slightly more sensitive to Δ^9-THC than the Y-1 cells.

Inhibition by CBD

Unlike the lack of inhibitory activity seen with CBD against Lewis lung cells, this drug dramatically inhibited steroidogenesis. The inhibition of steroidogenesis was slightly greater than that caused by Δ^9-THC (compare Tables 28.5 and 28.6). Furthermore, CBD also decreased steroidogenesis to below basal levels (Table 28.6), a situation not routinely seen with Δ^9-THC.

Stimulus-induced steroidogenesis

Cycloheximide and actinomycin D

Functional mouse adrenal cells (Y-1) can be stimulated by several secretagogues (ACTH, cholera toxin, cyclic AMP) to synthesize steroids [3,5,30]. These agents all increase steroidogenesis, although presumably through different receptors, and all are inhibited by Δ^9-THC (unpublished observations). Table 28.7 shows that cycloheximide, an agent which inhibits protein synthesis [6,29] and has been shown to inhibit steroid synthesis [25], also inhibits steroidogenesis in tissue culture. Cycloheximide (0.1 mM) also inhibits (95 percent) the incorporation of ^{3}H-amino acids into

Table 28.7 Effects of cycloheximide and actinomycin D on steroidogenesis[a]

		Stimulated		
Stimulant	*Basal rate*	*No inhibitors*	*+ Cycloheximide*	*+ Actinomycin D*
ACTH	4.9	10	3.5	11
	3.9	12	3.9	12
	0.9	1.8	0.6	—
Cholera toxin	5.2	18	4.3	16
cAMP	2.9	8.7	2.4	—

[a] Cells were preincubated for 15 min with cycloheximide (1×10^{-1}mM), actinomycin (2.5×10^{-4}mM), or in the absence of any drug. ACTH (125 μIU/ml), cholera toxin (50 ng/ml), or cAMP (1 mM) was added to appropriate plates and incubated 2 hr. Each data point is the mean of duplicate incubation.

protein. Actinomycin D (Act D), an inhibitor of RNA synthesis [24], has no effect on Y-1 steroidogenesis (Table 28.7) or on ^{3}H-amino acid uptake into protein; Δ^{9}-THC ($10^{-5}M$) had no effect on ^{3}H-amino acid uptake (acid-soluble or insoluble radioactivity) into protein (unpublished observations).

Discussion

The evaluation of macromolecular synthesis, transport, and steroidogenesis in the presence of some of the cannabinoids reveals the complexity of the interaction of these compounds with cellular processes. The *in vivo* antitumor activities of several of the cannabinoids reported by Munson *et al.* are consistent with our *in vitro* observations. The series of compounds tested *in vitro* indicates that there is no relationship between CNS activity and the inhibition of macromolecular synthesis since abn Δ^{8}-THC and CBN, which are not psychoactive [7], are potent inhibitors of *in vitro* DNA synthesis. From a comparison of Δ^{8}- and abn Δ^{8}-THC, both of which are potent compounds, it appears that the relative positions of the alkyl and phenolic groups in the C-ring are not important for *in vitro* activity. Opening the B-ring as in CBD or abn CBD inactivates the compound.

In addition, Munson *et al.* [18] reported that CBD increased the rate of tumor growth *in vivo* and shortened the animals' survival time. Several of our experiments (data not shown) indicated that CBD stimulates (whereas Δ^{9}-THC inhibits) the rate of incorporation of ^{3}H-thymidine into DNA in Lewis lung cells *in vitro.* Some alterations in the A-ring appear to be incompatible with *in vitro* activity, as evidenced by the relative inactivity of cannabichromene, 8β,11-diOH-Δ^{9}-THC, and cannabicyclol.

One conclusion that can be gleaned from the *in vitro* tumor studies is that the position of the double bond in the A-ring (Δ^{9}-, Δ^{8}-THC) is not important for activity, although we have not yet tested Δ^{8}-THC. One of the cell lines we evaluated *in vitro* is isolated normal bone marrow cells. The effects of cannabinoids on these cells might prove useful in predicting *in vivo* toxicity problems (bone marrow suppression). Δ^{9}-THC was the only active cannabinoid tested that had a much smaller effect on bone marrow in comparison to tumor cells, indicating that Δ^{9}-THC has a high degree of selective toxicity.

Levy and Munson (personal communication) have shown that animals treated with up to 200 mg/kg Δ^{9}-THC showed a transient decrease in the number of peripheral leukocytes (first 3 days), but cell counts returned to control levels even after 10 days of treatment with Δ^9-THC (200 mg/kg). This indicates that Δ^9-THC is relatively nontoxic to the bone marrow.

Studies performed on isolated Lewis lung cells grown in tissue culture reinforce our *in vivo* and *in vitro* observations. These cells grow logarithmically and are killed within a few hours after adding 10^{-4} *M* Δ^9-THC, whereas cytosine arabinoside (10^{-6} *M*) and Act D (10^{-7}*M*) required cumulative doses over 2 days before a decrease in cell number was noticeable. Δ^9-THC produced a dose-dependent inhibition of DNA synthesis (acid-insoluble material), while decreasing only the radioactivity in the acid-soluble pool at a dose (10^{-4}*M*) we have shown to be cytocidal. Therefore, we conclude that the inhibition of DNA synthesis produced by Δ^9-THC at noncytodial levels is not due to an inhibition of precursor uptake (because there is no change in acid-soluble radioactivity) but occurs at some distal step.

The inhibition of steroid synthesis produced by Δ^9-THC is of major interest since Δ^9-THC apparently acts as a feedback inhibitor in the steroidogenic pathway. The dose-dependent inhibition of steroidogenesis was seen in both normal and malignant steroid-secreting cells and is independent of the type of stimulus used (e.g., ACTH, cyclic AMP, cholera toxin). This indicates that Δ^9-THC is not working at the ACTH receptor site, or that the inhibition was peculiar to the cell type or species used. The incorporation of radioactive amino acids into protein or into the acid-soluble fraction was unaffected by Δ^9-THC, but steroid synthesis was dramatically inhibited. Cycloheximide, an inhibitor of protein synthesis, decreased ^{3}H-amino acid incorporation into protein and abolished steroidogenesis. Actinomycin D, an inhibitor of RNA synthesis, did not affect steroidogenesis or ^{3}H-amino acid incorporation.

These results dovetail nicely with the results reported by Birmingham and Bartova [2], who showed that Δ^9-THC inhibited steroidogenesis in a manner compatible with feedback inhibition. However, in contrast to what was observed in tumors *in vitro,* CBD produced a dose-dependent inhibition of steroidogenesis similar to that of Δ^9-THC. These results indicate that there may be no single unifying mechanism by which the cannabinoids exert their many actions. Yet if one were to visualize a model based on available information, we feel that the structural similarities between the cannabinoids and steroids would lend themselves to some fair comparisons. Both classes of compounds contain members which produce CNS effects [10,22,27] that are immunosuppressive

[11,20,23], alter macromolecular synthesis (1,31), and can inhibit steroid synthesis probably allosterically. We are currently evaluating this type of model in the hope of delineating the mechanism(s) by which the cannabinoids exert many of their actions.

ACKNOWLEDGMENT

This investigation was supported in part by grants from the Department of Health, Education, and Welfare; DA 00490, CA 17840, and CA 17551.

REFERENCES

1. Ahsmore, J. and G. Weber (1968) Hormonal control of carbohydrate metabolism in liver. *Carbohydrate Metabolism and Its Disorders,* vol. I. (F. Dickens, P. I. Randle, and W. J. Whelan, eds.). New York: Academic Press, pp. 335–384.
2. Birmingham, M. K. and A. Bartova (1976) Effects of cannabinol derivatives on blood pressure, body weight, pituitary-adrenal function, and mitochondrial respiration in the rat. *Marihuana: Chemistry, Biochemistry and Cellular Effects* (G. G. Nahas *et al.,* eds.). New York: Springer-Verlag.
3. Birmingham, M. K., E. Kurlento, R. Lane, B. Muhlstock, and H. Traikov (1960) Effects of calcium on the potassium and sodium production by adenosine 3′,5′-monophosphate, and on the response of the adrenal to short contact with ACTH. *Can. J. Biochem. Physiol. 38:*1077–1085.
4. Carchman, R. A., L. S. Harris, and A. E. Munson (1975) Inhibition of DNA synthesis by cannabinoids. *Cancer Res.* (accepted for publication).
5. Carchman, R. A., S. D. Jaanus, and R. P. Rubin (1971) The role of adrenocorticotropin and calcium in adenosine cyclic 3′,5′-phosphate production and steroid release from the isolated perfused cat adrenal gland. *Mol. Pharmacol. 7:*491–499.
6. Colombo, B., L. Felicetti, C. Baglioni (1965) Inhibition of protein synthesis by cycloheximide in rabbit reticulocytes. *Biochem. Biophys. Res. Commun. 18*(3):389–395.
7. Dewey, W. L., L. S. Harris, and J. S. Kennedy (1972) Some pharmacological and toxicological effects of 1-trans-Δ^8 and 1-trans-Δ^9 tetrahydrocannabinol in laboratory rodents. *Arch. Int. Pharmacodyn. Ther. 196:*133–145.
8. Graham, F. L. and G. F. Whitamore (1970) Studies in mouse L-cells on the incorporation of 1-β-D-arabinosylcytosine into DNA and on the inhibition of DNA polymerase by 1-β-D-arabinosylcytosine-5′-triphosphate. *Cancer Res. 30:*2636–2644.
9. Harris, L. S., A. E. Munson, and R. A. Carchman (1975) Antitumor properties of cannabinoids. *Pharmacology of Cannabis.* New York: Raven Press (in press).
10. Henken, R. I., R. E. McGlone, R. Daly, and F. C. Bartter (1967)

Studies on auditory thresholds in normal man and in patients with adrenal cortical insufficiency: the role of adrenal cortical steroids. *J. Clin. Invest. 46:*429–435.

11. Johnson, R. T. and V. Wiersma (1974) Repression of bone marrow leukopoiesis by Δ^9-tetrahydrocannabinol (Δ^9-THC). *Res. Comm. Chem. Pathol. Pharmacol.* 7:613–616.
12. Kolodny, R. C., W. H. Masters, R. M. Kolodner, and T. Gelson (1974) Depression of plasma testosterone levels after chronic intensive marihuana use. *N. Engl. J. Med. 290:*872–874.
13. Kowal, J. and R. Fiedler (1968) Adrenal cells in culture. *Arch. Biochem. Biophys. 128:*406–421.
14. Leuchtenberger, C., R. Leuchtenberger, and U. Ritter (1973) Effects of marijuana and tobacco smoke on DNA and chromosomal complement in human lung explants. *Nature 242:*403–404.
15. Leuchtenberger, C., R. Leuchtenberger, and A. Schneider (1973) Effects of marijuana and tobacco smoke on human lung physiology. *Nature 241:*137–139.
16. Litchfield, J. T. and F. Wilcoxin (1949) A simplified method for evaluating dose-effect experiments. *J. Pharmacol. Exp. Ther. 96:*99–113.
17. Merari, A., A. Barak, M. Plaues (1973) Effects of $\Delta^{1(2)}$ tetrahydrocannabinol on copulation in the male rat. *Psychopharmacologia 28:* 243–46.
18. Munson, A. E., L. S. Harris, M. A. Friedman, W. L. Dewey, and R. A. Carchman (1975) Anti-neoplastic activity of cannabinoids. *J. Natl. Cancer Inst.* (in press).
19. Murphy, B. E. P. (1969) Protein binding and the assay of nonantigenic hormones. *Recent Prog. Horm. Res. 25:*563–610.
20. Nahas, G. G., N. Suciu-Foca, J. P. Armand, and A. Morishima (1974) Inhibition of cellular immunity in marihuana smokers. *Science 183:*419–420.
21. Nir, I., D. Ayalon, A. Tsafiri, T. Cordoua, and H. R. Lindner (1973) Suppression of the cyclic surge of lutenizing hormone secretion and of ovulation in the rat by Δ^1-tetrahydrocannabinol. *Nature 243:* 470–471.
22. Paton, W. D. M. (1975) Pharmacology of marijuana. *Annu. Rev. Pharmacol. 15:*191–220.
23. Raffel, S. (1961) *Immunity.* 2nd Edition. New York: Appleton-Century-Crofts, pp. 279–331.
24. Reich, E. (1963) Biochemistry of actinomycin. *Cancer Res. 23:*1248–1441.
25. Rubin, R. P., S. D. Jaanus, R. A. Carchman, and M. Puig (1973) Reversible inhibition of ACTH-induced corticosteroid release by cycloheximide: evidence for an unidentified cellular messenger. *Endocrinology 93:*575–580.
26. Rubin, R. P. and W. Warner (1975) Nicotine-induced stimulation of steroidogenesis in adrenocortical cells of the cat. *Br. J. Pharmacol. 53:*357–362.
27. Singer, A. J. (1971) Marihuana: chemistry, pharmacology and patterns of social use. *Ann. N.Y. Acad. Sci. 191:*3–261.
28. Stenchever, M. A., T. J. Kunysz, and M. A. Allen (1974) Chromosome breakage in users of marihuana. *Am. J. Obst. Gynecol. 118:*113.

29. Wettstein, F. P., H. Noll, and S. Penman (1964) Effect of cycloheximide on ribosomal aggregates engaged in protein synthesis in vitro. *Biochim. Biophys. Acta* 87:525–528.
30. Wolff, J., R. Temple, and G. H. Cook (1973) Stimulation of steroid secretion in adrenal tumor cells by choleragen. *Proc. Natl. Acad. Sci. USA* 70:2741–2744.
31. Zimmerman, A. M. and D. K. McClean (1973) Action of narcotic and hallucinogenic agents on the cell cycle. *Drugs and The Cell Cycle* (A. M. Zimmerman *et al.*, eds.). New York: Academic Press.

Marihuana: Biochemical and Cellular Effects

Interactions with Neurotransmitters

29

A Comparison of the Subcellular Distribution of Cannabinoids in the Brains of Tolerant and Nontolerant Dogs, Rats, and Mice After Injecting Radiolabeled Δ^9-Tetrahydrocannabinol

WILLIAM L. DEWEY, BILLY R. MARTIN,
JACQUELINE S. BECKNER, AND LOUIS S. HARRIS

Introduction

A number of papers have appeared which contain evidence that laboratory animals develop tolerance to many of the effects of Δ^9-tetrahydrocannabinol (Δ^9-THC). For example, previous work from this laboratory [5] has shown that dogs develop tolerance to the behavioral effects of Δ^9-THC, the tolerance has a short onset, a long duration, and a large magnitude. A number of investigators have shown that rats develop tolerance to the behavioral effects of Δ^9-THC [1,2,12]. Tolerance to the behavioral effects of Δ^9-THC in mice has been reported [16] but has not been confirmed or extended before this study. The results of many of these and other studies were considered in other review articles concerned with Δ^9-THC tolerance in laboratory animals which were published from this laboratory [6,10,11]. Two of the review articles [10,11] were concerned primarily with characterizing the phenomenon of the tolerance observed in many laboratory species. The other review [6] contained the results of a number of studies in pigeons and dogs which were directed toward elucidating the mechanism or mechanisms responsible for the development of tolerance to this drug.

The whole-body (autoradiography) or organ distribution of radioactivity in animals after acute treatment with a radiolabeled sample of Δ^9-THC has been studied in many species. The results of these experiments indicate that the distribution of the cannabinoids is similar from one species to another. It was clear from previous studies that the tolerance to the behavioral effects of Δ^9-THC in pigeons was not due to altered metabolism [13] or to decreased uptake of cannabinoids into brain [7]. It has also been demonstrated

Marihuana: Chemistry, Biochemistry, and Cellular Effects, edited by Gabriel G. Nahas,

that the distribution of radioactivity in peripheral organs and brains of tolerant and nontolerant dogs was similar after ^{3}H-Δ^{9}-THC injection. However, quantification of radioactivity in subfractions of brain cells yielded a significant decrease in the concentration of radioactivity in the synaptic vesicle fraction of tolerant dogs as compared to the same fractions from acutely treated animals [9]. There were no other significant differences in the distribution of radioactivity in the brain subfractions of tolerant and nontolerant dogs. Relatively high concentrations of radioactivity were found in the synaptic vesicle fractions of both tolerant and nontolerant dogs. This observation is worthy of further study in that it suggests that the Δ^{9}-THC might be interacting with the neurotransmitters in these cell structures, and this might relate to the drug's mechanism of action.

The present study was intended to compare the subcellular distribution of Δ^{9}-THC in the brains of tolerant and nontolerant rats and mice in an attempt to determine the meaningfulness of the significant decrease in radioactivity in the synaptic vesicle fraction of tolerant as compared to nontolerant dogs. A second purpose of this study was to investigate the subcellular distribution of Δ^{9}-THC in the brains of rodents to ascertain whether the subcellular distributions in these species were similar to that observed and reported previously in the dog [9].

Methods

Behavioral measurements

Δ^{9}-THC and other cannabinoids that produce psychomimetic effects in man have been found to produce characteristic changes in the overt behavior of dogs; these changes are unique to these drugs and can be semiquantitated using the rating scale described previously [5,15]. The dog experiments discussed in this paper for comparison have been reported previously [9]. One group of 4 dogs (tolerant group) was injected intravenously with 0.5 mg/kg Δ^{9}-THC each day for 6 days, and on the 7th day the dog was given an IV injection of 0.5 mg/kg ^{3}H-Δ^{9}-THC (70 μCi/mg). The other group (acute group) of 4 dogs was given only the injection of 0.5 mg/kg ^{3}H-Δ^{9}-THC (70 μCi/mg). The dogs were observed for changes in overt behavior, a blood sample was taken 25 min after the injection, and they were sacrificed with an IV injection of 100 mg/kg pentobarbital 30 min after the injection of ^{3}H-Δ^{9}-THC.

The behavioral measure used to study the development of

tolerance to the effects of Δ^9-THC in rats in this study was the decrease in spontaneous activity observed after its acute injection. The spontaneous activity of Sprague-Dawley rats (200–250 gm) was determined by placing each animal in a round black glass container that was mounted on an activity platform. The activity platform was connected to an animal activity monitor, and the activity of each rat for 10-min sessions was measured before the first injection. Two groups of 6 rats each were injected daily with either Δ^9-THC or vehicle, and activity was measured 55 min after injection on both days 1 and 6. On day 7, the group of rats that was treated with the cannabinoid was injected intraperitoneally with 10 mg/kg of ^{3}H-Δ^9-THC (5 μCi/mg) and sacrificed 1 hr later. Two additional groups of rats ($n = 6$) were injected with either Δ^9-THC (10 mg/kg) or vehicle for 19 days. Spontaneous activity was measured on days 1, 12, and 19. On day 20, the drug-treated rats were injected with ^{3}H-Δ^9-THC (5 μCi/kg) 1 hr before sacrifice. A third group of rats were injected with ^{3}H-Δ^9-THC (10 mg/kg, IP; 5 μCi/mg) and sacrificed 1 hr later. These animals served as the acutely treated animals in this study. The animals were sacrificed by decapitation, and blood from the cervical wound was collected in heparinized centrifuge tubes.

The development of tolerance to Δ^9-THC in mice was quantitated using the propensity for Δ^9-THC to interfere with the ability of mice to stay on a rotating rod (6 rpm) for 3 min. In this experiment, animals were placed on a laboratory-fabricated roto-rod apparatus in which a 2.5-cm-diameter wooden dowel was being rotated by a kymograph motor. Mice were screened for their ability to stay on this rotating rod for 3 min before being accepted for this study. Mice that met the criteria outlined above were injected intraperitoneally with 50 mg/kg Δ^9-THC and placed behind the roto-rod for the 3-min test 1 hr after injection. All mice fell off the roto-rod within this 3-min period after the initial injection of Δ^9-THC. Three groups of mice were used in these studies. Each mouse in group 1 was injected with 50 mg/kg ^{3}H-Δ^9-THC (7.75 μCi/mg) and was sacrificed by decapitation 1 hr after the injection. Mice in group 2 were injected daily for 6 days with 50 mg/kg Δ^9-THC and tested on the roto-rod 55 min after the injection on days 1 and 6. On day 7, each mouse was given an IP injection of 50 mg/kg ^{3}H-Δ^9-THC (7.75 μCi/mg) and sacrificed 1 hr later. Each mouse in the third group was injected each day with unlabeled Δ^9-THC for 19 days and was tested on the roto-rod 55 min after the injection on day 19. On day 20, these animals received an IP injection of 50 mg/kg ^{3}H-Δ^9-THC (7.75 μCi/mg) as group 2 received on day 7. All mice were sacrificed by decapitation 1 hr after injection of the radiolabeled cannabinoid, and blood from the cervical wound was collected in heparinized centrifuge tubes.

Preparation of Δ^9-THC for injection

The Δ^9-THC used in these studies was received from the National Institute of Drug Abuse. The radiolabeled Δ^9-THC was tritiated on the α and β carbons of the pentyl side chain, and its radioactivity and chemical purity were verified in our laboratory by thin-layer and gas chromatographic techniques. The labeled and unlabeled Δ^9-THC were prepared in a vehicle combination of emulphor EL-620, ethanol, and saline (5:5:90), as described by Olson *et al.* [14]. Animals used for the acute portion of the rat and mice studies were injected with vehicle on each day that the test animals were injected with unlabeled Δ^9-THC, thus controlling for acute or chronic vehicle effect.

Subfractionation techniques

The brains were removed, weighed, and placed in cold immediately after sacrifice. The subfractionation procedure for the dog brains was described in detail in a previous communication from this laboratory [5]. Each rat brain was homogenized in total, and 6 mouse brains were combined, homogenized, and subfractionated according to the method of DeRobertis *et al.* [3,4], which is the same as that used in the dog studies. Essentially, the brain tissue was homogenized in 0.32 *M* sucrose (plus 10 μM Ca^{2+}) at 400 rpm for 2 min at 0–4°C. Each homogenate was diluted (1 gm/10 ml), and 10 percent of the homogenate was removed and stored. The remaining homogenate was centrifuged at 900*g* for 10 min in a Sorvall RC-2B centrifuge (0°C). The supernatant was decanted, and the crude nuclear (CN) pellet was resuspended twice in 2.0 ml of 0.32 *M* sucrose (10 μM Ca^{2+}) and recentrifuged. The CN supernatant and washes were combined and spun at 11,400*g* for 20 min. The supernatant was decanted and the sediment was washed once. The final pellet was the crude mitochondrial (CM) pellet. The CM supernatant was centrifuged in the Beckman L3-50 ultracentrifuge at 124,000*g* for 30 min. The final soluble supernatant (S) was decanted leaving the microsomal (MS) pellet. The CM pellet was resuspended in 0.32 *M* sucrose (10 μM Ca^{2+}) equivalent to one-third of the original homogenate volume. All other pellets were resuspended in less than 4.0 ml of 0.32 *M* sucrose.

The CM fraction was subfractionated by two methods: (1) discontinuous sucrose density gradient, and (2) osmotic shock. Discontinuous sucrose density gradient was prepared by layering successively 2.0 ml of 2.0 *M* sucrose and 3.0 ml of 1.4 *M*, 1.2 *M*, 1.0 *M*, and 0.8 *M* sucrose in ⅝-inch by 4-inch cellulose nitrate tubes. A 2.0-ml aliquot of the CM fraction was layered on the top, and the tubes were centrifuged in the Beckman L3-50 ultracentrifuge at 80,000*g* for 2 hr, which resulted in five distinct bands. Bands were marked A through E from the top to the bottom of the tube, with each band containing the following: (A) primarily myelin sheaths from nerve fibers; (B) myelin fragments, curved membranes, and small fragments of nerve endings; (C) primarily pinched-off cholinergic nerve endings, some curved membranes, and unidentified dense bodies; (D) pinched-off noncholinergic nerve endings; and (E) free mitochondria.

Osmotic shock of nerve endings and isolation of synaptic vesicles of the CM fraction were performed by diluting 2-ml aliquots of the CM fraction with 10 μM $CaCl_2$ to make a final 0.032 *M* sucrose solution. The diluted CM fraction was rehomogenized and then centrifuged at 11,400*g* for 20 min. The supernatant was decanted, and the remaining sediment (M_1) contained small myelin fragments, swollen mitochondria, and ruptured nerve endings. The M_1 supernatant was spun at 124,000*g* for 30 min, which yielded a synaptic vesicle pellet (M_2) and the final supernatant (M_3).

Duplicate aliquots of all samples, ranging in volumes from 0.2 to 2.0 ml, were placed in combustion cups filled with absorbant tissue paper and oxidized in a Packard Tri-Carb Sample Oxidizer (recovery $>$ 95 percent). Samples were then counted for radioactivity in a Beckman liquid scintillation counter, and quench was corrected for by external standardization. Radioactivity was expressed as nanograms of ^{3}H-Δ^9-THC plus metabolites per gram of tissue for subcellular fractions and subfractions, and as nanograms of ^{3}H-Δ^9-THC plus metabolites per milliliter for plasma and RBC samples. The radioactivity found in each sample was converted to total cannabinoids by dividing the dpm by the specific activity of the injected radiolabeled drug. The data presented in Tables 29.1–29.7 are the mean $\pm$ SE of the total cannabinoids (Δ^9-THC plus metabolites) in that particular brain fraction. Comparisons among groups were made by analysis of variance, with individual comparisons performed using Dunnet's modification of the *t*-test [15].

Results

Tolerance to the behavioral effects of Δ^9-THC in dogs, rats, and mice

The initial injection of either Δ^9-THC or ^{3}H-Δ^9-THC produced similar changes in overt behavior of dogs. Generally, within 30

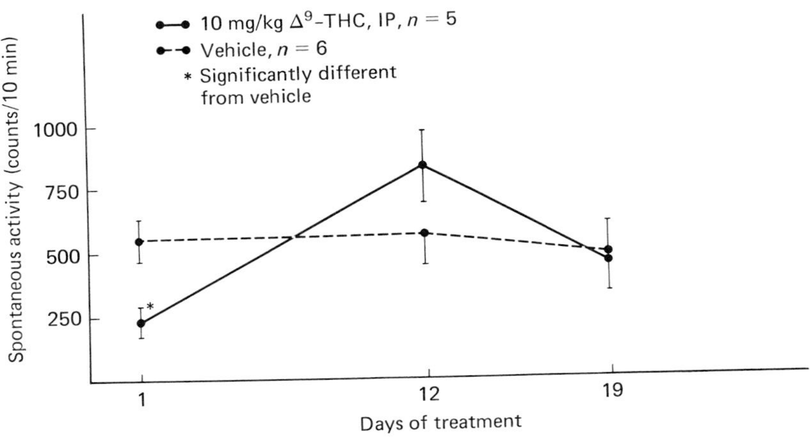

Figure 29.1. Development of tolerance to the hypoactivity caused by Δ^9-THC in rats.

min after administration of Δ^9-THC, the dogs were swaying from side to side and forward and backward (static ataxia), their tails were tucked between their hind legs, they were prancing, and were hyperreactive to a swinging hand or object. The dogs developed pronounced tolerance to these effects on overt behavior by the fifth daily injection of 0.5 mg/kg Δ^9-THC. Slight depression of activity and minimum static ataxia were the only changes observed at this time [5,9].

Tolerance to the overt behavioral effects of cannabinoids in rodents has been difficult to establish. High doses of Δ^9-THC and other cannabinoids are needed to produce a significant reproducible effect on the overt behavior of rats. In the present experiments, 10 mg/kg Δ^9-THC produced a significant reduction in spontaneous activity of rats. Tolerance had not developed to the hypoactivity when the rats were treated daily for 6 days but was observed when the injections were carried out for either 12 or for 19 days as shown in Figure 29.1. A significant reduction in activity was observed on day 1, but there was no difference between the activity of controls and treated rats on day 12 and day 19.

An IP injection of 50 mg/kg Δ^9-THC caused each mouse to lose its ability to stay on the rotating rod for 3 min when tested 55 min after drug administration. Tolerance had developed to this effect by the sixth daily IP injection and was also present after 19 daily injections. The degree of tolerance observed at either time was 100 percent; that is, although none of the animals could stay on the bar for 3 min after the first injection, they all could stay on for 3 min after either the sixth or nineteenth injection. In conclusion, significant tolerance to the effects of Δ^9-THC was observed in each of the three species used in these studies.

Concentration of cannabinoids in blood and brain of dogs, rats, and mice

The concentrations of cannabinoids (Δ^9-THC plus metabolites) in brain homogenates, plasma, and red blood cells after the injection of ^{3}H-Δ^9-THC to dogs, rats, and mice are presented in Table 29.1. Higher concentrations of cannabinoids were found in plasma than red blood cells when the ^{3}H-Δ^9-THC was given as either an acute injection or after chronic treatment with unlabeled Δ^9-THC in all three species. The ratios of the brain to plasma concentrations for each group of animals are also presented in Table 29.1. As can be seen, the brain to plasma ratio was significantly higher in acutely treated rats than in acutely treated dogs or mice. The ratio of the concentration of cannabinoids in brain to plasma was also significantly higher in the rats than in dogs or mice given 6 daily injections of unlabeled drug before injecting ^{3}H-Δ^9-THC. Although still higher, the differences in the ratios of brain to plasma concentration of cannabinoids in rats versus mice was not significant when the ^{3}H-Δ^9-THC was given after 19 daily injections of unlabeled drug.

As mentioned previously, different doses of Δ^9-THC were given to each species in these studies. This was necessary to obtain a reproducible effect to which tolerance could be demonstrated. For example, 50 mg/kg Δ^9-THC was administered intraperitoneally to the mice, and the brain and plasma concentrations of Δ^9-THC plus metabolites were much higher than those found in the dogs that were injected intravenously with 0.5 mg/kg or in rats injected intraperitoneally with 10 mg/kg Δ^9-THC.

The concentrations of cannabinoids (Δ^9-THC plus metabolites) found in plasma, red blood cells, and brain of dogs and rats were of the same order of magnitude. The concentrations in mice were generally 10 times higher. Approximately 0.2 percent of the total administered dose of Δ^9-THC was found in the whole brain of the dogs, and 0.1 percent of the administered dose was in the brain of mice, whereas only 0.036 percent of the total dose administered to rats was found in the brain. Even though the smallest percentage of the administered dose was found in the brains of the rats, they had a higher ratio of brain to plasma concentration of cannabinoids than either the dogs or mice.

Table 29.1 Concentration (ng/gm or ng/ml) of cannabinoids (Δ^9-THC plus metabolites) in plasma, red blood cells, and brain homogenates of tolerant and nontolerant dogs, rats, and mice

	Dogs		*Rats*			*Mice*		
Number of treatments	*1*	*7*	*1*	*7*	*20*	*1*	*7*	*20*
Plasma (ng/ml)	612 ± 62[a]	498 ± 72	468 ± 42	832 ± 176	671 ± 98	2665 ± 238	6567 ± 319[b]	3779 ± 240[d]
Red blood cells (ng/ml)	91 ± 13	150 ± 32	184 ± 9	282 ± 75	234 ± 33	1722 ± 214	2586 ± 295[e]	2131 ± 210
Brain homogenate (ng/gm)	344 ± 15	286 ± 2[e]	476 ± 27	658 ± 32[b]	495 ± 41[c]	1475 ± 123	3306 ± 257[b]	2367 ± 140[b,c]
Ratio of brain to plasma	0.57 ±0.04	0.61 ±0.08	1.07 ±0.14[f]	0.91 ±0.13[g]	0.79 ±0.10	0.56 ± .02	0.50 ± .03[h]	0.63 ± .04

[a] Results expressed as mean ± SE.

[b] Significantly different from day 1, $p < 0.005$.

[c] Significantly different from day 7, $p < 0.005$.

[d] Significantly different from day 1, $p < 0.025$.

[e] Significantly different from day 1, $p < 0.01$.

[f] Significantly different from dogs and mice on day 1, $p < 0.005$.

[g] Significantly different from dogs on day 7, $p < 0.05$.

[h] Significantly different from rats on day 7, $p < 0.01$.

Table 29.2 Δ^9-THC and metabolites (ng/gm brain) in the subcellular fractions of rat brain[a]

	Treatment days		
Subcellular fraction	*1*	*7*	*20*
Homogenate (H)	476 ± 27[b] —	726 ± 125[c] —	534 ± 19[d] —
Crude nuclear (CN)	119 ± 7 (25)	202 ± 45 (27)	130 ± 13 (24)
Crude mitochondrial (CM)	233 ± 17 (49)	359 ± 59 (47)	265 ± 20 (50)
Microsomal (MS)	40 ± 3 (8)	62 ± 7[e] (8)	63 ± 3[e] (12)
Supernatant (S)	37 ± 1 (8)	61 ± 7[e] (8)	92 ± 4[e,f] (17)

[a] On the treatment day indicated, rats were injected IP with 10 mg/kg of ^{3}H-Δ^9-THC and sacrificed 1 hr later. Six rats per group except day 20, $n = 5$.

[b] Results were expressed as mean ± SE. Numbers in parentheses indicate % of homogenate.

[c] Significantly different from day 1 at $p < 0.025$.

[d] Significantly different from day 7 at $p < 0.05$.

[e] Significantly different from day 1 at $p < 0.005$.

[f] Significantly different from day 7 at $p < 0.005$.

The subcellular distribution of cannabinoids in the brains of tolerant and nontolerant dogs has been described in detail elsewhere [9] and will be referred to here only for comparisons among the species. The distribution of radioactivity in the subcellular fractions of rat brains is presented in Table 29.2. The distribution of cannabinoids among the various fractions was similar in each group of rats and was similar to that reported previously for the distribution of cannabinoids in subcellular fractions of dog brains after acute or chronic treatment with Δ^9-THC. That is, the highest concentration was found in the CM fraction, followed by the CN fraction, with little in the MS or supernatant fractions. However, a number of significant differences were detected among treatment groups in homogenate, microsomal, and supernatant fractions of rat brains (Table 29.2). In each of these fractions, those from animals treated with only the labeled Δ^9-THC contained significantly less cannabinoids than the corresponding fractions from rats treated chronically with Δ^9-THC prior to the injection of the labeled cannabinoid.

Table 29.3 Δ^9-THC and metabolites (ng/gm brain) in the crude mitochondrial subfractions of rat brain[a]

	Treatment day		
Subfraction	*1*	*7*	*20*
Myelin (A)	58 ± 5[b] (12)	91 ± 16 (12)	69 ± 6 (13)
Membrane fragments (B)	41 ± 2 (9)	55 ± 12 (7)	42 ± 3 (8)
Cholinergic synaptosomes (C)	73 ± 8 (15)	129 ± 21[c] (17)	91 ± 9 (17)
Noncholinergic synaptosomes (D)	79 ± 18 (16)	80 ± 13 (11)	55 ± 9 (10)
Free mitochondria (E)	11 ± 2 (2)	12 ± 2 (2)	19 ± 3[d,e] (4)

[a] On the treatment day indicated, rats were injected IP with 10 mg/kg of ^{3}H-Δ^9-THC and sacrificed 1 hr later. Six rats per group except day 20, $n = 5$.

[b] Results were expressed as mean ± SE. Numbers in parentheses indicate the % of homogenate.

[c] Significantly different from day 1 at $p < 0.01$.

[d] Significantly different from day 1 at $p < 0.025$.

[e] Significantly different from day 7 at $p < 0.05$.

Table 29.4 Δ^9-THC and metabolites (ng/gm brain) in the synaptic vesicles of rat brain[a]

	Treatment day		
Subfraction	*1*	*7*	*20*
Myelin (M_1)	169 ± 9[b] (35)	192 ± 28 (25)	169 ± 16 (32)
Synaptic vesicles (M_2)	58 ± 8 (12)	63 ± 12 (8)	59 ± 7 (11)
Supernatant (M_3)	39 ± 2 (8)	72 ± 15[c] (9)	73 ± 5[c] (14)

[a] On the treatment day indicated, rats were injected IP with 10 mg/kg of ^{3}H-Δ^9-THC and sacrificed 1 hr later. Six rats per group except day 20, $n = 5$.

[b] Results were expressed as mean ± SE. Numbers in parentheses indicate the % of homogenate.

[c] Significantly different from day 1 at $p < 0.025$.

The CM fractions from the rat brains were subfractionated by ultracentrifugation on a discontinuous sucrose density gradient. This was done to separate the cholinergic and noncholinergic synaptosomes from the remainder of this fraction. The majority of the cannabinoids in the CM faction were found to be in these synaptosome subfractions as shown in Table 29.3. There were few significant differences in the quantity of radioactivity in any subfraction among the three treatment groups.

The CM fraction was also subfractioned by exposing an aliquot of this fraction to osmotic shock followed by ultracentrifugation to separate the synaptic vesicles from other components of this fraction. The concentrations of cannabinoids in each of these subfractions for each treatment group are presented in Table 29.4. There were no significant differences in the quantity of cannabinoids in any of these subfractions among the three treatment groups, except for an increase in the supernatant on days 7 and 20. From 8 to 12 percent of the total cannabinoids in the whole-brain homogenate was associated with the synaptic vesicle fraction.

The distribution of cannabinoids in the subcellular fractions of mouse brains is presented in Table 29.5. The distribution of can-

Table 29.5 Δ^9-THC and metabolites (ng/gm brain) in the subcellular fractions of mouse brain[a]

	Treatment days		
Subcellular fraction	*1*	*7*	*20*
Homogenate (H)	1475 ± 123[b]	3306 ± 257[c]	2367 ± 140[c,d]
Crude nuclear (CN)	384 ± 46	648 ± 93[e]	457 ± 31[f]
Crude mitochondrial (CM)	609 ± 52	1621 ± 130[c]	1296 ± 75[c,g]
Microsomal (MS)	320 ± 32	273 ± 14	189 ± 9[c,g]
Supernatant (S)	109 ± 11	264 ± 21[c]	180 ± 8[c,d]

[a] On the treatment day indicated, mice were injected IP with 50mg/kg of ^{3}H-Δ^9-THC and sacrificed 1 hr later. Six groups of 6 mice each were used per determination.

[b] Results are expressed as mean ± SE. Numbers in parentheses indicate % of homogenate.

[c] Significantly different from day 1 at $p < 0.005$.

[d] Significantly different from day 7 at $p < 0.005$.

[e] Significantly different from day 1 at $p < 0.01$.

[f] Significantly different from day 7 at $p < 0.05$.

[g] Significantly different from day 7 at $p < 0.025$.

Table 29.6 Δ^9-THC and metabolites (ng/gm brain) in the crude mitochondrial subfractions of mouse brain[a]

Subfraction	Treatment day 1	7	20
Myelin (A)	124 ± 14[b] (8)	435 ± 42[c] (13)	259 ± 14[c,d] (11)
Membrane fragments (B)	68 ± 5 (5)	393 ± 31[c] (12)	169 ± 12[c,d] (7)
Cholinergic synaptosomes (C)	196 ± 19 (13)	603 ± 44[c] (19)	272 ± 7[d] (12)
Noncholinergic synaptosomes (D)	132 ± 19 (8)	391 ± 41[c] (12)	332 ± 20[c] (14)
Free mitochondria	22 ± 4 (2)	68 ± 23[e] (4)	49 ± 10 (2)

[a] On the treatment day indicated, mice were injected IP with 50 mg/kg of ^{3}H-Δ^9-THC and sacrificed 1 hr later. Six groups of 6 mice each were used per determination.

[b] Results are expressed as mean ± SE. Numbers in parentheses indicate % of homogenate.

[c] Significantly different from day 1 at $p < 0.005$.

[d] Significantly different from day 7 at $p < 0.005$.

[e] Significantly different from day 1 at $p < 0.025$.

Table 29.7 Δ^9-THC and metabolites (ng/gm brain) in the synaptic vesicles of mouse brain[a]

Subfraction	Treatment day 1	7	20
Myelin (M_1)	339 ± 17[b] (24)	1171 ± 98[c] (35)	838 ± 23[c,d] (36)
Synaptic vesicles (M_2)	54 ± 7 (4)	265 ± 18[c] (8)	181 ± 25[c,e] (8)
Supernatant (M_3)	68 ± 5 (5)	178 ± 19[c] (6)	153 ± 14[c] (6)

[a] On the treatment day indicated, mice were injected IP with 50 mg/kg of ^{3}H-Δ^9-THC and sacrificed 1 hr later. Six groups of 6 mice each were used per determination.

[b] Results are expressed as mean ± SE. Numbers in parentheses indicate % of homogenate.

[c] Significantly different from day 1 at $p < 0.005$.

[d] Significantly different from day 7 at $p < 0.005$.

[e] Significantly different from day 7 at $p < 0.01$.

nabinoids throughout the subcellular fractions was similar in all groups. The pattern of distribution of cannabinoids throughout the subcellular fractions of the mouse brains was similar to that found in the rat experiments described above and in the dog studies previously reported [9]. The amount of cannabinoids in the total homogenate was significantly higher after chronic treatment than after a single injection of Δ^9-THC in mice. Obviously, this was also observed in the fractions of the homogenate. Significantly more Δ^9-THC and metabolites were in the brain when the ^{3}H-Δ^9-THC was given after 6 injections than after 19 injections of the unlabeled drug. Similarly, the distribution of cannabinoids in the subfractions of the CM fractions derived by ultracentrifugation on a discontinuous sucrose density gradient (Table 29.6) or after osmotic shock (Table 29.7) was similar to that seen in the same subfractions of rat and dog brains. Considerably higher concentrations of cannabinoids were found in the subfractions of the CM fraction of mouse brains when the ^{3}H-Δ^9-THC was given after 6 injections than after 19 injections of unlabeled drug, which in turn were higher than those in the brains of mice given only the single injection of ^{3}H-Δ^9-THC. Table 29.8 shows a comparison of the distribution of cannabinoids in the various fractions and subfractions of the three species in terms of percentage of total homogenate. As

Table 29.8 Percentage of whole-brain homogenate in fractions and subfractions of dog, rat, and mouse brain

	Dogs		*Rats*			*Mice*		
Number of treatments	*1*	*7*	*1*	*7*	*20*	*1*	*7*	*20*
Fraction								
Crude nuclear (cn)	22	31	25	27	24	25	19	20
Crude mitochondrial (cm)	46	44	49	47	50	41	49	55
Microsomal (ms)	12	10	8	8	12	21	9	8
Supernatant (s)	15	14	8	8	17	7	8	8
Subfraction (sucrose density)								
Myelin (A)	29	29	12	12	13	8	13	11
Membrane fragments (B)	3	3	9	7	8	5	12	7
Cholinergic synaptosomes (C)	7	6	15	17	17	13	19	12
Noncholinergic synaptosomes (D)	6	6	16	11	10	9	12	14
Free mitochondria (E)	1	2	2	2	4	2	4	2
Subfraction (osmotic shock)								
Myelin (M_1)	32	32	35	25	32	24	35	36
Synaptic vesicles (M_2)	7	4	12	8	11	4	8	8
Supernatant (M_3)	7	5	8	9	14	5	6	7

can be seen in this table, the distribution was similar in all three species after either acute or chronic treatment.

Discussion

The evidence is convincing that laboratory animals develop tolerance to the effects of Δ^9-THC. The development of tolerance to the daily injection of Δ^9-THC in dogs, rats, and mice in the present study confirms and extends previous reports [10]. The mechanism responsible for this phenomenon is unknown. Previous reports from our laboratory have shown that the development of tolerance to the effects of Δ^9-THC in pigeons was not due to an alteration in metabolism [13] or to distribution of the parent compound or its metabolites into brain tissues [7]. The results of experiments in dogs [9] demonstrated that the tolerance which developed in that species could not be accounted for on the basis of altered metabolism or distribution in peripheral organs or into any of 27 different areas of the brain.

However, the amount of radioactivity was significantly decreased in the synaptic vesicles of dogs treated for 6 days with unlabeled Δ^9-THC before injecting ^{3}H-Δ^9-THC; this decrease was more than that observed in the synaptic vesicle fraction from dogs given only a single dose of radiolabeled Δ^9-THC. It was hypothesized at that time that the development of tolerance might be due to this difference in the subcellular distribution of the radioactivity in the brains of tolerant versus nontolerant dogs. The results of these experiments in rats and mice do not support this hypothesis. Although tolerance developed in each of these species prior to the injection of ^{3}H-Δ^9-THC, the percentage of the total radioactivity in the whole-brain homogenate in the synaptic vesicle fraction in the tolerant animals was not less than that found in the nontolerant rodents. However, different degrees of tolerance were observed in each species. Complete tolerance was observed in the mice, approximately 50-percent tolerance was observed in dogs, but no tolerance was observed in rats after 6 daily injections of Δ^9-THC.

A number of differences exist between the experiments in dogs and those in rodents. The dose of Δ^9-THC needed to produce a pronounced effect in each species was different. A small dose of 0.5 mg/kg produced pronounced overt behavioral effects in dogs, but not in rats or mice. A dose of 10 mg/kg Δ^9-THC caused a decrease in spontaneous activity in rats, but this test has been somewhat inconsistent when Δ^9-THC was tested for its effects in the mouse in our laboratory. However, a consistent, pronounced effect on the behavior of mice was seen at the very high dose of 50 mg/kg in the roto-rod test.

The second difference in the experiments was the route of administration. The rodents were injected with Δ^9-THC intraperitoneally, whereas a much lower dose of Δ^9-THC was given intravenously to the dogs. Since the lower dose was given intravenously, it is doubtful that the route of administration could be an important factor contributing to the higher levels of cannabinoids found in the tolerant rodent brains as compared to that found in the tolerant dog brains.

The route of administration may have been indirectly responsible for the third difference in the experiments—the time of sacrifice after the injection of the ^{3}H-Δ^9-THC. The dogs were sacrificed 30 min and the rodents 1 hr after the injection. Blood levels were considerably higher in mice than in either dogs or rats at the time of sacrifice.

The effects of Δ^9-THC in dogs is complex. Although a syndrome unique to this type of drug is observed, some generalized central nervous system depression also is seen. Dogs develop tolerance to the cannabinoid syndrome (static ataxia and hyperexcitability) very rapidly, but they develop tolerance slowly, if at all, to the generalized depression. This depression is probably similar to or responsible for the hypoactivity seen in most species and quantitated in the present experiments in rats. The degree of tolerance to the hypoactivity in rats was not as impressive or consistent as that seen to the behavioral effects in mice and dogs. The mice had to coordinate motor function to stay on the rotating rod. The effect of Δ^9-THC interfered with their ability to perform this function. Tolerance to this effect of Δ^9-THC was different from that observed in dogs and rats, in which the effect of the cannabinoids was to interfere with natural movement.

The distribution of cannabinoids (Δ^9-THC plus metabolites) in the subcellular fractions of the brains of the three species was similar. The highest quantity of radioactivity was found in the crude mitochondrial fraction, and very little was found in the supernatant. This differs significantly from the subcellular distribution of most other psychomimetic agents, which tend to be found in high quantities in the supernatant. Considerable quantities of cannabinoids were found in the synaptosomes and synaptic vesicle subfractions. These results suggest that Δ^9-THC may be interacting with that portion of the neuron involved in storing the neurotransmitters. The possibility that the mechanism of action of Δ^9-THC can be attributed to its interaction with neurotransmitter systems of the brain could be supported by these findings. However, little convincing evidence has appeared to suggest that the pharmacological effects of Δ^9-THC and other cannabinoids are associated with one or another of the purported neurotransmitters. Unlike many CNS-acting drugs, Δ^9-THC must be given in much higher doses than is necessary to produce significant alterations in behavior or in brain levels or turnover rates of norepinephrine, dopamine, serotonin, or acetylcholine. Certainly, one could not postulate the involvement of one specific neurotransmitter to explain the tolerance that laboratory animals develop to Δ^9-THC without first demonstrating the involvement of this amine in the mechanism of action of cannabinoids.

Generally, the concentrations of cannabinoids in the brains of tolerant pigeons [13] and dogs [9] were lower than in the brains of animals treated acutely with labeled Δ^9-THC. The concentration of cannabinoids was consistently higher after chronic administration in the rodents than was observed after acute administration. These differences may be due to a qualitative or quantitative difference in the metabolism of Δ^9-THC in rodents as compared to the other species. As mentioned previously, Δ^9-THC was administered intravenously in the dog experiments, exposing the brain and other organs of the body to the parent compound before its passage through the liver and its resultant metabolism. The pigeons were injected intramuscularly. Little drug administered by this route goes to the liver prior to the heart. Δ^9-THC was administered intraperitoneally in the rodent experiments. Considerable quantities of the drug were taken into the liver and metabolized before it entered the systemic circulation. The evidence presented to date suggests that the metabolic pathway of Δ^9-THC in the various species is similar; however, an exhaustive investigation into the comparative metabolism of this drug in pigeons, dogs, rats, and mice has not been reported. Little data have appeared on the metabolism of this drug or most other drugs in pigeons or mice. We will continue to attempt to elucidate the mechanisms responsible for these differences in brain levels of cannabinoids and their possible role in the development of tolerance to Δ^9-THC.

ACKNOWLEDGMENT

This work was supported by USPHS Grant Number DA-00490.

REFERENCES

1. Carden, B. and J. Olson (1973) Learned behavioral tolerance to marihuana in rats. *Pharmacol. Biochem. Behav. 1*:73–76.
2. Carlini, E. A. (1968) Tolerance to chronic administration of *Cannabis sativa* (marihuana) in rats. *Pharmacology 1*:135–142.

3. DeRobertis, E., D. A. Pellegrino, D. A. G. Rodriguez, and L. Salganicoff (1962) Colinergic and noncholinergic nerve endings in rat brain. *J. Neurochem.* *9:*23–25.
4. DeRobertis, E., D. A. G. Rodriguez, L. Salganicoff, D. A. Pellegrino, and L. M. Zieher (1963) Isolation of synaptic vesicles and structural organization of the acetylcholine system within brain nerve endings. *J. Neurochem.* *10:*225–235.
5. Dewey, W. L., J. Jenkins, T. O'Rourke, and L. S. Harris (1972) The effects of chronic administration of *trans*-Δ^9-tetrahydrocannabinol on behavior and the cardiovascular system of dogs. *Arch. Int. Pharmacodyn. Ther.* *198:*118–131.
6. Dewey, W. L., B. R. Martin, and L. S. Harris (1975) Chronic effects of Δ^9-THC in animals: tolerance and biochemical changes. *The Pharmacology of Marihuana.* New York: Raven Press.
7. Dewey, W. L., D. E. McMillan, L. S. Harris, and R. T. Turk (1973) Distribution of radioactivity in brain of tolerant and nontolerant pigeons treated with ^{3}H-Δ^9-tetrahydrocannabinol. *Biochem. Pharmacol.* *22:*399–405.
8. Gill, E. W., W. D. M. Paton, and R. G. Pertwee (1970) Preliminary experiments on the chemistry and pharmacology of cannabis. *Nature* *228:*134–136.
9. Martin, B. R., W. L. Dewey, L. S. Harris, and J. S. Beckner (1975) ^{3}H-Δ^9-tetrahydrocannabinol tissue and subcellular distribution in the central nervous system and tissue distribution in peripheral organs of tolerant and nontolerant dogs. *J. Pharmacol. Exp. Ther.* (in press).
10. McMillan, D. E. and W. L. Dewey (1972) On the mechanism of tolerance to Δ^9-THC. *Current Research in Marijuana.* (M. F. Lewis, ed.). New York: Academic Press, pp. 94–114.
11. McMillan, D. E., W. L. Dewey, and L. S. Harris (1971) Characteristics of tetrahydrocannabinol tolerance. *Ann. N.Y. Aca. Sci.* *191:*83–99.
12. McMillan, D. E., R. D. Ford, J. M. Frankenheim, R. A. Harris, and L. S. Harris (1972) Tolerance to active constituents of marihuana. *Arch. Int. Pharmacodyn. Ther.* *198:*132–144.
13. McMillan, D. E., W. L. Dewey, R. T. Turk, L. S. Harris, and J. H. McNeil, Jr. (1973) Blood levels of ^{3}H-Δ^9-tetrahydrocannabinol and its metabolites in tolerant and nontolerant pigeons. *Biochem. Pharmacol.* *22:*383–397.
14. Olson, J. L., M. Makhani, K. H. Davis, and M. E. Wall (1973) Preparation of Δ^9-tetrahydrocannabinol for intravenous injection. *J. Pharm. Pharmacol.* *25:*344.
15. Spaulding, T. C., R. Ford, W. L. Dewey, D. E. McMillan, and L. S. Harris (1972) Some pharmacological effects of phenitrone and its interaction with delta-9-THC. *Eur. J. Pharmacol.* *19:*310–317.
16. Winer, B. (1972) *Statistical Principles in Experimental Design.* New York: McGraw-Hill.

30

Sites of Neurochemical Action of Δ^9-Tetrahydrocannabinol: Interaction with Reserpine

BENG T. HO AND KENNETH M. JOHNSON

Introduction

The psychological and physiological effects of marihuana are of considerable interest to many researchers, and the syntheses of Δ^9-tetrahydrocannabinol (Δ^9-THC), the major active constituent in marihuana, and its metabolite 11-hydroxy-Δ^9-THC have facilitated the study of the neurochemical and behavioral effects of this plant material. At present, the literature is somewhat controversial regarding the possible mechanism of action of Δ^9-THC on the brain. Studies of the changes caused by Δ^9-THC on the concentration and turnover of the two biogenic amines, serotonin (5-HT) and norepinephrine (NE), are inconsistent. Leonard [21] has shown no changes in the levels of 5-HT and NE and their major metabolites—5-hydroxyindoleacetic acid (5-HIAA) and normetanephrine (NM)—in the brain of rats receiving Δ^9-THC, but Sofia, Dixit, and Barry [26] reported an increase in 5-HT in the whole brain and in some areas of rat brain. Elevations of 5-HT after Δ^9-THC administration were also shown in mouse brain by Holtzman *et al.* [18] and by Welch *et al.* [29].

In our laboratories, the effects of Δ^9-THC on mouse brain 5-HT were found to be dose-dependent. Small doses resulted in an increase of NE with a concomitant decrease in 5-HT, whereas the reverse was seen with high doses of Δ^9-THC [14]. In monkeys, Δ^9-THC caused a decrease in 5-HT and NE in various brain areas, but whole-brain concentrations were not significantly altered [14]. Using low doses of Δ^9-THC, Gallager *et al.* [10] showed no alteration in cerebral 5-HT turnover. Leonard also studied the rate of depletion (turnover rate) of 5-HT and NE after inhibiting their synthesis with *p*-chlorophenylalanine and *α*-methyl-*p*-tyrosine, respectively, and he concluded that Δ^9-THC does not affect the rate of neuroamine depletion (21). In contrast to this, Sofia *et al.* [26]

Marihuana: Chemistry, Biochemistry, and Cellular Effects, edited by Gabriel G. Nahas,

showed a 50-percent decrease in the turnover rate of 5-HT after blocking monoamine oxidase.

In examining the effects of Δ^9-THC on the release and metabolism of NE, Schildkraut and Efron [25] injected ^{3}H-NE intracisternally before giving large IP doses of Δ^9-THC. They found that Δ^9-THC decreased the retention of ^{3}H-NE and produced an increase in both 0-methylated and deaminated 0-methylated metabolites of NE. In other related studies, investigators found that Δ^9-THC attenuated the disappearance of radioactive NE from rat brain [28], whereas an enhancement in formation of ^{3}H-NE and ^{3}H-dopamine (^{3}H-DA) in rat brains was seen after IV administration of ^{3}H-tyrosine [23].

The results of one of our studies showed no change in the levels of brain 5-HT and NE in rats after inhalation of Δ^9-THC smoke, although decreases in 5-HIAA and NM were evident between the 7–21-day period [13]. In another study [16], chronic administration of Δ^9-THC altered the metabolism of intracisternally injected ^{3}H-5-HT and ^{3}H-NE by decreasing the formation of ^{3}H-5-HIAA and increasing ^{3}H-deaminated metabolites of NE. The opposite effect on the turnover of the two neuroamines was suggested as a basis for the psychoactive property of Δ^9-THC. Using both chronic and acute IV injection of Δ^9-THC, Englert *et al.* [8] studied the depletion of 5-HT and NE in reserpinized rats to determine if the storage mechanism was involved. The depletion of 5-HT by reserpine was significantly inhibited in animals pretreated with Δ^9-THC, whereas NE was not affected. The effects of chronic Δ^9-THC treatment on the major enzymes involved in neuroamine synthesis were determined by Ho and Englert [15]. The activity of tyrosine hydroxylase was increased, but no significant changes were observed in the activities of tryptophan hydroxylase and dopa decarboxylase.

Sofia *et al.* [27] found that the uptake of ^{14}C-5-HT by rat brain homogenates was inhibited by Δ^9-THC in concentrations as low as 0.1 μM. Inhibition of ^{3}H-5-HT, ^{3}H-NE, and ^{3}H-DA uptake in synaptosomes from rat forebrain was also observed by Johnson and Ho [20]. Howes and Osgood [19] examined the effects of Δ^9-THC on both uptake and release of ^{14}C-DA in crude synaptosomes from mouse striatum. They reported a dose-related decrease in the uptake of ^{14}C-DA and a small but significant release of the neuroamine by Δ^9-THC.

The effect of Δ^9-THC on rat brain acetylcholine (ACH) has been studied by Askew and Ho [2]. Although somewhat less effective than the Δ^8-THC, Δ^9-THC caused a depletion of ACH, and the authors suggested that the depletion was primarily due to a release of the neuroamine from the storage vesicles. In contrast to us, Domino [7] reported an increase of ACH in mouse brain by large doses of Δ^9-THC. Using intraventricular administration of hemicholinium-3, the same author observed a slight but significant increase in the steady-state levels of ACH in rat brain after an IP injection of Δ^9-THC. Large doses of Δ^9-THC were also found to decrease neocortical release of ACH [7].

The effects of Δ^9-THC on brain levels of cyclic adenosine 3′,5′-monophosphate (AMP) have been determined in both mice [6] and rats [3]. Low doses of Δ^9-THC caused a significant elevation of cAMP, whereas higher doses depressed the cyclic nucleotide level [6]. The overall biphasic effect of Δ^9-THC on cAMP was correlated with known changes in biogenic amines, temperature regulation, and behavior. In rats, Δ^9-THC [3] had little effect on the cAMP level in several brain areas studied; however, Δ^8-THC increased the cyclic nucleotide significantly.

A decrease in vanillylmandelic acid (VMA or MHPA) excretion was reported in humans receiving large oral doses of Δ^9-THC [17]. A decrease in catecholamine (CA) turnover or a shift in the degradative pathway of CA from the oxidative to the reductive route was suggested.

In view of current limited knowledge of Δ^9-THC's mechanism of action on the brain, we have chosen to study the interaction of Δ^9-THC with reserpine to determine the sites of action of some neurochemical effects of Δ^9-THC.

Methods

Effects of Δ^9-THC on the subcellular distribution of endogenous 5-HT

Male Sprague-Dawley rats (averaging 160 gm) in groups of 4 were used. Each rat was given an IV injection of 1 mg/kg of Δ^9-THC in 4 percent Tween 80-saline suspension and decapitated 4, 7, or 19 hr later. The brains were homogenized in two parts 0.025 *M* sucrose containing 1.5 m*M* of ethylenediaminetetraacetic acid (EDTA) and 2 m*M* of tranylcypromine. The homogenate was centrifuged at 100,000*g* for 20 min as described by Giarman, Freedman, and Schanberg [11]. The supernatant and particulate fractions were separated and the pH adjusted to 2 with dilute HCl to give a total volume of 3 ml. 5-HT was first extracted into *n*-butanol and then returned to 1.5 ml of 0.1 *N* HCl containing 1 percent cysteine according to a modified procedure of Curzon and Green [5]. Internal standards of 5-HT were added to the whole-brain homogenates and run through the extraction procedure. Duplicate 0.5-ml aliquots were taken and assayed for 5-HT by reacting with *o*-phthalaldehyde (OPT). Fluorescence of the product was measured on an Aminco-Bowman spectrophotofluorometer (activation: 360 nm; fluorescence: 470 nm).

Release of ^{3}H-5-HT from the preloaded synaptosomes by Δ^9-THC

The rats (averaging 250 gm) were decapitated and the brain removed. The forebrain was dissected from the brain stem by a section passing between the anterior border of the superior colliculi and the anterior border of the mammillary bodies, and it was then homogenized with a Thomas grinding vessel and a Teflon pestle in 9 volumes of ice cold 0.32 *M* sucrose previously equilibrated with 5 percent CO_2–95 percent O_2. The homogenate was centrifuged at 1,000*g* for 10 min. After gently stirring the supernatant to obtain a uniform suspension of synaptosomes, we added a 0.2-ml aliquot to a flask containing 3.8 ml of Krebs–Henseleit bicarbonate medium (pH 7.4) with glucose (11 m*M*), half-strength calcium (1.3 m*M*), ascorbic acid (0.2 mg/ml), disodium EDTA (0.05 mg/ml), and pargyline (125 μM). Then 0.1 ml of ^{3}H(G)-5-HT creatinine sulfate (500 mCi/mmole) or L-leucine-4,5-^{3}H(N) (31.5 Ci/mM) was added, and the mixture was incubated at 37°C for 15 min under 5 percent CO_2–95 percent O_2. The reaction was terminated by placing the flasks in an ice bath, and the samples were transferred to centrifuge tubes and centrifuged at 20,000*g* for 20 min at 4°C. After suspension with ice-cold K–H buffer and centrifugation, the pellets were resuspended in 2 ml of the buffer and incubated at 37°C for 5 min. Δ^9-THC or its vehicle, 10 percent polyvinylpyrrolidone (PVP) in saline [9], was added in a volume of 0.1 ml and the incubation was continued for an additional 15 min. PVP as vehicle for all *in vitro* studies provided better solubility of Δ^9-THC in aqueous medium than Tween 80-saline. After the reaction was terminated in ice and centrifugation at 20,000*g* for 20 min, the pellets were washed with ice cold saline. The saline was aspirated and each pellet was dissolved after a 40-min incubation at 50°C with 0.7 ml of NCS solubilizer. Radioactivity was determined by liquid scintillation spectrometry in the presence of 2,5-diphenyloxazole (PPO) and 1,4-bis[2-(5-phenyloxazolyl)benzene] (POPOP).

The protein content, determined by a modified procedure of Lowry *et al.* [22], of the 0.2-ml aliquot of the synaptosomal preparation was found to vary no more than 5 percent between aliquots (between 1.6 and 1.8 mg).

Subcellular distribution of ^{3}H-Δ^9-THC in various brain areas

Rats were injected intravenously with 2 mg/kg of ^{3}H-Δ^9-THC (46 mCi/mM). The brains were removed and dissected into cortex, cerebellum, medulla-pons, midbrain-hypothalamus, striatum, and septum. The individual areas were pooled and homogenized in 9 volumes of ice cold 0.32 *M* sucrose. The homogenates were then subjected to differential centrifugation [1] as follows. Centrifugation at 1000*g* for 10 min yielded P_1 (nuclei and broken cell fragments) and S_1. S_1 was centrifuged at 10,000*g* for 15 min yielding P_2 (myelin, synaptosomes, and mitochondria) and S_2. S_2 was further centrifuged at 100,000*g* for 30 min to give P_3 (microsomal) and S_3 (supernatant). Unchanged ^{3}H-Δ^9-THC was extracted from P_1, P_2, P_3, and S_3 using petroleum ether. Recovery of ^{3}H-Δ^9-THC using this solvent is 90 percent or better. After evaporating the petroleum ether, we assayed the radioactivity in each sample by liquid scintillation spectrometry.

Effects of reserpine on the binding of ^{3}H-Δ^9-THC to synaptosomes

The 1,000*g* supernatant (as described directly above) was used as the source of synaptosomes. The synaptosomal preparation in the Krebs–Henseleit buffer was preincubated for 15 min with varying concentrations (0.1–100 μM) of reserpine before adding 1.6 μM of ^{3}H-Δ^9-THC (46 mCi/mM) in PVP-saline suspension. The incubation was continued for another 15 min. After the binding of ^{3}H-Δ^9-THC was terminated in ice and the pellets were washed (as described above), the unchanged ^{3}H-Δ^9-THC was extracted with 5 ml of petroleum ether. Aliquots of the petroleum ether were evaporated to dryness and the radioactivity was assayed.

Effects of Δ^9-THC on the binding of ^{3}H-reserpine to synaptosomes and other subcellular fractions

In a fashion similar to that described above, the synaptosomal preparation was preincubated with varying concentrations of Δ^9-THC before the addition of 1.74 or 1.34 μM of ^{3}H-reserpine (labeled on the trimethoxyphenyl ring, 133.9 mCi/mM). At the end of the experiment, ^{3}H-reserpine was extracted from pellets by the procedure of Alpers and Shore [1] as follows. The pellets were homogenized in 1.5 ml of 0.01 *N* HCl. To a 1.5-ml aliquot of the homogenate, we added 0.5 ml of 0.25 *M* borate buffer, pH 9. If necessary, 0.1 *N* NaOH was added to adjust the pH to 9. The homogenate was then extracted with 5 ml of toluene containing 1.5 percent of isoamyl alcohol (v/v). The toluene layer was separated from the aqueous layer by centrifugation, and a 4-ml aliquot was assayed for radioactivity.

Similar experiments were carried out as described in the above paragraph except that various subcellular fractions were assayed for radioactivity in place of whole crude synaptosomal preparations. The P_2 fraction (see Subcellular distribution of ^{3}H-Δ^9-THC in various brain areas) was separated into its component parts by layering it on a two-step discontinuous sucrose gradient (0.8 and 1.2 *M*) [12]. The tubes placed in an SW 50.1 swinging bucket rotor were centrifuged at 27,500*g* for 90 min. Myelin (P_2A) was layered at the 0.32–0.8 *M* interface, synaptosomes (P_2B) at the 0.8–1.2 *M* interface, and mitochondria (P_2C) were at the bottom. The individual layers were removed with a disposable pipette and solubilized in NCS for assaying radioactivity.

Results

Effects of Δ^9-THC on 5-HT

The effects of intravenously injected Δ^9-THC on the rat brain 5-HT are shown in Table 30.1. Although the total concentration of brain 5-HT remained unchanged, the drug caused a shift of 5-HT from the particulate or "bound" fraction to the supernatant or "free" fraction. Figure 30.1 presents the results of *in vitro*

Table 30.1 Effect of Δ^9-THC on the subcellular distribution of 5-HT in the rat brain[a]

	µg/gm			*Change from controls (%)*	
Treatment	*Total*	*Particulate (P)*	*Supernatant (S)*	*P*	*S*
Control (vehicle)	0.49	0.34 ± 0.01	0.15 ± 0.01	—	—
Δ^9-THC (1 mg/kg)					
4 hr	0.42	0.24 ± 0.01[b]	0.18 ± 0.01	−29.3	+20.0
7 hr	0.51	0.30 ± 0.01	0.21 ± 0.01[b]	−11.8	+40.0
19 hr	0.49	0.29 ± 0.03	0.20 ± 0.02	−14.7	+33.3

[a] Each value represents the mean ± SE of 4 animals.

[b] $p < 0.05$ (*t*-test).

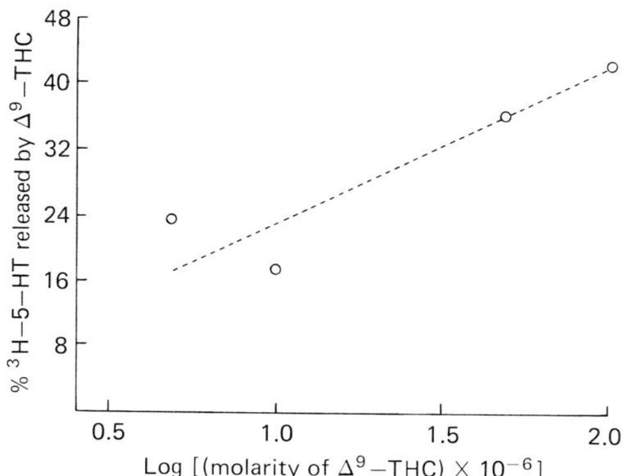

Figure 30.1. The release of ^{3}H-5-HT from synaptosomes by Δ^9-THC. After the synaptosomal pellets were preloaded by incubating them in 0.25 μM of ^{3}H-5-HT for 15 min, the percentage of ^{3}H-5-HT released by Δ^9-THC was determined by measuring the radioactivity remaining in pellets as follows:

$$\text{Percentage} = 100 \times \frac{^3\text{H-dpm (PVP)-}^3\text{H-dpm }(\Delta^9\text{-THC})}{^3\text{H-dpm (PVP)}} .$$

experiments in which Δ^9-THC was shown to release ^{3}H-5-HT from the preloaded synaptosomes in a dose-dependent fashion. However, Δ^9-THC failed to release ^{3}H-leucine from the preloaded synaptosomes. Although there was a 14.7-percent release by $^9\Delta$-THC of this amino acid, which is not stored in the synaptic vesicle, the value is not statistically different from the control.

Synaptosomes preloaded with ^{3}H-5-HT were also incubated at both 2° and 37°C. Since the vesicular 5-HT pump is an energy-requiring process, it can be assumed that at 37°C, ^{3}H-5-HT would "label" both the vesicular and nonvesicular pools, whereas very little of ^{3}H-5-HT would be taken up into the storage vesicles at 2°C; instead it would readily "label" the intraneuronal nonvesicular pool by passive diffusion. The data in Table 30.2 show that about twice as much ^{3}H-5-HT was released by Δ^9-THC when the preloading of the labeled amine was into both the vesicular and nonvesicular 5-HT pools, compared to nonvesicular loading only.

Thirty minutes after the intravenous injection of ^{3}H-Δ^9-THC, the radioactive compound, which amounted to 0.3 percent of the administered dose, was distributed more or less evenly throughout the brain (Table 30.3). Amounts in cerebellum and midbrain were lower than in other areas; however, this difference is not

Table 30.2 Temperature-dependent "labeling" of the synaptic vesicles and subsequent release of ^{3}H-5-HT by Δ^{9}-THC[a]

Δ^{9}-THC (μM)	^{3}H-5-HT (μM)	2°C			37°C			
		A: 5-HT taken up (ng)	B: 5-HT remaining (ng)	A/B[b]	C: 5-HT taken up (ng)	D: 5-HT remaining (ng)	C/D[b]	$\frac{C/D^{c}}{A/B}$
100	0.48	2.66 ± 0.34	2.15 ± 0.32	1.24	10.51 ± 0.50	4.51 ± 0.38	2.33	1.87
60	0.42	2.01 ± 0.34	1.23 ± 0.23	1.63	10.87 ± 0.61	3.31 ± 0.08	3.28	2.01

[a] Each value represents the mean ± SE from three determinations. The incubation time for ^{3}H-5-HT uptake or release by Δ^{9}-THC was 15 min.

[b] A direct indicator of the percentage of ^{3}H-5-HT released by Δ^{9}-THC.

[c] An indicator of the potency of Δ^{9}-THC to release ^{3}H-5-HT taken up at the 2 temperatures.

Table 30.3 The subcellular distribution of ^{3}H-Δ^{9}-THC in various brain areas

Subcellular fraction	Percentage of total ^{3}H-Δ^{9}-THC[a] Cerebellum	Pons-medulla	Midbrain-hypothalamus	Septum	Striatum	Cortex
	16.7 (1.31)[b]	10.5 (1.66)	14.5 (1.25)	5.4 (1.52)	9.5 (1.49)	43.4 (1.60)
P_1	24.0	24.9	24.7	23.0	27.2	17.3
P_2	37.6	34.6	31.9	41.9	35.8	40.7
P_3	25.2	25.1	26.4	19.6	22.4	28.3
S_3	13.2	15.4	17.1	15.5	15.2	13.7

[a] Each value is the mean of two independent experiments in which two rats received an injection of ^{3}H-Δ^{9}-THC (2 mg/kg,IV). The animals were sacrificed 30 min postinjection.

[b] Values in parentheses represent nM/gm of brain tissue.

statistically significant. An examination of the subcellular distribution of the drug reveals that the synaptosomal fraction (P_2) contains more ^{3}H-Δ^{9}-THC than any of the other fractions of all the six brain areas examined. This is particularly evident in the septum and cortex, which have a high density of nerve endings.

Table 30.4 The effect or reserpine pretreatment *in vivo* on the ability of Δ^{9}-THC to release ^{3}H-5-HT *in vitro*

$[K^+]$ in K–H buffer (mM)	Percentage of total ^{3}H-5-HT released[a] Vehicle pretreatment	Reserpine pretreatment	Diminution of effect by reserpine (%)
4.5	25.6	15.4	40.0
60.0	20.9	9.0	57.1

[a] Two rats were pretreated with reserpine (5 mg/kg, IV) or vehicle 16 hr before to sacrifice. The percentage of total ^{3}H-5-HT released by Δ^{9}-THC in a 20-min *in vitro* incubation was calculated from the radioactivity in pellets as follows:

$$\frac{[^{3}\text{H-dpm (0 min)}-{}^{3}\text{H-dpm (20 min, }\Delta^{9}\text{-THC)}]-[^{3}\text{H-dpm (0 min)}-{}^{3}\text{H-dpm (20 min, PVP)}]}{^{3}\text{H-dpm (0 min)}}.$$

Values at each time point were determined by triplicate observations.

Δ^9-THC–reserpine interaction

The extent of Δ^9-THC's involvement in releasing ^{3}H-5-HT from preloaded synaptosomes of the reserpinized rats was evaluated. As seen in Table 30.4, with the use of the synaptic vesicles, the storage capacity of which was being diminished by the reserpine treatment, the release of ^{3}H-5-HT by Δ^9-THC was less than with those vesicles obtained from animals receiving the vehicle instead of reserpine. The reduction of release was 40 and 57 percent, de-

Table 30.5 Effects of Δ^9-THC on the subcellular distribution of brain 5-HT in reserpine-treated rats

	μg/gm[b]			*Percentage change from reserpine control*	
Treatment[a]	*Total*	*Particulate (P)*	*Supernatant (S)*	*P*	*S*
Δ^9-THC pretreatment					
Reserpine (15 mg/kg)					
3 hr	0.12	0.06 ± 0.01	0.06 ± 0	—	—
6 hr	0.11	0.05 ± 0.01	0.06 ± 0	—	—
18 hr	0.23	0.10 ± 0.01	0.13 ± 0.01	—	—
Δ^9-THC (1 mg/kg) 1 hr before reserpine					
3 hr	0.29	0.10 ± 0.01[c]	0.18 ± 0.02[d]	+ 66	+200
6 hr	0.34	0.15 ± 0.02[d]	0.19 ± 0.01[d]	+200	+217
18 hr	0.47	0.25 ± 0.02[d]	0.22 ± 0.02[d]	+150	+ 69
Reserpine prior to Δ^9-THC					
Reserpine (15 mg/kg)					
3 hr	0.19	0.09 ± 0.02	0.10 ± 0	—	—
6 hr	0.25	0.12 ± 0.01	0.13 ± 0.01	—	—
18 hr	0.26	0.13 ± 0.01	0.13 ± 0.01	—	—
Δ^9-THC (1 mg/kg) 3 hr after reserpine					
3 hr	0.18	0.10 ± 0.01	0.08 ± 0.01	+ 11	+ 20
6 hr	0.15	0.07 ± 0.01[c]	0.08 ± 0.01[e]	− 42	− 39
18 hr	0.20	0.10 ± 0.01	0.10 ± 0.01	− 23	− 23

[a] Δ^9-THC was injected *i.v.* 1 hr before the IP administration of reserpine or 3 hr after reserpine as indicated; 5-HT concentration was determined 3, 6, or 18 hr after reserpine.

[b] Each value represents the mean ± SE of 4 animals.

[c] $p < 0.01$.

[d] $p < 0.001$.

[e] $p < 0.02$ (t-test).

Table 30.6 The effect of reserpine preincubation on the *in vitro* binding of ^{3}H-Δ^9-THC to synaptosomes

Reserpine (μM)	*ng* ^{3}*H-*Δ^9*-THC*[a] (*bound pellet*)
0	380 ± 43.2
0.1	373 ± 27.4
1.0	354 ± 31.8
10	358 ± 21.4
100	386 ± 26.4

[a] Each value represents the mean ± SE of three determinations. No significant differences exist between any of the groups. ^{3}H-Δ^9-THC in the incubation medium is 1.6 μM.

pending on the potassium concentration of the buffer. This result indicates that the 5-HT pool from which Δ^9-THC affects release is also affected by reserpine.

In the *in vivo* experiment, when Δ^9-THC was injected intravenously to rats 3 hr after the IP administration of reserpine, an enhancement in the depletion of brain 5-HT was observed (Table 30.5). Before the injection of Δ^9-THC, the 5-HT concentration was reduced in both the particulate and supernatant fractions as early as 3 hr after reserpine administration. Thereafter, Δ^9-THC further depleted 5-HT in both fractions to approximately the same extent from 6 to 18 hr. An antagonism, rather than the potentiation described above, of reserpine-induced depletion of 5-HT occurs if the sequence of administering the two drugs is reversed. Pretreatment with Δ^9-THC 1 hr before reserpine elicited a reversal of 5-HT reduction in both fractions; this effect was highly significant at all time intervals studied but was most pronounced at 6 hr (Table 30.5).

The mutual influence on binding to synaptosomes between reserpine and Δ^9-THC was determined *in vitro*. Table 30.6 shows that varying concentrations of reserpine in the incubation medium had no effect on the binding of ^{3}H-Δ^9-THC to the synaptosomal preparation. On the contrary, the binding of ^{3}H-reserpine was found to be affected by the presence of Δ^9-THC: at a concentration of Δ^9-THC near 10^{-4} *M*, the increase of ^{3}H-reserpine binding was 25–90 percent (Figure 30.2). When the enhancement of ^{3}H-reserpine binding by Δ^9-THC was examined in the subcellular location, Δ^9-THC caused a shift in ^{3}H-reserpine from the supernatant to the particulate fraction (Table 30.7). More specifically,

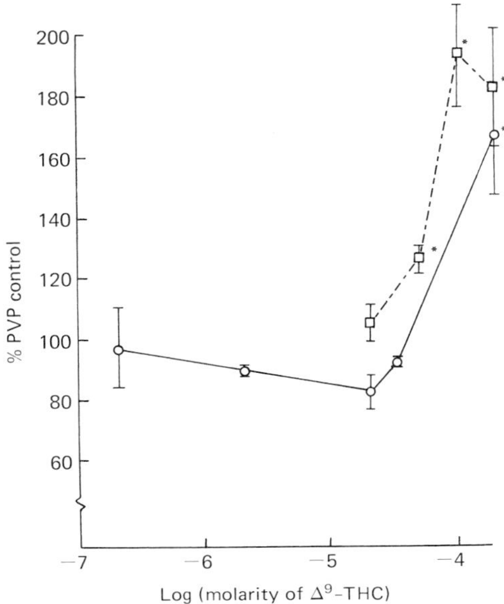

Figure 30.2. The effect of Δ^9-THC preincubation on the binding of ^{3}H-reserpine to synaptosomes. Each point represents the mean ± SE of 3 determinations. The values of ^{3}H-reserpine in experiments I (○——○) and II (□-----□) are 1.74 and 1.34 μM, respectively. $^*p < 0.01$ (t-test).

Table 30.7 The effect of Δ^9-THC preincubation on the *in vitro* binding of ^{3}H-reserpine to various subcellular fractions of the rat brain

	ng ^{3}H-reserpine/fraction[a]				
Treatment	P_2	S_2	P_2 (A)	P_2 (B)	P_2 (C)
PVP control	1141 ± 25	1672 ± 48	345 ± 23	200 ± 16	77 ± 16
Δ^9-THC (0.1 mM)	1602 ± 71[b] (140.4)	1369 ± 98[b] (81.9)	350 ± 22 (101.4)	553 ± 46[b] (276.5)	365 ± 41[b] (474.1)

[a] ^{3}H-reserpine = 1.93 μM. The various fractions are defined as follows: P_2, "synaptosomal" pellet; S_2, microsomes and supernatant; P_2 (A), myelin; P_2 (B), synaptosomes; P_2 (C), mitochondria. Values in parentheses represent percentage of radioactivity in samples with Δ^9-THC relative to the PVP control.

[b] $p < 0.01$ (t-test).

the bulk of this increased ^{3}H-reserpine binding was found in the mitochondrial fraction of the synaptosomal preparation.

Discussion

The results shown in Table 30.3 on the subcellular distribution of IV injected ^{3}H-Δ^9-THC in various brain areas suggest that some of the effects of Δ^9-THC can be related to the apparent preferential localization of the drug in the synaptosomal fraction. Although our data have been verified by a recent work of Martin *et al.* [24], they vary to some extent from those reported by Colburn *et al.* [4], who, using different extraction and fractionation techniques, found about 51 percent of Δ^9-THC and metabolites in the nuclear fraction (P_1), and only 25 percent in the synaptosomal fractions (P_2 A,B,C). The antagonistic effect of Δ^9-THC on the depletion of 5-HT (Table 30.5) by reserpine further indicated that this particular action of Δ^9-THC is on the presynaptic storage vesicles. This presumption is strengthened by the observation that Δ^9-THC alone causes a shift of 5-HT from the "bound" to the "free" form (Table 30.1), pointing to an effect of Δ^9-THC in releasing 5-HT from storage. The release of 5-HT by Δ^9-THC from the synaptic vesicles is further substantiated from the following *in vitro* observations: (1) most ^{3}H-Δ^9-THC was bound to the P_2 synaptosomal fraction (Table 30.3); (2) the Δ^9-THC–induced release of ^{3}H-5-HT was diminished in preloaded synaptosomes prepared from reserpinized animals (Table 30.4); (3) Δ^9-THC was not effective in releasing preloaded ^{3}H-leucine from the nonvesicular component of synaptosomes; (4) Δ^9-THC was twice as effective in releasing ^{3}H-5-HT when the labeled neuroamine was preloaded into both the vesicular and nonvesicular 5-HT pools rather than into the nonvesicular pool only (Table 30.2).

Although reserpine does not affect the binding of ^{3}H-Δ^9-THC to the synaptosomes (Table 30.6), the binding of ^{3}H-reserpine is enhanced in the presence of Δ^9-THC (Figure 30.2). The subcellular study (Table 30.7) reveals that the increased binding of reserpine occurs mostly on the mitochondria. The blockade by Δ^9-THC of reserpine binding at the synaptic vesicles by shifting to the secondary site may account for the observed attenuation of reserpine's depletion of 5-HT (Table 30.5). This reversal of the neurochemical effect of reserpine was also found to correlate with the prevention of reserpine-induced hypothermia in rats (8), and the involvement of 5-HT in the thermoregulation is established from the finding that cinanserin (2′-3–dimethylaminopropylthiocinnamanilide), a 5-HT antagonist, was able to prevent Δ⁹-THC from blocking the reserpine hypothermia [8]. Because of reserpine's lack of effect on the binding of ³H-Δ⁹-THC (Table 30.6), the findings, resulting from the injection of Δ⁹-THC after reserpine, on the enhancement of reserpine-induced depletion of 5-HT (Table 30.5) and the potentiation of reserpine hypothermia [8] can therefore be attributed to the synergistic effect of Δ⁹-THC in releasing the neuroamine.

Our studies based on the interaction between Δ⁹-THC and reserpine have established the ability of Δ⁹-THC to release brain 5-HT from its storage sites. In a related study, we reported the inhibition of synaptosomal uptake of 5-HT by Δ⁹-THC, possibly on the neuronal membrane [20]. Although the levels of brain 5-HT are unchanged after repeated inhalation of the Δ⁹-THC smoke by rats [13] and there is no difference in the concentrations of intracisternally injected ³H-5-HT in brains found between animals chronically injected with Δ⁹-THC and the vehicle [16], elevation of brain 5-HT has been reported in several acute studies [18,26,29]. Releasing of 5-HT as well as blocking the reuptake of the neuroamine may account for the increased neuroamine in brains. The blockade of 5-HT reuptake may also explain the decrease in brain 5-HIAA during two chronic studies [13,16].

REFERENCES

1. Alpers, H. S. and P. A. Shore (1969) Specific binding of reserpine–association with norepinephrine depletion. *Biochem. Pharmacol. 18:*1363.
2. Askew, W. E. and B. T. Ho (1974) Effect of tetrahydrocannabinols on brain acetylcholine. *Brain Res. 69:*375.
3. Askew, W. E. and B. T. Ho (1974) Effect of tetrahydrocannabinols on cyclic AMP levels in rat brain areas. *Experientia 30:*879.
4. Colburn, R. W., L. K. Y. Ng, L. Lemberger, and I. J. Lopin (1974) Subcellular distribution of Δ⁹-tetrahydrocannabinol in rat brain. *Biochem. Pharmacol. 23:*873.
5. Curzon, G. and A. R. Green (1970) Rapid method for the determination of 5-hydroxytryptamine and 5-hydroxyindoleacetic acid in small regions of the rat brain. *Br. J. Pharmacol. 39:*653.
6. Dolby, T. W. and L. J. Kleinsmith (1974) Effects of Δ⁹-tetrahydrocannabinol on the levels of cyclic adenosine 3′,5′-monophosphate in mouse brain. *Biochem. Pharmacol. 23:*1817.
7. Domino, E. F. (1971) Neuropsychopharmacological studies of marijuana: some synthetic and natural THC derivatives in animals and man. *Ann. N.Y. Acad. Sci. 191:*166.

8. Englert, L. F., B. T. Ho, and D. Taylor (1973) The effects of (-)-Δ^9-tetrahydrocannabinol on reserpine induced hypothermia in rats. *Br. J. Pharmacol. 49:*243.
9. Fenimore, D. C. and P. R. Loy (1971) Injectible dispersion of Δ^9-tetrahydrocannabinol in saline using polyvinylpyrrolidone. *J. Pharm. Pharmacol. 23:*310.
10. Gallager, D. W., E. Sandres-Bush, and F. Sulser (1972) Dissociation between behavioral effects and changes in metabolism of cerebral serotonin following Δ^9-tetrahydrocannabinol. *Psychopharmacologia 26:*337.
11. Giarman, N. J., D. X. Freedman, and S. M. Schanberg (1964) Drug-induced changes in the subcellular distribution of serotonin in rat brain with special reference to the action of reserpine. *Progress in Brain Research—Brain Amines* (H. E. Himmich and W. A. Himmich (eds.). Amsterdam: Elsevier, pp. 72–80.
12. Gray, E. G. and V. P. Whittaker (1962) The isolation of nerve endings from brain: an electron microscopic study of cell fragments derived from homogenization and centrifugation. *J. Anat. 96:*79.
13. Ho, B. T., D. Taylor, L. F. Englert, and W. M. McIsaac (1971) Neurochemical effect of *l*-Δ^9-tetrahydrocannabinol in rats following repeated inhalation. *Brain Res. 31:*233.
14. Ho, B. T., D. Taylor, G. E. Fritchie, L. F. Englert, and W. M. McIsaac (1972) Neuropharmacological study of Δ^9- and Δ^8-*l*-tetrahydrocannabinols in monkeys and mice. *Brain Res. 38:*163.
15. Ho, B. T., D. Taylor, and L. F. Englert (1973) The effect of repeated administration of (-)-Δ^9-tetrahydrocannabinol on the biosynthesis of brain amines. *Res. Commun. Chem. Pathol. Pharmacol. 5:*851.
16. Ho, B. T., D. Taylor and L. F. Englert (1974) Effects of Δ^9-tetrahydrocannabinol on the metabolism of ^{3}H-5-hydroxytryptamine and ^{3}H-norepinephrine in the rat brain. *Res. Commun. Chem. Pathol. Pharmacol. 7:*645.
17. Hollister, L. E., F. Moore, S. Kanter, and E. Noble (1970) Δ^1-tetrahydrocannabinol, synhexyl and marijuana extract administered orally in man: catecholamine excretion, plasma corticol levels and platelet serotonin content. *Psychopharmacologia 17:*354.
18. Holtzman, D., R. A. Lovell, J. H. Jaffe, and D. X. Freedman (1969) *l*-Δ^9-Tetrahydrocannabinol: neurochemical and behavioral effects in the mouse. *Science 163:*1464.
19. Howes, J. and P. Osgood (1974) The effect of Δ^9-tetrahydrocannabinol on the uptake and release of ^{14}-C-dopamine from crude striatal synaptosomal preparations. *Neuropharmacology 13:*1109.
20. Johnson, K. M. and B. T. Ho (1975) Characterization of the inhibition of synaptosomal serotonin uptake by (-)-Δ^9-tetrahydrocannabinol. *Brain Res.* (in press).
21. Leonard, B. E. (1971) The effect of $\Delta^{1,6}$-tetrahydrocannabinol on biogenic amines and their amine acid precursors in the rat brain. *Pharmacol. Res. Commun. 3:*1139.
22. Lowry, D. H., N. J. Rosenbrough, A. L. Farr, and R. J. Randall (1951) Protein measurement with the folin phenol reagent. *J. Biol. Chem. 193:*265.
23. Maitre, L., M. Staehelin, and H. Bain (1970) Effect of an extract of

cannabis and some cannabinols on catecholamine metabolism in rat heart and brain. *Agents Actions 1:*136.

24. Martin, B. R., W. L. Dewey, L. S. Harris, and J. S. Beckner (1974) Subcellular localization of ^{3}H-Δ^{9}-tetrahydrocannabinol in dog brain after acute or chronic administration. *Pharmacologist 16:*260.
25. Schildkraut, J. J. and D. Efron (1971) The effects of Δ^{9}-tetrahydrocannabinol on the metabolism of norepinephrine in the rat brain. *Psychopharmacologia 20:*191.
26. Sofia, R. D., B. N. Dixit, and H. Barry, III (1971) The effect of Δ^{1}-tetrahydrocannabinol on serotonin metabolism in the rat brain. *Life Sci. 10(1)*:425.
27. Sofia, R. D., R. J. Ertel, B. N. Dixit, and H. Barry, III (1971) The effect of Δ^{1}-tetrahydrocannabinol on the uptake of serotonin by rat brain homogenates. *Eur. J. Pharmacol. 16:*257.
28. Truitt, E. B. and S. M. Anderson (1971) Biogenic amine produced in the brain by tetrahydrocannabinols and their metabolites. *Ann. N.Y. Acad. Sci. 191:*68.
29. Welch, B. L., A. S. Welch, F. S. Messiha, and H. J. Berger (1971) Rapid depletion of adrenal epinephrine and elevation of telencephalic serotonin by (-)-trans-Δ^{9}-tetrahydrocannabinol in mice. *Res. Commun. Chem. Pathol. Pharmacol. 2:*382.

31

Effects of Δ^9-Tetrahydrocannabinol on the Homosynaptic Depression in the Spinal Monosynaptic Pathway: Implications for Transmitter Dynamics in the Primary Afferents

RADAN ČAPEK AND BARBARA ESPLIN

Introduction

The research effort directed toward delineating the effects of cannabinoids on neurotransmitters [20,21] stems undoubtedly from the generally accepted assumption that these compounds, like other drugs acting on the central nervous system, act primarily by affecting the synaptic transmission. The conventional direct approach of studying neurotransmitter mechanisms, in particular, the turnover, requires detailed knowledge of the transmitter and its metabolism, involving isolation and estimation of the transmitter and its precursors or metabolites. Despite the elegance and accuracy of these direct methods, there is a need for indirect methods, in which the transmitter dynamics are inferred from the characteristics of the postsynaptic response. The indirect methods may be of value to supplement the direct ones, and the former remain the only possibility when dealing with unidentified transmitters. Such an approach is best exemplified by the studies at the neuromuscular junction [4,13]; it has been also used in the sympathetic ganglia [2,19] and in the spinal cord [12].

The present study concerns the effects of Δ^9-tetrahydrocannabinol (Δ^9-THC) on the depression of the spinal monosynaptic reflex responses following the repetitive stimulation of the afferents of the same pathway, the homosynaptic depression of Beswick and Evanson [3]. It was suggested that it is attributable to the exhaustion of the excitatory neurotransmitter [7,9]. The pattern of decline of the monosynaptic responses evoked by short trains of stimuli at moderate frequencies was used to describe transmitter dynamics in the primary afferents because it reflects the depletion of the transmitter (each incoming volley releasing a constant fraction of the

Marihuana: Chemistry, Biochemistry, and Cellular Effects, edited by Gabriel G. Nahas,

transmitter available for release), while the transmitter store is being replenished at a constant fraction of the depleted part per second. The procedure used was recently described in greater detail [6].

The spinal cord has provided a convenient testing ground for many drugs acting on the central nervous system. It was used in these experiments as a model synaptic system and not because any of the multiple pharmacological effects of THC appear to be primarily linked to this structure. A relatively simple neural network, the spinal monosynaptic pathway was considered a subsystem, a paradigm or analog of a larger and more complex whole. In the case of THC, this parent whole remains rather poorly defined; our present knowledge about the locus of action of this drug is limited.

Methods

Experiments were done on spinalized cats of either sex weighing 2.5–4.5 kg. The anesthesia was induced by ethyl chloride and continued by ether. The trachea was cannulated, the spinal cord sectioned at the atlantooccipital junction, the anesthetic discontinued, and the preparation artificially respired. Ischemic decerebration was achieved by ligating the carotid and clamping the vertebral arteries. The mean blood pressure in the carotid artery and the CO_2 concentration in the expired air were continuously monitored. The cephalic vein was cannulated for drug injection. Gallamine triethiodide was used for paralysis in doses of 3 mg/kg IV. A laminectomy was performed in the lumbosacral region and the spinal cord covered by mineral oil. An infrared lamp, thermostatically controlled by a subdural probe, maintained the temperature of the spinal cord at 36°C.

The ventral roots (VR) L7 and S1 were severed on one side of the cord. The nerve to the biceps semitendinosus (BST) muscle was dissected, cut from the muscle in the ipsilateral hindlimb, and placed on platinum hook electrodes for stimulation. The monosynaptic reflex responses were recorded monophasically from the cut ventral root S1 or L7. The corresponding dorsal root was placed on another recording electrode to monitor the incoming volley to the spinal cord.

The potentials were displayed on an oscilloscope interfaced with a PDP 8/S computer. For input-output determination, the averaged incoming volleys and the monosynaptic responses were traced on a strip chart recorder, and the average peak-to-peak amplitudes of both responses were determined. The amplitudes of individual responses were also measured by the computer on line, typed out, and stored on a paper tape for further analysis. Δ^9-THC was dissolved in polyethylene glycol (PEG) 400 in a concentration of 10 mg/ml and was injected intravenously.

Results

Effect of THC on transmission of repetitive impulses

The monosynaptic responses evoked after a period of rest by a train of 10 supramaximal stimuli at 2, 5, or 10 Hz decline in a characteristic pattern. The decrease in their amplitudes is steep initially, but within a few impulses a plateau is reached (Figure 31.1a). To obtain better characteristics of this pattern, we delivered the train of 10 stimuli at a given frequency every 60 sec to the motor nerve. The amplitudes of all the first, second, and subsequent responses were averaged and expressed as fractions of the averaged first response. The resulting time course of the decline obtained in a representative experiment is shown in Figure 31.1(b).

The plateau level varied inversely with the frequency of stimulation (Table 31.1), as has been described by others [14,18].

The same sequence of stimulation was repeated after the administration of THC in doses ranging from 2–12 mg/kg IV. Typically, the plateau was lower and the decline steeper than before

Table 31.1 The change in plateau levels produced by THC[a]

		THC[c]			
	Control[b]	*5–30 min*	*31–60 min*	*61–90 min*	*>90 min*
n:	*8*	*8*	*7*	*7*	*2*
2	63 ± 3.5	− 8.8 ± 2.0	− 7.6 ± 2.3	− 4.5 ± 3.1	−3.4
5	56 ± 5.0	−11.6 ± 3.1	−11.1 ± 2.6	−10.9 ± 2.2	+0.1
10	53 ± 5.4	−11.3 ± 2.8	−10.5 ± 2.5	− 9.4 ± 2.8	+0.8

[a] This is a summary of *n* determinations, such as those shown in Figure 31.1. The level of plateau was determined from the average amplitudes of the last 5 responses and expressed as percentage of the first response.

[b] Means ± SE of the plateau level.

[c] Means ± SE of the differences in plateau levels after THC administration (5 mg/kg IV) at time intervals indicated.

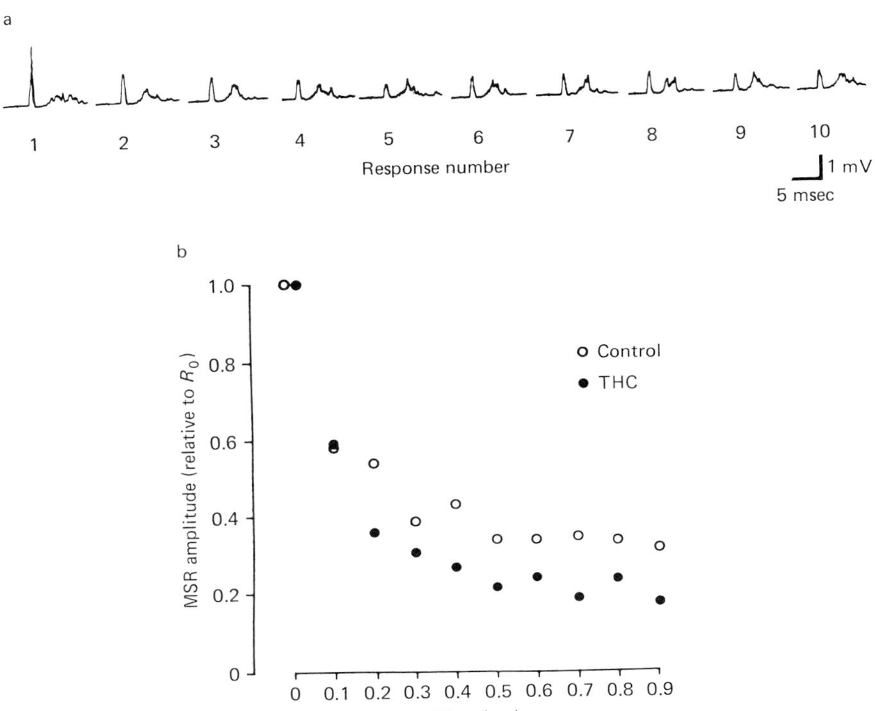

Figure 31.1 (a). Sample recording of the monosynaptic responses evoked by 10 supramaximal stimuli delivered to the BST nerve at 5 Hz. (b) The pattern of decline of the monosynaptic responses. Ordinate, averaged monosynaptic response amplitudes expressed as fractions of the averaged first one, R_0; abscissa, time; stimulation 10 Hz, BST nerve; ○ before, ● 30 min after THC (5 mg/kg IV) administration.

the drug administration (Figure 31.1a). The results of repeated measurements in eight experiments subjected to further analysis are summarized in Table 31.1. The THC-induced deepening of the decline was demonstrable for about 90 min after the administration of 5 mg/kg of THC. In experiments followed beyond this time interval, the plateau levels tended to return to the initial values. No changes in the pattern of decline were seen after the administration of the solvent.

The decline of the monosynaptic response elicited by repetitive stimuli is a consequence of the long synaptic recovery in this pathway. Thus, the data presented indicate that THC prolongs this recovery and thereby deepens the depression of monosynaptic responses evoked at moderate frequencies of stimulation.

Available experimental evidence allows further interpretation. The depression of monosynaptic responses is clearly related to the presynaptic mechanism: it is demonstrable at intervals between the successive volleys much longer than the recovery of motoneuron excitability [8,22]. Significantly, the amount of the excitatory transmitter of the primary afferents released by successive volleys decreases [7,16]. But before one can attempt to relate the effects of THC to this unidentified transmitter, the relation between the amplitude should be established.

Conversion from the monosynaptic response amplitude to the relative amount of transmitter

The extent of the postsynaptic discharge, reflected by the amplitude of the monosynaptic response, is directly related to the number of active afferent fibers, assessed by the amplitude of the presynaptic volley. In turn, the number of active afferent fibers is directly related to the amount of excitatory transmitter released, since it was shown that group Ia fibers of different conduction velocities release on the average the same amount of transmitter [17]. It follows that the input–output relation also represents the relation between the amount of transmitter and the number of motoneurons discharged.

As shown in Figure 31.2, the input–output line in the spinal monosynaptic pathway does not pass through the origin, indicating that a certain critical amount of transmitter, critical input, Q_c, is necessary to generate a detectable response. A given monosynaptic response represents this relative critical amount plus the appropriate fraction of the relative quantity above it. Thus, the amount of transmitter, Q_t, by which response of given amplitude, R_t, is evoked is given by

$$Q_t = Q_c + R_t(1 - Q_c). \qquad (31.1)$$

In this equation, all values are expressed relative to the maximum response and the corresponding input volley, both being equal to unity.

Determination of the fractional release and fractional replenishment rate of the transmitter

The basic assumption underlying the calculation of transmitter turnover parameters is that each incoming volley releases a constant fraction, p, of the transmitter, Q, in the readily releasable pool.

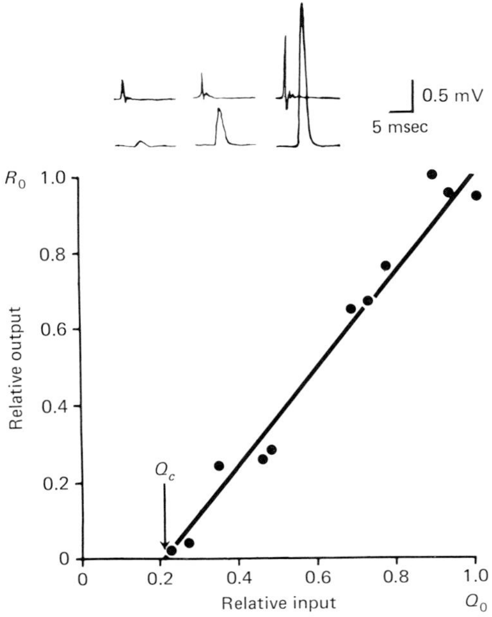

Figure 31.2. Ordinate, amplitude of the monosynaptic response as a fraction of the maximum response; abscissa, amplitude of the afferent volley relative to that producing the maximum output. Each point was obtained by averaging 4 afferent volleys and corresponding monosynaptic responses evoked by the same stimulus intensity at 0.1 Hz. The solid line was calculated by the least square method; Q_c is the critical input. Inset shows sample of averaged afferent volleys and corresponding monosynaptic responses at 3 stimulus intensities.

The decline in transmitter release is then the consequence of depletion of this store. The replenishment of this store depends on the degree of depletion; a constant fraction, r, of the depleted part at any time is replenished per second.

At time 0, before the first volley arrives, the quantity of transmitter in the pool is $Q_0 = 1$. The first volley releases instantaneously a fraction of the store, p, and still at time 0, but just after the first volley, the depleted store is

$$Q'_0 = 1 - p. \qquad (31.2)$$

The depletion initiates replenishment, which is a first-order process, so that at time, τ, that is, at the arrival of the second volley, the quantity, Q_τ, in the store is

$$Q_\tau = 1 - pe^{-r\tau}, \qquad (31.3)$$

and at time $n\tau$, when $n + 1$ volley arrives, the amount in the store is given as

$$Q_{n\tau} = 1 - [1 - Q_{(n-1)\tau}(1 - p)]e^{-r\tau}. \qquad (31.4)$$

The Q values in these equations represent the amount of transmitter in the readily releasable store, but because of the assumed constancy of the fraction released by each volley, they also reflect the quantities of transmitter released, relative to that released by the first volley. The time course of the changes in transmitter quantity in the store assumed by this model is shown in Figure 31.3.

To determine the turnover parameters, we converted the averaged relative amplitudes of the monosynaptic responses to the relative amounts of transmitter and fit the resulting time course to the described model. The quantity released by each volley at the end of the train, that is, at the steady state, when $Q_n\tau = Q_{(n-1)}\tau = Q_{SS}$, and that released by the second volley Q_τ were used to determine the values p and r by using Equations (31.3) and (31.4). The adequacy of the fitting procedure is illustrated in Figure 31.4 by comparison of the experimental time course and the time course calculated from the determined values p and r.

Figure 31.3. Changes in the relative amounts of transmitter in the apparent readily releasable store of the nerve terminals, calculated by equations 2–4 from parameters p and r given during stimulation at 2 Hz. The dotted line connects the points that can be determined experimentally.

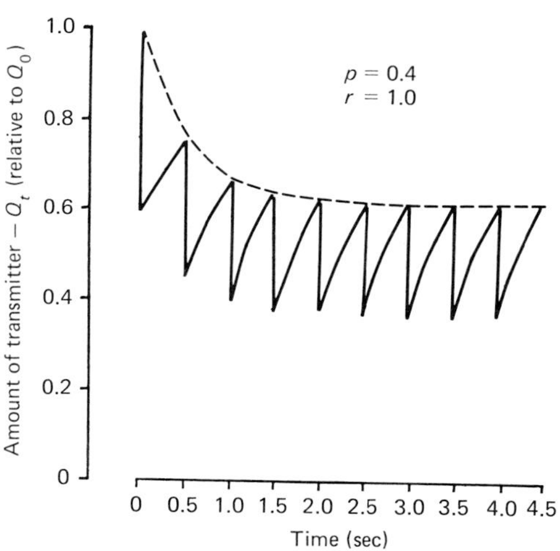

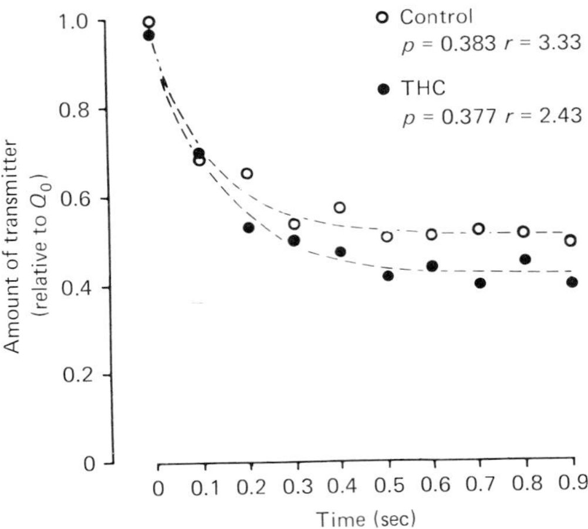

Figure 31.4. The decline of the relative amounts of transmitter released by 10 successive volleys of 10 Hz. Ordinate, the amounts of transmitter as fractions of that released by the first volley, Q_0, obtained from experiment in Figure 31.1(b); abscissa, time. ○ experimentally determined time course before THC administration; ● 30 min after THC (5 mg/kg IV) administration; the dotted line connects the relative amounts of transmitter calculated from the determined parameters *p* and *r*.

Effects of THC on the parameters of transmitter turnover

The values of transmitter turnover parameters determined before the administration of THC are summarized in Table 31.2. The fractional release per volley does not depend on the frequency of stimulation. However, the fractional replenishment per second is clearly frequency dependent, being higher at higher frequencies of stimulation.

The relative changes in *p* and *r* values induced by THC are shown in Figure 31.5. They were obtained from the experiments summarized in Table 31.1 and 31.2.

The effect of the drug on the fractional release per volley was not consistent. At some time intervals and at certain frequencies of stimulation, the mean value was increased of this parameter, but the increase was not uniform enough to reach statistical significance. The fractional replenishment per second was decreased at most time intervals. Further, the mean values were more decreased at higher frequencies of stimulation, indicating that the extent of the drug-induced change depended on the frequency of stimulation.

Table 31.2 Transmitter turnover parameters at various stimulation frequencies before drug administration[a]

Frequency (Hz)	*p*	*r*
2	0.354 ± 0.055	1.09 ± 0.07
5	0.321 ± 0.067	2.20 ± 0.30
10	0.330 ± 0.038	4.30 ± 0.57

[a] *p*, initial release as a fraction of the instant amount of transmitter in the apparent readily releasable pool per volley; *r*, replenishment as a fraction of the instant depleted part of this transmitter pool per sec. The values are means ± SE determined in 8 experiments.

The regression line and the correlation coefficient, r_{12}, in Figure 31.5 characterize this relation.

It was noted that at any given stimulation frequency, the magnitude of THC-induced change depended on the control value of *r;* the decrease was more pronounced when the control *r* was higher.

Figure 31.5. THC-induced changes in parameters *p* and *r*. The means of the differences of the values determined before and after drug administration were calculated and expressed as % of the control value. The time after THC administration (5 mg/kg IV) indicates the end of the interval in which the determinations were made. * Significantly different from 0 for $p < 0.05$.

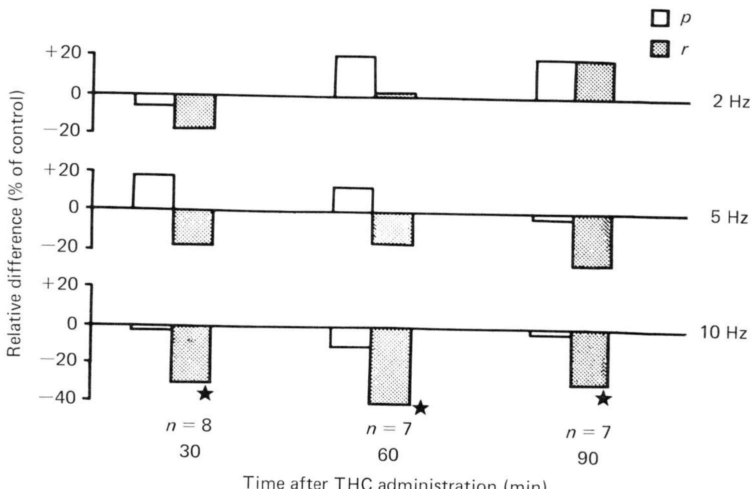

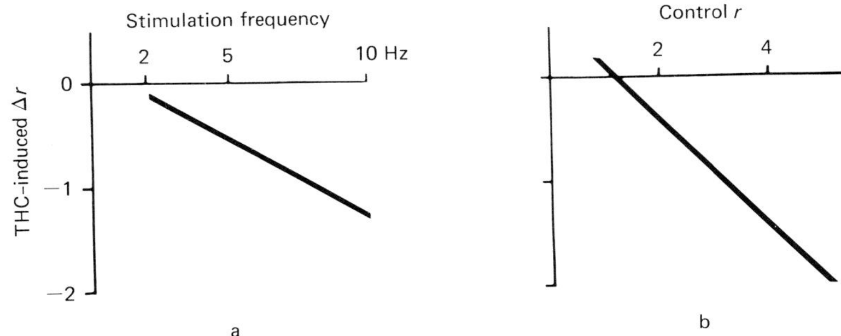

Figure 31.6. (a) Correlation $r_{12} = -0.45$ between stimulation frequency and the THC-induced change in the fractional replenishment rate, Δ*r*. (b) Correlation $r_{23} = -0.84$ between the fractional replenishment rate before drug administration, control *r*, and the THC-induced change in this parameter, Δ*r*. The number of pairs was 24 in both cases, including values obtained before and 30 min after THC administration (5 mg/kg IV) summarized in Figure 31.5. The multiple correlation R = 0.94.

As the regression line and the correlation coefficient, r_{23}, in Figure 31.6 indicate, this association was highly significant over the whole range of stimulation frequencies.

Since the *r* value depends directly on the frequency of stimulation (see Table 31.2), the obvious question arises: does the correlation of the extent of THC-induced change with the frequency of stimulation, r_{12}, merely reflect the fact that control levels are higher at higher frequencies of stimulation? This appears not to be the case. The absolute value of the multiple correlation, R, is distinctly higher than the value of correlation, r_{23}, between the control replenishment rate and the THC-induced change of this parameter. Hence, the THC-induced change in the fractional replenishment per second is related to the frequency of stimulation also independently.

Discussion

Which of the multiple pharmacological effects of THC the depression of transmission in the spinal monosynaptic pathway during repetitive stimulation could be related to is open for speculation. Such an effect would limit the upper frequency of impulses a given synaptic system is able to transmit, and the consequences would depend on the function of that system.

The described effect is not unique to THC. Trimethadione [11], benzodiazepines [23], and ethosuximide [5] were tested by comparable techniques and showed similar effect. Diazepam was also found to prolong synaptic recovery in the spinal monosynaptic pathway by a different test [22]. Like the above drugs, THC also displays anticonvulsant activity. The described synaptic action and anticonvulsant activity appear to be related. So far, all the drugs that were effective in this test were also clinically effective in petit mal epilepsy. However, the anticonvulsant profile of THC in animal tests differs from that of the mentioned anti-*petit mal* agents. Significantly, THC was not effective against minimal seizures produced by pentylenetetrazol [15], which is still probably the best available model for petit mal [24].

In the present study, we attempted to relate this type of action to transmitter dynamics. We used an indirect approach based on several assumptions. The discussion of their validity, which is beyond the scope of this chapter, was given in another communication [6].

It is assumed that the decline of the monosynaptic response on repetitive stimulation reflects the decreasing release of the excitatory transmitter by successive volleys. This decrease in transmitter release is entirely the consequence of the depletion of the apparent transmitter store available for release, the fraction of the store released by each afferent volley remaining constant. In terms of this model, the plateau represents an equilibrium when the amount of transmitter in the pool does not decline because the release and replenishment are equal. Thus, a lower plateau, such as that after THC administration, could be caused by an increase in the fractional release per volley or a decrease in the fractional replenishment per second.

The analysis of our data indicated that the fractional release was enhanced on some occasions, contributing to the observed effect, but it certainly was not the main factor. In this respect THC differed from ethosuximide, the only drug analyzed by this method [5]. Not only was the depression of repetitive impulses after ethosuximide administration clearly more profound and more uniform, but an increase in the fractional release appeared to be the main contributing factor to this activity.

The fractional rate of replenishment was decreased after THC administration on most occasions. The drug-induced decrease in the r value was more pronounced when this parameter was higher before drug administration. It was also more prominent at higher frequencies of stimulation. Thus, after drug administration the value *r* was less frequency dependent. The *r* value was also less dependent on the frequency of stimulation when the temperature of the spinal cord was 32°C rather than at 36°C (Esplin and Čapek, unpublished observation).

The replenishment of the releasable pool of the transmitter might be by mobilization from the depot pool, as at the neuromuscular junction [10]; by neuronal reuptake, as in the sympathetic nerve terminals [1]; by synthesis; or by a combination of these processes. Hopefully, neurochemical data on the identity and metabolism of the unknown excitatory transmitter of the primary afferents will be forthcoming to resolve this question.

ACKNOWLEDGMENT

We wish to express our thanks to Hana Bouček for excellent technical assistance and Humphrey Brown for solving all our computer-related problems. THC was obtained through the courtesy of the Non-Medical Use of Drugs Directorate, Health and Welfare, Canada. This research was supported by the Non-Medical Use of Drugs Directorate and the Medical Research Council of Canada, Grant DA-14.

REFERENCES

1. Bennett, M. R. (1973) An electrophysiological analysis of the uptake of noradrenaline at sympathetic nerve terminals. *J. Physiol. 229:*533.
2. Bennett, M. R. and E. M. McLachlan (1972) An electrophysiological analysis of the storage of acetylcholine in preganglionic nerve terminals. *J. Physiol. 221:*657.
3. Beswick, F. B. and J. M. Evanson (1957) Homosynaptic depression of the monosynaptic reflex following activation. *J. Physiol. 135:*400.
4. Čapek, R., D. W. Esplin, and S. Salehmoghaddam (1971) Rates of transmitter turnover at the frog neuromuscular junction estimated by electrophysiological techniques. *J. Neurophysiol. 34:*831.
5. Čapek, R. and B. Esplin (1973) Ethosuximide induced depression of repetitive transmission in the spinal monosynaptic pathway. *Pharmacologist 15:*161.
6. Čapek, R. and B. Esplin (1975) Homosynaptic depression and the transmitter turnover in the spinal monosynaptic pathway. *J. Neurophysiol.* (in press).
7. Curtis, D. R. and J. C. Eccles (1960) Synaptic action during and after repetitive stimulation. *J. Physiol. 150:*374.
8. Decandia, M. and L. Provini (1966) Motoneurone excitability during repetitive stimulation of group I afferent fibres. *Experientia 22:*187.
9. Eccles, J. C. (1953) Discussion of the paper by Jefferson and Schlapp. *The Spinal Cord* (J. L. Malcolm and J. A. B. Gray, eds.). Boston: Little, Brown and Company, p. 118.

10. Elmqvist, D. and D. H. J. Quastel (1965) A quantitative study of end-plate potentials in isolated human muscle. *J. Physiol. 178:*505.
11. Esplin, D. W. and E. M. Curto (1957) Effects of trimethadione on synaptic transmission in the spinal cord; antagonism of trimethadione and pentylenetetrazol. *J. Pharmacol. Exp. Ther. 121:*457.
12. Esplin, D. W. and B. Zablocka-Esplin (1971) Rates of transmitter turnover in spinal monosynaptic pathway investigated by electrophysiological techniques. *J. Neurophysiol. 34:*842.
13. Hubbard, J. I., R. LLinás, and D. M. J. Quastel (1969) *Electrophysiological Analysis of Synaptic Transmission.* London: Edward Arnold.
14. Jefferson, A. A. and W. Schlapp (1953) Some effects of repetitive stimulation of afferents on reflex conduction. *The Spinal Cord* (J. L. Malcolm and J. A. B. Gray, eds.). Boston: Little, Brown and Company, pp. 99–119.
15. Karler, R., W. Cely and S. A. Turkanis (1974) Anticonvulsant properties of Δ^9-tetrahydrocannabinol and other cannabinoids. *Life Sci. 15:*931.
16. Kuno, M. (1964) Mechanism of facilitation and depression of the excitatory synaptic potential in spinal motoneurones. *J. Physiol. 175:*100.
17. Kuno, M. and J. T. Miyahara (1969) Analysis of synaptic efficacy in spinal motoneurones from "quantum" aspects. *J. Physiol. 201:*479.
18. Lloyd, D. P. C. and V. J. Wilson (1957) Reflex depression in rhythmically active monosynaptic reflex pathways. *J. Gen. Physiol. 40:*409.
19. McCandless, D. L., B. Zablocka-Esplin and D. W. Esplin (1971) Rates of transmitter turnover in the cat superior cervical ganglion estimated by electrophysiological techniques. *J. Neurophysiol. 39:*817.
20. Nahas, G. G. (1973) *Marihuana-Deceptive Weed.* New York: Raven Press.
21. Paton, W. D. M. (1975) Pharmacology of marihuana. *Ann. Rev. Pharmacol. 15:*220.
22. Schlosser, W. (1971) Action of diazepam on the spinal cord. *Arch. Int. Pharmacodyn. Ther. 194:*93.
23. Swinyard, E. A. and A. W. Castellion (1966) Anticonvulsant properties of some benzodiazepines. *J. Pharmacol. Exp. Ther. 151:*369.
24. Woodbury, D. M. (1972) Applications to drug evaluation. *Experiperimental Models of Epilepsy* (D. P. Purpura, J. K. Penry, D. Tower, D. M. Woodbury, and R. Walter, eds.). New York: Raven Press, pp. 557–583.

32

Effects of Cannabinoids on Isolated Smooth Muscle Preparations

SUNE ROSELL, STIG AGURELL, AND
BILLY MARTIN

Introduction

To investigate the mechanisms of action of the psychoactive cannabinoids, one can use isolated peripheral tissues as test preparations, provided that there is a close chemical relationship between the acute behavioral actions and the effects on the isolated organ. In addition, the cannabinoids should be active in concentrations that produce the behavioral effects. To find such a tissue, we have tested the effects of cannabinoids on a number of isolated preparations.

Eight cannabinoids have been studied: (—)-Δ^1-tetrahydrocannabinol (Δ^1-THC) and its Δ^6-THC isomer, (—)-7-hydroxy-Δ^1-tetrahydrocannabinol (7-OH-Δ^1-THC) and its 7-OH-Δ^6-THC isomer. As regards 7-OH-Δ^1-THC and Δ^6-THC, the (—) as well as the (+) isomers were tested. The other two cannabinoids were cannabidiol (CBD) and cannabinol (CBN). The substances were dissolved in 10–100 μl 10 percent ethanol which, in the concentrations used, had no effects.

The 7-OH derivative of Δ^6-THC (4–400 ng/ml) did not affect the spontaneous contractions of the innervated rabbit jejunum suspended in Krebs solution at 37°C or the responses to sympathetic nerve stimulation. The sympathetic nerves in the mesentery were stimulated every 10 min at 5 msec, 20 V, and 2–25 Hz for 30 sec, causing both an inhibition of the spontaneous pendular contractions and a decrease in tone. Likewise, Δ^6-THC and 7-OH-Δ^6-THC (25 ng/ml bath fluid) did not influence the responses to motor nerve stimulation (0.2 Hz, 5 msec, and 5 V) on the rat phrenic nerve–diaphragm preparation, which parallels the finding by Layman and Milton [7] that neither Δ^1-THC nor CBD had any effect on that preparation.

In contrast to these negative results, the isolated guinea pig ileum

Marihuana: Chemistry, Biochemistry, and Cellular Effects, edited by Gabriel G. Nahas, © 1976 by Springer-Verlag New York Inc.

was found to be very sensitive to cannabinoids, especially to the 7-OH derivatives. In low concentrations they inhibit the twitch responses produced by electric field stimulation. Our results indicate that the guinea pig ileum may be suitable material in which the mechanisms of action of cannabinoids can be investigated.

The terminal portion was used after the 5 cm nearest the ileocecal junction had been discarded. The isolated ileum was suspended in Krebs solution (5 ml) bubbled with 95 percent O_2–5 percent CO_2. The temperature was 36–37°C. Rectangular electrical pulses of 0.5 msec duration, supramaximal strength (50 V), and 0.1 Hz were applied to the electrodes. Isometric or isotonic contractions were recorded by transducers (Grass FT. 03 and Harvard Apparatus, respectively) and displayed on a Rika Denki ink writer.

Monohydroxylated Tetrahydrocannabinoids

The (—)-7-OH-cannabinoids were found to be the most effective inhibitors of the twitch responses produced by electric field stimulation. Therefore, the effects of these compounds will be described first, even though (—)-Δ^1-THC and in some marihuana samples small amounts of (—)-Δ^6-THC are the main active principles from natural products.

7-OH-Δ^6-THC reduced the twitch response at a concentration in the bath of approximately 1 ng/ml or higher (Figure 32.1) [10]. A 50-percent inhibition was obtained with about 5 ng/ml (Figure 32.2). The effect was noted within 2 min and was maximal within 10–15 min. Despite repeated washings, the inhibition persisted for about an hour after 1–5 ng/ml were given. Because of the high lipid solubility of the cannabinoids, this may not be unexpected. In some experiments, we stimulated the ileum with acetylcholine, histamine, substance P, or 5-hydroxytryptamine (5-HT). 7-OH-Δ^6-THC reduced the twitches evoked by 5-HT, but those evoked by acetylcholine, substance P, or histamine were not at all or very little affected (Figures 32.1 and 32.3). These data indicate that the inhibition of the twitch is of presynaptic origin. Both histamine and acetylcholine act directly on the smooth muscle. This is presumably also the case with substance P, whereas 5-HT acts primarily by stimulating the nervous structures of the intestinal wall [9]. 7-OH-Δ^1-THC was found to have approximately the same activity as 7-OH-Δ^6-THC on the isolated guinea pig ileum.

Of the optically active isomers, the naturally occurring (—)-7-

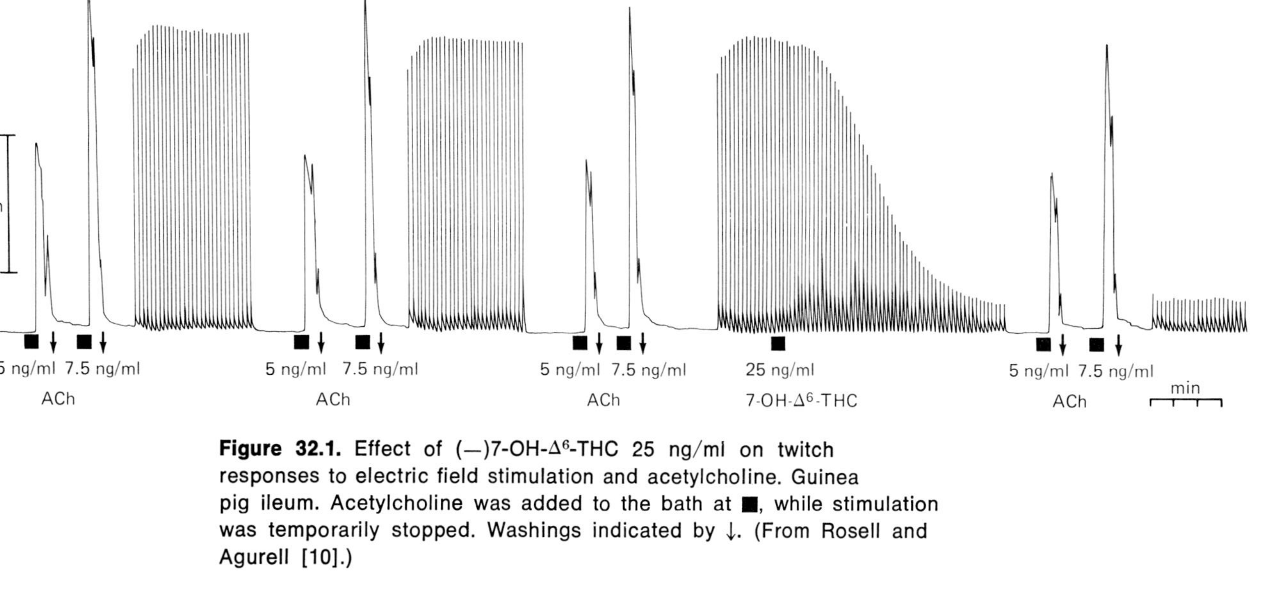

Figure 32.1. Effect of (—)7-OH-Δ^6-THC 25 ng/ml on twitch responses to electric field stimulation and acetylcholine. Guinea pig ileum. Acetylcholine was added to the bath at ■, while stimulation was temporarily stopped. Washings indicated by ↓. (From Rosell and Agurell [10].)

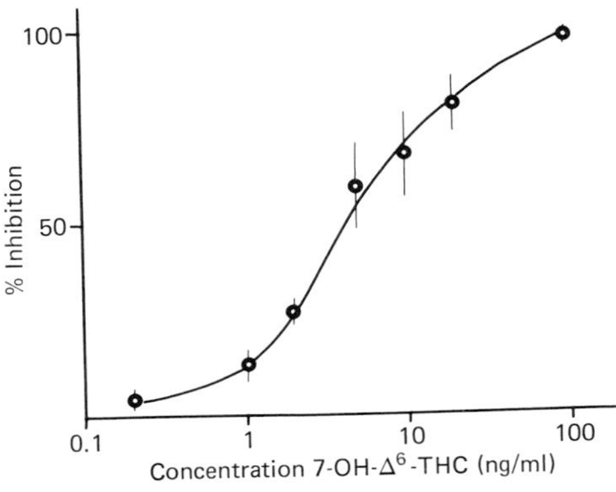

Figure 32.2. Inhibition of twitch responses by (—)7-OH-Δ^6-THC. The twitch responses were induced by electric field stimulation of the guinea pig ileum. The concentration of the drug in the bath is given on the abscissa.

OH-Δ^1-THC was found to be the most active compound. Thus, 25 ng/ml of (+)-7-OH-Δ^1-THC had hardly any detectable inhibitory effect on the twitches (Figure 32.4), and it was found that the (+) isomer is at least twenty times less active than the naturally occurring (—) isomer. The difference in activities may be even greater since the (+) isomer may have been contaminated with the (—) isomer, although this may not be more than 5 percent. However, this would represent 5 ng/ml at a concentration of 100 ng/ml of (+)-7-OH-Δ^1-THC, which inhibits the response by 20–30 percent. As already indicated, 5 ng/ml of the (—)

Figure 32.3. Effect of (—)7-OH-Δ^6-THC, 20 ng/ml, on histamine (Hi) and 5-hydroxytryptamine (5-HT) responses of guinea pig ileum. Numbers indicate concentrations in the bath in ng/ml.

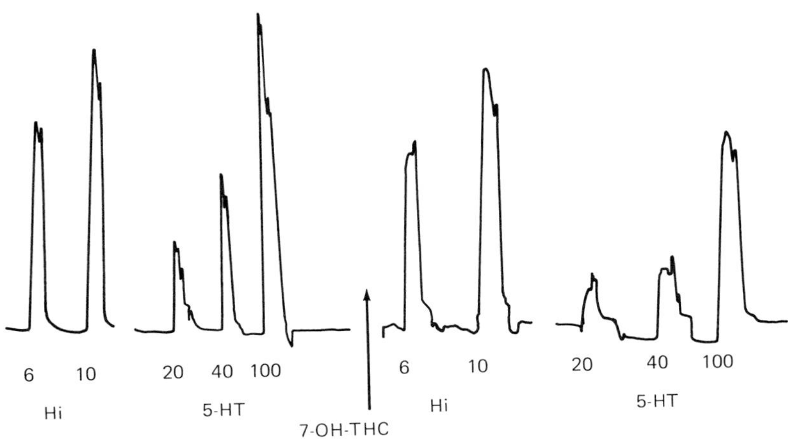

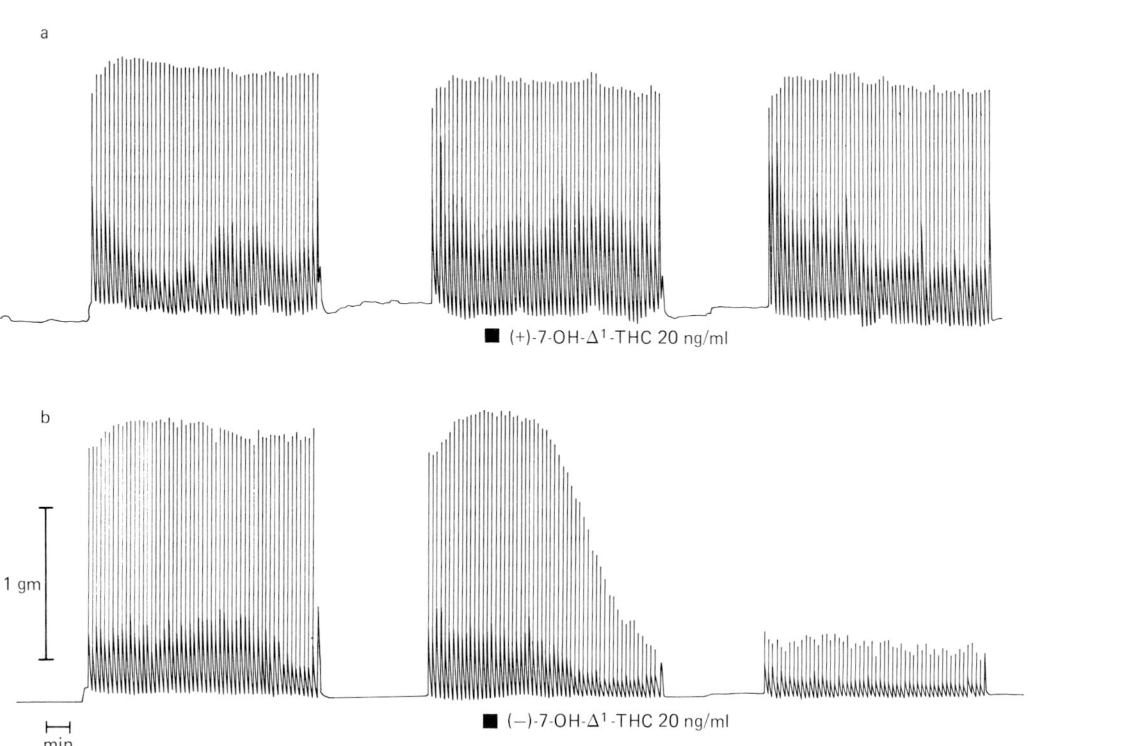

Figure 32.4. Effects of (+)-7-OH-Δ^1-THC (a) and (—)-7-OH-Δ^1-THC (b) on twitch responses after electric field stimulation. Guinea pig ileum.

isomer causes a 50-percent inhibition. Thus, the action of (—)-7-OH-Δ^1-THC on the electrically induced twitches is stereospecific. Presumably, this is true also for the Δ^6-isomer. These findings parallel the observation by Edery *et al.* [2] that (—)-Δ^1-THC and (—)-Δ^6-THC elicited behavioral effects in the rhesus monkey, whereas the (+) isomers were inactive.

Nonhydroxylated Tetrahydrocannabinoids

Δ^6-THC also inhibited the electrically induced twitches, but it was five to ten times less potent than 7-OH-Δ^6-THC. Furthermore, the inhibition was much more gradual in onset (Figure 32.5). CBD and CBN were without effect at concentrations up to 100 ng/ml; this corresponds to the finding of Layman and Milton [7]. Δ^1-THC had approximately the same potency as Δ^6-THC. (+)-Δ^6-THC was inactive at concentrations up to 100 ng/ml. Higher concentrations were not tested.

The order of potency of the different cannabinoids on the guinea pig ileum seems to be the same as their psychopharmacological activity. Even though the quantitative contribution of the 7-OH metabolites of Δ^6- and Δ^1-THC toward the psychopharmacological activity of THC in man is still unresolved, the 7-OH compounds are equally as active as (if not more than) their nonhydroxylated analogs (cf. [1,4,6]). CBD and CBN are thought to be much less active [3]. Δ^6-THC is about as active as Δ^1-THC [3] and appears to have similar psychological effects in man [5].

On the basis of brain concentrations in the mouse, Gill, Jones, and Lawrence [4] calculated that 7-OH-Δ^1-THC is 7.1 times more potent than Δ^1-THC in producing behavioral changes. This ratio is in excellent agreement with our results on the guinea pig ileum.

Discussion

The present results indicate that the isolated guinea pig ileum is a suitable organ in which to study the mechanism of action of cannabinoids. Thus, the inhibition of the twitch responses seems to be stereospecifically produced at concentrations comparable to those that may be achieved while smoking cannabis. Cannabis smokers may absorb 1–10 mg of Δ^1-THC to achieve psychic effects [1]. Assuming that this amount is evenly distributed in the whole body, which admittedly is a great oversimplification, the

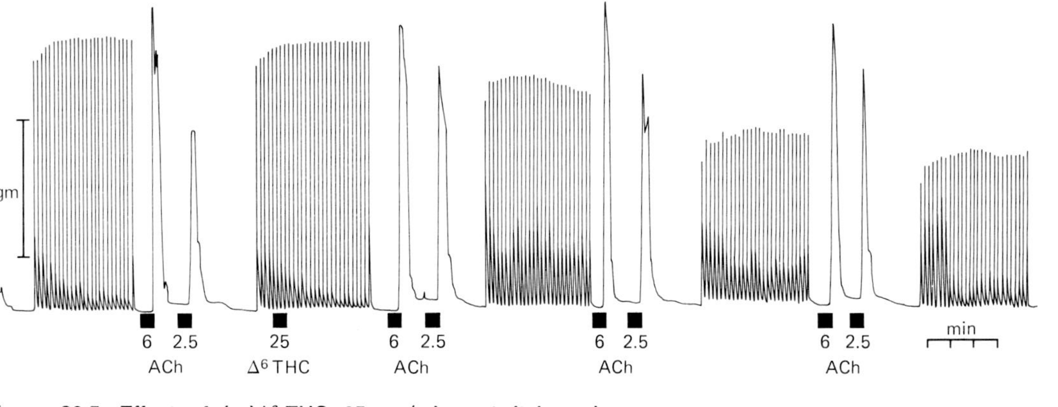

Figure 32.5. Effect of (—)Δ^6-THC 25 ng/ml on twitch and acetylcholine responses of guinea pig ileum. The numbers indicate concentrations in the bath in ng/ml.

From Rosell and Agurell [10].

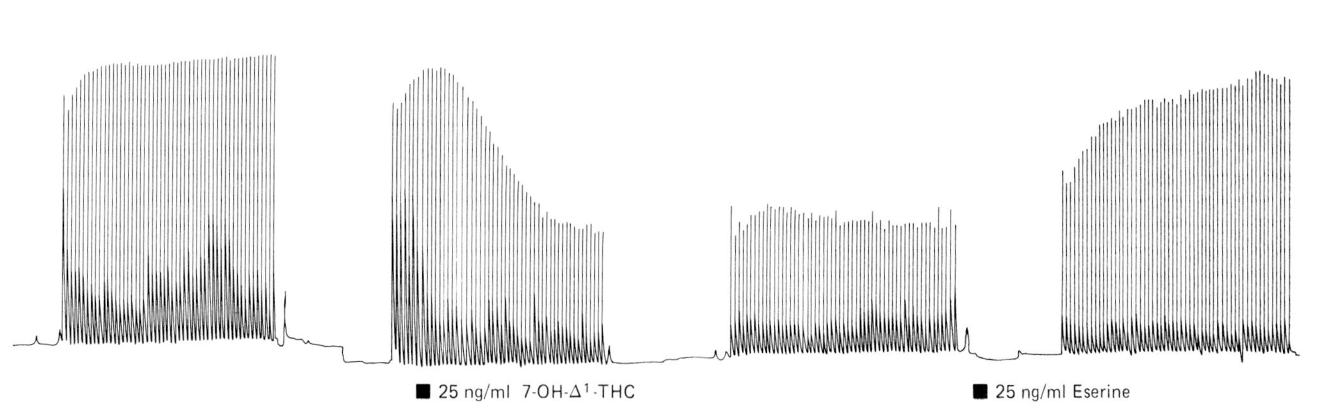

Figure 32.6. Effect of physostigmine (eserine) on the response of the guinea pig ileum to electric field stimulation and exposure to 7-OH-Δ^1-THC (25 ng/ml).

concentration of Δ^1-THC and its metabolites would be in the order of 50 ng/ml. Thus, the isolated guinea pig ileum is affected by THC in concentrations that may have psychoactive effects in man.

The inhibition of the twitch responses is a presynaptic effect, as indicated by the fact that the twitches produced by smooth muscle–stimulating agents such as acetylcholine, histamine, and substance P are not blocked. This opinion is further substantiated by the finding that eserine antagonizes the action of THC (Figure 32.6). Evidently eserine blocks the inactivation of acetylcholine and thus potentiates the cholinergic neurons, which constitute the final common neuronal pathway for the electrically evoked twitches of the ileum.

Presumably, the inhibitory action of THC compounds on the twitch response after electrical stimulation of the guinea pig ileum is due to interaction with some neurotransmitter including acetylcholine, 5-HT, or catecholamines.

The finding that cannabinoids did not affect the sympathetic nerve activity in the innervated rabbit jejunum preparations indicates that adrenergic mechanisms may not be involved primarily. Likewise, neuromuscular transmission processes seem to be unaffected since the motor activity in the rat phrenic nerve–diaphragm preparation did not change in the presence of cannabinoids. An interesting finding is that Δ^1-THC produces a slow, long-lasting inhibition of acetylcholine output from the guinea pig ileum [8]. This effect was demonstrated on resting longitudinal strips of guinea pig ileum exposed to 5 μg/ml Δ^1-THC, a concentration about 200 times higher than that which caused a 50-percent inhibition of the twitch response in the present experiments. Therefore, it is difficult to determine whether the inhibition of acetylcholine output was due to a specific effect or to unspecific actions of Δ^1-THC. Our finding that eserine counteracts the inhibition favors the former alternative.

ACKNOWLEDGMENTS

This investigation was supported by the Swedish Medical Research Council (No. 3518, 2724).

We gratefully acknowledge the technical assistance of Lotta Malmström and Ivan Sandell.

REFERENCES

1. Braude, M. and S. Szara (1976) *The Pharmacology of Cannabis*. New York: Raven Press (in press).
2. Edery, H., Y. Grunaeld, Z. Ben-Zvi, and R. Mechoulam (1971)

Structural requirements for cannabinoid activity. *Ann. N.Y. Acad. Sci. 191:*40–53.

3. Edery, H., Y. Grunfeld, G. Porath, Z. Ben-Zvi, A. Shani, and R. Mechoulam (1972) Structure-activity relationships in the tetrahydrocannabinol series. *Arzneim. Forsch. 22:*1995–2003.
4. Gill, E. W., G. Jones, and D. K. Lawrence (1973) Contribution of the metabolite 7-hydroxy-Δ^1-tetrahydrocannabinol in mice. *Biochem. Pharmacol. 22:*175–184.
5. Hollister, L. E., and K. H. Gillespie (1973) Δ^8- and Δ^9-tetrahydrocannabinol: comparison by oral and i.v. administration. *Clin. Pharmacol. Ther. 14:*353–357.
6. Jones, G., M. Widman, S. Agurell, and J. E. Lindgren (1974) Monohydroxylated metabolites of Δ^1-tetrahydrocannabinol in mouse brain. *Acta Pharm. Suec. 11:*283–294.
7. Layman, J. M., and A. S. Milton (1971) Some actions of Δ^1-tetrahydrocannabinol and cannabidiol at cholinergic junctions. *Proc. Br. Pharmacol. Soc. 41:*379P–380P.
8. Paton, W. D., R. G. Pertwee, and D. Temple (1972) The general pharmacology of cannabinoids. *Cannabis and Its Derivatives* (W. D. Paton and J. Crown, eds.). London: Oxford University Press.
9. Rocha E. Silva, M., J. R. Valle, and Z. P. Picarelli (1953) A pharmacological analysis of the mode of action of serotonin (5-hydroxytryptamine upon the guinea pig ileum). *Br. J. Pharmacol. 8:*378–388.
10. Rosell, S., and S. Agurell (1975) Effects of 7-hydroxy- Δ^6-tetrahydrocannabinol and some related cannabinoids on the guinea pig isolated ileum. *Acta Physiol. Scand. 94:*142–144.

33

Effects of Δ^9-Tetrahydrocannabinol and Cannabinol on Rat Brain Acetylcholine

EDWARD F. DOMINO

Introduction

It is well documented that Δ^9-tetrahydrocannabinol (Δ^9-THC) in man has a biphasic effect of initial elation and the feeling of being "high" followed by sedation and sleepiness [7,12]. Studies in animals also tend to bear out a "stimulant" action, although a "depressant" effect is far more readily apparent. Whether the "stimulation" is merely due to behavioral disinhibition is not known. Neurochemical studies in animals that bear on these behavioral effects have been sparse. There is evidence that the monoaminergic systems are affected, especially with large doses of Δ^9-THC [11].

Our interests have been focused on an interaction of Δ^9-THC with acetylcholine (ACH). The evidence involving ACH is conflicting. Layman and Milton [10] studied the effects of Δ^9-THC and cannabidiol (CBD) at several peripheral cholinergic sites. Δ^9-THC in a concentration of 1.59×10^{-7} M reduced the twitch response of the transmurally stimulated guinea pig ileum 50 percent for several hours. Cannabidiol in concentrations of 3.18×10^{-6} M had no effect. In some experiments both compounds reduced the response of the guinea pig ileum to ACH as well as to histamine.

On the other hand, Gill *et al.* [6] found that Δ^9-THC had either no effect on or enhanced the actions of ACH on the guinea pig ileum. Layman and Milton [10] also reported that both cannabinoids reduced the spontaneous release of ACH from the guinea pig ileum, but had no effect on the rat phrenic nerve–diaphragm preparation, ACH-induced contractions of the frog rectus abdominus muscle, or on the pre- or postganglionically stimulated cat nictitating membrane.

Our preliminary studies [2] on the effects of Δ^9-THC indicated that very large (50 mg/kg) coma-producing doses given IP

Marihuana: Chemistry, Biochemistry, and Cellular Effects, edited by Gabriel G. Nahas,

elevated total brain ACH in mice. Doses of 10 mg/kg IP of Δ^9-THC also elevated brain ACH and reduced its utilization in rats. The effects of IV Δ^9-THC on ACH release from the cat neocortex seemed to be biphasic. Small doses (0.5 mg/kg) in 2 of 3 pretrigeminal brainstem–transected cats enhanced ACH release, but larger doses (1–6 mg/kg) clearly depressed ACH release. In these studies ACH was measured using the frog rectus abdominus and leech muscle assays.

Subsequently, Askew *et al.* [1] studied the effects of Δ^9-THC, Δ^8-THC, and its metabolite 11-OH-Δ^8-THC given IV on rat brain ACH using two different enzymatic assays of ACH. They reported that 1 hr after IV administration of 5 mg/kg of either Δ^8- or Δ^9-THC, rat brain ACH was reduced. In the same dose, 11-OH-Δ^8-THC had no effect. The ACH content of rat brain synaptosomes isolated 1 hr after 5 mg/kg of Δ^8-THC IV also showed 50 percent decreased ACH. Brain choline acetyltransferase activity was not affected, although acetylcholinesterase activity was slightly reduced ($p < 0.05$) in the Δ^8-THC–treated animals. Askew *et al.* suggested that their data were consistent with an increased release of ACH.

In as much as 5 mg/kg of these THC derivatives produces obvious behavioral depression in rats, their findings seemed incompatible with our previous results. Hence, we decided to reinvestigate the problem. This chapter describes some additional data that support our initial findings of an elevation in brain ACH with large doses of Δ^9-THC.

Methods

Male Holtzman rats approximately 28–32-days old were used in groups of 8–15 per treatment. They were maintained on an *ad libitum* diet with a light cycle of 7 AM to 12 midnight and a dark cycle from 12 AM to 7 AM. The animals were decapitated 30 min after various pretreatments approximately 2 hr into the light cycle (9:00 AM). Logarithmic doses of Δ^9-THC or cannabinol (CBN) were given IP in Tween 20 in doses of 3.2, 10, and 32 mg/kg. In addition, the effects of 100 mg/kg IP of CBN after 30 min, 5 mg/kg IV, and 10 mg/kg IP of Δ^9-THC after 60 min were studied. In order to measure brain ACH utilization, we gave another series of animals 1 μg of acetylseco hemicholinium-3 (acetylseco HC-3) intraventricularly (IVT) under diethyl ether anesthesia 30 min before decapitation. We have previously reported the pharmacology of this cholinergic antisynthesis agent [3]. When given in small doses IVT, acetylseco HC-3 lowers brain ACH. Increases or decreases in the lowered level of brain ACH can be used as an indirect measure of brain ACH turnover. We have used the term "brain ACH utilization" to describe this measure. It is not a direct measure of brain ACH turnover but only an indirect means of estimating it.

The mean data $\pm$ SE were calculated, and a group comparison Student's t test was used for determining statistical significance.

Results

Effects of Δ^9-THC on rat brain ACH and its utilization

The mean nmol $\pm$ SE of ACH/gm rat brain for 12 control animals given no injection was 25.3 $\pm$ 0.8. Thirty minutes after Tween vehicle alone was given to 11 rats, brain ACH was 26.4 $\pm$ 1.3 nmol/gm. This value was not significantly different from that achieved after no injection.

After we administered 1 μg of acetylseco HC-3 in 13 animals, brain ACH was reduced to 20.3 $\pm$ 0.9 nmol/gm. This decrease was highly significant ($p < 0.001$). These data are plotted in Figure 33.1, in which the mean ACH $\pm$ SE of the no treatment controls is plotted as the lightly stippled upper horizontal bar (control), and the acetylseco HC-3–treated animals as the darkly stippled lower horizontal bar.

When Δ^9-THC was given alone in doses of 3.2, 10, and 32 mg/kg IP 30 min later, only the largest dose caused a significant increase in brain ACH above control ($p < 0.05$). Doses of Δ^9-THC of 5 mg/kg IV and 10 mg/kg IP 1 hr later also did not significantly affect total brain ACH (see Figure 33.1). On the other hand, in animals pretreated with acetylseco HC-3, doses of 10 and 30 mg/kg of Δ^9-THC significantly elevated brain ACH to control levels ($p < 0.001$), indicating that ACH utilization was reduced.

Effects of CBN on rat brain ACH and its utilization

The effects of CBN on rat brain ACH are summarized in Figure 33.2. The mean brain ACH $\pm$ SE of the controls given the vehicle alone for 15 rats was 26.7 $\pm$ 0.8 nmol/gm. After 1 μg of acetylseco HC-3 was given to another 13 rats, it was reduced to 20.4 $\pm$ 0.7 nmol/gm ($p < 0.001$). In general, CBN was relatively ineffective in altering rat brain ACH in contrast to Δ^9-THC. Doses of 10 and

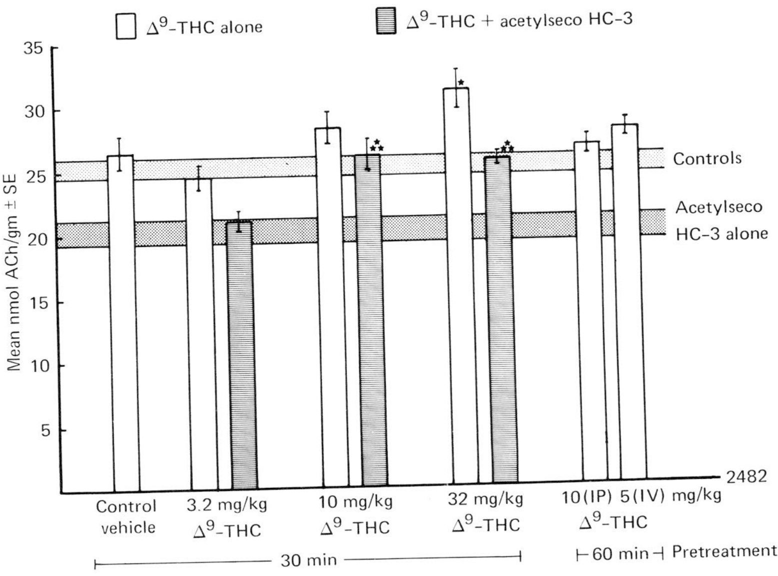

Figure 33.1. Effects of Δ^9-THC on rat brain. ACH. The upper lightly stippled horizontal bar represents the mean ± SE brain ACH of control rats, and the lower darkly stippled bar the brain ACH of rats given 1 μg of acetylseco HC-3 IVT. The height of each vertical bar represents the mean nM ACH/gm, and the small verticle line represents this value ± SE. The graph shows the effects of Δ^9-THC alone as well as of Δ^9-THC plus acetylseco HC-3 after various doses of Δ^9-THC 30 and 60 min after IP or IV injection. All data at 30 min were obtained after IP injection. $^*p < 0.05$, $^{***}p < 0.001$. Student t-test group comparison. Each bar represents the mean of 8–13 animals per group. Symbols are the same in this and subsequent figures.

100 mg/kg IP had no significant effect. Surprisingly, a dose of 32 mg/kg IP to 9 rats elevated brain ACH to 29.6 ± 0.9 nmol/gm, and with acetylseco HC-3 in 8 rats to 22.9 ± 0.6 nmol/gm. These results were statistically significant ($p < 0.05$), indicating that CBN has a pharmacological action on the brain cholinergic system that is much weaker than the effect of Δ^9-THC.

Effects of Δ^9-THC plus CBN on rat brain ACH and its utilization

As illustrated in Figure 33.3, the combination of Δ^9-THC plus CBN had much less effect on rat brain ACH than either drug alone. Only after 100 mg/kg IP of each compound was rat brain ACH

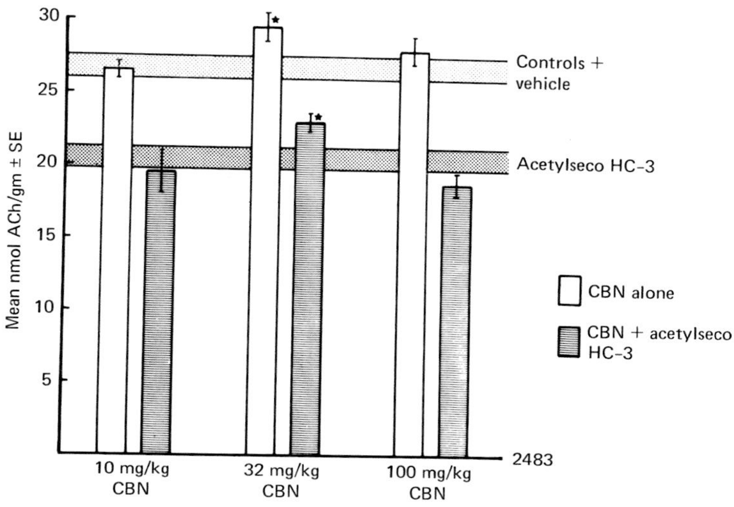

Figure 33.2. Effects of CBN on brain ACH. Note that CBN elevated brain ACH significantly ($p < 0.05$) only at 32 mg/kg IP, in contrast to the effects of Δ^9-THC (see Figure 33.1).

utilization reduced ($p < 0.001$). In this series, the mean ± SE of brain ACH for the vehicle control animals ($n = 9$) was 27.5 ± 1.0 nmol/gm, and after acetylseco HC-3 it was 19.0 ± 0.5 nmol/gm ($n = 12$).

Discussion

The present data provide additional evidence that large doses of Δ^9-THC elevate rat brain ACH and reduce its utilization. As might be expected, CBN is much less effective. Inasmuch as doses of 3.2 mg/kg of Δ^9-THC already depress acquisition of one-way rat shuttle box behavior [2], the failure of this dose to affect rat brain ACH indicates a dissociation of total brain ACH and Δ^9-THC behavioral effects. Regional brain ACH studies are indicated to determine whether the elevation in rat brain ACH results from massive doses of Δ^9-THC unrelated to more subtle behavior-altering effects. It is well known that sedatives elevate rat brain ACH and reduce its utilization [4]. Hence, the present findings may merely reflect the CNS depression produced by these cannabinoids.

The most surprising finding is that in equal massive IP doses,

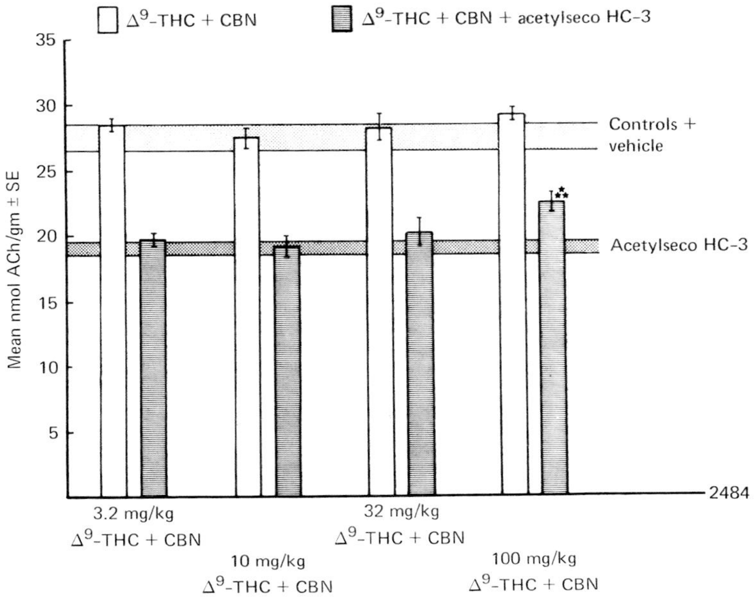

Figure 33.3. Effects of equal doses of Δ^9-THC and CBN on brain ACH. Note that CBN antagonized the effects of 10 and 32 mg/kg of Δ^9-THC. After 100 mg of Δ^9-THC was administered, steady-state ACH levels were not affected. However, there was a significant ($p < 0.001$) reduction in ACH utilization, as evidenced by the elevation of brain ACH in the acetylseco HC-3–treated animals.

CBN and Δ^9-THC are antagonistic. Previous literature on this subject is most confusing. Krantz *et al.* [9] reported that IP injection of Δ^9-THC in mice prolonged pentobarbital sleeping time. CBN was much less effective in this regard, in agreement with our rat brain ACH data. When both agents were given intraperitoneally, CBN blocked the effects of Δ^9-THC on pentobarbital-induced sleeping time, a finding also in agreement with our rat brain ACH data. Fernandes *et al.* [5] also reported that CBN given intraperitoneally selectively blocked the prolongation by Δ^9-THC of hexobarbitone sleeping time in the rat, in contrast to cannabidiol, which further enhanced the effects of Δ^9-THC. However, Hollister and Gillespie [8] reported that orally 20 mg of Δ^9-THC had the same mental and physical effects in man as the same dose of Δ^9-THC with 40 mg of either CBN or CBD. Both cannabinoids were in the stomach and the intestines together in this human study. In the animal studies quoted, both compounds were together intraperitoneally. The reason for the marked differences in rodents versus man is not apparent. Route, species, chemical batch, and dosage are obvious variables. Further studies to unravel these disturbing discrepancies are indicated. The results reported in the present study are certainly to be regarded as preliminary and in need of further confirmation.

ACKNOWLEDGMENTS

The author would like to acknowledge the efforts of Ms. Ann Wilson in these studies.

This work was supported in part by grant DA 001001–02, USPHS.

REFERENCES

1. Askew, W. E., A. P. Kimball, and B. T. Ho (1974) Effect of tetrahydrocannabinols on brain acetylcholine. *Brain Res. 69:*375–378.
2. Domino, E. F. (1971) Neuropsychopharmacologic studies of marijuana—some synthetic and natural THC derivatives in animals and man. *Ann. N.Y. Acad. Sci. 191:*166–191.
3. Domino, E. F., M. E. Mohrman, A. E. Wilson, and V. B. Haarstad (1973) Acetylseco hemicholinium-3, a new choline acetyltransferase inhibitor useful in neuropharmacological studies. *Neuropharmacology 12:*549–561.
4. Domino, E. F. and A. E. Wilson (1972) Psychotropic drug influences on brain acetylcholine utilization. *Psychopharmacologia 25:*291–298.
5. Fernandes, M., A. Schabarek, H. Coper, and R. Hill (1974) Modification of Δ^9-THC actions by cannabinol and cannabidiol in the rat. *Psychopharmacologia 38:*329–338.
6. Gill, E. W., W. D. M. Paton, and R. G. Pertwee (1970) Preliminary experiments on the chemistry and pharmacology of cannabis. *Nature 228:*134–136.
7. Hollister, L. (1974) Structure-activity relationships in man of cannabis constituents, and homologs and metabolites of Δ^9-tetrahydrocannabinol. *Pharmacology 11:*3–11.
8. Hollister, L. E. and H. Gillespie (1975) Interactions in man of *delta*-9-tetrahydrocannabinol. II. Cannabinol and cannabidiol. *Clin. Pharm. Ther. 18:*80–83.
9. Krantz, J. C., Jr., H. J. Berger, and B. L. Welch (1971) Blockade of (−)-trans-Δ^9-tetrahydrocannabinol depressant effect by cannabinol in mice. *Am. J. Pharmacol 143:*149–152.
10. Layman, J. M. and A. S. Milton (1971) Some actions of Δ^1-tetrahydrocannabinol and cannabidiol at cholinergic junctions. *Br. J. Pharmacol. 41:*379P.
11. Mechoulam, R., ed. (1973) *Marijuana.* New York: Academic Press.
12. Paton, W. D. M. (1975) Pharmacology of marijuana. *Annu. Rev. Pharmacol. 15:*191–200.

34

Cannabinoids and the Inhibition of Prostaglandin Synthesis

J. F. HOWES AND P. F. OSGOOD

Introduction

During the last decade, there has been a rapid expansion of interest in both prostaglandins and cannabinoids. Prostaglandins are being recognized as basic to many physiological or pathological functions, and it is not surprising that many drugs interact with them. Evidence is accumulating that Δ^9-tetrahydrocannabinol (Δ^9-THC) and other cannabinoidlike agents affect prostaglandin synthesis. For this to be a viable hypothesis, it is necessary to indicate clear physiological changes caused by Δ^9-THC that are attributable to inhibition of prostaglandin synthesis.

The evidence that we review or present here provides a strong indication that the hypothesis is valid, and although a great deal of experimental evidence still has to be gathered, we feel that it provides a useful guideline to potential therapeutic areas for cannabinoids.

The first section of this chapter outlines circumstantial data indicating an involvement of prostaglandins in the actions of Δ^9-THC, and the second outlines more direct evidence from our laboratories and that accumulated by other workers.

Indirect Pharmacological Evidence

Cardiovascular system

Δ^9-THC has a variety of actions on the cardiovascular system, including tachycardia and hypotension in humans. Effects in animals are varied and depend largely on the state of the animal. One reproducible effect that we have reported [31] is potentiation of the actions of epinephrine and norepinephrine on the cardiovascular system of the dog (Table 34.1). It has been reported [19] that norepinephrine (NE) elicits PGE_2 release from the kidney,

Marihuana: Chemistry, Biochemistry, and Cellular Effects, edited by Gabriel G. Nahas,

Table 34.1 Cardiovascular response to Δ^1-THC and SP-111[a]

Treatment	*Response*	*p*
Change in mean arterial blood pressure (mmHg)		
Δ^1-THC	-34.0 ± 5.2	
(SP-111)	-18.0 ± 6.5	<0.2
PR to 2 μg/kg of epinephrine (mmHg)		
Before Δ^1-THC	43 ± 5.2	
After Δ^1-THC	73 ± 11.3	<0.05
Before (SP-111)	22 ± 2.3	
After (SP-111)	38 ± 4.3	<0.02
PR to 2 μg/kg of norepinephrine (mmHg)		
Before Δ^1-THC	43 ± 5.3	
After Δ^1-THC	78 ± 9.2	<0.02
Before (SP-111)	26 ± 5.8	
After (SP-111)	42 ± 8.9	<0.1
Change in duration of PR (%)		
Epinephrine after Δ^1-THC	$+32.6 \pm 3.1$	
Epinephrine after (SP-111)	$+21.9 \pm 3.0$	<0.1
Norepinephrine after Δ^1-THC	$+36.5 \pm 3.5$	
Norepinephrine after (SP-111)	$+28.7 \pm 2.8$	<0.3

[a] Four dogs were used in each determination. The dose of Δ^1-THC was 2 mg/kg, IV. The dose of SP-111 was 3 mg/kg, IV; PR, pressor response. Data from Zitko *et al* [31]. Copyright 1972 American Association for the Advancement of Sciences.

which counteracts the pressor effects of NE. If prostaglandin synthesis is inhibited, the pressor effect of NE is potentiated. A similar situation occurs with angiotensin II. This also causes renal PGE_2 production which offsets the pressor effect. Inhibition of PGE synthesis markedly enhances the pressor effect of angiotensin II. Preliminary experiments in our laboratory indicate that Δ^9-THC potentiates the effect of angiotensin II.

The mechanism described may explain the effect of Δ^9-THC on the pressor actions of epinephrine and norepinephrine. The kidney may not be the only site of action. It has been reported that treatment of isolated cat spleen [10] or rabbit heart [22] with eicosatetraenoic acid (ETA) resulted in a potentiation of the adrenergic response of these tissues. Similarly, indomethacin had a potentiating effect on the cat spleen [7]. Zimmerman *et al.* [30] demonstrated that both indomethacin and ETA potentiated the effects of norepinephrine and of adrenergic nerve stimulation in the dog paw perfusion experiment.

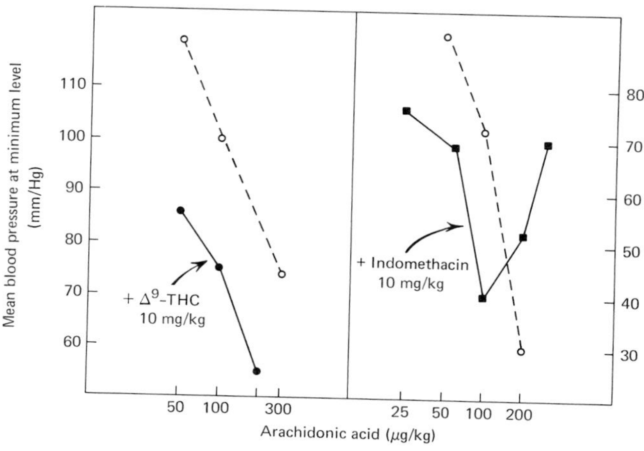

Figure 34.1. The effects of Δ^9-THC and indomethacin on the hypotensive activity of arachidonic acid in the rat.

In our laboratories, we have demonstrated that indomethacin potentiates the hypotensive activity of arachidonic acid in the anesthetized rat blood pressure experiment. Δ^9-THC caused a similar shift in the dose response curve (Figure 34.1). If the potentiation of arachidonic acid by indomethacin is due to inhibition of its conversion to prostaglandins, a similar mechanism could be invoked for Δ^9-THC. Definitive proof must come from assay of prostaglandin after arachidonic acid administration.

Pulmonary system

The importance of the prostaglandins in the pulmonary system and in asthmatic conditions is becoming well recognized [16]. The lung contains large amounts of prostaglandins. $PGF_{2\alpha}$ is a potent bronchoconstrictor. Δ^9-THC has exhibited some bronchodilator activity [28], which could be due to an inhibition of prostaglandin synthesis. Anti-inflammatory drugs such as aspirin are known to reduce the bronchoconstrictor effects of arachidonic acid and $PGF_{2\alpha}$. The relationship here is tenuous but seems worthy of further investigation since some useful advance in asthma therapy could result.

Central nervous system

Once again, several pieces of rather tenuous evidence indicate the involvement of prostaglandins in the actions of Δ^9-THC. One of us has reported [13] that Δ^9-THC at high dose levels potentiates the psychomotor stimulation, stereotypies, and aggregated toxicity seen with amphetamine. Amphetamine is an indirect-acting amine, many of the actions of which are due to release of dopamine or norepinephrine centrally. If the prostaglandins modulate the action of these amines centrally as they appear to do peripherally, then inhibition of prostaglandin synthesis might explain these actions of Δ^9-THC. We have shown that Δ^9-THC inhibits PGE synthesis in tissue derived from the corpus striatum (see section on "Direct pharmacological evidence").

PGE_1 antagonizes the convulsant activity of pentylenetetrazole, and Δ^9-THC lowers the threshold for minimal seizures [26,27]. This action of Δ^9-THC is in line with the concept that Δ^9-THC inhibits prostaglandin synthesis.

Analgesic, antipyretic and anti-inflammatory effects

Two groups of investigators [17,24] showed that Δ^9-THC was active in the Randall-Sellito procedure even though the values for the ED50 differed. But whereas Kosersky's group claimed that Δ^9-THC possessed antipyretic activity but no anti-inflammatory activity in the carrageen-induced edema test, Sofia *et al.* found activity in the carrageen test, but no antipyretic activity. Sofia and coworkers [23] also demonstrated that Δ^9-THC was active against adjuvant-induced arthritis, and they also showed in a later publication [25] that Δ^9-THC was active against edema produced by carrageen, dextran, formalin, kaolin, and sodium urate.

The analogy with aspirin and other anti-inflammatory agents is evident.

Luteinizing hormone secretion

Δ^9-THC at a dose of 2 mg per rat suppresses the secretion of luteinizing hormone (LH) from the anterior pituitary. 7-oxa-13-prostynoic acid, a prostaglandin antagonist, also prevented the luteinizing hormone releasing factor (LHRH)-stimulated release of LH.

The prostaglandins are involved in the release of other anterior pituitary hormones, but as yet the effects of Δ^9-THC have not been studied on hormones such as growth hormone. If the hypothesis is valid, one would expect a decreased synthesis and/or release of growth hormone after Δ^9-THC administration.

Direct Pharmacological Evidence

The eye

Glaucoma is an eye disease characterized by increased ocular pressure. There are various forms of glaucoma, including secondary glaucoma, which occurs as a sequel to preexisting ocular disease or injury. Prostaglandin formation is known to be involved in the inflammatory response to injury. The IV infusion of prostaglandins into rabbits [5] and dogs [20] was reported to increase intraocular pressure, and, more recently, Green and Podos [9] have shown that an increase in intraocular pressure was produced in rabbits by infusion of arachidonic acid, the precursor of PGE_2. In the latter instance, Δ^9-THC reduced intraocular pressure, which was interpreted as being due to inhibition of PGE_2 synthesis in the eye. In man, marihuana smoking or the administration of Δ^9-THC has been reported to reduce intraocular pressure [8,11].

Δ^9-THC and other cannabinoids may therefore possess useful therapeutic activity as antiglaucoma agents. They would be likely to have utility in the treatment of secondary glaucoma involving injury, inflammation, and prostaglandin synthesis.

In vitro prostaglandin biosynthesis

Burstein and Raz [4] demonstrated that Δ^9-THC inhibited the formation of prostaglandins in bovine seminal vesicle preparations. In a subsequent paper, Burstein *et al.* [3], showed that Δ^9-THC and other cannabinoids inhibited prostaglandin synthesis in bovine seminal vesicle preparations. These data correlate well with the anti-inflammatory activity described by Sofia *et al.* [23] (see Table 34.2).

Using a rabbit renal medulla acetone powder preparation and measuring the formation of PGE_2 and $PGF_{2\alpha}$ from [1-^{14}C]-arachidonic acid, Crowshaw and Hardman [6] showed that Δ^9-THC and 11-OH-Δ^9-THC at concentrations of 100 μg/ml inhibited prostaglandin E_2 formation by 32 percent and 48 percent, respectively. No inhibition of $PGF_{2\alpha}$ formation was observed.

In our own laboratories, we have studied the formation of PGE_1 from ^{14}C-8,11,14-eicosatrienoic acid. A preliminary report of this work was published [15]. We discovered a dose-related inhibition of PGE_1 synthesis in the presence of Δ^9-THC, a water-soluble analog, SP-111,[1] and indomethacin (Figure 34.2). Our concentrations of cannabinoids were much less than those used in previous

[1] SP-111 is (−)-*trans*-Δ^9-THC-4-(morpholino) butyrate hydrochloride.

Table 34.2 Anti-inflammatory activity of cannabinoids and inhibition of prostaglandin synthesis

Substance	*Anti-inflammatory*[a] *activity* ED50 (95% CL)	*Inhibition of* PGE_1 *synthesis*[b] ID50 ($M \times 10^{-4}$)
Indomethacin	1.2 (0.6–2.1)	0.008
Cannabinol	20.0 (12.7–31.6)	0.70
Olivetol	22.8 (13.3–39.2)	1.00
Cannabidiol	15.1 (8.0–28.4)	2.20
Δ^9-Tetrahydro-cannabinol	5.9 (3.1–11.2)	3.18
p-Cymene	>1600	>7.36
α-Limonene	>1600	>7.35

[a] Carragen-induced fluid paw edema in the rat. Data from Sofia *et al.* (1973); copyright PJD Publications, Westbury, New York.

[b] Inhibition of PGE_1 synthesis in bovine seminal vesicles. Data from Burstein *et al.* (1973); copyright Pergamon Press Ltd., Oxford, England.

reports, and, surprisingly, both the cannabinoids were more potent than indomethacin. This agrees with the already established phenomenon of differing sensitivities of prostaglandin synthetase samples from different tissues.

In the whole-brain tissue of the rat, adenosine diphosphate (ADP) stimulates PGE_1 synthesis [1]. In our striatal preparations, ADP also gave a dose-related increase in PGE_1 synthesis (Figure 34.3). In the presence of $10^{-6}M$ Δ^9-THC, there was a parallel shift to the right of the dose-effect curve, whereas with SP-111 there was a nonparallel shift in the same direction.

In previous work [14,21], we have demonstrated an effect of Δ^9-THC on striatal dopamine disposition. Both dopamine and PGE_1 affect the enzyme adenyl cyclase. Walker and Walker [29] have shown that dopamine stimulates the formation of cyclic AMP in rat striatal tissue. McAfee and Greengard [18] have suggested that in sympathetic ganglia, dopamine released from interneurons increases the formation of cyclic AMP, which brings about hyperpolarization of the postganglionic neuron. They have demonstrated that PGE_1 blocks dopamine-induced hyperpolarization. Bergstrom and coworkers [2] have found that PGE_2 decreases stimulation-induced overflow of dopamine in slices of rat striatum. This last finding is in agreement with many other studies suggesting that PGE prevents release of neurotransmitter at the prejunctional sympathetic nerve ending [10].

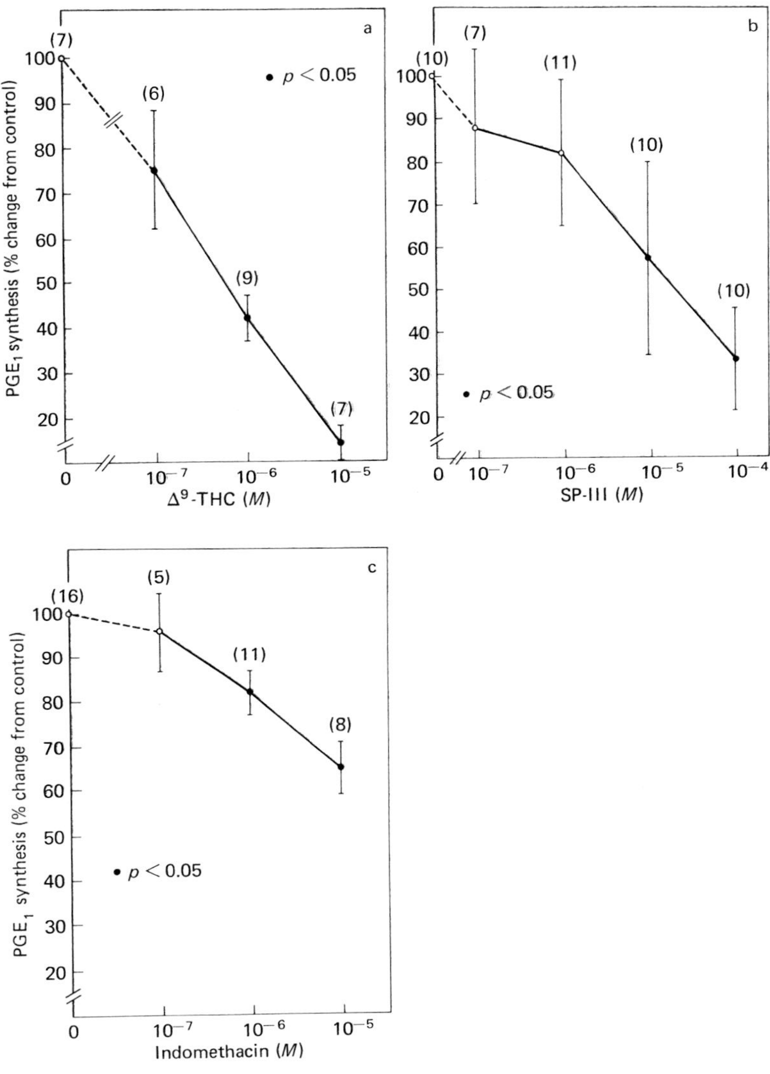

Figure 34.2. Effects of (a) Δ^9-THC, (b) SP-111, and (c) indomethacin on the formation of PGE_1 by rat striatal synaptosomes.

Thus, some of the observed central nervous system effects of Δ^9-THC could be explained on the basis of prostaglandin synthesis inhibition and removal of the modulating effects of the prostaglandins on dopamine.

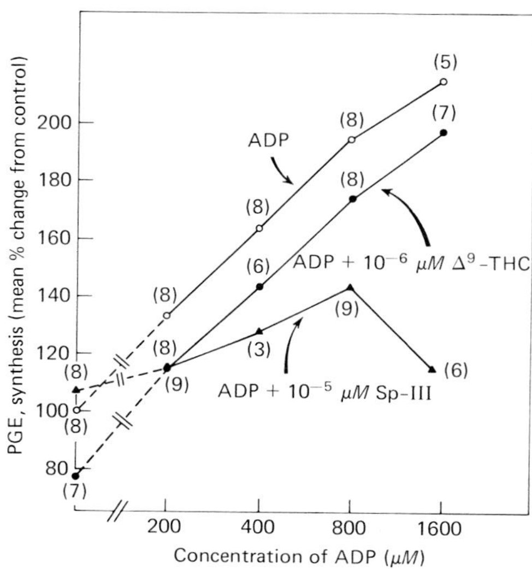

Figure 34.3. Effects of Δ^9-THC and SP-111 on ADP-stimulated synthesis of PGE_1 in rat striatal synaptosomes.

Conclusions

We have proposed a hypothesis that some of the actions of Δ^9-THC and other cannabinoids could be explained on the basis of inhibition of prostaglandin synthesis. In support of this hypothesis, we have shown that in several *in vitro* systems Δ^9-THC inhibits prostaglandin synthesis. Further, it has been demonstrated that Δ^9-THC can block the increase in intraocular pressure brought about by arachidonic acid. These data are of particular interest since they point to a potential therapeutic use of Δ^9-THC. Consistent with this hypothesis is the finding that Δ^9-THC is active as an anti-inflammatory agent. Once again, this could point to a potential therapeutic use of cannabinoids.

The similarity between the effects of Δ^9-THC and indomethacin on the cardiovascular system, as well as the effects of minimal convulsive seizures, are consistent with the hypothesis stated above, although they provide no direct evidence for it. The effects of Δ^9-THC on luteinizing hormone secretion are also consistent with the hypothesis. It would be interesting to see the effect of Δ^9-THC on growth hormone secretion.

If our hypothesis is valid, then one could predict useful therapeutic activities for the natural and synthetic cannabinoids.

REFERENCES

1. Abdulla, Y. H. and E. McFarlane (1972) Control of prostaglandin biosynthesis in rat brain homogenates by adenine nucleotides. *Biochem. Pharmacol. 21:*2841.
2. Bergstrom, S., L. Farnebo and K. Fuxe (1973) Effect of prostaglandin E_2 on central and peripheral catecholamine neurons. *Eur. J. Pharmacol. 21:*362.
3. Burstein, S., E. Levin and C. Varanelli (1973) Prostaglandins and cannabis II: inhibition of biosynthesis by the naturally occurring cannabinoids. *Biochem. Pharmacol. 22:*2905.
4. Burstein, S. and A. Raz (1972) Inhibition of prostaglandin E_2 synthesis by Δ^1-tetrahydrocannabinol. *Prostaglandins 2:*369.
5. Chiang, T. S. and R. P. Thomas (1972) Effects of progesterone and epinephrine on the ocular hypertensive response to intravenous infusion of prostaglandin E_1. 5th International Congress on Pharmacology, abstract No. 243.
6. Crowshaw, K. and H. F. Hardman (1974) Effect of Δ^9-tetrahydrocannabinol (Δ^9-THC) on prostaglandin (PG) synthesis and the relationship of this effect to the hypothermic response in mice. *Fed. Proc. 33:* abstract No. 1847.
7. Fereira, S. H. and S. Moncada (1971) Inhibition of prostaglandin synthesis augments the effects of sympathetic nerve stimulation on the cat spleen. *Br. J. Pharmacol. 43:*419P.
8. Frank, I. M., R. S. Hepler, L. Epps, J. T. Ungerleider and S. Szara (1972) Marihuana and delta-9-tetrahydrocannabinol: effects on intraocular pressure in young adults. 5th International Congress on Pharmacology, abstract No. 426.
9. Green, K. and S. M. Podos (1974) Antagonism of arachidonic acid-induced ocular effects by Δ^1-tetrahydrocannabinol. *Invest. Ophthalmol. 13:*422, 1974.
10. Hedqvist, P., L. Stjarne, and A. Wennmalm (1971) Facilitation of sympathetic neurotransmission in the cat spleen after inhibition of prostaglandin synthesis. *Acta Physiol. Scand. 83:*430.
11. Hepler, R. S. and I. M. Frank (1971) Letter to the editor, marihuana smoking and intraocular pressure. *J.A.M.A. 217:*1392.
12. Holmes, S. W. and E. W. Horton (1967) Prostaglandins and the central nervous system. *Prostaglandin Symposium of the Worcester Foundation for Experimental Biology* (P. W. Ramwell and S. E. Shaw, eds.). New York: Interscience Publishers, pp. 21–38.
13. Howes, J. F. (1973) The effect of Δ^9-tetrahydrocannabinoid on amphetamine induced lethality in aggregated mice. *Res. Commun. Chem. Pathol. Pharmacol. 6:*895.
14. Howes, J. F. and P. F. Osgood (1974) The effect of Δ^9-tetrahydrocannabinol on the uptake and release of ^{14}C-dopamine from crude striatal synaptosomal preparations. *Neuropharmacology 13:*1109.
15. Howes, J. F. and P. F. Osgood (1974) The effects of Δ^9-THC and a water soluble derivative on PGE_1 synthesis on the corpus striatum. *Pharmacologist 16:*abstract 389.
16. Kadowitz, P. J., P. D. Joinir, and A. L. Hyman (1975) Physiological and pharmacological roles of prostaglandins. *Annu. Rev. Pharmacol. 15:*285.

17. Kosersky, D. S., W. L. Dewey, and L. S. Harris (1973) Antipyretic, analgesic and anti-inflammatory effects of Δ^9-tetrahydrocannabinol in the rat. *Eur. J. Pharmacol. 24:*1.
18. McAfee, D. A. and P. Greengard (1972) Adenosine 3′5′-monophosphate: electrophysiological evidence for a role in synaptic transmission. *Science. 178:*310.
19. McGiff, J. C. (1975) Prostaglandins as regulators of blood pressure. *Hosp. Prac.* 101.
20. Nakano, J., A. C. K. Chang, and R. G. Fisher (1972) Effect of prostaglandins E_2 and $F_{2\alpha}$ on the carotid arterial blood flow, cerebrospirial fluid pressure and intraocular pressure in dogs. *Proc. Soc. Exp. Biol. Med. 140:*866.
21. Osgood, P. F. and J. F. Howes (1974) Cannabinoid induced changes in mouse striatal homovanillic acid and dehydroxyphenylacetic acid. The effects of amphetamine and *l*-dopa. *Res. Commun. Chem. Pathol. Pharmacol. 9:*621.
22. Samuelsson, B. and A. Wennmalm (1971) Increased nerve stimulation induced release of noradrenaline from the rabbit heart after inhibition of prostaglandin synthesis. *Acta Physiol. Scand. 83:*163.
23. Sofia, R. D., L. C. Knoblock, and H. B. Varsar (1973) The anti-edema activity of various naturally occurring cannabinoids. *Res. Commun. Chem. Pathol. Pharmacol. 6:*909.
24. Sofia, R. D., S. D. Nalepa, J. J. Harakal and H. B. Varsar (1973) Anti-edema and analgesic properties of Δ^9-tetrahydrocannabinol (THC). *J. Pharmacol. Exp. Ther. 186:*646.
25. Sofia, R. D., S. D. Nalepa, H. B. Varsar, and L. C. Knoblock (1974) Comparative antiphilogistic activity of Δ^9-tetrahydrocannabinol, hydrocortisone and aspirin in various rat paw edema models. *Life Sci. 15:* 251.
26. Sofia, R. D., T. A. Solomon, and M. Barry, III (1971) The anticonvulsant activity of Δ^1-tetrahydrocannabinol in mice. *Pharmacologist 13:* Abstract 309.
27. Turkanis, S., W. Cely, D. M. Olsen, and R. Karler (1974) Anticonvulsant properties of cannabidiol. *Res. Commun. Chem. Pathol. Pharmacol. 8:*231.
28. Vachon, L., M. X. Fitzgerald, N. H. Solliday, I. A. Gould and E. A. Gaensler (1973) Single dose effect of marihuana smoke. Bronchial dynamics and respiratory center sensitivity in normal subjects. *N. Engl. J. Med. 288:*985.
29. Walker, J. B. and J. P. Walker (1973) Neurohumoral regulation of adenylate cyclase activity in the rat striatum. *Brain Res. 54:*386.
30. Zimmerman, B. G., M. J. Ryan, S. Gomer, and E. Kraft (1973) Effect of the prostaglandin synthesis inhibitors indomethacin and eicosa-5,8,11,14-tetraenoic acid on adrenergic responses in dog cutaneous vasculature. *J. Pharmacol. Exp. Ther. 187:*315, 1973.
31. Zitko, B. A., J. F. Howes, R. K. Razdan, B. C. Dalzell, H. C. Dalzell, J. C. Sheehan, H. G. Pars, W. L. Dewey and L. S. Harris (1972) Water soluble derivatives of Δ^1-tetrahydrocannabinol. *Science 177:* 442.

35

Effects of Cannabinol Derivatives on Blood Pressure, Body Weight, Pituitary-Adrenal Function, and Mitochondrial Respiration in the Rat

M. K. BIRMINGHAM AND A. BARTOVA

Introduction

Interactions of cannabinoids with pituitary-adrenal functioning deserve a clearer delineation in order to define their relevance to the etiology of hypertension and because information available on this subject is scant. Barry *et al.* [1] reported raised circulating corticosterone levels in normotensive rats after the acute administration of Δ^9-THC, and Dewey *et al.* [6] observed a decrease in adrenal ascorbic acid. In this laboratory, chronic IP administration of Δ^9-tetrahydrocannabinol (Δ^9-THC) at a daily dose of 3 mg/kg for 1 week caused a slight and statistically not significant lowering of circulating corticosterone levels in rats with adrenal regeneration hypertension [3]. Such animals responded to this dose, which is moderate for the rat, by a statistically highly significant well sustained decline in blood pressure, suggesting neither accumulation nor habituation over the 1-week period of drug administration, or else a precise cancelling out of the two effects. Body weight was not affected (and food intake was not measured, in contrast to a citation of our work [10]).

The present study was undertaken in order to gain information regarding sites of action of cannabinol derivatives that could be pertinent to their antihypertensive potency. To this end, we assessed the effects of Δ^9-THC administered both *in vitro* and *in vivo* on adrenal function and on the mitochondrial metabolism of various tissues. The *in vivo* studies also include a comparison of the effects of Δ^8-THC with those of Δ^9-THC on blood pressure, body weight, and adrenal function in rats with adrenal regeneration hypertension.

Marihuana: Chemistry, Biochemistry, and Cellular Effects, edited by Gabriel G. Nahas,

Materials and Methods

All experiments were carried out on Wistar rats. The effects on blood pressure were determined on female rats rendered hypertensive by the technique of Skelton [16]. The treatment with cannabinol derivatives, initiated 4–8 months after adrenal enucleation, consisted of daily IP injections of Δ^8-THC or Δ^9-THC (Canadian Food and Drug Directorate) in 0.2 ml glycerol formol for 2 weeks at a dose of 3 mg/kg body weight. Vehicle and saline-injected animals served as control groups, 10 rats per group. The animals were weighed daily. Blood pressure was determined before beginning treatment and on the 8th and 13th days of treatment by the tail-cuff method in conditioned, unanesthetized animals.

The animals were decapitated between 10:30 and 11 AM; 24 hr after the last injection, blood was collected from the trunk into heparinized beakers, organs were removed and weighed, and plasma corticosterone levels were determined by fluorometry [18].

The study on the *in vivo* effects of Δ^9-THC on NADH-oxidase activity was conducted on normal male rats. The drug was administered daily in 0.2 ml vehicle at doses of 3 and 20 mg/kg IP for a maximum of 8 days. The vehicle consisted of 5 percent ethanol, 11 percent propylene glycol, and 13 percent Tween 80 in 0.9 percent saline. The animals, 10 rats per group, were decapitated between 1 and 2 PM, 1 hr after the 1st, 2nd, or 8th injection. Organs were weighed and plasma corticosterone levels were determined as described. NADH-oxidase was isolated by the method of Stoppani *et al.* [17] from pooled heart tissue of 3–4 animals, affording three samples per group, and by the method of De Robertis [5], from pooled brain parts of 10 animals, affording one sample per group. The pooled brain regions were composed of hypothalamus, medulla, and pons. The activity of the enzyme system was determined as described by Stoppani [17] in a Beckman DK-2 spectrophotometer, and the rate of NADH oxidation was measured by diminution of the absorbancy at 340 nm.

To assess the effects of Δ^9-THC on NADH-oxidase activity *in vitro,* we grouped the brain regions according to the method of Glowinski and Iversen [7] into four parts—cerebral cortex, hypothalamus plus thalamus plus midbrain, medulla plus pons, and cerebellum. Then we assessed the NADH-oxidase activity in the presence of 10^{-5} *M* Δ^9-THC, in a reaction mixture consisting of 0.13 *M* potassium buffer pH 7.35, 0.015 m*M* cytochrome c, and 0.125 m*M* NADH. Δ^9-THC was added to the reaction mixture in dioxane in a volume of 10 μl. Control preparations received dioxane as well.

To assess the effects of Δ⁹-THC on adrenal function *in vitro*, we quartered rat adrenals, preincubated them, and then incubated the adrenals for 2 hr with or without ACTH, 1 IU/100 mg tissue, and with or without Δ⁹-THC added to the incubation medium in 5 μl dioxane. Controls received dioxane as well. Corticosterone production was measured by fluorometry, the production of 18-hydroxydeoxycorticosterone (18–OH–DOC), by the Porter-Silber reaction.

Results

In vitro effects of Δ^9-THC

Adrenal steroid biogenesis

The effect of 10^{-5} *M* Δ^9-THC on the production of corticosterone and 18–OH–DOC by quartered adrenals from male rats is shown in Table 35.1. Δ^9-THC did not alter the production of corticosterone, nor did it affect the ACTH-stimulated output of 18–OH–DOC consistently. The unstimulated production of 18–OH–DOC was significantly reduced by an average of 42 percent ($p < 0.01$).

Oxygen uptake by mitochondrial preparations

Intact mitochondria. Δ^9-THC inhibited malate-glutamate–supported respiration of intact ADP-activated liver mitochondria from male rats at concentrations as low as 10^{-9} *M*. In 13 experiments

Table 35.1 *In vitro* effects of Δ^9-THC on the production of corticosterone and 18-hydroxydeoxycorticosterone by rat adrenal glands

Additions	*Corticosterone* (μg/100 mg/2 hr)	*18–OH–DOC* (μg/100 mg/2 hr)
None	2.87 ± 0.39[a]	3.67 ± 0.45
10^{-5} *M* Δ^9-THC	2.75 ± 0.36	2.11 ± 0.06[b]
ACTH, 1 IU/100 mg	14.0 ± 1.04	9.12 ± 0.61
THC ± ACTH	14.7 ± 1.60	8.30 ± 0.82

[a] ± SE; $n = 8$.

[b] $p < 0.01$.

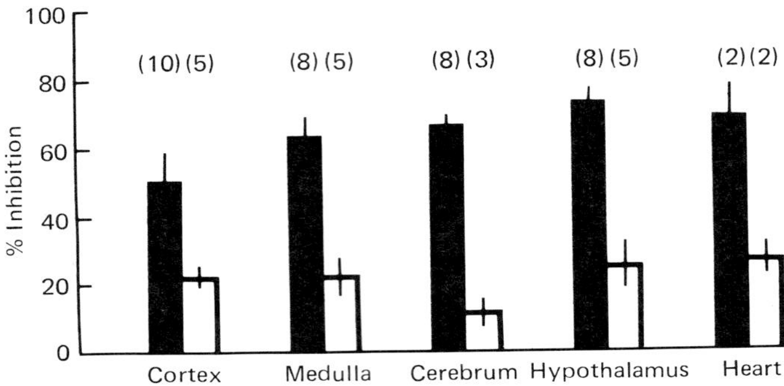

Figure 35.1. Effects of Δ^9-THC and DOC on NADH-oxidase activity of rat brain and heart mitochondria *in vitro.* The enzyme preparation (85 μg of enzyme protein) was diluted to 2.5 ml in a medium containing 0.13 *M* potassium phosphate buffer, pH 7.35, 0.015 m*M* cytochrome c, and 0.125 m*M* NADH. Δ^9-THC (*closed bars*) and DOC (*open bars*) in 10^{-5} *M* concentration were added in 10 μl of dioxane. The number of samples is given in brackets. Vertical lines denote SE. Control values: nM NADH oxidized/mg/min: cerebral cortex 81 $\mp$ 3; medulla + pons 90 $\mp$ 3; cerebellum 93 $\mp$ 11; hypothalamus plus thalamus plus midbrain 90 $\pm$ 2; heart 247 $\pm$ 4.

conducted in the presence of 10^{-9}—10^{-7} *M* Δ^9-THC, the inhibition averaged 39 $\pm$ 4 percent (range 17–60 percent). The inhibitory effect of Δ^9-THC on succinate-supported respiration was minimal, averaging 6 $\pm$ 1 percent (range 2–16 percent) in 14 experiments at concentrations of 10^{-8}–10^{-4} *M*.

NADH-oxidase activity. Figure 35.1 depicts the effects of 10^{-5} *M* Δ^9-THC and 10^{-5} *M* deoxycorticosterone (DOC) on the NADH-oxidase activity of heart and of four brain regions—hypothalamus plus thalamus plus midbrain, cerebellum, medulla oblongata plus pons, and cerebral cortex; all were obtained from male rats. The inhibitory action of Δ^9-THC greatly exceeded that of DOC, a classical inhibitor of this system, in all preparations. In the brain the most marked effect occurred in the hypothalamus plus thalamus plus midbrain region, the smallest in the cortex, and the regional difference between these two tissues was statistically significant.

The mixed nature of the inhibition was established by the Lineweaver-Burk plot. The effect was localized at the amytal-sensitive site of the electron transfer system, and it was found to be logarithmically related to dose ([2] and unpublished observations).

In vivo effects of Δ^8- and Δ^9-THC

Hypertensive female rats

Blood pressure, body weight, and organ weight. Figure 35.2 depicts changes in blood pressure and body weight of female adrenal hypertensive (ARH) rats during a 2-week period of daily IP administration of Δ^8- or Δ^9-THC at a dose of 3 mg/kg body weight. The blood pressure measurements were taken on day 1 before the onset of injection and on days 8 and 13 or 14, 22 hr after the last injection. Therefore, the values reflect chronic rather than acute effects. Both Δ^8- and Δ^9-THC caused a statistically significant reduction in blood pressure averaging 13 mmHg at the end of the first and 14.5 mmHg at the end of the second week in the Δ^8-THC–treated rats, and 18.5 and 13.5 mmHg in the Δ^9-THC–treated rats. No alterations in blood pressure were observed in the rats injected with saline, and the slight reduction found with the glycerol-formol vehicle was not statistically significant.

Periodic and synchronous fluctuations in body weight occurred

Figure 35.2. Effects of Δ^9-THC (●) and Δ^8-THC (▲) on blood pressure and body weights of female rats with adrenal regeneration hypertension. Rats injected with saline (○) or with vehicle (v) served as controls. Each group was composed of 10 animals. Vertical lines indicate SE.

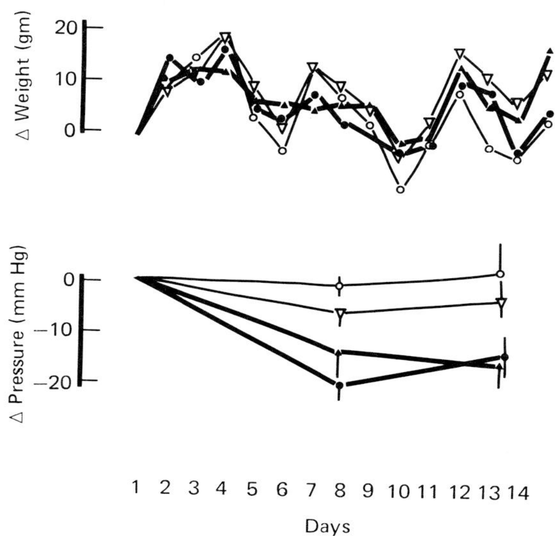

Table 35.2 Effects of chronic administration of Δ^8- and Δ^9-THC[a] on organ weights and peripheral corticosterone levels of female rats with adrenal regeneration hypertension

	Organ weight					*Body weight (gm)*	
Treatment	*Adrenal (mg)*	*Kidney (gm)*	*Thymus (mg)*	*Heart (gm)*	*Liver (gm)*	*Initial*	*Final*
Saline	32.9 ± 3.4 9	1.87 ± 0.06 10	311 ± 25 10	1.22 ± 0.04 10	9.83 ± 0.39 10	237 ± 8 10	239 ± 8 10
Vehicle	34.4 ± 3.7 9	1.82 ± 0.08 10	$208 \pm 18^{s}{}_{1}$ 9	1.12 ± 0.04 10	10.92 ± 0.41 10	243 ± 11 10	254 ± 7 10
Δ^8-THC	36.0 ± 3.3 10	1.73 ± 0.06 10	$184 \pm 16^{s}{}_{3}$ 10	$1.03 \pm 0.03^{s}{}_{2}$ 10	$11.06 \pm 0.40^{s}{}_{1}$ 10	218 ± 10 10	233 ± 9 10
Δ^9-THC	34.0 ± 5.2 8	1.88 ± 0.11 8	$132 \pm 27_{s3}^{v1}$ 8	$1.04 \pm 0.05^{s}{}_{2}$ 8	10.56 ± 0.45 8	221 ± 7 8	226 ± 9 8
		Organ weight/100gm final body weight				*Plasma corticosterone (µg/100 ml)*	
Saline	13.6 ± 1.51 9	0.80 ± 0.03 10	132 ± 12 10	0.52 ± 0.02 10	4.15 ± 0.20 10	64.3 ± 11.9 10	(54.7 ± 7.8)[b] 9
Vehicle	13.7 ± 1.65 9	$0.71 \pm 0.02^{s}{}_{1}$ 10	$83 \pm 9^{s}{}_{2}$ 9	$0.44 \pm 0.01^{s}{}_{1}$ 10	4.30 ± 0.09 10	52.9 ± 8.0 10	
Δ^8-THC	15.5 ± 1.78 10	0.74 ± 0.02 10	$81 \pm 9^{s}{}_{2}$ 10	$0.44 \pm 0.01^{s}{}_{1}$ 10	$4.76 \pm 0.11_{v_2}^{s_2}$ 10	52.9 ± 6.5 10	
Δ^9-THC	15.0 ± 2.08 8	0.84 ± 0.06 8	$59 \pm 11^{s}{}_{3}$ 8	0.46 ± 0.03 8	4.71 ± 0.20 8	46.2 ± 9.8 8	(38.0 ± 6.1)[b] 7

[a] Treatment 3 mg/kg IP for 2 weeks. Levels of significance compared to saline (s) and vehicle (v) injected rats are indicated by subscripts: 1, $p < 0.05$; 2, $p < 0.01$ or 0.02; 3, $p < 0.001$.

[b] Omitting a value that exceeded 3 SD of the mean.

in the four groups, but no changes attributable to the cannabinol derivatives could be discerned (Figure 35.2). Thymus weight was decreased by 59 percent in Δ^9-THC–treated rats, by 41 percent in the Δ^8-THC–treated rats, and by 31 percent in rats injected with the vehicle (Table 35.2). Per unit body weight, Δ^8-THC caused a highly significant enlargement of the liver, whereas Δ^9-THC had only a marginally significant effect ($0.05 < p < 0.1$).

Plasma corticosterone. The peripheral corticosterone levels were high and varied greatly within groups. The lowest average was in the Δ^9-THC–treated animals, but none of the differences between groups was statistically significant.

Normal rats—chronic effects

Body and organ weights. Only the effects of Δ^9-THC have been studied so far, and two doses—3 and 20 mg/kg IP—were tested. Rats exposed for 8 days to the lower dose continued to grow at exactly the same rate as the rats injected with the vehicle. The dose of 20 mg/kg, however, caused a highly significant (38 percent) retardation of the growth rate (Figure 35.3).

The low dose of Δ^9-THC increased the weight of the adrenals, the kidneys, and, per unit body weight, the liver (Table 35.3). By

Figure 35.3. Effects of Δ^9-THC (*heavy line and solid dots*) on body weights of normal male rats. (a) Daily dose 3 mg/kg body weight, initial body weight 200 gm. (b) Daily dose 20 mg/kg body weight, initial body weight 180 gm. Each group was composed of 10 rats. Vertical lines indicate SE.

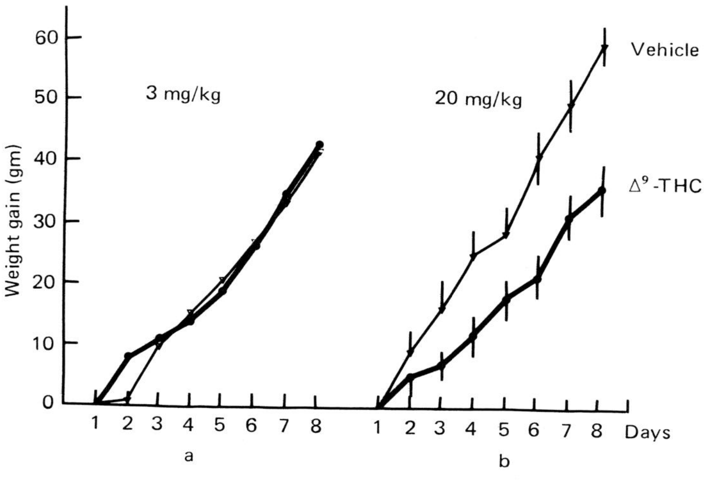

Table 35.3 Effects of chronic administration of Δ^9-THC on organ weights and peripheral corticosterone levels of normal male rats[a]

	Treatment 3 mg/kg IP *for 8 days*						
	Organ weights					*Body weight (gm)*	
	Adrenals (mg)	*Kidney (gm)*	*Thymus (mg)*	*Pituitary (mg)*	*Liver (gm)*	*Initial*	*Final*
Vehicle	36.6 ± 0.81 10	2.20 ± 0.09 10	588 ± 4.0 10	—	10.79 ± 0.42 10	198 ± 1 10	240 ± 6 10
Δ^9-THC	42.1 ± 2.0^{v_1} 10	2.765 ± 0.078^{v_3} 10	544 ± 43 10	—	12.06 ± 0.49 10	203 ± 3 10	245 ± 5 10
	Organ weights/100 gm final body weight					*Plasma corticosterone (μg/100 ml)*	
Vehicle	15.3 ± 0.48 10	0.91 ± 0.02 10	245 ± 15 10	—	4.45 ± 0.09 10	19.4 ± 1.38 10	
Δ^9-THC	17.2 ± 0.72^{v_1} 10	1.13 ± 0.03^{v_3} 10	221 ± 11 10	—	4.91 ± 0.14^{v_3} 10	23.6 ± 1.74 10	
	Treatment 20 mg/kg IP *for 8 days*						
Vehicle	37.3 ± 1.8 10	1.93 ± 0.04 10	638 ± 29 10	6.5 ± 0.3 10	11.49 ± 0.20 10	177 ± 4 10	237 ± 3 10
Δ^9-THC	38.2 ± 2.6 4	1.88 ± 0.04 10	550 ± 13^{v_2} 10	6.6 ± 0.5 10	9.31 ± 0.27^{v_3} 10	181 ± 2 10	218 ± 4^{v_3} 10
	Organ weight/100 gm final body weight					*Plasma corticosterone (μg/100 ml)*	
Vehicle	15.7 ± 0.75 10	0.82 ± 0.02 10	269 ± 12 10	2.73 ± 0.12 10	4.85 ± 0.08 10	23.8 ± 3.7 10	
Δ^9-THC	17.6 ± 1.22 4	0.86 ± 0.02 10	253 ± 19 10	2.85 ± 0.29 10	4.28 ± 0.13^{v_3} 10	55.0 ± 10.7^{v_2} 10	

[a] See footnote to Table 35.2.

contrast, liver weight decreased with exposure to the high dosage, and this effect was highly significant expressed in both absolute terms and per unit body weight. The higher dose also induced thymus involution.

Plasma corticosterone. The concentration of corticosterone in the peripheral plasma of these normal males was much lower and less variable than that found in the female hypertensive rats bearing regenerated adrenal glands. The average for the rats treated with 3 mg/kg was slightly but not significantly greater than that of the controls ($0.05 < p < 0.1$). However, at the higher dose, a highly significant increase to more than twice the normal value was observed (Table 35.4).

NADH-oxidase activity. NADH oxidase isolated from the heart and a region of the brain composed of hypothalamus plus medulla plus pons was, if anything, slightly more active in the tissue derived from the animals treated chronically with the low dose of Δ^9-THC, compared to the vehicle-treated group (Figure 35.4).

Normal rats—acute effects

Plasma corticosterone. Plasma corticosterone levels rose 5-fold 1 hr after the first injection of 3 mg/kg on day 1, and 3-fold 1 hr after the second injection on day 2 (Table 35.4). At the higher

Table 35.4 Acute and chronic effects of Δ^9-THC on plasma corticosterone levels of normal male rats

	μg/100 ml, 1 hr after injection (n = *10*)		
	Day 1	*Day 2*	*Day 8*
Vehicle	17.8 ± 1.7	15.8 ± 2.9	19.4 ± 1.4
Δ^9-THC 3 mg/kg IP	87.3 ± 13.9[a]	50.6 ± 11.8[b]	23.6 ± 1.7[c]
Vehicle	16.4 ± 1.0	19.8 ± 3.6	23.8 ± 3.7
Δ^9-THC 20 mg/kg IP	123.9 ± 3.2[d]	103.1 ± 5.1[e]	55.0 ± 10.7[f]

[a] $p < 0.001$ versus vehicle.

[b] $p = 0.01$ versus vehicle; <0.02 versus day 1.

[c] $p < 0.1$ versus vehicle; <0.05 versus day 2.

[d] $p < 0.02$ versus low dose; <0.001 versus vehicle.

[e] $p < 0.001$ versus low dose; <0.001 versus vehicle; <0.01 versus day 1.

[f] $p < 0.001$ versus low dose; <0.02 versus vehicle; <0.001 versus day 2.

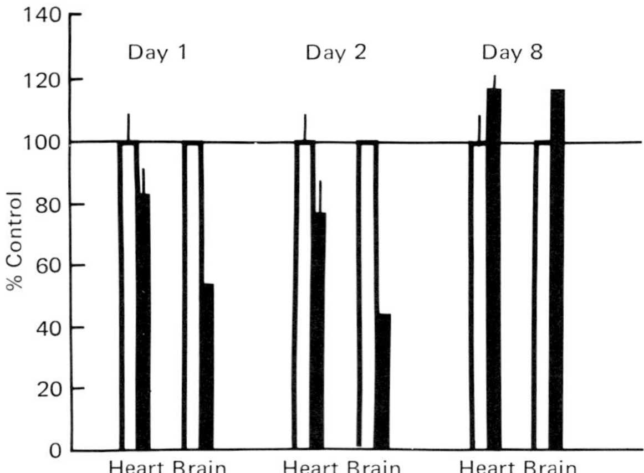

Figure 35.4. Effects of Δ^9-THC on NADH oxidase of rat brain and heart mitochondria *in vivo.* The animals received daily IP injections of 3 mg Δ^9-THC/kg body weight, and the enzyme preparation (72–112 μg enzyme protein) was diluted to 2.5 ml in a medium containing 0.13 *M* potassium phosphate buffer, pH 7.35, 0.015 m*M* cytochrome c, and 0.125 m*M* NADH. Open bars: vehicle-treated rats; closed bars: rats injected with Δ^9-THC. Vertical lines denote SE. Control values (nM NADH oxidized/mg/min): heart 375 $\pm$ 30; brain 106 $\pm$ 4.

dose, the levels were raised 8-fold on day 1 and 5-fold on day 2. These increases were highly significant as were the differences between the two doses and the decline in response with time.

NADH-oxidase activity. The dose of 3 mg/kg caused a statistically not significant lowering of the average activity in the enzyme system isolated from the hearts of the animals after the first and the second injection (Figure 35.4). The average activity in the enzyme system of the brain preparation was reduced to less than half the activity of the control preparation, but this effect must await validation since it was established with only 1 sample per group.

Discussion

Treatment of adrenal-enucleated hypertensive rats for 2 weeks with Δ^9-THC at a daily dose of 3 mg/kg IP induced a sustained reduction in blood pressure, had no effect on body weight, and caused a statistically not significant decline in the concentration of circulating corticosterone, thus replicating the results obtained in earlier work in which the treatment was confined to 1 week [3]. Chronic treatment with a similar dose of Δ^8-THC caused a sustained reduction in blood pressure as well, without affecting body weight or plasma corticosterone levels. The weight gain of normal male rats was also completely unaffected by IP administration of Δ^9-THC at a dose of 3 mg/kg, as opposed to the highly significant retardation in growth elicited by 20 mg/kg.

In contrast to our findings, Nahas *et al.* reported a progressive weight loss accompanied by only transient changes in the blood pressure of spontaneously hypertensive rats upon oral administration of Δ^9-THC at daily doses of 5–25 mg/kg [10]. Differences in animal model, dosage, and the route and duration of administration at any one dose (3–5 days only) may account for the discrepancy. Dewey *et al.* found no significant effect on growth rate with 5 mg/kg IP of Δ^9-THC [6]. Sjödén, Järbe, and Henriksson observed no effect with 2.5 mg/kg IP of Δ^9-THC but a significant effect with double that dose of Δ^8-THC [15], as did Manning and coworkers with a dose of 4 mg/kg IP of Δ^9-THC [8]. This suggests that conditions and precise dosage are critical. Furthermore, our observations indicate that a change in dose may reverse the nature of a response since an increase in liver weight occurred upon chronic administration of the cannabinoids in both hypertensive and normotensive rats at the low dose, whereas a high dose decreased liver size.

Striking differences between acute and chronic effects on pituitary-adrenal function were reflected in the plasma corticosterone levels, which rose excessively at both doses 1 hr after the first administration, slightly—but significantly—less after the second administration, and returned to normal by the 8th day at the lower dose. The acute changes are in accord with the results reported by other investigators [1,6]. The extent to which the waning response reflects a refractoriness to the stimulus or increased peripheral usage and detoxification remains to be assessed. The pronounced lipophilic properties of the cannabinol derivatives would favor the central nervous system as a target site. Our limited *in vivo* studies on the acute effects of Δ^9-THC, which point to a greater inhibitory action on the mitochondrial enzyme preparations from brain than from heart tissue, compared to equivalent potency *in vitro,* are suggestive of a preferential access of the drug to the central nervous system. The hypertrophy of liver and kidney noted at the low dose suggests that enhanced detoxification may contribute to the normalization of circulating plasma or corticosterone levels with time. Dewey *et al.* observed no decline in the ascorbic acid–depleting response after the 5th day of chronic daily IP administration of 1 or 5 mg/kg [6].

In normal rats, the levels of corticosterone rose 5-fold 1 hr after the first injection of 3 mg/kg, i.e., when the blood pressure in female ARH rats drops precipitously by 40 mmHg [3]; the rise in corticosterone levels then declines with time as does the acute, 1-hr response in blood pressure. Thus, these two parameters are inversely related, assuming that female ARH rats respond to acute doses in the same manner as normal rats; this may not be entirely the case since the plasma levels of ARH rats were higher to start with and tended to decline below normal values after chronic administration of Δ^9-THC. If this latter tendency is a true effect, the chronic decrease in blood pressure could be favored by a lowered secretion of adrenal steroids, including 18–OH–DOC, a mineralocorticoid shown to be hypertensive in the rat and the dog [11,14,-12] and to be seen in hypertensive disease in rat and man [13,9]. A direct inhibitory effect on the basal secretion of 18–OH–DOC at the adrenal level, noted by us *in vitro,* could then be of functional significance.

Summary and Conclusions

Chronic IP administration of Δ^8- and Δ^9-THC for 2 weeks at a dose of 3 mg/kg evokes a sustained reduction in the blood pressure without affecting body weight of rats suffering from adrenal regeneration hypertension. A dose of 20 mg/kg causes marked growth retardation in normal male rats. Δ^9-THC elicits a dramatic increase in plasma corticosterone levels after the first administration, but the response becomes attenuated and appears to be abolished by the 8th day in animals injected with 3 mg/kg/day. *In vitro* studies indicate a potent inhibitory effect of Δ^9-THC on brain metabolism at an amytal-sensitive site; the extent of inhibition varies with the location within the central nervous system. Preliminary experiments suggest that a similar inhibition is also associated with the acute response to Δ^9-THC *in vivo.* The basal production of 18–OH–DOC by the rat adrenal *in vitro* is significantly inhibited by 10^{-5} M Δ^9-THC, but a relationship between the antihypertensive effects of cannabinols and pituitary-adrenal function, if it exists, remains elusive.

ACKNOWLEDGMENTS

It is a pleasure to acknowledge the expert assistance of J. Duhaimes and M. Anger for the experiments on hypertensive rats, and of H. Traikov, I. Truffin, S. and A. D. Duby, Wah-Tung Hum, and K. Sudarshan for the *in vitro* studies and experiments comparing chronic and acute effects of THC.

The research was supported by the Non-Medical Use of Drugs Directorate, Department of Federal Health and Welfare, Canada, and by the Medical Research Council of Canada.

REFERENCES

1. Barry III, H., J. L. Perhach, and R. K. Kubena (1970) Δ^1-tetrahydrocannabinol activation of pituitary adrenal function. *Pharmacologist 12:*323.
2. Bartova, A. and M. K. Birmingham (1974) Site of Δ^9-tetrahydrocannabinol (Δ^9-THC) inhibition in the electron transport chain. *Proc. Can. Fed. Biol. Soc. 17:*18.
3. Birmingham, M. K. (1973) Reduction by Δ^9-tetrahydrocannabinol in the blood pressure of hypertensive rats bearing regenerated adrenal glands. *Br. J. Pharmacol. 48:*169.
4. Birmingham, M. K., M. L. MacDonald and J. G. Rocheford (1968) Adrenal function in normal rats and in rats bearing regenerated adrenal glands. *Functions of the Adrenal Cortex* (K. W. McKerns, ed.) Vol. 2. New York: Appleton-Century-Crofts, pp. 647–689.
5. De Robertis, E., A. P. De Iraldi, G. R. De Lores, A. Salganicoff, and L. Salganicoff (1962) Cholinergic and non-cholinergic nerve endings in rat brain-I. *J. Neurochem. 9:*23.
6. Dewey, W. L., T.-C. Peng, and L. S. Harris (1970) The effect of 1-trans-Δ^9-tetrahydrocannabinol on the hypothalamo-hypophyseal-adrenal axis of rats. *Eur. J. Pharmacol. 12:*382.
7. Glowinski, J. and L. L. Iversen (1966) Regional studies of catecholamines in the rat brain-I. *J. Neurochem. 13:*655.
8. Manning, F. J., J. H. McDonough, T. F. Elsmore, C. Saller and F. J. Sodetz (1971) Inhibition of normal growth by chronic administration of Δ^9-tetrahydrocannabinol. *Science 174:*424.
9. Melby, J. C., S. L. Dale, and T. E. Wilson (1971) 18-hydroxydeoxycorticosterone in human hypertension. *Circ. Res. 28*(II):143.
10. Nahas, G. G., I. W. Schwartz, J. Adamec, and W. M. Manger (1973) Tolerance to Δ^9-tetrahydrocannabinol in the spontaneously hypertensive rat. *Proc. Soc. Exp. Biol. Med. 142:*58.
11. Oliver, J. T., M. K. Birmingham, A. Bartova, M. P. Li, and T. H. Chan (1973) Hypertensive action of 18-hydroxydeoxycorticosterone. *Science 182:*1249.
12. Oliver, J. T., P. Frei, S. Levy, and M. K. Birmingham (1976) The role of 18-hydroxylated steroids in the etiology of hypertension. Comparison of the effects of 18-hydroxydeoxycorticosterone, deoxycorticosterone and aldosterone on blood pressure, saline intake and serum electrolyte levels in intact dogs. *Symposium on the Physiopath-*

ology of Adrenal Cortex. 8th Panamerican Congress of Endocrinology, Buenos Aires, 1974 (in press).

13. Rapp, J. P. and L. K. Dahl (1972) Possible role of 18-hydroxydeoxy-corticosterone in hypertension. *Nature 237:*338.
14. Rapp, J. P., D. K. Knudsen, J. Iwai and L. K. Dahl (1973) Genetic control of blood pressure and corticosterone production in rats. *Circ. Res. 32*(I):139.
15. Sjödén, P.-O., T. U. C. Järbe, and B. Henriksson (1973) Influence of tetrahydrocannabinols (Δ^8-THC and Δ^9-THC) on body weight, food and water intake in rats. *Pharmacol. Biochem. Behav. 1:*395.
16. Skelton, F. R. (1955) Development of adrenal regeneration hypertension and cardiovascular renal lesions during adrenal regeneration in the rat. *Proc. Soc. Exp. Biol. Med. 90:*342.
17. Stoppani, A. O. M., C. M. C. De Brignone, and J. A. Brignone (1968) Structural requirements for the action of steroids as inhibitors of electron transfer. *Arch. Biochem. Biophys. 127:*463.

Marihuana: Biochemical and Cellular Effects

Organic and Developmental Effects

36

The Immune Response and Marihuana

HARRIS ROSENKRANTZ

Introduction

The fermenting fervor of dispute related to contrary marihuana findings continues to diminish the credibility of research efforts in this field. No doubt scientific and public communities desire a rapid resolution of discrepancies in order to assume rational positions on legal aspects of marihuana use. Unfortunately, the pendulum of evidence swings erratically through an arc of harmful to not harmful in critical areas of cannabinoid research. The questions of mental performance, teratogenicity, endocrine dysfunction, and immunological impairment potentially induced by marihuana have at the moment not yielded uniformly conclusive answers. The issues remain of paramount importance since the number of users steadily increases, and the quality of illicit cannabinoid agents is constantly being improved [21].

The contrary results reported for the effects of marihuana and pure cannabinoids on immunological defense mechanisms are being examined. Even before the announcements of an apparent marihuana suppression of the cell-mediated immune response [22,23], several ancillary factors suggested that marihuana might interfere with immunological mechanisms: (1) tobacco smoking was an immunosuppressant of both humoral [6,24,34] and cellular [33,35] immune pathways; (2) marihuana, like tobacco, stimulated the pituitary-adrenal axis [3,21], which could initiate involution of the thymus [3,28], a primary organ of the immune system; (3) cannabinoids have a remarkable affinity for lung tissue [7,28], a major organ of phagocytosis, providing prolonged exposure of drug to macrophages irrespective of route of administration of cannabinoids [7,28]; (4) marihuana has influenced alveolar macrophage structure, function, and mobilization [7,20]; (5) cannabis use has evoked allergic reactions [18,30]; (6) cannabinoids might perform as haptenes because of their nearly complete binding to plasma proteins [3,21]; and (7) cannabinoids have repressed bone marrow

Marihuana: Chemistry, Biochemistry, and Cellular Effects, edited by Gabriel G. Nahas, © 1976 by Springer-Verlag New York Inc.

leukopoiesis [3,13]. Perhaps other indirect evidence exists that has escaped attention.

Of course, despite possible prediction of a physiological or biochemical effect of a drug that has not been tested in a specific cellular process, a direct demonstration of cause and effect is mandatory. However, when direct evidence is obtained and then is unconfirmed or refuted, the resolution of the discrepancy is often difficult. This is the present situation for proof of the interaction of cannabinoids and the immune mechanisms as documented in Table 36.1. Using blood lymphocytes from marihuana users and two types of *in vitro* tests—T-cell rosette formation or incorporation of tritiated thymidine in the presence of a mitogen or particulate antigen—some investigators [4,22] found inhibition of cell-mediated immunity, but others did not [14,36]. A skin test was also negative [32]. On the other hand, mouse skin allografts survived longer [17] and splenic lymphocytes were inhibited by Δ^9-tetrahydrocannabinol (Δ^9-THC) [17]. When the *in vitro* influence of cannabinoids on cellular-mediated immunity was tested, thymidine incorporation into lymphocytes and T-cell rosette formation were suppressed [1,4,5]. The humoral immune response of the blood lymphocytes of marihuana users was not affected. [4,36]. In contrast, splenic lymphocytes from rodents given Δ^9-THC were impaired as determined by three different methods [16,17,27].

The review of the above investigations disclosed a distinction between human and animal studies in that the findings on rodents were consistent. Although immunosuppression of the humoral response was observed after oral administration of Δ^9-THC, it was important to substantiate this finding for marihuana smoke. The present investigation evaluated this potential interaction of marihuana with the humoral immune pathway under conditions simulating marihuana smoking in man through use of an automatic inhalator. The immunosuppression obtained by the inhalation route was similar to that obtained by corresponding oral doses of Δ^9-THC in the same strain of rat.

Methods and Materials

The inhalation and oral studies were independently conducted at different times but employing the same personnel and environmental factors. Fischer rats weighing approximately 110–140 gm were housed in pairs of the same sex in wire suspension cages $7 \times 9.5 \times 7$ inches. Both sexes were used in the inhalation study,

Table 36.1 Cannabinoid effects on the cellular-mediated and humoral immune responses

Cannabinoid	Dose (mg/kg)	Route	Species	Cell type and source	Mitogen or antigen: Route	Mitogen or antigen: Type	Methodology	Finding	Reference
Cellular-mediated immune response									
Marihuana	4 ×/wk[a]	Lungs	Man	Lymphocyte, blood	*In vitro*	SRBC[b]	T-cell rosette	Inhibition	4
	4 ×/wk	Lungs	Man	Lymphocyte, blood	*In vitro*	PHA; MLC[b]	^{3}H-thymidine incorp.	Inhibition	22
	3 ×/wk	Lungs	Man	Lymphocyte, blood	*In vitro*	PHA	^{3}H-thymidine incorp.	No change	36
	3 ×/wk	Lungs	Man		intraderm.	2,4-DNCB[b]	Skin test	No change	32
	1 ×/wk	Lungs	Man	Macrophage, alevoli	none	None	Morphology	Change	20
Marihuana ext.	2 μg/ml	*In vitro*	Man	Leukocyte, blood	none	None	Migration	Inhibition[c]	31
Δ^9-THC	2–22 μM	*In vitro*	Man	Lymphocyte, blood	*In vitro*	PHA	^{3}H-thymidine incorp.	Inhibition	1
		In vitro	Rat	Lymphocyte, spleen	*In vitro*	PHA	^{3}H-thymidine incorp.	Inhibition	1
	$9 \times 10^{-7}M$	*In vitro*	Man	Lymphocyte, blood	*In vitro*	SRBC	T-cell rosette	Inhibition[d]	4
	$2 \times 10^{-4}M$	*In vitro*	Man	Lymphocyte, blood	*In vitro*	PHA; MLC	^{3}H-thymidine incorp.[e]	Inhibition[f]	5
	210 × 14 days	Oral	Man	Lymphocyte, blood	*In vitro*	PHA	^{3}H-thymidine incorp.	No change	14
	$1.6 \times 10^{-5}M$	*In vitro*	Mouse[g]	Lymphocyte, spleen	*In vitro*	Δ^9-THC	^{3}H-thymidine incorp.	Stimulation	23
	50–200	Oral	Mouse	Lymphocyte, spleen	*In vitro*	PHA	^{3}H-thymidine incorp.	Inhibition	17
	50–200	Oral	Mouse		skin	Allograft	Graft survival	Increased	17
	0.3–1.3	IP	Rat	Macrophage, perit.	intraderm.	Adjuvant	Migrat. inhib. factor	Suppressed	8
Humoral immune response									
Marihuana	4 ×/wk	Lungs	Man	Lymphocyte, blood	*In vitro*	SRBC-hemolysin[h]	B-cell rosette	No change	4
	3 ×/wk	Lungs	Man	Lymphocyte, blood	*In vitro*	Pokeweed	^{3}H-thymidine incorp.	No change	36
Δ^9-THC	140	IP	Mouse	Lymphocyte, spleen	IP	SRBC	Plaque formation	Inhibition	16
	25–200	Oral	Mouse	Lymphocyte, spleen	*In vitro*	Lipopoly. B[i]	^{3}H-thymidine incorp.	Inhibition	17
	1–10	Oral	Rat	Lymphocyte, spleen	IP	SRBC	Plaque formation, Serum antibodies	Inhibition	27

[a] Time since last use of marihuana variable.
[b] SRBC = sheep red blood cells; PHA = phytohemagglutinin; MLC = mixed lymphocyte culture (allogeneic cells); 2,4-DNCB = 2,4-dinitrochlorobenzene.
[c] Leukocytes from both marihuana smokers and nonsmokers responded similarly.
[d] Inhibition also induced by cannabinol and cannabidiol.
[e] A decreased incorporation of ^{3}H-leucine and ^{3}H-uridine was also seen.
[f] Inhibition also obtained with various cannabinoids and 11-OH metabolites.
[g] Sensitized to Δ^9-THC.
[h] Trypsinized sheep red blood cells coated with antisheep hemolysin for detection of B-cell C_3 receptor.
[i] *E. coli* lipopolysaccharide B.

but only females were tested in the oral trial. All animals were fed commercial rat chow and water *ad libitum* and were in a room regulated for a 12-hr dark/light circadian cycle and maintained at $23 \pm 2°C$.

Cannabinoid materials and doses

Marihuana cigarettes contained approximately 2.1 percent Δ^9-THC, 0.17 percent cannabidiol, and 0.15 percent cannabinol; corresponding maximum values for marihuana placebo cigarettes were 0.05 percent, 0.01 percent, and 0.01 percent, respectively. Oral preparations were solutions of 96 percent pure synthetic (—)-*trans* Δ^9-THC in USP grade sesame oil; the latter served as vehicle control. All cannabinoids were supplied by the National Institute on Drug Abuse and were stored at 5°C. Before use, cigarettes were maintained at 60 percent humidity and 23°C for 24–48 hr.

The Δ^9-THC doses for both routes of administration were selected to be relative to those consumed by man. This was determined, as outlined in Table 36.2, by expressing doses on the basis of body

Table 36.2 Relevancy of Δ^9-tetrahydrocannabinol doses and routes of administration used in animals as compared to man

	mg/kg Δ^9-THC (marihuana, 1% THC; hashish, 5% THC)		
Route[a]	*Man*[b]	*Rat*[c]	*Mouse*[c]
Inhalation, 1 cig/day	0.1–0.5	0.7–3.5	1–6
3 cigs/day	0.3–1.5	2–10	4–18
6 cigs/day	0.6–3.0	4–20	7–36
Approx. LD50	[d]	36–42	40–60[e]
Oral	0.3–1.5	2–10	4–18
	0.9–4.5	6–30	10–54
	1.8–9.0	12–63	20–100
Approx. LD50	[d]	800–1200	1400–2200

[a] In man, oral route requires 3 times the inhalation dose.

[b] Assumes 50 kg mean body weight and 50% loss of THC during smoking.

[c] Dose based on body surface area; conversion factor of 7 and 12 for rat and mouse, respectively.

[d] As a guide, IV LD50 in monkey was about 100 mg/kg and orally it was estimated to be approximately 15,000 mg/kg.

[e] N value; however, IV and inhalation values in rat shown to be nearly identical.

surface area and encompassing the Δ^9-THC dose range for an average quality of marihuana (1 percent THC) and of hashish (5 percent THC) [26,28]. An average human body weight of 50 kg has been assumed to represent the spectrum of weights of young to older marihuana users. Several investigators have shown that 50 percent of the Δ^9-THC in marihuana is destroyed and/or entrapped in the residual butt during smoking [3,26]. Therefore, 1 percent Δ^9-THC (10 mg/gm) marihuana and 5 percent Δ^9-THC (50 mg/gm) hashish would provide 5 and 25 mg THC, respectively, or 0.1–0.5 mg/kg body weight for each gram of cannabis preparation smoked.

The oral dose in man is approximately 3 times the inhalation dose. Body surface area conversion factors from man to rat and mouse are 7 and 12, respectively. Data are given for these two rodents because they, in addition to man, have been used for immunological studies with marihuana and Δ^9-THC. The relationship of LD50 values to these calculated Δ^9-THC doses in man and actual Δ^9-THC doses used in rodents are included as reference points of efficacy and safety [26]. On the basis of the above considerations, it was decided to use Δ^9-THC inhalation doses of 0.7, 2, and 4 mg/kg and intragastric doses of 1, 5, and 10 mg/kg.

Treatment protocols

The three prerequisites for obtaining meaningful data on the potential interaction of Δ^9-THC and the humoral immune response were: (1) approximation of the type of human smoking conditions; (2) administration of known doses of the drug; and (3) maintenance in the animal model of identical environmental surroundings for the two routes of administration used by man. To achieve these objectives, we compared smoking conditions in the automatic inhalator with smoking procedures used by man, as outlined in Table 36.3. Tobacco users (U.S. brands) generally inhale a 30–40-ml puff volume of 2-sec duration and retain smoke in their lungs for approximately 15 sec before expelling it. A fresh puff is consumed each minute. Tobacco investigators have used the tobacco reference cigarette (University of Kentucky) to calibrate their smoking machines accordingly [26]. The naive marihuana smoker inhales and expires the marihuana smoke similarly to the tobacco smoker. However, the experienced cannabis consumer deviates from these conditions by inspiring approximately a 50–200-ml puff for 8–10 sec and retaining the smoke for 30–60 sec before exhaling [26]. For the present rat inhalation study, a 150-ml puff volume (50 ml from each of 3 cigarettes) was automatically

Table 36.3 Simulation of human marihuana use in rats exposed to marihuana smoke in an automatic smoking machine

Parameter	*Marihuana (NIDA)*	*Placebo (NIDA)*	*Tobacco (Ky ref.)*	*Tobacco (U.S. brands)*
Cigarette weight (gm)	1011 ± 19	861 ± 17	1114 ± 13	1100 ± 15
Total particulates (mg/8 puffs)	24 ± 3	18 ± 3	26 ± 3	2 − 31
Butt length (mm)	33 ± 4	31 ± 2	35 ± 2	35 ± 3
Puff volume (ml/cig)	35 − 200[a]	50 ± 2[b]	35 ± 2	30 − 40
Puff duration (sec)	2 − 15[a]	2 ± 0.1[b]	2 ± 0.1	2 ± 0.1
Exposure interval (sec)	15 − 45[a]	30 ± 0.2[b]	15 ± 0.1	10 − 20
Purge period (sec)	15 − 30[a]	30 ± 0.2[b]	43 ± 0.1	40 − 50

[a] Naive marihuana smoker at lower end and experienced smoker at higher end.

[b] Conditions selected for the rat were a 50-ml puff simultaneously from each of 3 marihuana or placebo cigarettes over a 2-sec puff duration for a 30-sec exposure interval, followed by 30 sec of fresh air each min [7,26].

delivered to a constant-volume smoke chamber by simultaneously smoking 3 marihuana (or placebo) cigarettes. Each minute the cigarettes were puffed for 2 sec, the smoked retained in the inhalator for 30 sec, followed by displacement of the smoke with fresh air for 30 sec. The cycle of events was repeated each minute. The smoking apparatus permitted simultaneous exposure of 8–10 rats [26].

The estimation of Δ^9-THC doses relied on direct and indirect (recovery of Δ^9-THC from total particulates trapped on filter pads inserted between smoked cigarettes and the entrance to animal holders) gas chromatographic analyses of marihuana smoke. Several such determinations on different lots of marihuana cigarettes yielded Δ^9-THC concentrations in smoke of 0.6–0.9 μg/ml after 4 puffs, and 1.8–2.5 μg/ml after 8 puffs by both analytical approaches. No cigarettes were used for more than 8 puffs. When more than 8 puffs were used, additional fresh cigarettes were ignited to replace expended ones without interrupting the automatically controlled smoking sequence. Since the concentration of Δ^9-THC in smoke was known for 4 and 8 puffs, summation of values afforded estimates of smoke Δ^9-THC concentrations in those instances where 12 or 16 puffs were employed. Variation of the puff number permitted variation of Δ^9-THC dose during inhalation.

The Δ^9-THC concentration in smoke was converted to the usual expression of dose (mg/kg) by consideration of the following facts: (1) the rat tidal volume was approximately 0.8 ml; (2) the rat respiration rate was 40–80/30 sec (lower level adjusts for Δ^9-THC–induced hypopnea) (26); (3) each exposure period lasted 30 sec; (4) there were 4, 8, or 16 exposure periods (4, 8, or 16 puffs); and (5) the mean Δ^9-THC smoke concentration was 0.7, 2, and 4 μg/ml for 4, 8, and 16 puffs, respectively. Since the tidal volume was taken as 0.8 ml, the concentration of inspired Δ^9-THC was 0.6, 1.6, and 3.2 μg/ml for 4, 8, and 16 puffs, respectively. Therefore, the concentration of Δ^9-THC in tidal air times the mean respiration rate per exposure times the number of exposures equals the quantity of Δ^9-THC entering the rodent nasal passages. For example, in the instance of 8 puffs, the equation would be 1.6 μg/ml $\times$ 60 respirations $\times$ 8 exposures $=$ 768 μg Δ^9-THC/rat. However, rodents are obligatory nasal breathers, and it has been shown that 50 percent of smoke particulates are filtered out in the rodent nasal turbinates [26]. Of the quantity (50 percent) that reaches the lungs, 80 percent is absorbed into the pulmonary circulation [26]. Therefore, the 768 μg Δ^9-THC/rat is reduced to 307 μg/rat or 0.3 mg/150 gm body weight. This value is converted to 2 mg/kg. Similar calculations for 4 and 16 puffs yield Δ^9-THC inhalation doses of 0.7 and 4 mg/kg, respectively.

The mechanical smoking sequence and doses outlined above were incorporated into the inhalation treatment protocol. Five rats of each sex, after conditioning to the inhalator, were simultaneously exposed once daily during the morning for 5 days to 4, 8, or 16 puffs of marihuana. Control rats were exposed to placebo smoke, while others were sham-treated (placed in the smoking machine but not given smoke). On the first day of exposure, each rat received a single IP injection of 0.5 ml of a 50-percent suspension of washed sheep red blood cells (SRBC) in isotonic saline.

Orally treated female rats (8 per group) received a daily Δ^9-THC dose of 1, 5, or 10 mg/kg, and control animals were given sesame oil (0.5/100 gm body weight) for 5 days. All rats were injected with SRBC in an identical manner to those used in the inhalation study. Δ^9-THC or vehicle was withheld from other control rats in the presence and absence of SRBC in order to estimate efficacy of antigenic stimulation and to determine background levels of functional splenic antibody cells, respectively. Five days after SRBC injection, the animals were decapitated and blood specimens were collected.

Preparation of cells

SRBC were obtained in Alsever's fluid from the same donor sheep for both studies. When used for immunization, SRBC were washed

3 times in isotonic saline. For serological use, SRBC were rinsed 3 times and diluted to a 1-percent suspension in 0.01 *M* phosphate-buffered saline (PBS) at pH 7.3. In the plaque formation test, a 20-percent suspension of washed SRBC in Medium 199 provided SRBC as indicator cells.

Splenic cells were obtained by fragmentation of each teased spleen, suspended in Medium 199, through a mesh-60 grid. Viable splenic lymphocytes were determined by dye exclusion of 0.2 percent trypan blue, and suspensions of 2×10^7/ml viable cells in Medium 199 were used for counting antibody-forming cells (AFC) in the localized hemolysis in gel (LHG) plaque formation test.

Hemochemical and physiological parameters

Medium 199 was used both as a diluent of cells and in the preparation of gels because it improved sensitivity of the LHG method [27]. Gel plates (100×15 mm) consisted of 7.5 ml of 1.2 percent agarose for the lower layer, and after this layer was solidified, the upper layer containing 0.1 ml of 20 percent SRBC and 0.1 ml of 2×10^7/ml viable splenic cells in 0.6 percent agarose was deposited on the lower layer. Gelation proceeded initially for 20 min at 23°C and then for 2 hr at 37°C. When gelation was completed, the surface of the gel was coated with 1 ml of 20 percent guinea pig complement, which had been absorbed with an equal volume of packed SRBC for 60 min at 4°C. After the complement was added, the gel plates were incubated for 50 min at 37°C and excess complement solution was then decanted. The specificity of AFC and the extent of background interference were estimated by preparing gel plates with SRBC or viable splenic cells alone and in the presence or absence of complement. Hemolytic plaques on experimental gel plates were corrected for those counted on control gel plates.

Serum antibody titers (expressed as the reciprocal) to SRBC were measured by a standard hemagglutination (HT) procedure using a microtiter apparatus [27]. Heat-inactivated (30 min at 56°C) sera were serially diluted in PBS, and each dilution received an equal volume of 1 percent SRBC in PBS. After gentle agitation for 50 sec, the reaction plates were incubated for 2 hr at 23°C and the highest dilution having definitive hemagglutination was noted.

A preliminary attempt was made to detect circulating antibodies with a rabbit antiserum to rat IgG in the sera of rats exposed to marihuana smoke. Standard double diffusion commercial gel plates were used.

In addition to the hemochemical procedures, we observed some behavioral and physiological changes. Animals were observed for signs of CNS inhibition or stimulation, and exploratory activity, rectal temperature, and respiration rate were measured. At the beginning of treatment and at autopsy, we recorded body weights and calculated the growth rate from the ratio of final body weight to initial body weight. During necropsy, animals were inspected for gross pathology and wet weights of spleen, thymus, and adrenals were measured.

Results

The experimental design permitted evaluation of the inductive phase of the primary immune response in coincidence with that period of time during which drug tolerance did not develop fully. The credibility of findings relies strongly on concomitant measurements of the number of AFC, HT, and splenic weights by the two routes of cannabinoid administration and at doses used by man. The behavioral and physiologic manifestations substantiated drug expression. The student *t*-test was applied for each parameter.

Behavioral and physiological findings

Generally, Δ^9-THC activity occurred sooner and with more intensity via the inhalation route than the oral route (Table 36.4). In addition, recovery from daily aberrations induced by drug took place more quickly by the inhalation route. After inhalation of marihuana smoke, both sexes displayed a dose-related CNS inhibition and reductions in exploratory activity and respiration rate. Ataxia and incoordination were commonly seen soon after removal from the smoking apparatus. A borderline hypothermia and decrease in growth rate were associated with the high dose. Daily changes were essentially reversed in 4–6 hr. No gross pathology was seen in any animals. A non–dose-related decrease (18–35 percent) in absolute and relative thymus weights occurred for both sexes. There was a 15-percent increase in female adrenal weights at the high dose. Also at the high dose, absolute and relative spleen weights diminished approximately 18 percent.

Intragastric administration of Δ^9-THC initiated behavioral changes 3–4 hr after treatment. The more intense CNS inhibition was expressed as ataxia and incoordination. Only at 10 mg/kg was there a fall in exploratory activity and respiration rate (Table 36.4). A slight increase in rectal temperature and a borderline decrease in growth rate occurred at the high dose. Abnormal signs disappeared

Table 36.4 Behavioral and physiological changes in rats exposed to marihuana smoke or treated orally with Δ^9-THC for 5 days[a]

Δ^9-THC (mg/kg)	CNS inhibition Day in study (left) Change (%) (right)		Exploratory activity Day in study (left) Change (%) (right)		Rectal temperature Day in study (left) Change (%) (right)		Respiration rate Day in study (left) Change (%) (right)		Growth Rate Day in study (left) Change (%) (right)	
Marihuana smoke inhalation										
Placebo	3	+10%	5	−31%[b]	5	±0%	5	−15%	6	− 3%
0.7	3	+ 5	5	−16	5	+4	5	−12	6	+ 4
2	2	+33[b]	3	−48[b]	3	+4	3	−25[b]	6	− 3
4	1	+72[b]	1	−60[b]	3	−3[b]	1	−28[b]	6	− 9[b]
Oral Δ^9-THC										
Vehicle										
1	5	+ 5	5	± 0	5	±0	5	± 0	6	+ 4
5	3	+20[b]	4	−10	5	+1	4	−10	6	+14
10	2	+50[b]	3	−25[b]	3	+5[b]	3	−25[b]	6	−10[b]

[a] Inhalation values were derived from a comparison of values during treatment with those measured before treatment on the same animals; in the oral study, treated values are compared to those of vehicle control.

[b] $p < 0.01$–0.05.

6–8 hr after gavage. No gross pathological changes were found. Thymic and adrenal weights were unchanged. Absolute and relative splenic weights were reduced 11–15 percent at both 5 and 10 mg/kg (Table 36.5).

Hemochemical findings

By and large, the results obtained with each sex exposed to marihuana smoke were similar; therefore, their respective hemochemical data have been combined for presentation in Table 36.5. However, female controls (placebo and sham-treated) tended to have a larger number of AFC than male control rats. In any case, for both sexes, there was a dose-related decline in AFC. The decrease was 61–74 percent in females and 24–75 percent in males as compared to the mean AFC values of placebo and sham-treated groups. The HT values for all control animals (placebo and sham-treated) of both sexes were in close agreement. A dose-related decrease of 22–44 percent was observed for males, but a similar decrement for females was independent of dose. An attempt to identify and quantitate the presence of serum IgG in treated rats using a rabbit antiserum to rat IgG was unsuccessful. In a group of untreated rats (neither sham treated nor exposed to marihuana or placebo smoke), the IgG precipitin reaction was clearly detectable up to serum dilutions of 1:32.

In the oral study, AFC was reduced 56–78 percent, and HT was decreased 48–66 percent at all doses (Table 36.5).

Discussion

Despite the discrepancy of findings on marihuana's influence on the immune processes in man, it has been demonstrated in this study by parallel changes in three parameters that relevant doses of marihuana and Δ^9-THC in the rat are immunosuppressant. By both preferred routes of administration used by human cannabinoid consumers, the primary immune response to SRBC was inhibited. As many precautions as possible were taken to obtain reliable results. The inbred Fischer rat strain meets the NIH standards of immunogenetic homogeneity (monitored at Charles River Breeding Laboratories by riciprocal skin homografting) and has a remarkably low incidence of pulmonary disease (essential for inhalation studies). The drug doses used were not lethal or intoxicating to the point of irreversible debilitation. The inhalation exposure conditions were reliably reproducible. The contribution of carbon monoxide toxicity

Table 36.5 Marihuana smoke inhalation and oral Δ^9-THC suppression of the humoral immune response in rats

Δ^9-THC (mg/kg)		*Antibody-forming cells ($\times 10^6$) (mean ± SD)*		*Hemagglutination titer (recip. of dil.) (mean ± SD)*		*Spleen weight) (mg/100 gm FBW (mean ± SD)*	
Inhalation	*Oral*	*Inhalation*	*Oral*	*Inhalation*	*Oral*	*Inhalation*	*Oral*
plac.	veh.	145 ± 41	189 ± 27	209 ± 52	185 ± 21	276 ± 29	297 ± 12
0	0	155 ± 23	165 ± 17	204 ± 49	184 ± 17	236 ± 23	303 ± 16
0.7	1	69 ± 35	57 ± 7[a]	147 ± 65	69 ± 9[a]	252 ± 25	311 ± 7
2	5	60 ± 40[a]	84 ± 12[a]	131 ± 52[a]	98 ± 11[a]	264 ± 28	266 ± 5[a]
4	10	34 ± 24[a]	43 ± 9[a]	123 ± 49[a]	63 ± 9[a]	227 ± 23[a]	255 ± 9[a]

[a] $p < 0.05$–0.01 as compared to controls; there were 8–10 rats per group (equal numbers of both sexes in the inhalation study).

was virtually eliminated by using a single daily exposure, by providing fresh air for one-half of each exposure cycle, and by restricting the number of marihuana puffs to a quantity that did not cause death when the tobacco reference cigarette was used. The immunity investigation was confined to 5 days, a time for optimal expression of AFC and HT responses to SRBC in the Fischer rat [27]. Finally, any criticism as to the use of SRBC as a suitable antigenic stimulant for B-cell proliferation and maturation may be countered by the recent report of similar findings of Δ^9-THC inhibition of the humoral response to *E. coli* lipopolysaccharide B [17].

Although the present study evaluated the inductive phase of the primary immune response, it has been demonstrated that the productive phase is also impaired by oral Δ^9-THC [27]. In order to interpret the suppression of both the inductive and productive phases of the humoral pathway, it would seem reasonable to infer that the early processing of antigenic information is implicated. At least, in part, the initial step of phagocytizing particulate antigen by lung, liver, and splenic macrophages may be involved. The macrophage processing of antigen is a prerequisite for stimulation of immunocyte maturation and proliferation. Cannabinoids could interfere with macrophage function through causing structural alterations, inhibiting biochemical pathways, or altering transport mechanisms. Others have reported structural and functional changes in alveolar macrophages in marihuana smokers and in rodents and lung explant cultures treated with cannabinoids [3,7,8,20,28]. It has been postulated that altered lysosomal integrity could explain reduced cellular immunity [12]. Cannabinoids have been shown to affect cell membranes and transport in erythrocytes, bull spermatozoa, iris cells, and ileal cells [9,10,15,25]. Mitochondrial energy metabolism during antigenic processing must be sustained. Although there is no direct evidence for changes in macrophage mitochondria, Δ^9-THC has impaired mitochondrial function in hepatocytes [2,19].

Whereas the administration of Δ^9-THC orally established a definitive situation of cause and effect, the inhalation of marihuana smoke presented a more complex situation. One must contend with both the cannabinoid content and the physicochemical properties of the pyrolytic products. Research findings on tobacco smoke have shown that the immune system is affected by noncannabinoid smoke ingredients. Cigarette smoke suppressed the cellular immune pathway and the primary and secondary immune humoral responses, depressed the number and function of splenic plaque-forming cells, and inhibited macrophage protein synthesis [6,11,24,29,33–35].

In many instances, chronic exposures were performed in the evaluation of both arms of the immune mechanism. However, in the present study, subacute exposure to placebo smoke did not inhibit the humoral response, implicating cannabinoids more strongly as immunosuppressants.

Perhaps it is appropriate to comment on the unresolved disagreement on a potential cannabinoid effect on man's immune systems. Clinical investigators have tried to establish the general health, use of noncannabinoid drugs, and frequency of marihuana consumption. On the other hand, the environmental setting, the Δ^9-THC content of the cannabis (a variation from a trace quantity to 3 percent depending upon country of origin), and actual previous use of marihuana remain questionable variables.

It seems reasonable to conclude that pure Δ^9-THC, at reasonable doses, is immunosuppressive in rodents and that cannabinoids in marihuana smoke have a similar effect since placebo marihuana smoke did not elicit an equivalent inhibition. The inability to detect a reduction in the release of IgG during the primary immune response may have been due, in part, to the fact that IgM is the first immunoglobulin to be released in the primary immune response. Documentation is sufficient to encourage continued investigation of cannabis constituents in the area of immunobiology and immunochemistry. The important consideration of the role of immunosuppression in relationship to tolerance and other adaptive processes seen for other physiological parameters during prolonged treatment with Δ^9-THC or marihuana smoke must be entertained.

ACKNOWLEDGMENTS

The author expresses his appreciation to Dr. Henry J. Esber, Dr. Miasnig Hagopian, Andrew J. Miller, Rosa A. Sprague, and Jeffrey Grant for collaborative efforts. Special thanks are extended to Dr. Monique C. Braude and the National Institute on Drug Abuse for supplies of cannabinoids and financial support under NIH Grant No. DA 00932–01.

REFERENCES

1. Armand, J.-P., J. T. Hsu, and G. G. Nahas (1974) Inhibition of blastogenesis of T lymphocytes by delta-9-THC. *Fed. Proc. 33:*539.
2. Bino, T., A. Chari-Bitron, and A. Shahar (1972) Biochemical effects and morphological changes in rat liver mitochonchia exposed to Δ^1-tetrahydrocannabinol. *Biochim. Biophys. Acta 288:*195–202.
3. Braude, M. C. and S. Szara (eds.) (1975) *The Pharmacology of Marihuana.* New York: Raven Press.

4. Cushman, P. and R. Khurana (1975) Effects of marihuana smoking and tetrahydrocannabinol on T-cell rosettes. *Fed. Proc. 34:*783.
5. DeSoize, B., J. Hsu, G. G. Nahas, and A. Morishima (1975) Inhibition of human lymphocyte transformation in vitro by natural cannabinoids and olivetol. *Fed. Proc. 34:*783.
6. Esber, H. J., F. F. Menninger, Jr., A. E. Bogden, and M. M. Mason (1973) Immunological deficiency associated with cigarette smoke inhalation by mice: primary and secondary hemagglutinin response. *Arch. Environ. Health 27:*99–104.
7. Fleischman, R. W., R. A. Sprague, D. W. Hayden, M. C. Braude, and H. Rosenkrantz (1975) Chronic marihuana inhalation toxicity in rats. *Toxicol. Appl. Pharmacol 34:*467–478.
8. Gaul, C. C. and A. Mellors (1975) Delta-9-tetrahydrocannabinol and decreased macrophage migration inhibition activity. *Res. Commun. Chem. Pathol. Pharmacol. 10:*559–564.
9. Gibermann, E., S. Gothilf, A. Shahar, and T. Bino (1975) Effects of Δ^9-tetrahydrocannabinol on the membrane permeability of bull spermatozoa to potassium. *J. Reprod. Fertil. 42:*389–390.
10. Green, K. and J. E. Pederson (1973) Effect of Δ^1-tetrahydrocannabinol on aqueous dynamics and ciliary body permeability in the rabbit. *Exp. Eye Res. 15:*499–507.
11. Holt, P. G. and D. Keast (1973) Cigarette smoke inhalation: Effects on cells of the immune series in the murine lung. *Life Sci. 12:*377–383.
12. Irvin, J. E. and A. Mellors (1975) Δ^9-Tetrahydrocannabinol-uptake by rat liver lysosomes. *Biochem. Pharmacol. 24:*305–306.
13. Johnson, R. J. and V. Wiersema (1974) Effects of a Δ^9-tetrahydrocannabinol (Δ^9-THC) metabolite on bone marrow myelopoiesis. *Res. Commun. Chem. Pathol. Pharmacol. 8:*393–396.
14. Lau, R. J., C. B. Lerner, D. G. Tubergen, N. Benowitz, E. F. Domino and R. T. Jones (1975) Non-inhibition of phytohemagglutinin (PHA) induced lymphocyte transformation in humans by Δ^9-tetrahydrocannabinol (Δ^9-THC). *Fed. Proc. 34:*783.
15. Laurent, B., P. E. Roy, and L. Gailis (1974) Inhibition by Δ^1-tetrahydrocannabinol of a sodium-potassium ion transport ATPase from rat ileum. *Can. J. Physiol. Pharmacol. 52:*1110–1113.
16. Lefkowitz, S. S. and C. Yang (1975) Drug induced immunosuppression of the plaque forming cell response. 75th Meeting, Am. Soc. Microbiol., p. 81.
17. Levy, J. A., A. E. Munson, L. S. Harris, and W. L. Dewey (1975) Effects of Δ^9-THC on the immune response of mice. *Fed. Proc. 34:* 782.
18. Liskow, B., J. L. Liss, and C. W. Parker (1971) Allergy to marihuana. *Ann. Intern. Med. 75:*571–573.
19. Mahoney, J. M. and R. A. Harris (1972) Effect of Δ^9-tetrahydrocannabinol on mitochondrial processes. *Biochem. Pharmacol. 21:* 1217–1226.
20. Mann, P. E. G., A. B. Cohen, T. N. Finley, and A. J. Ladman (1971) Alveolar macrophages. Structural and functional differences between non-smokers and smokers of marijuana and tobacco. *Lab. Invest. 25:*111–120.

21. *Marihuana and Health.* (1974) Fourth Report to the U.S. Congress, Department of Health, Education and Welfare Publ. No. (ADM) 75–181, pp. 1–152.
22. Nahas, G. G., N. Sucia-Foca, J.-P. Armand, and A. Morishima (1974) Inhibition of cellular mediated immunity in marihuana smokers. *Science 183:*419–420.
23. Nahas, G. G., D. Zagury, I. W. Schwartz and M.-D. Nagel (1973) Evidence for the possible immunogenicity of Δ^9-tetrahydrocannabinol (THC) in rodents). *Nature 243:*407–408.
24. Nulsen, A., P. G. Holt, and D. Keast (1974) Cigarette smoking, air pollution, and immunity. Model system. *Infect. Immun. 10:*1226–1229.
25. Raz, A., A. Schurr, and A. Livne (1972) The interaction of hashish components with human erythrocytes. *Biochim. Biophys. Acta 274:* 269–272.
26. Rosenkrantz, H. and M. C. Braude (1974) Acute, subacute and 23-day chronic marihuana inhalation toxicities in the rat. *Toxicol. Appl. Pharmacol. 28:*428–441.
27. Rosenkrantz, H., A. J. Miller, and H. J. Esber (1976) Δ^9-Tetrahydrocannabinol suppression of the primary immune response in rats. *J. Toxicol. Environ. Health 1:*119–125.
28. Rosenkrantz, H., R. A. Sprague, R. W. Fleischman, and M. C. Braude (1975) Oral Δ^9-tetrahydrocannabinol toxicity in rats treated for periods up to six months. *Toxicol. Appl. Pharmacol. 32:*399–417.
29. Roszman, T. L., L. H. Elliott, and A. S. Rogers (1975) Suppression of lymphocyte function by products derived from cigarette smoke. *Am. Rev. Respir. Dis. 111:*453–456.
30. Schapiro, C. M., A. R. Orlina, P. Unger, and A. A. Billings (1974) Antibody response to cannabis. *J.A.M.A. 230:*81–82.
31. Schwartzfarb, L., M. Needle, and M. Chavez-Chase (1974) Dose-related inhibition of leukocyte migration by marihuana and Δ^9-tetrahydrocannabinol (THC) in vitro. *J. Clin. Pharmacol. 14:*35–41.
32. Silverstein, M. J. and P. J. Lessin (1974) Normal skin test responses in chronic marijuana users. *Science 186:*740–741.
33. Thomas, W. R., P. G. Holt, and D. Keast (1973) Cellular immunity in mice chronically exposed to fresh cigarette smoke. *Arch. Environ. Health 27:*372–375.
34. Thomas, W. R., P. G. Holt, and D. Keast (1973) Effect of cigarette smoking on primary and secondary humoral responses in mice. *Nature 243:*240.
35. Thomas, W. R., P. G. Holt, and D. Keast (1974) Recovery of immune system after cigarette smoking. *Nature 248:*358–359.
36. White, S. C., S. C. Brin, and B. W. Janicki (1975) Mitogen-induced blastogenic responses of lymphocytes from marihuana smokers. *Science 188:*71–72.

37

Teratologic Effects of Cannabis Extracts in Rabbits: A Preliminary Study

ETIENNE FOURNIER, EDY ROSENBERG,
NOAH HARDY, AND GABRIEL NAHAS

Introduction

During the past decade, several research groups have investigated the teratogenic effects of marihuana extracts in animals. Miras [14] reported that rats that had consumed food containing cannabis extract at a concentration of 0.2 percent for several months had diarrhea and a reduced growth rate. He further stated that these animals, upon being bred, showed a significant reduction in fertility. However, their offspring appeared normal in all aspects through the first 90 days. Persaud and Ellington [19] reported that *C. sativa* resin 4.2 mg/kg body weight produced teratogenic effects in rats when administered in days 1 to 6 of gestation. They observed a high incidence of malformed fetuses, increase of fetal resorption, decrease of fetal weight and size, and a high incidence of abnormalities: syndactyly, encephalocele, phocomelia, amelia, and abdominal viscera eventration. Gerber and Schramm [3] administered doses of cannabis extracts of 250 or 500 mg/kg to guinea pigs and rabbits, and they also reported various congenital malformations. Pace, Davis, and Borgen [18] studied the effects of Δ^9-tetrahydrocannabinol (Δ^9-THC) on rats and guinea pigs injected subcutaneously with 0.1–100 mg/kg. They found no teratogenic effects due to THC in the rats or guinea pigs. Using tagged Δ^9-THC, they also observed its passage through the placenta. Their study was confirmed by that of Idänpään-Heikkilä *et al.* [6], who reported that Δ^9-THC passes through the placental membrane 30 min after its intraperitoneal administration. These authors suggested that the marihuana extracts might include other teratogenic substances besides THC. They also stated that similar experimental tests should be conducted on the rabbit.

Marihuana: Chemistry, Biochemistry, and Cellular Effects, edited by Gabriel G. Nahas, © 1976 by Springer-Verlag New York Inc.

Because of these conflicting reports, the U.S. National Institute on Drug Abuse (NIDA) conducted studies with pregnant rats and rabbits with levels of THC markedly lower than those used in previous experiments, but at a range 10–100 times the "effective human dose."

At those levels, the NIDA studies confirmed the finding that marihuana did not appear to have serious deleterious effects during pregnancy on the fetus or the mother, or, after birth, on the newborn [4,10]. In a recent review of this data, Rosenkrantz and Braude [20] reaffirmed the generally negative findings of reproductive damage to the offspring of experimental animals given behaviorally "effective dose levels." However, Mantilla-Plata, Clewe, and Harbison [12] reaffirmed that at high dose levels, marihuana was teratogenic in mice and rabbits and suggested that such information made it essential to establish parameters for the possible production of abnormality in man based on similar animal experiments. Thomas [22] reported teratological effects on the zebra fish (*Brachidanio rerio*) embryo exposed to 2 ppm of Δ^9-THC. Sassenrath and Chapman [21] reported that two of the offspring of macaques treated daily with 2.4 mg/kg orally for 1 yr were abnormal: both were small; one female infant died at birth with hydrocephalus and myocardial degeneration; and the surviving male had persistent behavioral hyperactivity.

This chapter reports the initial results of our investigation of the teratogenic effects of cannabis extracts in the rabbit.

Methods

Capsules of cannabis resin extract containing 44 mg THC were administered orally. Chromatographic analysis of the unesterified oil indicated a mixture of Δ^8- and Δ^9-THC in a 5:1 proportion. One or two capsules per day, corresponding to 15 or 30 mg/kg body weight, of THC were administered to 2 groups of ten 6-month-old rabbits of 3 kg average weight. A third group of 20 rabbits served as control. The females were mated with 2 different untreated males. THC treatment was begun 5 days after copulation, when egg implantation had already occurred. The females were treated for 8 days, from the 5th through the 12th day after copulation, according to the technique described by Tuchman-Duplessis [23]. Throughout gestation, the animals' weight and food consumption were measured and the rabbits were frequently observed. Urine was collected and analyzed for detection of cannabis products.

On day 28, half the animals in each group were sacrificed after the fetuses had been delivered by cesarean section. The other half were left to deliver spontaneously. In the group of animals in which cesarean section was performed, we noted the number and position of macerated, living, and dead fetuses, as well as those of resorption nodules and of corpora lutea in the ovaries. The weights of the fetuses and of the placentas were also recorded. All the fetuses were observed macroscopically, and a third of them were examined histologically according to Wilson's method [25]. The carcasses of the remaining two-thirds were examined by coloration with alizarine red and decoloration with glycerin.

For the animals born normally, we observed the number of living and dead offspring at birth, the degree of cannibalism, the number of offspring that died after birth, and the average weights on days 4 and 30. On day 21 after birth, dorsoventral and lateral x-ray films of the offspring were taken.

Cannabis detection in the rabbits' urine

Twenty four hour urine collection was made in the animals treated with cannabis. A 5-ml aliquot was extracted in petroleum ether and ethyl ether for THC and cannabinol detection. THC is largely metabolized into 7-OH-THC, which is extractable by ether in the presence of acid pH and is turned into cannabinol by sulfonic paratoluene acid. Cannabinol is then revealed by thin-layer chromatography.

Results

Congenital abnormalities in control group of test animals

Since this study involves only one species of animal, we will first recall our observations on *fauve de Bourgogne* rabbits collected from 25 series of teratological examinations, conducted on a total of 1850 control females, which constitute our fundamental laboratory statistical references (Tables 37.1 and 37.2).

We observed three categories of abnormalities with the following incidence:

1. Variants with no pathological character	*Percent*
Stunted central ossification	5.5
Stunted interparietal ossification	9.6
Stunted suboccipital ossification	9.3

Table 37.1 Percentage of abnormalities in offspring of reference groups of rabbits

After cesarean section of 925 pregnant animals

	Normal fetuses	*Resorption nodules*	*Deaths at birth*	*Abnormalities observed*
Total	7070 (8 per litter)	499	363	58
% of total		7.06	5.13	0.82

After normal delivery of 925 pregnant animals

	Normal offspring	*Deaths at birth*	*Cannibalism*	*Deaths after birth*	*Abnormalities observed*
Total	7361 (8 per litter)	307	539	830	12
% of total		4.20	4.32	11.28	0.16

Table 37.2 Abnormalities observed in 14,431 offspring of 1850 normal untreated rabbits

Minor		
Harelip	6	
Harelip with cleft palate	5	
Eventration	3	
Umbilical hernia	4	
Paw subluxation	15	
Spina bifida	4	
No tail	2	
Defective ear implantation	1	
Anus and bladder fistula	1	
Partial anonychia	2	
Total	43	0.3%
Major		
Partial lack of the dome of the skull with hernia of the cerebral substance	8	
Anencephalia	4	
Hydrocephalus	2	
Ateloprosopia	2	
Agenesis of the inferior maxilla with ateloglossia	2	
Phocomelia	1	
Atelorachidia + atelomyelia	2	
Diplomyelia	2	
Syndactyly	2	
Pulmonary atelectasia	1	
Atelostomia	1	
Total	27	0.2%

	Percent
Costal fusion	3.0
Existence of 13th rib	2.0
Slow-growing ossification of the sternum	60–70
2. Minor congenital abnormalities (Table 37.2)	0.3
3. Major congenital malformations (Table 37.2)	0.2

These basic observations allow us to evaluate the possible teratogenic effect of drugs. In addition, other factors observed are as important as the abnormalities for interpreting the teratogenic potential of a drug. These factors are total number and weight of fetuses per litter; and the presence and number of resorption nodules, macerated or dead fetuses, live fetuses, and animals living after parturition.

Rabbits treated with cannabis products

Effects of cannabis treatment on gestating animals

All the animals lost weight during the 7 first days of gestation (Figure 37.1). At fourteen days, they had resumed their former weights, and in all three groups, weight increase occurred from day 14 to day 28. The average weights of the treated animals and of the controls before parturition were comparable. The quantity of food consumed by the three groups of animals was the same. The treated animals did not present any observable neurological or behavioral abnormalities; however, they appeared to be a little drowsy in the first few days of treatment. Cannabinoid derivatives, especially

Figure 37.1. Mean weight change of pregnant rabbits (*fauve de Bourgogne*).

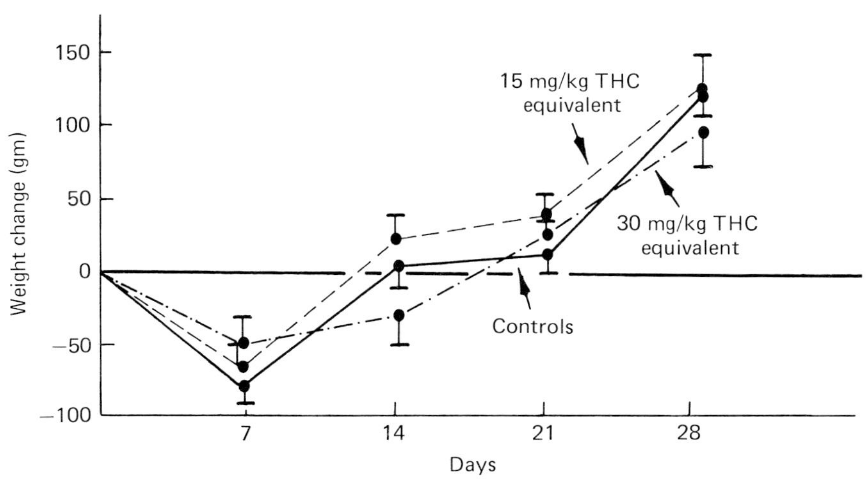

Table 37.3 Incidence of abnormalities in offspring of rabbits after cesarean section

	Control	*15 mg/kg THC*	*30 mg/kg THC*
Pregnant animals (no.)	10	10	10
Fetuses alive (no.)	74	73	60
Corpora lutea (no.)	91	95	77
Resorption nodules (no.)	5	7	6
Fetuses macerated (no.)	3	7	5
Dead fetuses (no.)	2	1	0
Average weights of fetuses (gm)	31.0	27.7	30.1
Average weights of placentas (gm)	5.6	5.3	6.0
Variations	50	45	43
Abnormalities	1	5	3

the 7-hydroxy cannabinol metabolite, were detected in the urine, during the treatment period, indicating intestinal absorption of the preparation used.

Malformations observed after cesarean section (Tables 37.3 and 37.4)

The number of living fetuses per litter was smaller in the 30-mg-THC–treated group. The number of corpora lutea was also smaller for this group of animals. The average fetal weights were comparable in all three groups, as were the average weights of their placentas (5.3–6 gm). The number of resorption nodules was increased in the groups treated with 15 or 30 mg/kg THC. The percentage of macerated fetuses was about 4–5 percent for both the

Table 37.4 Comparative percentage of abnormalities after cesarean section in 4 groups of rabbits

	Reference group	*Control group*	*15 mg/kg THC*	*30 mg/kg THC*
Fetuses alive per litter	8	7	7	6
Resorption nodules	7.1%	6.8%	9.6%	10.0%
Fetuses macerated	5.1%	4.1%	9.6%	8.3%
Abnormalities	0.8%	1.4%	6.9%	5.0%

reference controls and the experimental controls. In the animals treated with THC, the percentage of macerated fetuses was higher: 9.6 for the animals treated with 15 mg/kg, and 8.3 for those treated with 30 mg/kg THC.

Congenital defects at birth (Table 37.5)

In the control group, we noted only one minor congenital malformation: umbilical hernia. In the animals treated with 15 mg/kg THC, we noted a major abnormality (Figure 37.2): a fetus lacking the dome of the skull and the dorsal spine but still having a neural tube; the fetus also had a large eventration. Three other fetuses had important eventrations, and another one had a harelip with a cleft palate. In the rabbits treated with 30 mg/kg, 3 fetuses had congenital abnormalities: 2 had a hip subluxation and 1 a harelip.

These results show an increase of macerated fetuses in the THC-treated group and also a statistically significant increase in congenital malformations. In the 133 living fetuses, we noted 8 abnormalities, an average incidence of 5.3 percent, as compared to a 0.8-percent incidence in our laboratory reference control group. We noted a higher number of abnormalities in the 15 mg/kg THC-treated animals than in those treated with 30 mg/kg THC.

Table 37.5 Congenital malformations in rabbits after cesarean section

			Incidence
Controls	Rabbit 8—fetus 8:	umbilical hernia	1.4%
15 mg/kg THC	Rabbit 3—fetus 5:	lack of brain pan with hernia of the cerebral substance and persistence of the "neural tube"; large eventration	
	fetus 4:	eventration	5.6%
	fetus 5:	eventration	
	Rabbit 7—fetus 8:	harelip with cleft palate	
30 mg/kg THC	Rabbit 3—fetus 1:	harelip	
	Rabbit 7—fetus 5, fetus 6:	hip subluxation	5.0%

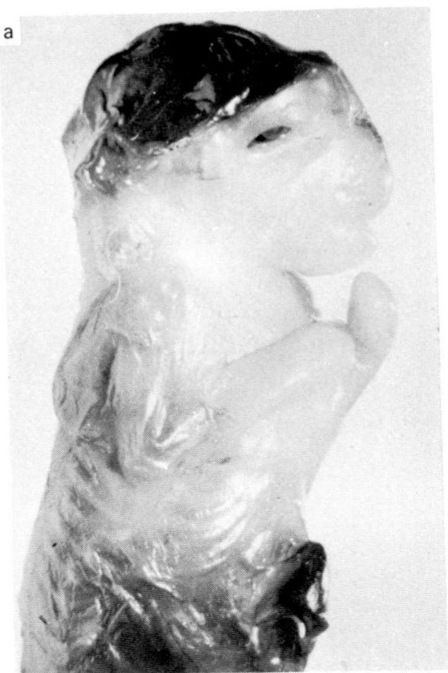

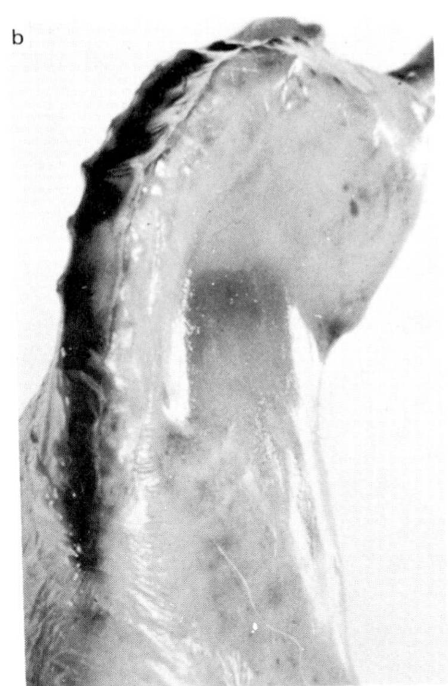

Figure 37.2. Major abnormalities of a fetus removed from a rabbit to which cannabis extract (15 mg THC equivalent per kg) was administered orally from day 5 to day 12 after implantation. Note (a) the absence of dome of skull and the presence of a large eventration; (b) note the absence of spine.

Results observed after normal parturition (Tables 37.6, 37.7, and 37.8)

There was a reduction of normal offspring per litter, especially significant for the treatment group (49), which received 30 mg/kg THC, compared with the control group (60).

Neonatal mortality was higher in the THC-treated group than in the control group. Cannibalism was similar in the different groups. Postnatal mortality was slightly higher in the treated groups.

No malformations were found in the control group, but in each of the treated groups a congenital malformation was observed: a spina bifida in one, and a harelip with a cleft palate in the other. The mean body weights of the pups taken 4 days after birth were 24 and 17 percent lower in the treated groups than in the control. After one month, this was still measurable in the treated groups: the 15- and 30-mg THC equivalent groups were 11.8 and 13.3 percent lighter than the control.

Table 37.6 Incidence of abnormalities in offspring of rabbits after normal delivery

	Controls	*15 mg/kg THC*	*30 mg/kg THC*
Pregnant females	10	10	10
Offspring	68	60	49
Dead at birth	3	7	5
Cannibalism	5	3	3
Dead after birth	7	10	7
Abnormalities	0	1	1
Average weight (gm) 4th day	71	54.3	59.5
Average weight after 1 month (gm)	580	511	503

Table 37.7 Comparative percentage of abnormalities after normal delivery in 4 groups of rabbits

	Reference group	*Control group*	*15 mg/kg*	*30 mg/kg*
Normal offspring per litter	8	7	6	5
Dead at birth	4.2%	4.4%	11.7%	10.2%
Cannibalism	7.3%	7.3%	5.0%	6.1%
Dead after birth	11.3%	10.2%	16.7%	14.3%
Abnormalities	0.1%	0.0%	1.7%	2.0%

Table 37.8 Congenital malformations in rabbits after normal birth

Controls	*Malformation*	*Incidence (%)*
THC 15 mg/kg	Rabbit 5—fetus 7: spina bifida	1.7
THC 30 mg/kg	Rabbit 4—fetus 2: harelip with cleft palate	2.0

Discussion

The mechanism of the teratological effects we observed might be attributed to the inhibitory effect of the natural cannabinoids and their metabolites on DNA, RNA, and protein anabolism [1,11,16]. Our observations confirm those of Mantilla-Plata *et al.* [12] but do not duplicate those of Rosenkrantz and Braude [20]. Such conflicting reports might be accounted for by methodological differences; therefore, uniform criteria should be established for performing and evaluating teratological tests.

The dose of 15–30 mg/kg of cannabinoids orally administered for 8 days to a 3-kg animal amounted to 360–720 mg. Such doses might be considered high when compared with casual human consumption. However, the dose administered did not induce any acute detectable toxic effect, confirming the low somatic toxicity of cannabis products. In addition, because of the rabbit's short gestation, the fetus was exposed to the drug only for relatively short periods of time. In man, exposure time could be increased ninefold. Because of the cumulative properties of the cannabinoids in body fat [9], cannabinoids could accumulate in the human fetus over such a period. Furthermore, since metabolism in small animals is faster than in man, drug doses higher than the human toxic dose are routinely administered in teratological tests.

If the doses administered in the present experiments are higher than those used by casual cannabis smokers, they fall well within the range consumed by habitual consumers. The older literature (WHO Report [1971]) mentions consumption of marihuana preparations of 10–24 gm/day, containing from 200–720 mg THC equivalent. More recent reports [8,13] describe marihuana smokers consuming 20–35 gm of cannabis products per day, equivalent to 400–700 mg of THC, without any toxic effect.

THC is 3 to 5 times [7] more active when absorbed by inhalation than by ingestion (15 mg THC *per os* is equivalent to 5 mg by inhalation). In that case, the highest dose (400–700 mg) that has been inhaled by a 70-kg man without any apparent ill effect would correspond to the ingestion of 1200–2100 mg THC (17–30 mg/kg). This dose, or the "maximal human dose" (dose that can be consumed in 1 day without any apparent toxic effect), is comparable to that which is administered orally to our experimental animals. Teratological tests of drugs intended for chronic use in man have been conducted with doses amounting to between 3 and 10 times the "maximal human dose."

Nevertheless, these experiments cannot be interpreted as direct evidence of the teratological effect of cannabis in man; they indicate only that such an effect is a possibility which should not be overlooked, and which can be documented only by longitudinal epidemiological studies.

ACKNOWLEDGMENTS

We wish to thank Professor Paris, of the Faculty of Pharmacy, for providing the cannabis extracts and for analyzing it for its THC content. These extracts were made available by NIDA (USA) through Professor Braenden, Chief, Technological Laboratory of Narcotics, Geneva, Switzerland.

REFERENCES

1. Blevins, R. D. and J. D. Regan (1976) Δ^9-Tetrahydrocannabinol: effect on macromolecular synthesis in human and other mammalian cells. *Marihuana: Chemistry, Biochemistry, and Cellular Effects* (G. G. Nahas *et al.*, eds.). New York: Springer-Verlag.
2. Desoize, B. and G. G. Nahas (1975) Effet inhibiteur du delta-9-THC sur la synthèse des protéines et des acides nucléiques. *C.R. Acad. Sci.* [D] (Paris) *281:*475.
3. Gerber, W. F. and L. C. Schramm (1969) Effect of marihuana extract on fetal hamsters and rabbits. *Toxicol. Appl. Pharmacol. 14:* 276–282.
4. Haley, S. L., P. L. Wright, J. B. Plank, M. L. Kiplinger, M. C. Braude, and J. C. Calandra (1976) The effect of natural and synthetic delta-9-THC on fetal development. *Toxicol. Appl. Pharmacol.* (in press).
5. Harbison, R. D. (1971) Maternal distribution and placental transfer of 14C delta-9-THC in pregnant mice. *Toxicol. Appl. Pharmacol. 19:*105.
6. Idänpään-Heikkilä, J., G. E. Fritchie, L. F. Englert, B. T. Ho, and W. M. McIsaac (1969) Placental transfer of tritiated delta-9-tetrahydrocannabinol. *N. Engl. J. Med. 281:*330.
7. Isbell, H., G. W. Gorodetsky, D. Jasinski, U. Claussen, F. Spulak, and F. Korte (1969) Effects of (-) delta-9-trans-tetrahydrocannabinol in man. *Psychopharmacologia 14:*115–123.
8. Jones, R. T. (1976) The 30-day trip: clinical studies of cannabis tolerance and dependence. *The Pharmacology of Cannabis* (M. Braude and S. Szara, eds.). Raven Press: New York.
9. Kreuz, D. S. and J. Axelrod (1973) Delta-9-THC: localization in body fat. *Science 179:*391–392.
10. Kiplinger, M. L., P. L. Wright, S. L. Haley, J. B. Plank, M. C. Braude, and J. C. Calandra (1976) The effect of natural and synthetic delta-9-THC on reproductive and lactation performance in albino rats. *Toxicol. Appl. Pharmacol.* (in press).
11. Leuchtenberger, C., R. Leuchtenberger, U. Ritter, and N. Inui (1973) Effects of marihuana and tobacco smoke on DNA and chromosomal complement in human lung explants. *Nature 242:*403–404.

12. Mantilla-Plata, B., G. L. Clewe, and R. D. Harbison (1973) Teratogenic and mutagenic studies of delta-9-tetrahydrocannabinol in mice. *Fed. Proc. 32:*746 abs.
13. Mendelsohn, J. H., J. C. Kuehnle, I. Greenberg, and N. K. Mello (1975) Marihuana use, work and motivation. *The Pharmacology of Cannabis* (M. Braude and S. Szara, eds.). New York: Raven Press.
14. Miras, C. J. (1965) Some aspects of cannabis action. *Hashish: Its Chemistry and Pharmacology* (G. E. W. Wolstenholme and J. Knight, eds.). Boston: Little, Brown and Company, p. 37.
15. Nahas, G. G. (1973) *Marihuana, Deceptive Weed.* New York: Raven Press.
16. Nahas, G. G., G. Desoize, J. P. Armand, J. Hsu, and A. Morishima (1975) Natural cannabinoids: apparent depression of nucleic acids and protein synthesis in cultured human lymphocytes. *Pharmacology of Cannabis* (S. Szara and M. Braude, eds.). New York: Raven Press.
17. Nahas, G. G., N. Sucia-Foca, J. P. Armand, and A. Morishima (1974) Inhibition of cellular mediated immunity in marihuana smokers. *Science 183:*419–420.
18. Pace, H. B., M. Davis, and L. A. Borgen (1971) Teratogenesis and marihuana. Marihuana: chemistry, pharmacology and patterns of social use. *Ann. N.Y. Acad. Sci. 191:*123.
19. Persaud, T. V. N. and A. C. Ellington (1967) Cannabis in early pregnancy. *Lancet II:*1306.
20. Rosenkrantz, H. and M. C. Braude (1975) Comparative chronic toxicities of delta-9-THC administered by inhalation or orally in rats. *The Pharmacology of Cannabis* (M. Braude and S. Szarra, eds.). Raven Press: New York.
21. Sassenrath, E. M. and L. F. Chapman (1975) Tetrahydrocannabinol-induced manifestations of the "marihuana syndrome" in group-living macaques. *Fed. Proc. 34:*1666–1670.
22. Thomas, R. J. (1975) The toxicologic and teratologic effects of delta-9-tetrahydrocannabinol in the zebrafish embryo. *Toxicol. Appl. Pharmacol. 32:*184–190.
23. Tuchman-Duplessis, H. (1972) Teratogenic drug screening—present procedures and requirements. *Teratology 5:*271–285.
24. Tuchman-Duplessis, H. (1973) Teratogenèse medicamenteuse. Interprétation clinique des résultats experimentaux. *Ann. Histochim. 18:* 13–18.
25. Wilson, J. (1965) *Teratology: Principle and Techniques.* Chicago: University of Chicago Press.

38

Alteration of Δ^9-Tetrahydrocannabinol–Induced Prenatal Toxicity by Phenobarbital and SKF-525A

BERNARDO MANTILLA-PLATA AND
RAYMOND D. HARBISON

Introduction

Delta-9-tetrahydrocannabinol (Δ^9-THC) produced embryotoxic and fetotoxic effects when administered to pregnant rats [17] and mice [11,13,18]. These studies showed that a dose-dependent increase in embryo fetotoxicity can be produced. Several other studies have been recently reviewed by Fleischman *et al.* [6]. When administered to pregnant mice at critical times of fetal organogenesis, THC has been shown to induce cleft palate in the fetus [12]. In contrast, a recent study of THC in mice showed no malformations [6]. The different types of vehicles, dosages, routes of administration, and gestational development periods used in these studies have complicated the interpretation and comparability of teratological data.

The alteration of experimental teratogenesis by inhibitors or stimulators of teratogen biotransformation has been a useful means of elucidating teratogenic mechanisms. Posner *et al.* [19] demonstrated that 2-diethylaminoethyl-2,2-diphenylvalerate hydrochloride (SKF-525A) administration reduced chlorcyclizine teratogenesis in rats by inhibiting the formation of its major metabolite, norchlorcyclizine. Harbison and Becker [10] demonstrated that phenobarbital pretreatment reduced and SKF-525A pretreatment increased the teratogenic effect of diphenylhydantoin in mice. Our previous studies have demonstrated that factors that apparently alter the metabolism of THC also influence THC-induced toxicity. Phenobarbital pretreatment antagonized and SKF-525A potentiated THC-induced mortality in mice [15]. These pretreatments also altered the distribution and excretion of THC.

Marihuana: Chemistry, Biochemistry, and Cellular Effects, edited by Gabriel G. Nahas,

The purpose of this study was to determine the influence of vehicle and route of administration on plasma concentration of THC and to determine the effect of phenobarbital and SKF-525A pretreatment on prenatal toxicity, teratogenicity, and placental transfer of THC in mice.

Methods and Materials

Swiss origin mice (ICR strain, Charles River, Wilmington, Massachusetts, or CFW strain, Carworth Farms, Webster, New City, New York) were housed in stainless-steel cages and allowed food (Purina Laboratory Chow) and tap water without restriction. Virgin female mice were housed overnight with males of the same strain, and copulation was ascertained by the presence of a vaginal plug or by the finding of sperm in the vaginal smear; this time was considered day 1 of gestation. Females were separated and housed in groups for treatment.

All drugs were made in a vehicle to deliver the appropriate dosage in a volume of 10 mg/kg of body weight. Control animals received the vehicle solution or no injection.

Phenobarbital-pretreated animals were injected intraperitoneally with phenobarbital sodium at a dosage of 60 mg/kg given twice a day for 4 days, and THC was administered 12–24 hr after the last injection. SKF-525A was administered intraperitoneally at a dosage of 40 mg/kg 1 hr before the injection of THC. Phenobarbital and SKF 525A were dissolved in isotonic saline.

THC (National Institute on Drug Abuse), as 97 percent Δ^9-THC, was mixed with [2,4-^{14}C]-THC to a final dosage of 5 mg (20 μCi)/kg. The plasma concentration of total radioactivity (THC–M) was compared in male mice after intraperitoneal and oral administration of THC in 10 percent Tween-80 and saline (Tween) or corn oil. To measure maternal plasma, placental, and fetal concentrations of THC–M, we suspended THC in Tween and administered it intravenously on gestational day 14. A Packard TriCarb Model 3320 liquid scintillation counter was used to measure radioactivity. Plasma and tissue samples for liquid scintillation counting were collected, prepared, and counted by a previously described method [11]. There is no evidence for metabolic disruption of the ^{14}C-THC molecule and loss of the ^{14}C fragments. Therefore, measurement of ^{14}C permitted quantitation of this moiety. However, no attempt was made to quantitate separately THC and metabolites in these tissues. Results are reported as dpm per 0.5 ml or 100 mg of plasma or tissue and are considered to be THC plus metabolites (THC–M).

To determine the role of drug interaction on THC-induced teratogenic effects, we suspended THC (97 percent Δ^9-THC) in Tween 1 hr before injection and administered it intraperitoneally on gestational days 10–11 or 12–13 at doses of 50 and 200 mg/kg to pregnant mice pretreated with SKF-525A and phenobarbital, respectively. Control pregnant animals received the vehicle solution, the appropriate pretreatment, THC alone, or no injection.

Female body weights were recorded on days of treatment and at the time of cesarean section. Laparotomy was performed on day 19 of gestation, and the following observations were recorded: total number of implantation sites, and number and position of live, dead, and resorbed fetuses. Fetuses were removed, sacrificed, dried on absorbent paper, and individually weighed on a balance, and the weight was expressed in milligrams.

Individual fetuses were examined for external anomalies. Each litter was divided into two subgroups. Fetuses in one subgroup were fixed in Bouin's solution, sectioned by hand with a razor blade, and examined with a dissecting microscope for internal anomalies by the method of Barrow and Taylor [1]. Fetuses in the other subgroup were fixed in 95 percent ethanol, then they were cleared and stained with alizarin red S by the method of Dawson [5]. Stained skeletons were examined under a dissecting microscope for skeletal defects.

Frequencies of anomalies and resorptions were evaluated by the binomial expansion method [8]. All other statistical evaluations were made by the two-tailed grouped t-test. The level of significance in all cases was $p < 0.05$.

Results

Effects of route of administration and vehicle on plasma concentration of THC

The vehicle and the route of administration affected the absorption of THC–M. THC administered in oil is less available than in Tween (Figure 38.1). Absorption after IP administration in Tween is rapid and plasma disappearance slow. The plasma disappearance of THC–M was similar after IP or oral administration of THC in corn oil. The IP route produced significantly higher THC–M concentrations than that after oral administration.

The effects of SKF-525A and phenobarbital pretreatment on

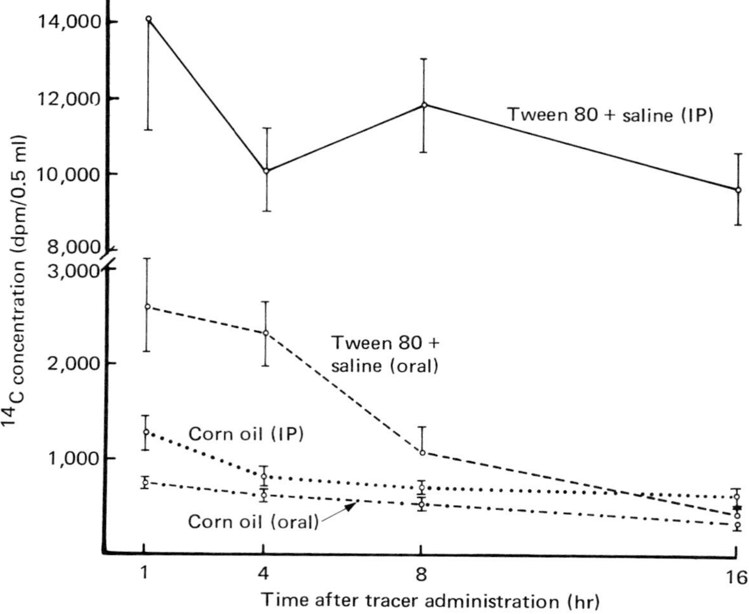

Figure 38.1. Effects of route of administration and vehicle on plasma concentration of THC plus metabolites. The dosage of ^{14}C-THC was 5 mg (20 μCi)/kg. Each point on the graph represents the mean of 10 male mice.

THC-induced teratogenesis are summarized in Table 38.1. In the dosages and pretreatment schedules used, THC was not lethal to any pregnant female.

Prenatal deaths

THC significantly increased the incidence of resorption over the control level when administered on gestational days 10–11 at a dosage of 50 mg/kg or after 200 mg/kg during gestational days 10–11 or 12–13 (Table 38.1). The vehicle control of Tween was administered on gestational days 8–13 and induced an 8-percent fetal resorption rate. SKF-525A administered under a similar treatment schedule induced 16 percent resorptions (Table 38.1). However, only the pretreatment control group received this subchronic treatment with SKF-525A. The test animals received a single injection of SKF-525A before THC administration. The pretreatment with SKF-525A potentiates THC-induced fetal resorption rates after treatment on gestational days 10–11 or 12–13. The

Table 38.1 Effects of SKF-525A and phenobarbital on THC-induced teratogenesis

Treatment	*THC (mg/kg)*	*Gestational age*[a]	*% resorption* ± SE[b]	*Mean fetal body weight (gm* ± SE)[c]	*% cleft palate* ± SE[d]
Vehicle	0	8–13	7.8 ± 1.4	1.22 ± 0.01	1.2 ± 0.8
SKF[e]	0	8–13	16.5 ± 1.9[g]	1.23 ± 0.01	1.3 ± 0.9
PB[f]	0	6–9	10.9 ± 2.6	1.22 ± 0.02	0
THC	50	10,11	23.0 ± 4.5[g]	1.05 ± 0.02[g]	5.9 ± 4.0
THC + SKF	50	10,11	66.7 ± 5.8[g,h]	1.04 ± 0.02[g]	10.0 ± 9.0[g]
THC	50	12,13	9.2 ± 2.9	1.15 ± 0.01[g]	0
THC + SKF	50	12,13	66.4 ± 4.0[g,h]	1.04 ± 0.03[g,h]	36.4 ± 10.2[g,h]
THC	200	10,11	33.6 ± 4.0[g]	1.09 ± 0.02[g]	0
THC + PB	200	10,11	35.4 ± 3.5[g]	1.17 ± 0.01[g,h]	8.2 ± 7.8[g,h]
THC	200	12,13	26.7 ± 6.6[g]	1.08 ± 0.02[g]	4.8 ± 2.7
THC + PB	200	12,13	37.5 ± 6.5[g]	1.12 ± 0.02[g,h]	76.5 ± 10.3[g,h]

[a] The day of treatment of the mother.

[b] Mean % of fetuses from 8–15 pregnant mice.

[c] Fetuses from 8–15 pregnant mice.

[d] Mean % of surviving fetuses examined for internal anomalies from 8–15 pregnant mice.

[e] SKF-525A, 40 mg/kg, 1 hr before THC administration.

[f] Phenobarbital, 60 mg/kg, twice a day for 4 days.

[g] Significant, $p < 0.05$, with respect to vehicle control.

[h] Significant, $p < 0.05$, with respect to THC-treated group.

in utero organism is more sensitive to this interaction during late organogenesis or gestational days 12–13. Pretreatment with phenobarbital did not modify the incidence of THC-induced fetal resorptions.

Fetal body weight

THC significantly reduced the body weight of surviving fetuses when compared to control groups (Table 38.1). Fetal body weight of the vehicle control group (1.22 gm) did not differ significantly from that of the control animals receiving no injection. Administration of SKF-525A or phenobarbital alone did not alter body weight when compared to control groups. Administration of THC, 50 mg/kg, on gestational days 10–11 or days 12–13 significantly reduced the fetal body weight to approximately 1.05 and 1.15 gm, respectively. SKF-525A pretreatment enhanced THC-induced reduction of fetal body weight. The greater response after this pretreatment was seen during late organogenesis, or gestational days 12–13. There was a 14-percent reduction in fetal body weight when compared to control group.

Phenobarbital pretreatment partially antagonized THC-induced reduction of fetal body weight seen after THC administration at 200 mg/kg on gestational days 10–11 or 12–13 (Table 38.1). The body weights of these groups were 1.09 gm and 1.08 gm, respectively. The greater protection after phenobarbital pretreatment was seen during gestational days 10–11. The body weight of this group was 1.17 gm (2.7 percent lower than the vehicle control). Thus, phenobarbital pretreatment antagonized and SKF-525A enhanced THC-induced reduction of fetal body weight.

Anomalies

The skeltons of surviving fetuses showed no defects that could be attributed to THC or its interaction with either SKF-525A or phenobarbital.

Administration of THC at a dosage of 50 mg/kg on gestational days 12–13 or at a dosage of 200 mg/kg on days 10–11 did not induce cleft palate. However, THC 50 mg/kg administered on days 10–11 and THC 200 mg/kg administered on days 12–13 did produce a 5–6-percent incidence of cleft palate (Table 38.1). Administration of SKF-525A or phenobarbital alone failed to induce cleft palate. SKF-525A pretreatment on days 10–11 increased the incidence of THC-induced cleft palate from about 6 percent to 10 percent. On days 12–13, although the incidence of cleft palate in the groups receiving THC alone was negligible, pretreatment with SKF-525A potentiated the incidence of THC-induced cleft palate from 0 to 36 percent (Table 38.1). Phenobarbital pretreatment on days 10–11 increased the incidence of cleft palate from 0 to 8 percent. Treatment on days 12–13 significantly potentiated the incidence of THC-induced cleft palate from 5 percent to 77 percent (Table 38.1). Conversely to the effect on acute toxicity, both phenobarbital and SKF-525A pretreatment potentiated the teratogenicity of THC.

Distribution of THC

The effects of phenobarbital and SKF-525A on plasma concentration of THC-M are shown in Figure 38.2. EKF-525A pretreatment resulted in statistically significantly higher plasma con-

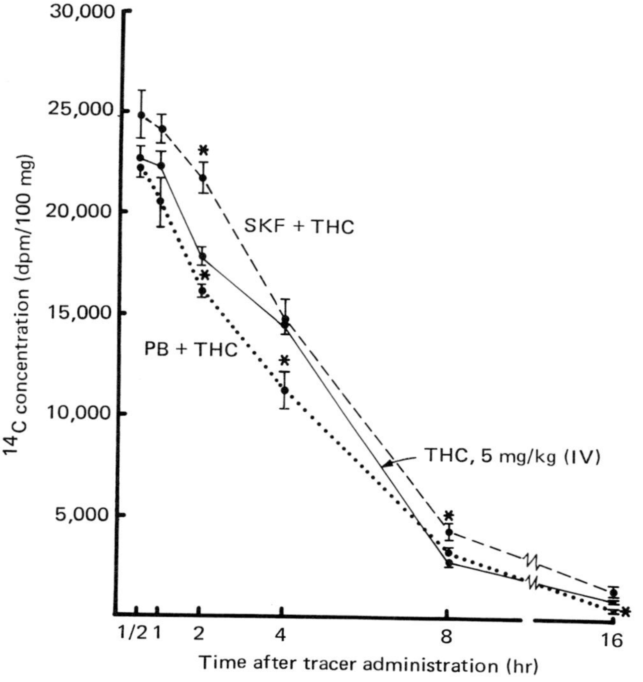

Figure 38.2. Effects of SKF-525A and phenobarbital on plasma concentrations of THC-M. Each point on the graph represents the mean of 6–8 pregnant mice. Asterisk indicates a significant difference ($p < 0.05$) from THC alone.

centrations of THC-M at 1, 2, and 8 hr after THC administration; on the other hand, phenobarbital pretreatment significantly reduced the plasma concentration of THC-M at 2, 4, and 16 hr after THC administration when compared to untreated animals. These data demonstrate that phenobarbital and SKF-525A can alter the total plasma concentration of THC plus metabolites.

The distribution of THC to the placenta is shown in Figure 38.3. SKF-525A pretreatment increased the concentration and prolonged the disappearance of THC-M from placental tissue. Conversely, phenobarbital pretreatment increased the disappearance and decreased the concentration of THC-M in placental tissue. The level of THC-M in placental tissues affected the transfer of THC-M to the fetus.

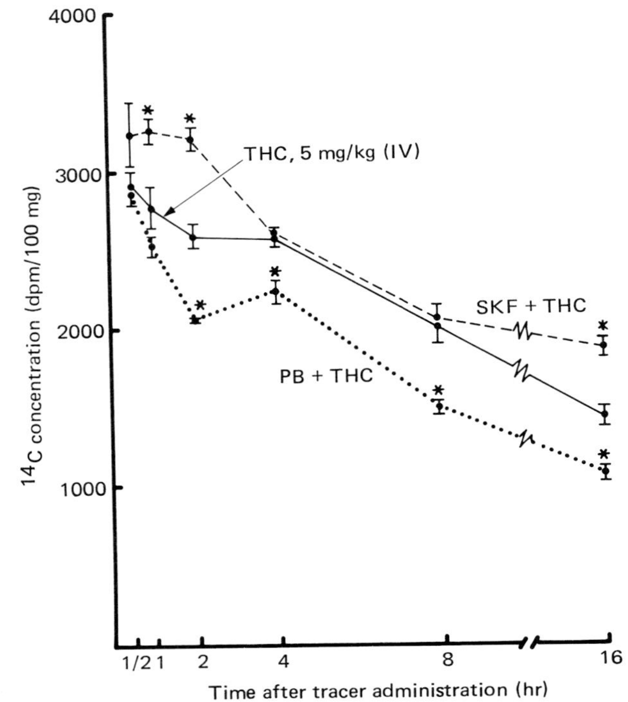

Figure 38.3. Effects of SKF-525A and phenobarbital on the concentration of THC–M in placenta. Each point on the graph represents the mean of 6–8 pregnant mice. Asterisk indicates a significant difference ($p < 0.05$) from THC alone.

The level of THC-M found in the fetus is shown in Figure 38.4. Approximately 10 times less carbon-14 was found in fetal tissues when compared to placenta. SKF-525A pretreatment significantly increased the concentration of THC-M in the fetus. Phenobarbital pretreatment significantly decreased the concentration of THC-M in the fetus. SKF-525A pretreatment prolonged and phenobarbital pretreatment increased the disappearance of THC-M from the fetus. THC also was measured in amnionic fluid. Phenobarbital pretreatment reduced the level of THC-M. No significant differences in THC-M were seen in the amnionic fluid after SKF-525A pretreatment.

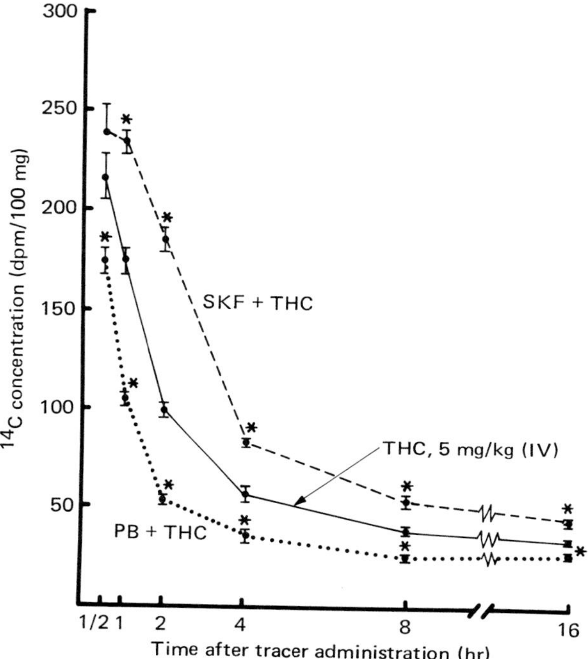

Discussion

The vehicle and route of administration were critical in determining the quantity of THC absorbed, and, consequently, its biological effects. THC was poorly absorbed from oil solutions after IP or oral administration. The toxicity of THC has been found to depend on its rate of absorption [15,20]. The IP route of administration remains as the alternative in studies concerning dose-related THC-induced biological effects. A similar observation was noted in a previous study [14]. Thus, comparisons of dose-related THC-induced teratological effects can be valid only when the same vehicle, route of administration, and treatment schedules have been used.

THC and its primary metabolite, 11-OH-THC, are psychoactive compounds. In mice, Christensen *et al.* [4] found that 11-OH-THC is rapidly converted to the inactive metabolite, 8,11-diOH-THC. Gill and Jones [7] reported that SKF-525A pretreatment (25 mg/kg 25 min before THC administration) only slightly inhibited THC hydroxylation, but it markedly inhibited the further metabolism of 11-OH-THC. Accordingly, if the second enzymatic conversion is more sensitive than the first, then 11-OH-THC might accumulate, in the case of the inhibitor studies, or be metabolized faster, in the case of the stimulator studies. Thus, the effect of inhibitors (i.e., SKF-525A) or stimulators (i.e., phenobarbital) could be exerted at both enzymatic steps.

The present study suggests that factors which apparently alter THC metabolism also influence THC-induced teratogenesis. Pretreatment of pregnant mice with SKF-525A apparently inhibited the metabolism of THC, significantly increased plasma levels of THC plus metabolites, and potentiated THC-induced teratogenicity. Placental transfer of THC-M is possibly the rate-limiting step of THC-induced *in utero* deaths. Essentially any drug may cross the placenta, but this is of importance only if the drug crosses rapidly enough to achieve toxic concentrations in embryo or fetal blood and tissues at a critical period when development may be affected. The drugs transferred most rapidly appear to be molecules with high lipid solubility [16]. Our studies show that relatively small amounts of THC-M are found in placental tissue. Only one-tenth of the THC-M found in the placental tissue was measured in fetal tissue. SKF-525A pretreatment significantly increased the placental transfer of THC-M, exposing the fetus to a higher concentration of THC-M. Also, the finding of THC-M in amnionic fluid indicates that amnionic fluid may store THC-M and continuously expose the fetus to this compound. Further, there were no significant differences in the amount of THC-M found in amnionic fluid after SKF-525A pretreatment.

On the other hand, phenobarbital pretreatment exerted a series of mixed effects. Plasma concentration and placental transfer of THC-M were reduced. There was a significant decrease in THC-M amounts measured in fetal tissues and amnionic fluid. The reduction in the THC-M levels in the fetus may explain the antagonistic effect in relation to fetal body weight. However, phenobarbital pretreatment potentiated THC-induced teratogenicity. This is in contrast to the antagonistic effect seen in relation to THC-induced toxicity in male mice [15]. The nature of the metabolites probably determines their toxic activity, and the nature of the metabolite as well as its concentration influence the teratogenic response. Phenobarbital probably alters qualitatively the THC metabolites produced. The finding of an epoxide, 9,10-epoxy-hexahydrocannabinol, during the biotransformation of THC in two species, squirrel monkey [9] and rabbit [3], suggests that this metabolic pathway may also exist in the mouse. Even more, an aldehyde intermediate, 11-oxo-THC, has been reported in rats [2]. A reactive intermediate metabolite could explain phenobarbital-induced potentiation of cleft palate induction.

The data presented in this study should be extrapolated to humans with caution since human beings would not usually employ a dose as large as that administered in these studies. However, the possibility of adverse reproductive consequences under some circumstances, especially with multiple drug use, or accumulative effects, cannot be ruled out.

ACKNOWLEDGMENTS

Supported in part by USPHS, NIH Grant DA00141 and ES00267. We gratefully acknowledge the technical assistance of Ms. Geralyn L. Clewe. SKF-525A was generously supplied by Smith Kline and French Laboratories, and the cannabinoids by the National Institute on Drug Abuse.

REFERENCES

1. Barrow, M. V. and W. T. Taylor (1969) A rapid method for detecting malformations in rat fetuses. *J. Morphol. 127:*291–305.
2. Ben-Zvi, Z. and S. Burstein (1974) 7-Oxo-delta 1-tetrahydrocannabinol: a novel metabolite of delta 1-tetrahydrocannabinol. *Res. Commun. Chem. Pathol. Pharmacol. 8:*223–229.
3. Ben-Zvi, Z. and S. Burstein (1975) Transformation of Δ^1-tetrahydrocannabinol (THC) by rabbit liver microsomes. *Biochem. Pharmacol. 24:*1130–1131.
4. Christensen, H. D., R. J. Freudenthal, J. T. Gidley, R. Rosenfeld, G. Boegli, L. Testino, D. E. Brine, C. G. Pitt, and M. E. Wall (1971) Activity of delta-8 and delta-9 tetrahydrocannabinol and related compounds in the mouse. *Science 172:*165–167.
5. Dawson, A. B. (1926) A note on the staining of the skeleton of cleared specimens with alizarin red S. *Stain Technol. 1:*123–124.
6. Fleischman, R. W., D. W. Hayden, H. Rosenkrantz, and M. Braude (1975) Teratologic evaluations of Δ^9-tetrahydrocannabinol in mice, including a review of the literature. *Teratology 12:*47–50.
7. Gill, E. W. and G. Jones (1972) Brain levels of Δ^1-tetrahydrocannabinol and its metabolite in mice—correlation with behavior and the effect of the metabolic inhibitors SKF-525A and piperonyl butoxide. *Biochem. Pharmacol. 21:*2237–2248.

8. Goldstein, A. (1964) *Biostatistics, An Introductory Text.* New York: Macmillan, pp. 91–101.
9. Gurny, O., D. E. Maynard, R. G. Pitcher, and R. W. Kierstead (1972) Metabolism of (-)-Δ^9- and (-)-Δ^8-tetrahydrocannabinol by monkey liver. *J. Am. Chem. Soc. 94:*7928–7939.
10. Harbison, R. D. and B. Becker (1970) Effect of phenobarbital and SKF-525A pretreatment on diphenylhydantoin teratogenicity in mice. *J. Pharmacol. Exp. Ther. 175:*283–288.
11. Harbison, R. D. and B. Mantilla-Plata (1972) Prenatal toxicity, maternal distribution and placental transfer of tetrahydrocannabinol. *J. Pharmacol. Exp. Ther. 180:*446–453.
12. Mantilla-Plata, B., G. L. Clewe, and R. D. Harbison (1975) Δ^9-Tetrahydrocannabinol-induced changes in prenatal growth and development of mice. *Toxicol. Appl. Pharmacol. 33:*333–340.
13. Mantilla-Plata, B., G. L. Clewe and R. D. Harbison (1973) Teratogenic and mutagenic studies of Δ^9-tetrahydrocannabinol in mice. *Fed. Proc. 32:*746.
14. Mantilla-Plata, B. and R. D. Harbison (1976) Distribution studies of [^{14}C] delta-9-tetrahydrocannabinol in mice: effect of vehicle, route of administration and duration of treatment. *Toxicol. Appl. Pharmacol.* (in press).
15. Mantilla-Plata, B. and R. D. Harbison (1974) Effects of phenobarbital and SKF-525A pretreatment, sex, liver injury and vehicle on Δ^9-tetrahydrocannabinol toxicity. *Toxicol. Appl. Pharmacol. 27:*123–130.
16. McKechnie, F. B. and J. G. Converse (1955) Placental transmission of thiopental. *Am. J. Obstet. Gynecol. 70:*639–644.
17. Pace, H. B., W. M. Davis, and L. A. Borgen (1971) Teratogenesis and marihuana. *Ann. N.Y. Acad. Sci. 191:*123–131.
18. Phillips, R. N., R. F. Turk, and R. B. Forney (1971) Acute toxicity of delta-9-tetrahydrocannabinol in rats and mice. *Proc. Soc. Exp. Biol. Med. 136:*260–263.
19. Posner, H. S., A. Graves, C. T. G. King, and A. Wilk (1967) Experimental alteration of the metabolism of chlorcyclizine and the incidence of cleft palate in rats. *J. Pharmacol. Exp. Ther. 155:*494–505.
20. Rosenkrantz, H., I. A. Heyman, and M. Braude (1974) Inhalation, parenteral and oral LD_{50} values of Δ^9-tetrahydrocannabinol in Fischer rats. *Toxicol. Appl. Pharmacol. 28:*18–27.

39

Pharmacogenetic Studies on Cannabis and Narcotics: Effects of Δ^1-Tetrahydrocannabinol and Morphine in Developing Mice

SIMONE RADOUCO-THOMAS, F. MAGNAN, AND C. RADOUCO-THOMAS

Introduction

Because marihuana is often used chronically by young people [24,27], pharmacological studies of Δ^1-tetrahydrocannabinol (Δ^1-THC) in animals should obviously include chronic drug regimens in young growing animals.

On the other hand, effects of THC varying from no obvious response up to psychotic episodes in different individuals have been reported [7,30]. These unusually wide variations in effect indicate that genetic factors may be involved in modulating the effects of THC at moderate doses. It thus seemed urgent to explore genetic differences by testing the effect of THC among selected inbred strains of mice.

Finally, in view of the persistent controversy concerning the relationship between the use of THC and the use of morphine, it was decided to compare the effects of both drugs in the same strains. The use of morphine also served as a pharmacological control condition to assure that THC-strain differences were unique to THC and were not an artifact of nonspecific strain differences.

This report describes acute and chronic behavioral effects of THC in young mice of three highly inbred strains, DBA/2J, A/J, and C57 BL/6, which differ markedly in general arousal level, emotionality, and avoidance learning [3]. Comparative data are presented concerning the effect of morphine in the same experimental conditions.

Marihuana: Chemistry, Biochemistry, and Cellular Effects, edited by Gabriel G. Nahas,

Methods

Animals

Male mice of three inbred strains, DBA/2J, A/J, and C57 BL/6, were used. They were obtained from the Jackson Laboratories, Bar Harbor, Maine. After weaning at 20 days, the animals were randomly housed in groups of 8–10 in plastic cages. Food and water were available *ad libitum* at all times.

Drugs

The THC solution was prepared by diluting the alcoholic standard solution with propylene glycol and a solution of 1 percent Tween saline. Morphine sulfate was dissolved in saline. All experimental animals received an IP injection (20 μl/gm body weight) of the drug solution or of the corresponding vehicle. In both acute and chronic experiments, we used a constant dose: 10 mg/kg for THC and 30 mg/kg for morphine.

Procedure

Acute studies were carried out on experimental groups of 5–10 mice. The gross behavior of the mice was carefully observed, recorded, and compared to that of their controls before, during, and after the drug injection. Particular attention was given to locomotor activity, social behavior, and aggressiveness.

Chronic studies were carried out in young mice from the 20th up to the 60th postnatal day. The drugs were administered daily, 7 days a week, at the end of the morning in order to allow systematic observations of the preinjection behavior. Each experimental group included 20 mice, from which 10 would be submitted to a distributed and 10 to a massed avoidance shock conditioning test at the end of drug treatments. The body weight was recorded every 7 days.

Apparatus

Shock avoidance was evaluated in an automatic two-way grid-shock shuttlebox. During each trial, the conditioned stimulus was given 5 sec before an electric shock was delivered to the grid floor. The intertrial interval was 60 sec. A total of 250 trials was given in one session only (massed avoidance conditioning) or in five consecutive sessions, each daily session consisting of 50 trials (distributed avoidance conditioning). The statistical analysis of the results is given in detail elsewhere [15].

The motor activity of the mice was evaluated by means of an

Animex activity meter, which allows the use of the home cage during measurements.

Results

Behavioral effects of chronic dosing of THC

Behavioral changes observed during the chronic treatment

During the period of administration, i.e., from the 20th up to the 60th postnatal day, the behavior of the treated mice and of their controls was carefully observed and recorded before and 1–2 hr after the daily injection of 10 mg/kg THC. Clear differences were noted among the three strains. Specific pharmacological profiles differentially characterized the three strains.

In DBA mice, the first injection of THC did not induce any significant modification of the gross observable behavior. However, after 3 days, the daily dose elicited some excitation. After 7 days only, a clear-cut response was obtained: a 5 min period of greater locomotor activity followed by a shorter period of immobility. During this period, the mice had their eyes half-closed and stayed huddled together. They seemed to aggregate with each other for warmth. During the third and fourth weeks, the duration of this biphasic response decreased progressively to a few minutes and then remained unchanged until the end of the treatment. Some manifestations of fear, aggressiveness, or both appeared progressively among all treated mice, whereas control mice became more and more tame. Thus, random running and fleeing were elicited in the drugged mice by the approach of the experimentor, and they struggled and tried to bite during the injection. After the injection, they were highly reactive to external stimuli, particularly during the phase of immobility. Both types of behavior—aggressiveness and hyperreactivity—became particularly evident at the third week of treatment. They were still present but less evident at the end of the treatment.

In the A/J mice, the first dose of THC was followed immediately by a 2-min period of random hyperactivity and a depression of about 1 hr. During the next days, the excitatory phase increased in duration (2–10 min) and in intensity (running and jumping), while the depression, or immobility phase, remained unchanged. The mice also began to show a strong agitation before and during the injection. This behavioral pattern remained almost unchanged during the following 2 weeks. From the fifth week, two new responses were accompanying the initial random running: a dragging of the hind legs apparent in 75 percent of the population, and an almost generalized Straub-like reaction. At that time, the duration of the depressive phase was decreased to 30 min.

In the C57 strain, the first injection of THC immediately elicited a strong biphasic response. During the initial excitatory phase, the mice ran and showed the Straub reaction. Some mice even exhibited a jumping topography similar to naloxone-induced withdrawal jumping. After about 5–10 min, this excitement went into a catalepticlike state, which lasted about 1 hr. In the following days, the excitation period was characterized by some bounds and jumps. Some mice showed an ataxic gait. During the consecutive depressive phase, the mice stayed huddled together with their heads hidden under the wood chip bedding material. They appeared to be strongly sedated when undisturbed. However, when exposed to slight tactile stimulation, they responded immediately with the Straub tail reaction. During the second week, the excitation period lasted for only 5 min, whereas the depression increased to 90 min. From the third up to the sixth week of treatment, the duration and

Figure 39.1. Post-treatment effect of chronic THC doses on the distributed conditioning avoidance in 3 inbred strains of mice.

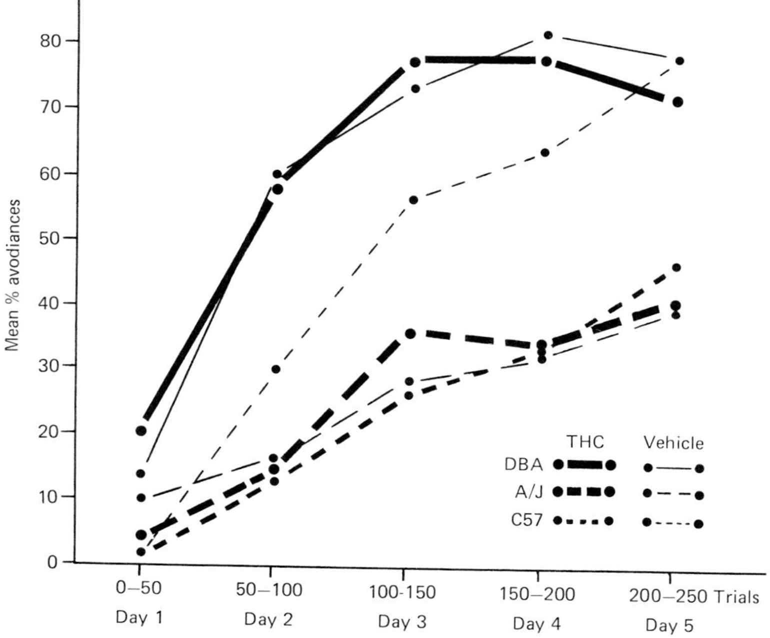

intensity of the depressive phase receded in an orderly fashion. On the other hand, a dragging of the hind legs became evident in about 25 percent of the population in the middle of treatment but was observed in only 10 percent of the population at the end of the treatment.

Some particular features that were common to all the three strains are to be mentioned. During the treatment period, the treated groups became progressively more hyperexcitable before the daily injection. Furthermore, a higher spontaneous activity of all drugged groups was still evident a few weeks after cessation of the treatment. On the other hand, a diminution of self-grooming and of grooming other mice was also observed in all drugged groups; the mice became more recognizable by their nonglossy coat. Also, in the black-haired C57 strain, white hairs began to appear in the drugged group immediately after cessation of the treatment and were always more numerous in the previously drugged than in the control mice during the following months.

Behavioral modifications observed after the chronic treatment

The shuttlebox behavior of the chronically treated mice was observed 1 day after the treatment was stopped. Two different schedules—massed and distributed avoidance conditionings—were used.

In the distributed avoidance conditioning (Figure 39.1), no dif-

Figure 39.2. Post-treatment effect of chronic THC doses on the massed conditioning avoidance in 3 inbred strains of mice.

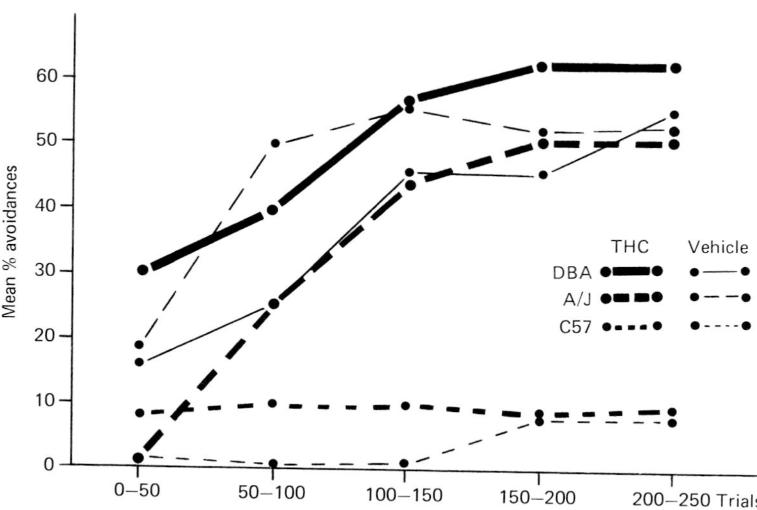

ference was found between the THC-treated mice and the controls, neither in the low-scoring A/J strain nor in the high-scoring DBA strain. However, the performance of the C57 mice was significantly inhibited.

In the massed avoidance conditioning (Figure 39.2), the performance of the C57 mice was unaffected, whereas that of the DBA and of the A/J mice was significantly modified by the previous THC treatment. However, in these two strains the previous THC treatment resulted in opposite modifications of the performance. This opposition was particularly evident during the first part of the conditioning session when the performance of the treated mice was strongly ameliorated in the DBA strain and strongly inhibited in the A/J mice.

Differential effects of THC and morphine

Acute effects of THC and morphine in the three inbred strains

The acute effect of morphine and THC were compared in 60-day-old mice of the three strains. In some cases, the drug was injected daily on a few consecutive days in order to obtain a well-developed response. Generally speaking, the acute response of these mice to THC was a biphasic one that resembled the initial response of the 20-day-old mice (see above). The effect of morphine was monophasic in all three strains.

In the DBA mice, the first injection of THC had no pharmacological effects. Only at the sixth day was a significant effect of THC demonstrated by a strong hyperexcitability of the mice before the injection. The THC injection elicited a 5-min running and jumping stage followed by a shorter period of immobility. The first injection of morphine also did not induce any significant behavior modification. However, on the next day, the morphine injection elicited a state of deep sedation for about 2 hr.

The A/J mice responded to THC, after 4 days, with a period of excitation (running and jumping) followed by a short period of rest. The acute effect of THC in the A/J mice was thus almost the same as in the DBA mice, with a predominance of the excitatory components. The effect of morphine in the A/J mice was also similar to its effect in the DBA mice. As a matter of fact, morphine elicited immediately on the first day a period of deep sedation for about 2 hr. The Straub tail reaction was present.

The C57 mice responded immediately to the first injection of THC and of morphine. THC induced a 10-min stage of hyperactivity followed by a long-lasting (1 hr) period of catalepsy and ataxia. During this deep depression period, any tactile stimulation induced a Straub-like reaction in the corresponding mouse. On the other hand, the first injection of morphine elicited the classical "running fit," which lasted more than 2 hr. The Straub tail reaction was observed in most of the animals.

Chronic effects of THC and morphine in the C57 strain

The chronic effects of THC and of morphine were compared only in C57 young mice, which were submitted to daily drug injections from their 20th up to the 60th postnatal day. As was true for the acute doses, the effect of THC was found to be the opposite of that of morphine on many parameters. At the beginning of the treatment, the THC mice showed, after a short period of excitation, a deep and long-lasting depression, whereas the morphine-treated mice ran for over 2 hr at this stage. At the end of the treatment, the depressive effect of THC was reduced but the morphine-induced running fit was not (Figure 39.3).

Surprisingly, the Straub tail reaction, which was elicited as early as the first day by THC, was induced only after 10 days by

Figure 39.3. Effect of chronic doses of morphine on the spontaneous motor activity of C57 BL6 mice. Locomotor activity (counts) before (B) and after (A) the daily injection at the 3rd and 5th weeks of treatment.

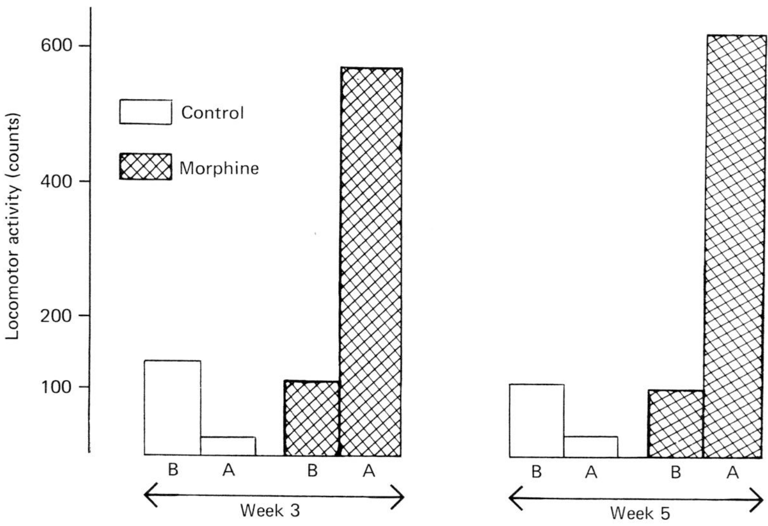

Table 39.1 Post-treatment effect of chronic morphine doses on the distributed and massed conditioning avoidance in C57 BL6 mice

Avoidance during trial (%)	*Distributed practice*		*Massed practice*	
	Morphine	*Control*	*Morphine*	*Control*
0–50	6.2	5.2	8.4	2.2
50–100	12.8	18.4	11.2	0.9
100–150	46.3	43.4	15.2	1.4
150–200	63.0	56.4	15.0	1.0

morphine. On the other hand, whereas the THC mice showed increasingly more intense aggressive agitation, the behavior of the morphine mice remained, in the interinjection periods, very similar to that of the control mice. No sign of aggressiveness was recorded in the morphine group.

Four days after treatment was stopped, two types of avoidance trial procedures were carried out to eliminate possible interferences due to eventual withdrawal symptoms or to a long-lasting metabolism. In the distributed avoidance practice, the performance of the treated mice was inhibited by the previous THC treatment but not by the morphine treatment. On the other hand, the massed avoidance performance was ameliorated by morphine as it was by THC (Table 39.1). This improvement could be related to anxiety-decreasing properties of morphine [2].

Finally, a common consequence of the chronic treatment was found in both treated groups after the treatment was stopped, i.e., the less glossy appearance of the hair and the earlier than normal appearance of white hairs. This effect seemed to be irreversible since 1 yr after cessation of the treatment, the treated mice of both drug regimens were still differentiated from their controls by the appearance of their hair, which was whiter and more lusterless.

Discussion

Behavioral effects of chronic doses of THC

The results of these experiments support and extend the data of the literature concerning the effects of THC in mice [20]. The biphasic time response curve of THC is well known, as is the THC-induced hypersensitivity to tactile and auditory stimuli. The ability of THC to induce the Straub tail-raising phenomenon and the dragging of the hind legs is less frequently documented, although these effects have been described in male albino Cox mice after IV injections of toxic doses of THC [21] and in some CFW mice after IP doses of 50 mg/kg THC [5]. Our observation that chronic THC treatment induces progressively a state of aggressive agitation is consistent with Carlini's speculation [4] that, although acute administration of THC may reduce aggression, chronic administration actually increases aggression.

Of greatest interest in terms of the objectives of this study is the observation that these various THC effects were distributed unequally among the three strains. Such results suggest genetic differences in the response to THC. Quantitative differences are obvious. The DBA mice were the least sensitive and the C57 mice the most sensitive to THC. As a matter of fact, in the DBA mice the intensity of various effects elicited by THC was lower than in other mice, and in both young and adult mice a latency period of a few days was seen before THC elicited an overt pharmacological response.

These differences in sensitivity may result from genetic differences in the rate of penetration of THC or in other pharmacokinetic parameters. The higher tolerance of the C57 strain to alcohol has been correlated with a genetically determined higher activity of alcohol dehydrogenase [25]. They could also result from genetic variations in the regional neurochemical substratum to THC (see below).

The responses of the three strains also differed qualitatively. The adrenergic component appears more predominant in the response of the C57 mice to THC. Several of the characteristics of the THC effects in the C57 mice strongly resemble the behavioral effects of dopa, which has been shown to induce in large doses an aggressive excitation and the Straub tail phenomenon and in doses lower than 400 mg/kg hypokinesia with hyperexcitability to external stimuli [29]. C57 mice have been recently shown by Mandel and coworkers [13] to have higher norepinephrine levels in the whole brain, particularly the pons medulla.

An additional aspect to be considered is tolerance [17]. Quantitative and qualitative differences in tolerance to the excitatory and to the inhibitory effects of THC have also been observed among the three strains. It would appear rational to detect and evaluate the tolerance to the pharmacological effects of THC via the locomotor activity. However, direct analysis of the evolution of the behavioral response to THC during the treatment from the 20th to the 60th postnatal day cannot be interpreted only in terms of tolerance. As a matter of fact, a reduction in locomotor excitatory response could correspond not only to a development of tolerance but also to an enhancement of responsiveness to the locomotor inhibitory effect of THC [6]. Furthermore, given our experimental conditions, the reduction of the effect could also result from a progressive maturation of the blood-brain barrier. This would presumably produce decreasing penetration of THC into the brain. Therefore, it would be premature to speculate about the magnitude of tolerance to THC during development.

The analysis of the shuttlebox performance of the three strains after stopping treatment also demonstrates strain-specific responses. Our data concerning the controls (nontreated mice) confirm that the three strains differ in their rate of avoidance response in a shuttlebox [3]. The performance level of the C57 mice is somehow higher than that generally attributed to this strain. This difference may be related to the animals' age. In our experimental conditions, their performance was also higher than that of 80-day-old C57 mice [15,23].

On the other hand, our data concerning the treated mice demonstrate that the chronic administration of THC from the 20th to the 60th postnatal day results in strain-dependent modifications of shuttlebox avoidance behavior. The performance of the C57 mice was strongly inhibited in the distributed avoidance condition, whereas performances of the DBA and A/J mice were modified—but in opposite directions—in the massed avoidance condition. Obviously, the differences observed between the three strains may be related to motivational and emotional factors as well as to avoidance learning or memory differences.

It is worthwhile to emphasize that DBA mice have been ranked very high on emotionality scales and that, in our experimental conditions, the performance of previously THC-treated DBA mice was significantly increased on the first day of the distributed avoidance condition (Figure 39.1) and more intensively in the 1-day massed avoidance condition (Figure 39.2). In both cases, anxiety may decrease the performance of the "naive" animal. The higher level of performance of the THC-treated DBA mice could suggest a long-lasting inhibitory effect of THC on emotional factors for this strain.

The C57 mice showed a strong inhibition of the performance during the distributed avoidance condition. The cholinergic system has been implicated in the avoidance retention process. Furthermore, C57 mice have been demonstrated to have less active acetylcholine metabolism in the temporal cortex than DBA mice [16]. A long-lasting inhibitory effect of THC on this system is not to be excluded.

In all strains, the described avoidance differences within a strain, i.e., between treated and control mice, were reversible as within-strain differences were no longer recorded in the shuttlebox avoidance evaluations carried out 100 and 200 days later [15]. However, when the mice were treated from the 60th to the 80th postnatal day, irreversible modifications of the shuttlebox behavior were observed [23]. Similar residual learning deficits after prolonged treatment with cannabis and alcohol have also been described in rats [9,14].

Differential effects of THC and morphine

Our results concerning the effect of morphine in mice are in accordance with the data of Oliverio and coworkers [19] and of Shuster *et al.* [26], who have shown that the DBA and A/J strains exhibited little or no running response to THC in doses up to 25 mg/kg, whereas C57 mice showed a strong response.

The comparison of the effects of THC and morphine in the three strains leads to several statements which are, for clarity, separated as follows.

First, a close inspection of these results indicates that THC produced a biphasic activity effect in all three strains, although the predominant overall effect was either stimulation or depression, depending on the strain. However, morphine produced only a monophasic effect, each strain demonstrating only excitation or inhibition, but never both together.

Second, in each strain the locomotor activity of the mice was modified in two diametrically opposed directions by THC and by morphine. Thus, in the C57 strain, morphine elicited a strong running response, whereas the THC pattern was predominantly depressive. For the DBA and A/J mice, the effect of THC was predominantly excitatory, whereas that of morphine was sedative.

Finally, a relationship was noted between the strain and the magnitude of the pharmacological responses to both THC and morphine. For example, the C57 mice showed a marked behavioral response to THC and to morphine, whereas DBA and A/J mice showed a mild response to both drugs. The C57-specific high sensitivity to THC and morphine does not reflect a strain-specific hypersensitivity to drugs in general, as C57 mice have been demonstrated to be hyposensitive to barbiturates. They responded to pentobarbital with a longer latency and a shorter duration than other strains, DBA included [18].

The two opposite behavioral responses of C57 mice to THC and to morphine could involve a common neurochemical mechanism. The similarities between the time response curve of THC and the dose response curve of dopa are impressive (see above). On the other hand, the narcotic-induced running fit has been shown to be mediated by the adrenergic system [12]. Both drugs thus seem to act via the adrenergic system. The norepinephrine concentration and turnover have been shown to be significantly higher in the brains of C57 mice compared with DBA [13]. With this in mind, one could interpret the selective common hypersensitivity of C57 mice to opposite behavioral effects of THC and morphine as the response of strain-specific hyperactive adrenergic synapses to drug-specific differences in the target structures of THC and morphine in the brain.

The importance of this selective high sensitivity of the C57 strain to both morphine and THC is not to be underestimated. It is perhaps more than coincidental that this strain has also been demonstrated to have a high alcohol preference [9] and a high susceptibility to morphine addiction [8].

Studies carried out in self-administering morphine-dependent conventional rats have shown great individual variability in the daily morphine intake [11,22]. Molecular studies on opiate receptors [28] carried out on these animals have also shown a high variability in narcotic binding [10].

For investigators to obtain a better understanding of sensitivity to narcotics and cannabis, our results on the progenitor strains—C57 BL/6 and DBA/2J—will be completed by behavioral and molecular studies on their reciprocal F_1 hybrids and their recombinant-inbred lines (RI). The importance of using this technique in genetic studies has been emphasized by Bailey [1] and by Eleftheriou *et al.* [26]. It is hoped that these studies will represent a valuable approach toward a better understanding of the possible role of genetic factors in pharmacodependence.

ACKNOWLEDGMENTS

This work was supported by the Health and Welfare Grant 605–23–8 of the Non-Medical Use of Drug Directorate (NMUDD) and the Medical Research Council Grant MA-5084.

The authors are grateful to Mrs. E. D. Baronet-Lacroix for the invaluable secretarial assistance and skillful preparation of the illustrations. Special thanks are also due to Miss D. Huot and Mr. G. Boutin for their assistance in preparing the manuscript.

Dr. R. A. Graham, Chief of Scientific Services, Health Protection

Branch, Ottawa, is gratefully acknowledged for the generous supply of Δ^1-THC. The authors express their sincere appreciation to Mr. Crépeau for his excellent collaboration on the experimental work during his summer research studentship. They are also indebted to R. N. Grove for reading the manuscript and for his very helpful comments and suggestions.

REFERENCES

1. Bailey, D. W. (1971) Recombinant inbred strains. *Transplantation 11:*325.
2. Boissier, J. R. (1962) La morphine est-elle un tranquillisant? *Thérapie 17:*519.
3. Bovet, D., F. Bovet-Nitti, and A. Oliverio (1969) Genetic aspects of learning and memory in mice. *Science 163:*139.
4. Carlini, E. A. (1974) Cannabis sativa and aggressive behavior in laboratory animals. *Arch. Invest. Med. (Mex.) 5* (suppl. 1): 161.
5. Cutler, M. G., J. H. Mackintosh, and R. A. Chance (1975) Effects of cannabis resin on social behaviour in the laboratory mouse. *Psychopharmacologia 41:*271.
6. Davis, W. M., J. M. Holbrook, and M. Babbini (1973) Differential effects of morphine on active avoidance as a function of pre-drug performance. *Pharmacol. Res. Commun. 5:*47.
7. Deniker, P. (1974) Pharmacologie humaine des drogues psychodysleptiques. *Pharmacology, Toxicology and Abuse of Psychotomimetics (Hallucinogens)* (Simone Radouco-Thomas, A. Villeneuve, and C. Radouco-Thomas, eds.). Quebec: Les Presses de l'Université Laval, pp. 153–171.
8. Eriksson, K. and K. Kiianmaa (1971) Genetic analysis of susceptibility to morphine addiction in inbred mice. *Ann. Med. Exp. Biol. Fenn. 49:*73.
9. Freund, G. (1970) Impairment of shock avoidance learning after long-term alcohol ingestion in mice. *Science 168:*1599.
10. Garcin, F., S. Radouco-Thomas, P. Singh, and C. Radouco-Thomas (1975) Behavioural models of morphine dependence in rat and narcotic ligand/pharmacoreceptor interactions. Abstracts Sixth Int. Congress Pharmacol. No. *725:*308.
11. Garcin, F., Simone Radouco-Thomas, R. Grove, and C. Radouco-Thomas (1974) Relapse to morphine dependence. Effect of narcotic antagonists (naloxone). *Proc. Can. Fed. Biol. Soc. 17:*158.
12. Hollinger, M. (1969) Effect of reserpine, α-methyl-p-tyrosine, p-chloro-phenylalanine and pargyline on levorphanol-induced running activity in mice. *Arch. Int. Pharmacodyn. Ther. 179:*419.
13. Kempf, E., J. Greilsamer, G. Mack, and P. Mandel (1974) Correlation of behavioural differences in three strains of mice with differences in brain amines. *Nature 247:*483.
14. Fehr, K. A., H. Kalant, A. E. Leblanc, and G. V. Knox (1976) Permanent learning impairment after chronic heavy exposure to cannabis or ethanol in the rat. *Marihuana: Chemistry, Biochemistry, and Cellular Effects* (G. G. Nahas *et al.*, eds.). New York: Springer-Verlag.

15. Magnan, F. (1976) Effet du Δ^1-tetrahydrocannabinol sur la mémoire et l'apprentissage après administration chronique, lors de la croissance, chez trois souches consanguines de souris. Thèse, Université Laval, Québec.
16. Mandel, P., A. Ebel, J. C. Hermetet, D. Bovet and A. Oliverio (1973) Etudes des enzymes du système cholinergique chez les hybrides F_1 de souris se distinguant par leur aptitude au conditionnement. *C. R. Acad. Sci. [D] (Paris) 276:*395.
17. Mechoulam, R., ed. (1973) *Marijuana. Chemistry, Pharmacology, Metabolism and Clinical Effects.* New York: Academic Press.
18. Meier, G. W., J. L. Hatfield, and D. P. Foshee (1963) Genetic and behavioral aspects of pharmacologically induced arousal. *Psychopharmacologia 4:*81.
19. Oliverio, A., C. Castellano, and B. E. Eleftheriou (1975) Morphine sensitivity and tolerance: a genetic investigation in the mouse. *Psychopharmacologia 42:*219.
20. Paton, W. D. M. and R. G. Pertwee (1973) The pharmacology of cannabis in animals. *Marijuana. Chemistry, Pharmacology, Metabolism and Clinical Effects* (R. Mechoulam, ed.). New York: Academic Press, pp. 192–285.
21. Phillips, R. N., R. F. Turk, and R. B. Forney (1970) Acute toxicity of Δ^9-tetra-hydrocannabinol in rats and mice. *Proc. Soc. Exp. Biol. Med. 136:*260.
22. Radouco-Thomas, C., Françoise Garcin, and Simone Radouco-Thomas (1974) Relapse to narcotics and effect of opioid antagonists. Intravenous self-administration model in ex-addict rats. *J. Pharmacol. 5* (suppl. 2): 81.
23. Radouco-Thomas, S., F. Magnan, R. N. Grove, P. Singh, Françoise Garcin, and C. Radouco-Thomas (1975) Effect of chronic administration of Δ^1 tetra-hydrocannabinol on learning and memory in developing mice. *Pharmacology of Cannabis* (S. Szara and M. C. Braude, eds.). New York: Raven Press.
24. Radouco-Thomas, S., A. Villeneuve, Françoise Garcin, and R. Michaud (1974) Student drug abuse survey in the Province of Quebec (Canada). *Pharmacology, Toxicology and Abuse of Psychotomimetics (Hallucinogens)* (S. Radouco-Thomas, A. Villeneuve, and C. Radouco-Thomas, eds.). Quebec: Les Presses de l'Université Laval, pp. 419–438.
25. Rodgers, D. A. (1966) Factors underlying differences in alcohol preference among inbred strains of mice. *Psychosom. Med. 28:*498.
26. Shuster, G. W., G. Y. Webster, and B. E. Eleftheriou (1975) A genetic analysis of the response to morphine in mice: analgesia and running. *Psychopharmacologia 42:*249.
27. Snyder, S. H. (1971) *Uses of Marijuana.* New York: Oxford University Press.
28. Snyder, S. H., C. B. Pert, and G. W. Pasternak (1974) The opiate receptor. *Ann. Intern. Med. 81:*534.
29. Strömberg, U. (1970) Dopa effects on motility in mice; potentiation by MK485 and dexchlorpheniramine. *Psychopharmacologia 18:*58.
30. Braude, C. and S. Szara, eds. (1976) *Pharmacology of Cannabis.* New York: Raven Press.

40

Permanent Learning Impairment After Chronic Heavy Exposure to Cannabis or Ethanol in the Rat

KEVIN A. FEHR, HAROLD KALANT,
A. EUGENE LEBLANC, AND GEORGE V. KNOX

It has been recognized for many years that advanced alcoholism may be accompanied by slowing and interruption of mental processes, difficulty with abstract thought, loss of memory, and impairment of learning [17]. Patients with these symptoms were often found to have diffuse or patchy cortical atrophy and dilatation of the cerebral ventricles. In recent years it has been possible to diagnose advanced alcoholism antemortem by means of pneumoencephalography. Although there has been some debate as to whether this picture is due primarily to malnutrition, head injury, hypoxia, a direct toxic effect of alcohol, or to all of these and possibly other factors in varying combinations, no one has seriously disputed its occurrence or its relation to alcoholism.

For well over a century, clinical reports from India, Brazil, the Middle East, and North Africa have described a similar state, usually referred to as "dementia," in long-term heavy users of the more potent preparations of cannabis designated by such names as charas, hashish, and kif [4,12]. As in the case of alcoholic dementia, it is impossible to separate, in retrospect, the effects of cannabis from those of malnutrition, injury, intercurrent illness, and use of other drugs.

Within the past 10 years, clinical descriptions of a similar picture have appeared in North America, the United Kingdom, and western Europe. The subjects have been mainly adolescents and young adults of middle- and upper-class origin, often university students, who have used cannabis for relatively short periods but very intensively. The symptoms range from mild impairment of verbal memory [6] to the full-blown picture described above, and it has been suggested that this picture, like that in alcoholics, may in some cases represent an organic brain syndrome [9]. One group

Marihuana: Chemistry, Biochemistry, and Cellular Effects, edited by Gabriel G. Nahas,

has reported finding air encephalographic evidence of enlargement of the ventricles and cortical atrophy in a small group of such patients [1].

These reports and suggestions have been the subject of heated controversy. One reason is that the cannabis users in question are often multiple drug users. Also, despite their middle- or upper-class origins, they often choose a life style in which malnutrition, infection, and other factors confound the interpretation of drug effects. Another reason is that heavy use of cannabis in Western society has not existed for long enough to permit the accumulation of an adequate body of radiologic and histopathologic evidence to establish whether organic damage occurs. Lastly, similar symptoms may occur as a manifestation of chronic intoxication with cannabis, and it is not always clear whether the clinical observations have been made long enough after the last drug use to permit a differentiation between intoxication and residual cell damage.

Therefore, we have examined the effects of cannabis in the rat on the learning and performance of a food-motivated maze test, during acute and chronic intoxication, and also at various times after the end of chronic intoxication. We have also extended the latter study to include a different learning task involving shock avoidance and motor coordination. For comparison, we have used rats treated chronically with intoxicating doses of alcohol as well as drug-free controls. The results suggest strongly that permanent impairment can be produced by prolonged *heavy* dosage with either drug.

Methods

The cannabis preparation was an organic solvent extract of marihuana leaf material provided by Health and Welfare Canada and known to contain 1 percent Δ^9-tetrahydrocannabinol (Δ^9-THC) by weight. The extract was activated by heat [5] to convert all the tetrahydrocannabinolic acid to THC. After the THC content was assayed by gas-liquid chromatography [20], the active extract was dissolved in olive oil for administration to the rats.

Performance in the Hebb–Williams closed-field maze has been shown to be sensitive to cortical ablation and to drug-induced learning deficits. For our study, we used the Rabinovitch and Rosvold modification [15]. Partially food-deprived rats were trained until they ran through the simplest maze problems nine times with a

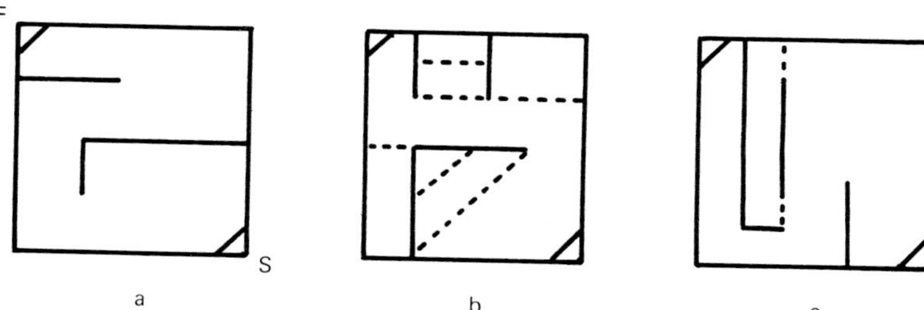

Figure 40.1. Examples of maze problems used in the learning study. (a) Training problem; S indicates starting box, F is food box (the goal). (b) Simple problem (No. 1 of the series of 12 graded problems); (c) difficult problem (No. 12). Solid lines indicate the barriers; broken lines indicate the limits of error zones.

combined time of less than 60 sec. At the goal box, they obtained a reward of mashed rat food and sugar.

When trained to criterion, they were tested on a series of 12 problems arranged in order of increasing difficulty (Figure 40.1). Every time the front feet crossed a dotted line, the rat was charged with an error. Problem 12 (Figure 40.1) was difficult because of the open alley; the main error was to run in circles around the center barrier. The rats were given 9 trials on each problem. The first trial on each problem was regarded as a "learning trial" and not scored. The next 8 trials were scored for the total number of errors committed from start to finish.

Acute and Subacute Cannabis Effects

For the acute experiment, 18 animals were reduced to 80 percent of their free feeding weight and trained in the maze. They required 8 days of training to reach criterion. On test day 1, they were tested on the first 4 problems and assigned to 2 equal groups matched on the basis of their scores. On test day 2, one group was treated with cannabis extract (THC dose, 10 mg/kg) administered by stomach tube 1 hr before testing. The other group was treated with an equal volume of olive oil. During the next 2 hr, each rat was tested on problems 5–8 of the series. The scores of the 2 groups on the drug days are shown in Table 40.1.

The THC-treated animals made significantly more errors than

Table 40.1 Effects of acute and subacute treatment with cannabis extract (THC 10 mg/kg orally) on error scores in maze learning by rats

	Single dose		
	Problems 1–4 (no drug)	*Problems 5–12 (placebo or drug)*	*Daily dose for 14 days Problems 1–12*
Control	20.4 ± 1.2[a]	68.2 ± 4.8	77.6 ± 3.6
Treated	19.8 ± 1.7	87.6 ± 9.0 ($p < 0.05$)	144.0 ± 18.6 ($p < 0.01$)

[a] Mean ± SE; n = 9 per group for experiment A, and 5 per group for experiment B.

the controls. This impairment agrees with the findings of Carlini and Kramer [3] on a different type of maze test.

In a second experiment, 5 rats reduced in weight were treated with marihuana extract (THC, 10 mg/kg) daily for 14 days, while 5 others were given olive oil. On days 6–14, all animals were given a training session immediately before treatment. By day 14, all animals were adequately trained. These animals were then tested on problems 1–12 over the next 3 days, 1–3 hr after drug or placebo administration on each day.

After 6–7 days, the THC-treated animals became very irritable shortly after treatment. They exhibited backward circling and licking behavior and shrieked whenever handled. This is consistent with observations by Carlini *et al.* [2]. During testing they showed little interest in the problems and moved very slowly, often stopping to lick the plexiglass floor of the maze. When they finally reached the food box, however, they ate avidly. As shown in Table 40.1, they had much higher scores than the controls. The rats in this experiment did not become tolerant to the action of the drug; instead, the effect was more clearly evident than after a single dose.

Chronic Experiments

Thirty 50-day-old rats were randomly divided into 3 groups of 10, and each group was subdivided into 5 placebo-treated and 5 drug-treated animals. The drug animals in group 1 received the standard dose of cannabis extract (THC, 10 mg/kg) daily for 30 days, while the placebo animals received an equal dose of olive oil.

Table 40.2 Error scores in maze tests after chronic treatment with cannabis extract (THC 10 mg/kg)

Length of treatment (days)	*Test*		*Retest*	
	Treated	*Control*	*Treated*	*Control*
30	89.6 ± 12.2[a]	81.6 ± 15.1		
60	96.2 ± 9.2	108.4 ± 10.9	50.8 ± 2.8	54.8 ± 5.8
90	124.8 ± 6.1	113.6 ± 9.8	49.4 ± 2.3	48.2 ± 3.5

[a] Mean ± SE; $n = 5$ per group. No significant differences due to treatment.

The other two groups were treated similarly for 60 and 90 days, respectively.

The animals were then withdrawn from treatment for 2 weeks. During the second week they were coded randomly, reduced to 80 percent of their free feeding weight, and trained in the maze. After the end of the training period, they were tested on problems 1–12 over a period of 4 days, beginning 25 days after the end of drug or placebo treatment. In order to test for retention of learning, we retested the 60- and 90-day groups 2 weeks after the initial testing.

The scores over 12 problems for the 3 groups are shown in Table 40.2. Although there is a significant trend toward higher scores with increasing age ($p < 0.01$), an analysis of variance showed no significant difference between the scores of the treated and control animals. Retesting of groups 2 and 3 two weeks after the initial testing also showed no difference in scores.

A second experiment with greater exposure to cannabis was then conducted in which both the duration of treatment and the dose of cannabis were doubled. In addition, a second and unrelated learning task was employed, which included elements of shock avoidance and motor coordination. Since Walker and Freund [18] had reported lasting impairment of shuttlebox avoidance learning by rats after prolonged ethanol ingestion, an ethanol-treated group was added for comparison.

Twenty-six male rats weighing about 120 gm were randomly allocated to 3 groups: 8 controls, 8 cannabis treated, and 10 ethanol treated. The larger ethanol-treated group reflected our expectation of a higher mortality rate in this group. All animals received chow and tap water *ad libitum.* The cannabis group was treated daily with cannabis extract in olive oil at a dose equivalent to THC 20 mg/kg for 6 months. All animals survived the treatment period in good health with normal growth. The ethanol animals were intubated daily with a 25-percent (w/v) solution of ethanol in water. The initial dose, equivalent to 2 gm of absolute ethanol per kilogram, was gradually increased to 6 gm/kg over 2 weeks and maintained at this level for the balance of the 6-month period. One animal died of unknown causes during treatment, 2 were lost for other reasons, and 7 survived for testing. These animals grew rather poorly, gaining 50–100 gm less than those of both other groups. The controls were treated with a sucrose solution equal in calories to the daily dose of ethanol. All animals survived the treatment, but 1 died of a respiratory infection during maze testing.

After 6 months all treatment was stopped, and the animals were allowed to recover from drug effects for 1 month. Each rat was coded and reduced to 80 percent of its free feeding weight, and maze training was begun. This training took over 3 weeks, and it was necessary to substitute chocolate ice cream as the reward before the animals would perform satisfactorily. They were then tested on the same 12 problems that had been used in the earlier experiments. Two separate scoring criteria were used. One was the number of runs needed to reach a criterion of 3 out of 4 correct trials for each problem, to a maximum of 20 trials per problem. The other was the total error score on the second to ninth runs on each problem.

As shown in Table 40.3, the error score and runs-to-criterion score in the ethanol group were both significantly higher than in the controls. The mean error score of the cannabis group was also significantly higher than that of the controls, whereas the difference in runs-to-criterion score was marginal. These results are self-

Table 40.3 Results of maze tests after 6 months chronic treatment

Drug	*Error score*	*Runs to criterion (no.)*
Control	87.4 ± 6.4[a]	93.7 ± 6.0
Marihuana extract (THC 20 mg/kg)	106.5 ± 5.1 ($p < 0.025$)	104.3 ± 2.9 ($p < 0.075$)[b]
Ethanol	102.4 ± 5.3 ($p < 0.05$)	108.8 ± 4.3 ($p < 0.05$)

[a] Mean ± SE; $n = 8$ per group.

[b] p = significance of difference from control on a one-sided t-test.

contained and should not be compared with those in Tables 40.1 and 40.2 because the scores are clearly influenced by the size of the rat.

The same rats were then trained on the moving belt apparatus [10], which has previously been used as a sensitive measure of impairment by ethanol, pentobarbital, and meprobamate. The rat is trained to stay on a continuous motor-driven belt that runs over an electrified grid. If the rat puts one or more of its paws off the belt, it receives a small electric shock from the grid and simultaneously activates a cumulative timer. The error score is expressed as the number of seconds spent off the belt during a standard 2-min trial. Each rat was given 3 trials per day for up to 12 consecutive days. As the score of each rat reached criterion (no more than 1.2 sec, or 1 percent of the trial time, off the belt), it was eliminated from further training to prevent overtraining. The mean score for the 3 daily trials was calculated for each animal. The rats were then left for 2 months without further training, and they were then retrained in the same way after this period.

The raw error scores are shown in Figure 40.2. An analysis of variance performed on square root transformations of the scores showed a significant interaction among the 3 groups on both testing and retesting. A probit transformation resulted in linear learning curves over the training period. The slopes of the ethanol and control groups were significantly different ($p < 0.05$). The cannabis group presented a more complex picture. The initial learning appeared to be identical with that of the control group, mainly because of two very rapid learners that heavily influenced the mean score of the cannabis group. However, the group as a whole showed significantly poorer scores than the controls ($p < 0.05$) from day 8 to day 12.

In the retraining phase, the ethanol curve was again significantly different from that of the controls. Although the scores of the cannabis group were higher than those of the controls, the large variance prevented any conclusions from this phase of the experiment.

One year after the end of the period of prolonged drug exposure, the few surviving animals (1 control, 2 alcohol, and 2 marihuana rats) were chronically implanted with recording electrodes in the anterior neocortex, dorsal hippocampus, and mesencephalic reticular formation. No obvious EEG abnormalities were observable from visual inspection of the recordings from the control and alcohol groups. However, the hippocampal recordings from the marihuana animals showed "epileptiform" abnormalities con-

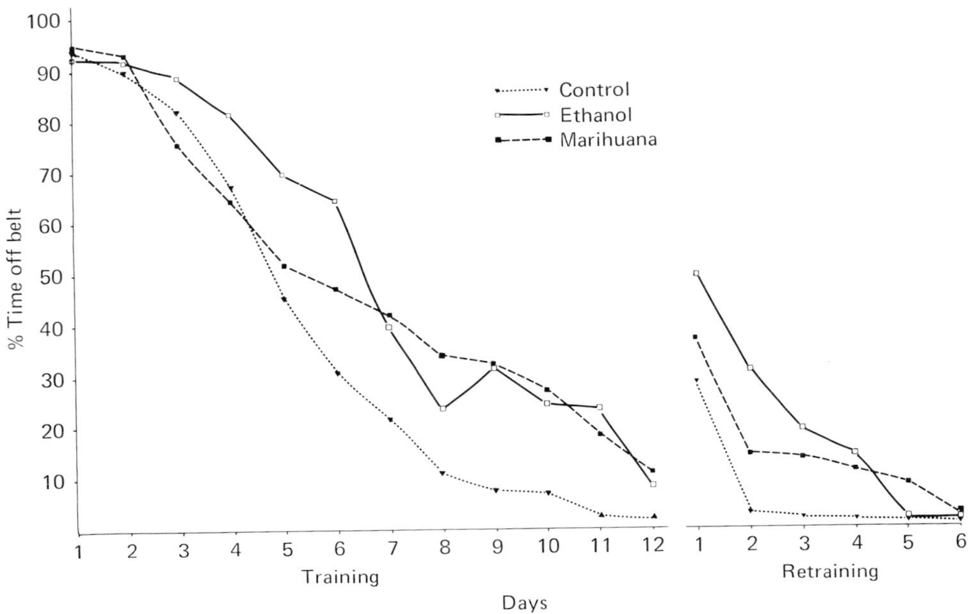

Figure 40.2. Group means of error scores on successive days during learning of the moving belt test. Training began approximately 2 months after the end of a 6-month treatment period with drugs or placebo, as indicated.

sisting of irregularly occurring high-voltage sharp waves. Neuronal damage has not yet been confirmed histologically.

Discussion

The results of the acute and 2-week cannabis treatments confirm the impairment of maze learning by cannabis [3] and suggest that tolerance to the impairing effects of THC does not develop within 14 days. In view of the long half-life and high lipid solubility of THC, the apparent absence of tolerance might conceivably reflect drug accumulation in the body on the dosage schedule used. However, the animals did develop tolerance to the anorexic effect of the drug very rapidly. This is consistent with reports of tolerance in other studies [4,8,11–13,16]. In other work, we have found that tolerance to THC, as measured by changes in its interaction with ethanol, is primarily a central nervous system phenomenon rather than a reflection of increased rate of drug metabolism [16]. It seems likely that the whole spectrum of tolerance mechanisms in relation to cannabis will prove to be rather complex.

After the 6-month treatment with high doses of either ethanol or cannabis extract, there was residual, and apparently permanent, impairment of learning on two different tasks. This confirms and extends the findings of Walker and Freund [18]. In the case of cannabis, one might wonder whether we are dealing with continuing chronic intoxication rather than residual damage. However, the half-life of the slow phase of THC elimination in the rat is about 24 hr [20], so that by the 30 days after the end of drug treatment the residual level of THC in the body should be only $(0.5)^{30}$ of the plateau value attained during chronic treatment. This suggests that the learning impairment observed then and at later times is indeed due to residual cellular change.

The connection between the learning deficit and organic brain damage requires further definition. It is well known that other chemically induced organic brain damage syndromes (e.g., those produced by lead or methyl mercury) are recognizable as behavioral impairment before histological damage becomes apparent [19]. The preliminary EEG changes in the present work tend to support the interpretation that we are indeed dealing with organic damage, and histological confirmation is now being sought in further experiments.

It should be noted that no residual impairment was found at a THC dose of 10 mg/kg daily for 3 months, so that a very high level of cumulative exposure seems necessary. Since a comparable experiment cannot ethically be done in humans, one naturally wonders whether these findings have any relevance to chronic heavy users of cannabis. The effective dose (THC 20 mg/kg) cannot be applied literally to humans for two major reasons. The first is that rodents are much more resistant than larger species to most drug effects on the central nervous system. The lowest IV dose of THC reported to produce significant effects on EEG recordings in the rat is 1 mg/kg [14]. The second is that the drug was given by stomach tube, and it is well known that much larger doses of cannabis are required by mouth than by IV or intrapulmonary administration to produce comparable effects [7]. In fact, despite receiving what sounds like a huge dose, the cannabis-treated animals were visibly intoxicated for only about 4 hr after each dose, gained weight normally, and were in good general health throughout the experiment. The 6 gm/kg dose of ethanol would also be lethal in humans, yet even though it produced greater general impairment of health in the rats, it was fairly well tolerated.

At the same time, the daily achievement of a substantial degree of intoxication is consistent with the levels of use described in clinical accounts of very heavy users in various countries. In the production of lasting impairment of learning, the degree of intoxication may be more important than the actual drug. The similarity of the residual impairment produced by cannabis and alcohol supports this conclusion.

The 6-month treatment period was necessary before impairment became evident. The necessity of long-term treatment is not surprising since alcoholics do not exhibit symptoms of organic damage until after 5–10 years of heavy drug use. This would be expected if the mechanism, as suggested for other neurotoxins [19], were a slight increase in the rate of attrition of brain cells with age. We conclude that animal studies of this type may be a reasonable model for damaging effects of *heavy* drug use in humans.

REFERENCES

1. Campbell, A. M. G., M. Evans, J. L. G. Thomson, and M. J. William (1971) Cerebral atrophy in young cannabis smokers. *Lancet 2:*1219.
2. Carlini, E. A., A. Hamaoui, and R. M. W. Märtz (1972) Factors influencing the aggressiveness elicited by marihuana in food deprived rats. *Br. J. Pharmacol. 44:*794.
3. Carlini, E. A. and C. Kramer (1965) Effects of cannabis sativa (marihuana) on maze performance of the rat. *Psychopharmacologia* 7:175.
4. C.I.N.M.U.D. (1972) Cannabis and its effects. *Cannabis, A Report of the Commission of Inquiry into the Non-medical Use of Drugs.* (G. LeDain, chairman.). Ottawa: Information Canada, chap. 2.
5. De Zeeuw, R. A., Th. M. Malingré, and F. W. H. M. Merkus (1972) Δ^1-Tetrahydro-cannabinolic acid, an important component in the evaluation of cannabis products. *J. Pharm. Pharmacol. 24:*1.
6. Entin, E. E. and P. J. Goldzung (1973) Residual effects of marihuana usage on learning and memory. *Psychol. Rec. 23:*169.
7. Isbell, H., C. W. Gorodetsky, D. R. Jasinski, V. Claussen, F. Von Spulak, and F. Korte (1967) Effects of (-)-Δ^9-trans-tetrahydrocannabinol in man. *Psychopharmacologia 11:*184.
8. Kalant, H. and A. E. LeBlanc (1974) Effect of acute and chronic pretreatment with Δ^1-tetrahydrocannabinol on motor impairment by ethanol in the rat. *Can. J. Physiol. Pharmacol. 52:*291.
9. Kolansky, H. and W. T. Moore (1971) Effects of marihuana on adolescents and young adults. *J.A.M.A. 216:*486.
10. LeBlanc, A. E., H. Kalant, R. J. Gibbins, and N. D. Berman (1969)

Acquisition and loss of tolerance to ethanol by the rat. *J. Pharmacol. Exp. Ther. 168:*244.

11. McMillan, D. E., L. S. Harris, J. M. Frankenheim, and J. S. Kennedy (1970) 1-Δ^9-trans-Tetrahydrocannabinol in pigeons: tolerance to the behavioral effects. *Science 169:*501.
12. Nahas, G. G. (1973) *Marihuana—Deceptive Weed.* New York, Raven Press, chap. 6.
13. Paton, W. D. M. and R. G. Pertwee (1973) The pharmacology of cannabis in animals. *Marihuana: Chemistry, pharmacology, metabolism and clinical effects* (R. Mechoulam, ed.). New York: Academic Press, p. 191.
14. Pirch, J. H., R. A. Cohn, P. R. Barnes, and E. S. Barratt (1972) Effects of acute and chronic administration of marijuana extract on the rat electrocorticogram. *Neuropharmacology 11:*231.
15. Rabinovitch, M. S. and H. E. Rosvold (1951) A closed-field intelligence test for rats. *Can. J. Psychol. 5:*122.
16. Siemens, A. J. and H. Kalant (1974) Metabolism of Δ^1-tetrahydrocannabinol by rats tolerant to cannabis. *Can. J. Physiol. Pharmacol. 52:*1154.
17. Victor, M. (1968) Alcohol and nutritional diseases of the nervous system. *J.A.M.A. 167:*65.
18. Walker, D. W. and G. Freund (1971) Impairment of shuttle-box avoidance learning following prolonged alcohol consumption in rats. *Physiol. Behav. 7:*773.
19. Weiss, B. and W. Simon (1972) Quantitative perspectives on the long-term toxicity of methyl mercury and similar poisons. Presented at the 5th Rochester International Conference on Environmental Toxicity, June.
20. Willinsky, M. D., H. Kalant, O. Meresz, L. Endrenyi, and N. Woo (1974) Distribution and metabolism in vivo of ^{14}C-tetrahydrocannabinol in the rat. *Eur. J. Pharmacol. 27:*106.

smoking dosage for monkeys (Δ^9-THC 48.4 mg/kg/month) equated with that consumed by a 75-kg man smoking about 160 gm/month of 5 percent hashish, below the average reported by Tennant and Groesbeck [15] for heavy smokers in their study.

Expressed in terms of joints, equivalents were as follows: (1) heavy-smoking monkeys, equivalent to 7 joints per day for man; (2) moderate-smoking monkeys, equivalent to 1 joint per day for man, 7 days a week, but smoked on a schedule of 3½ joints on each of 2 of 7 days; (3) light-smoking monkeys, equivalent to one-half joint per day for man.

Results

Immediate effects

The smoke of active marihuana in heavy and moderate dose levels and IV Δ^9-THC induced distinct and immediate (acute) changes in behavior. The monkeys responded less to all forms of sensory stimuli and tended to stare blankly into space.

In the four heavy- and moderate-smoking monkeys prepared with deep and surface electrodes, distinct changes occurred in many brain regions, but they were most consistent in the septal region, hippocampus, and amygdala (Figure 41.1). Changes in scalp recordings in these monkeys and in the 2 intact (without implanted electrodes) heavy-smoking monkeys were not significant. When they did occur, they were nonspecific and reflected alterations in level of awareness, such as drowsiness.

Changes in recordings of the 2 monkeys that received IV Δ^9-THC were more pronounced than those obtained from monkeys exposed to smoke of active marihuana. High-amplitude spiking or slow activity, or both, occurred at specific subcortical sites. When the monkeys displayed catatonic-like behavior, the recordings resembled those we had previously obtained from the septal region of severely disturbed psychotic patients [7,10,11]. At other times, when the monkeys behaved as if they might be hallucinating, recording changes were most pronounced in the sensory relay nuclei, and recordings from nuclei-containing cells for specific transmitter chemicals were also affected (Figure 41.2).

These behavioral and recording changes came on gradually in the smoking monkeys, being quite pronounced at the end of the smoke exposure, whereas they occurred within 1 min after IV administration of Δ^9-THC. There was then a gradual return to base line in 30–40 min.

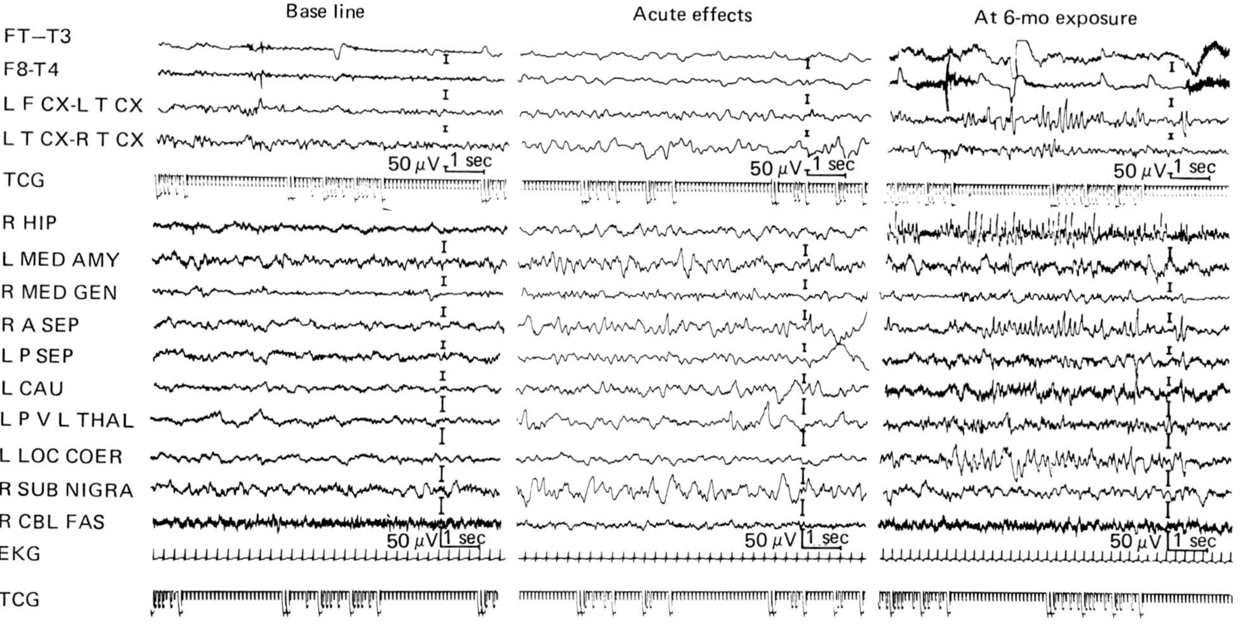

Figure 41.1. Sample EEGs obtained from an electrode array #2 monkey before (base line), 6 min after exposure to smoke of active marihuana (acute effects), and after 6 months' exposure at the heavy-smoking dose level. During the acute effects, there is generalized slower activity and distinct sharp waves in the amygdala, septal region, and substantia nigra in association with the animal's reduced awareness.

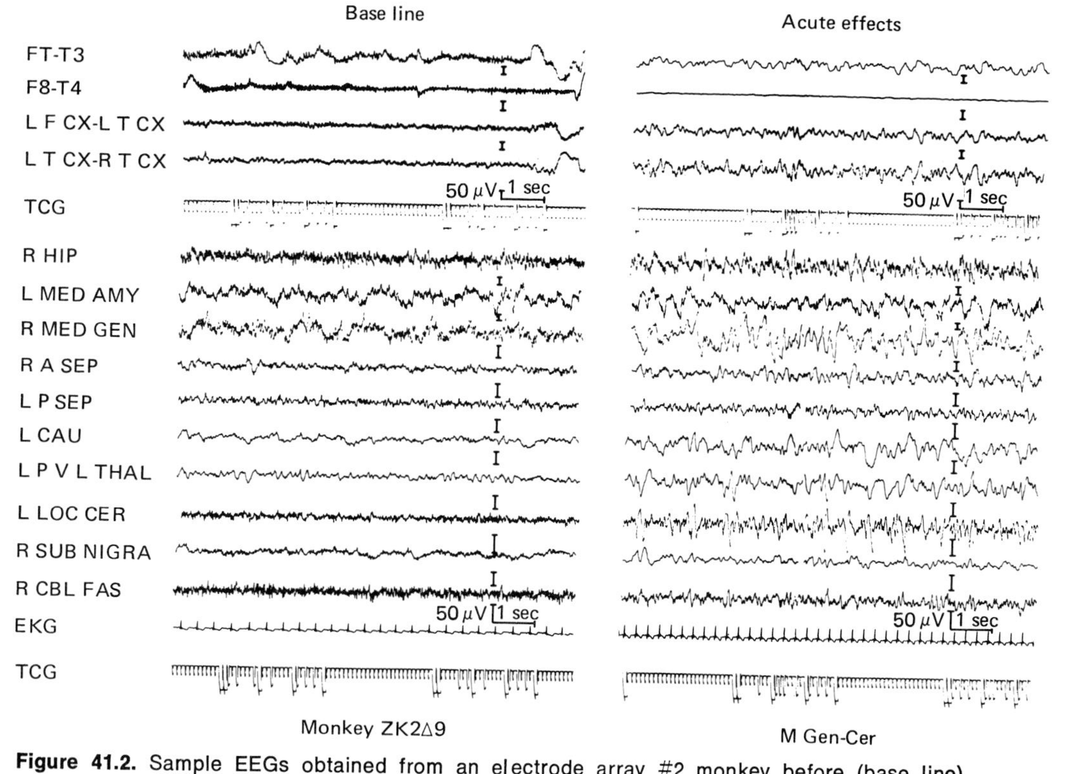

Figure 41.2. Sample EEGs obtained from an electrode array #2 monkey before (base line) and 5 min after (acute effects) IV administration of Δ^9-THC. There are generalized slowing; distinct spiking in the locus ceruleus, medial geniculate, and amygdala; and some sharp waves in septal leads.

These acute behavioral and recording effects were not seen in the light-smoking monkeys or in the heavy smokers of inactive marihuana.

Persistent effects

With the passage of time, there were persistent (chronic) changes in brain activity, with the septal region, hippocampus, and amygdala being most profoundly affected. In the monkeys termed moderate and heavy smokers of active marihuana, the chronic brain changes became apparent about 3 months after the study began. In the monkeys given injections of Δ^9-THC, the chronic changes were evident in 2–3 months after the beginning of the study. The recording changes outlasted the acute effects of the smoke or IV injection, persisting through the weekend when the monkeys were "rested." It was interesting that these distinct and persistent brain alterations were temporarily amended, being replaced by a different type of altered brain activity (more generalized) when the animals were again exposed to smoke or given an injection (Figure 41.3).

No changes appeared in the conventional scalp recordings of the 2 intact monkeys exposed to heavy smoking of active marihuana.

In those monkeys that were chronically exposed to light smoke of active marihuana or to smoke of inactive marihuana, no notable recording or behavioral alterations occurred.

Physical complications

Two monkeys, both in the heavy-smoking marihuana group (1 with electrodes and the other intact), died of respiratory complications during the study. One died 3.5 months after the study was begun, and the other after 5.5 months. The preliminary histopathologic report of the brains indicates minimal structural change in the cells in the septal region.

Postexposure effects

The remaining 11 monkeys were followed for 8 months after the 6 months' exposure to marihuana smoke or to IV Δ^9-THC. During this period, the electrodes of 3 of the monkeys had deteriorated so that meaningful deep recordings could not continue to be made. In 5 monkeys, however, electrodes continued to function well and recordings were obtained on a regular basis. Of this group, 1 monkey was a heavy marihuana smoker, 2 had received Δ^9-THC intravenously, and 2 had been exposed to smoke of inactive mari-

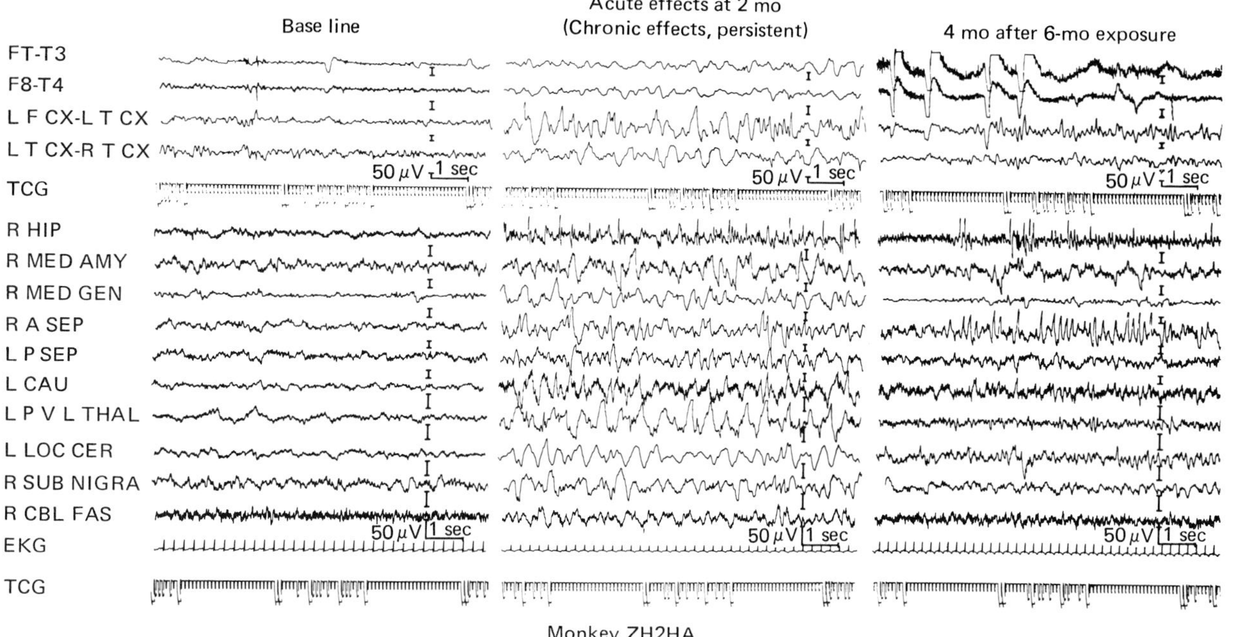

Figure 41.3. Sample EEGs obtained from an electrode array #2 monkey before (base line), during acute effects of exposure to smoke of active marihuana, and 4 months after the animal's 6 months' exposure. In the recording obtained during acute effects, there is marked generalized slowing with some sharp waves, most pronounced in the septal and hippocampal leads. These acute effects are superimposed on a record altered by 2 months of regular exposure to smoke of active marihuana. The recording obtained 4 months after the exposure period shows persistent altered activity, principally in the form of spikes and sharp activity in the septal region and hippocampus.

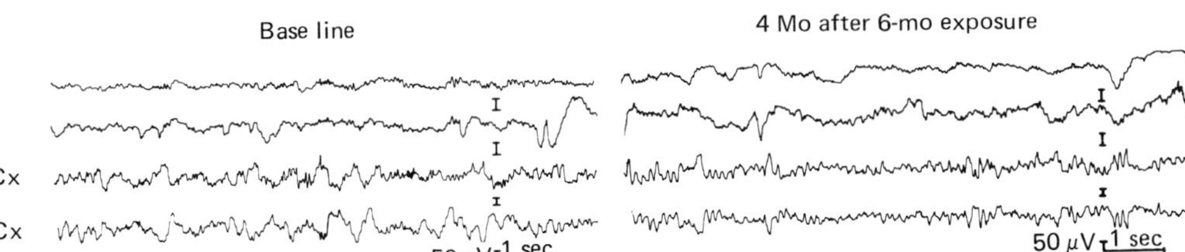

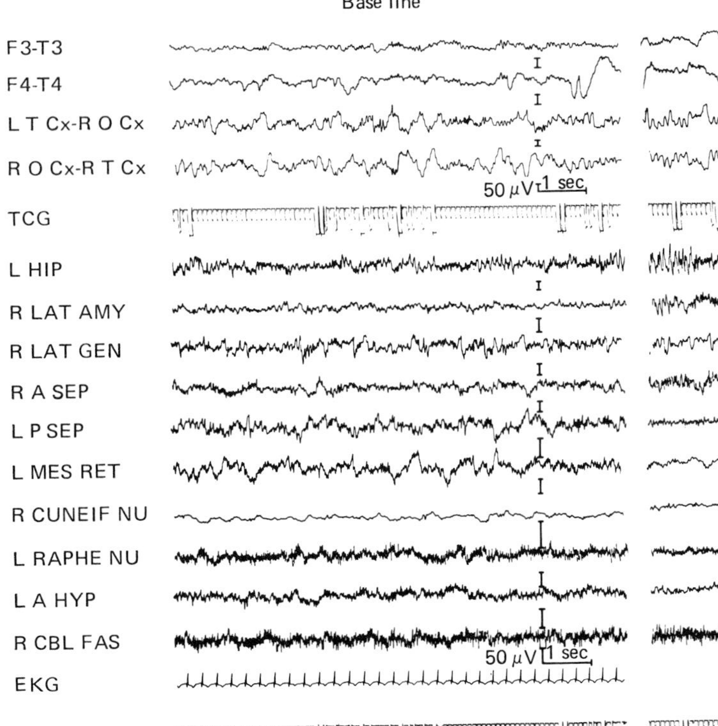

Figure 41.4. Sample EEGs obtained from an electrode array #1 monkey before (base line) and 4 months after its last IV injection of Δ^9-THC. Altered activity persists principally in the form of spike activity in the hippocampus and, to a lesser degree, in the septal region and lateral geniculate.

huana. In the heavy-smoking monkey and in the 2 that had received IV Δ^9-THC, EEG alterations recorded at the end of the 6 months' exposure period persisted essentially unchanged throughout the entire 8 months' postexposure observation period (Figures 41.3 and 41.4).

The 2 monkeys exposed to inactive marihuana smoke continued to have normal recordings.

Discussion

The results clearly indicate that irreversible brain changes can be induced in monkeys by prolonged administration of the active ingredients of *C. sativa* in amounts equivalent to those used by human subjects considered to be moderate to heavy marihuana smokers. Because of the nature of the controls used in the study, it is evident that the brain changes in the monkeys were not the result of exposure to heavy quantities of smoke per se or to the method by which it was delivered. Monkeys that smoked inactive marihuana by the same procedure and for the same length of time failed to develop changes. Further, 2 monkeys never exposed to smoke that were given one of the principal active derivatives, Δ^9-THC, by the IV route developed brain changes similar to those induced in monkeys smoking heavy and moderate amounts of active marihuana. Therefore, the critical statements made by some persons that the recording changes were the consequence of anoxia induced by smoke being forcibly pumped into the monkeys are invalid.

Others who have contended that the dose levels used in this study were excessive based their criticism on inaccurate information [1]. Even when the factor of Freireich *et al.* [5] is not used, and there are investigators who feel it should not be applied [2], the equated dose levels for the monkeys are still within dose ranges of marihuana used by many human subjects.

Studies in animals have an advantage over those in man in that numerous variables can be controlled. Nevertheless, there were some major problems with this study in monkeys that recent technical advances will alleviate in future studies. Since this study was conducted, we have developed a method for delivery of smoke to a monkey that more exactly simulates the smoking pattern of man. The development of a radioimmune assay for Δ^9-THC will now permit plasma dose levels of the active ingredient in monkeys to be adjusted to the same level as those found in human smokers.

With these advances, the criticisms raised by the present study should be settled beyond doubt.

ACKNOWLEDGMENTS

This study was supported by National Institute of Drug Abuse Grant N. 1–RO1–DA–00311–01. The *C. sativa* derivatives used in this study were obtained through the National Institute of Drug Abuse.

The author wishes to acknowledge the technical assistance of Charles J. Fontana and Herbert J. Daigle.

REFERENCES

1. Axelrod, J. (1974) Testimony during hearings before the subcommittee to investigate the administration of the Internal Security Act and other internal security laws of the committee on the judiciary, United States Senate, Ninety-third Congress, Second Session, May–June, 1974. Washington: U.S. Government Printing Office, p. 146.
2. Axelrod, J. Personal communication.
3. Bromberg, W. (1934) Marihuana intoxication: clinical study of cannabis sativa intoxication. *Am. J. Psychiatry 91:*303–330.
4. Campbell, A. M. G., M. Evans, J. L. G. Thomson, and M. J. Williams (1971) Cerebral atrophy in young cannabis smokers. *Lancet 2:*1219–1224.
5. Freireich, E. J., E. A. Gehan, D. P. Rall, L. H. Schmidt, and H. E. Skipper (1966) Quantitative comparison of toxicity of anticancer agents in mouse, rat, hamster, dog, monkey, and man. *Cancer Chemother. Rep. 50*(4):219–224.
6. Heath, R. G. (1954) Definition of the septal region. *Studies in Schizophrenia* (R. G. Heath and the Tulane University Department of Psychiatry and Neurology, eds.). Cambridge: Harvard University Press, pp. 3–5.
7. Heath, R. G. (1966) Schizophrenia: biochemical and physiologic aberrations. *Int. J. Neuropsychiatry 2:*597–610.
8. Heath, R. G. (1972) Physiologic basis of emotional expression: evoked potential and mirror focus studies in rhesus monkeys. *Biol. Psychiatry 5:*15–31.
9. Heath, R. G. (1975) Brain function and behavior. I. Emotion and sensory phenomena in psychotic patients and in experimental animals. *J. Nerv. Ment. Dis. 160:*159–175.
10. Heath, R. G., S. B. John, and C. J. Fontana (1968) The pleasure response: studies by stereotaxic technics in patients. *Computers and Electronic Devices in Psychiatry* (N. Kline and E. Laska, eds.). New York: Grune & Stratton, pp. 178–189.
11. Heath, R. G. and the Tulane University Department of Psychiatry and Neurology (1954) *Studies in Schizophrenia.* Cambridge: Harvard University Press.
12. Hollister, L. E. (1971) Marihuana in man: three years later. *Science 172:*21–28.

13. Kolansky, H. and W. T. Moore (1971) Effects of marihuana on adolescents and young adults. *J.A.M.A. 216:*486–492.
14. Rodin, E. A., E. F. Domino, and J. P. Porzak (1970) The marihuana-induced "social high." Neurological and electroencephalographic concomitants. *J.A.M.A. 213:*1300–1302.
15. Tennant, F. S. and C. J. Groesbeck (1972) Psychiatric effects of hashish. *Arch. Gen. Psychiatry 27:*133–136.
16. Tinklenberg, J. R., F. T. Melges, L. E. Hollister, and H. K. Gillespie (1970) Marijuana and immediate memory. *Nature 226:*1171–1172.

42

Marihuana's Effects on Human Gonadal Function

WYLIE C. HEMBREE III, PHILIP ZEIDENBERG, AND GABRIEL G. NAHAS

Introduction

Regulation of gonadal function in the human male begins *in utero* by the time a pregnancy can first be detected. Biochemical and morphological observations support the concept that the Y-bearing primitive germ cells are responsible for initiating the sequence of developmental events by which these gonocytes are enveloped by the Sertoli cells within seminiferous tubules. Thereafter, they are bathed by periodic surges of testosterone production by the peritubular Leydig cells. The dependence of this reproductive unit on hypothalamic-pituitary function becomes apparent during the perinatal period and is sustained until senescence.

It must be assumed that the regulatory mechanisms for this highly specialized germ cell environment have evolved in their present forms, in some measure, because of their success in assuring effective reproduction of the species by producing spermatozoa with the capacities required for normal fertilization and embryogenesis. Therefore, it is biologically appropriate to view the secretion of sufficient numbers of spermatozoa, capable of fertilization, as the primary function of the testis.

An increasing number, or perhaps an increasingly recognized number, of environmental perturbations limit or may destroy normal germ cell production. Their effect may be manifested as nonheritable chromosomal abnormalities, such as Klinefelter's syndrome and certain balanced translocations, which lead to absence or arrested development of the germinal epithelium. Other gene defects in testicular tissues result in abnormal enzyme or binding protein synthesis, such as the adrenogenital syndrome and testicular feminization, and these defects are also associated with absent sperm production. Ionizing radiation, nutritional deficiencies, viral infections, perhaps autosensitization, and a variety of synthetic and naturally

Marihuana: Chemistry, Biochemistry, and Cellular Effects, edited by Gabriel G. Nahas,

occurring chemicals alter the production of "fertile" spermatozoa. Three hundred years after the recognition of the spermatozoon as the testicular secretory product responsible for reproduction, the scientific community has now developed the technical and, more importantly, the conceptual framework within which the effects of certain naturally occurring pharmacologic agents—in this case, the psychoactive cannabinoid in marihuana—on male reproductive function might be critically examined.

Methods

The protocol for the initial phase of this study was part of a multidisciplinary evaluation of marihuana's effects in collaboration with Drs. Gabriel Nahas, Phillip Zeidenberg, and others. Immunologic, cytogenetic, psychological, and hormonal studies were carried out concurrently during four experimental periods (Figure 42.1). Five male volunteer subjects 20–27 years old were admitted to New York State Psychiatric Institute in the week of April 21–25, 1975. All had been previously screened by a trained psychiatrist to rule out any significant psychopathology. All volunteers were regular marihuana smokers, smoking at least 3–5 cigarettes per week. None was married and fertility had not been established in any.

Upon admission, each had a thorough physical examination, the results of which were within normal limits. Routine laboratory tests (SMA 6, SMA 12, CBC, urinalysis, etc.), chest x-ray films, EEGs, and EKGs were normal. All laboratory values remained within normal limits throughout the study, with the exception of creatinine phosphokinase (CPK). CPK levels were elevated on admission in each subject, returned toward normal during the study, but returned to within the normal range only in one subject.

All subjects underwent a 14–21-day drug-free period before smoking (period I), and a 2-week "wash-out" period after smoking (period IV). They were kept under constant observation throughout the study, and spot urine tests for other drugs were negative in all subjects throughout the study. After the initial 3-week "washout" period, subjects were allowed to smoke increasing amounts of marihuana cigarettes for a period of 4 weeks. All smoking was under direct observation, and subjects were checked repeatedly by the psychiatrist managing the project as to mental status and physical condition.

Subjects smoked increasing amounts of marihuana cigarettes, starting with 1 and increasing the number by 1 every other day

Table 42.1 Changes in sperm count, initial percentage of motility, and the percentage of motile sperm stimulated by theophylline in marihuana-smoking subjects

		Period			
Subject	*Parameter*	*I*	*II*	*III*	*IV*
A	Total count	284	243 ± 44[a]	279 ± 40	81 ± 16[b]
	Initial motility	62.4	80.3 ± 6.2	62.9 ± 9.3[c]	65.8 ± 3.5[c]
	Theophylline stimulation	10.9	13.8 ± 3.5	25.3 ± 5.5	26.4 ± 4.2[d]
B	Total count	290	228 ± 23	216 ± 25	104 ± 13[b]
	Initial motility	59.0	68.8 ± 2.7	68.4 ± 3.4	68.6 ± 3.3
	Theophylline stimulation	42.4	18.5 ± 6.0	20.9 ± 2.5	20.9 ± 1.5
C	Total count	150	106 ± 11	129 ± 21	47 ± 9[b]
	Initial motility	68.5	71.6 ± 2.3	61.2 ± 5.0	58.8 ± 2.3[d]
	Theophylline stimulation	20.0	14.6 ± 4.0	21.3 ± 3.0	28.3[c]
D	Total count	136	121 ± 22	124 ± 8	35 ± 2.5[b]
	Initial motility	53.4	71.1 ± 2.1	72.8 ± 6.2	35.1 ± 5.7[b]
	Theophylline stimulation	15.0	19.1 ± 1.4	19.7 ± 1.5	49.9 ± 14.0[c]
E	Total count	389	338 ± 37	224 ± 53	178 ± 24[d]
	Initial motility	62.1	67.7 ± 2.9	64.3 ± 2.1	62.5 ± 3.6
	Theophylline stimulation	16.4	18.9 ± 1.8	22.6 ± 4.7	25.6 ± 1.0[d]

[a] Mean ± 2 SE.

[b] $0.001 < p < 0.01$.

[c] $0.02 < p < 0.05$.

[d] $0.05 < p < 0.10$.

Discussion

Controversy exists concerning testosterone production during acute and chronic marihuana smoking. The seeming conflict between the published data of Mendelson *et al.* [14] and Schaeffer *et al.* [18] and that of Kolodny and coworkers [12] is illustrative of the difficulties inherent in defining changes in a single parameter after perturbing a multicomponent physiological system. Differences in assay reagents and methodology are of less importance than the validation of the performance of the assay in the hands of each investigator. The apparent conflict might also be more readily resolved if the hypothesis questioned were more precisely defined and the protocol employed analyzed as to its ability to yield data pertinent to the question.

For example, the usage of grouped data by each investigator, in both short-term and long-term studies, avoids the question of individual significance since sufficient data were not obtained to define, for each subject, the coefficient of variation of testosterone levels under control circumstances before marihuana use. The 100-percent difference between the minimum and maximum levels reported in 2 patients by Mendelson and the 175-percent range in the 36 samples obtained from Schaeffer's subjects make it unlikely that the 35-percent decrease reported by Kolodny would have been detected by these investigators. However, Kolodny's reports omit all individual data.

Multisample analysis is required to detect small changes in testosterone and gonadotropin levels [15]. Since only 1 ml of serum is required for these assays, the number obtained should be determined by the time during which the drug is anticipated to exert its effect.

In a short-term study, 15 values obtained at regular intervals on the day before and the day after the test day would serve as an adequate statistical base from which probabilities could be assigned to those values obtained during the period of marihuana use. Approximately 100 ml of whole blood would be required in such a design, and blood sampling could be repeated at judicious intervals without ill effects. In chronic studies, similar numbers of samples obtained at random during alternating periods of smoking and nonsmoking would also reveal decreases of greater than 50 percent. However, if persistent suppression of testosterone production is associated with chronic use, this question would be resolved most appropriately with isotopic measurement of urinary production rates of testosterone.

All reported studies have not included gonadotropin determinations, which would both corroborate and possibly explain the nature of the changes or lack of changes noted in testosterone levels. However, fluctuations in luteinizing hormone levels may be of greater magnitude and frequency than those of testosterone, further complicating the protocol followed and the minimum level of change that could be established.

High concentrations of intratesticular testosterone, 50–100 times peripheral levels, are found in men with normal spermatogenesis [19]. At least two mechanisms for intratubular concentration of androgens have been proposed for the mammalian testis [6]. However, it is not known what amount of intratesticular testosterone is required for normal sperm production, function, or both in the human. Peripheral testosterone values reported by Bonati *et al.* [1] in 2 cases of the so-called "fertile eunuch" syndrome were below the normal range for the assay used. These patients had normal sperm counts and were fertile according to their histories. None of the decreases in testosterone levels observed by Kolodny and his collaborators would be expected to result in eunuchoidism.

The hormonal results obtained in these studies suggest that heavy daily marihuana smoking in a hospital setting is not associated with significant decreases in pituitary gonadotropins or in serum testosterone levels. Our data neither confirm nor conflict with previously reported data. However, treatment of oligospermic patients with testosterone enanthate, 100 mg weekly, results in a 50–70-percent decrease in total sperm count within 4 weeks and is associated with a sustained decreased in serum LH and FSH of at least 60 percent within 1 week after the initial injection [8]. This degree of gonadotropin change would have been detected by this protocol and was not observed. Therefore, these data do not support a hormonally mediated (gonadotropin/testosterone) effect of marihuana upon gonadal function.

A simple dose-response relationship between testosterone production and sperm production has not been established and is unlikely in view of the multifactoral nature of the system. It can be reasoned that hormonal variations, if present, would be more significant if these changes were associated with or resulted in a decrease in sperm production. In addition, several cannabinoid effects proposed in somatic cell systems, if also manifested during spermatogenesis, could alter sperm production, function, or both in a manner unrelated to any hormonal changes. Data presented in this volume [10,13] suggest also that DNA synthesis in and content of testicular cells are altered after marihuana exposure in rodents. Alterations in germ cell replication in humans might result in decreased sperm production, without changes in sperm function. However, of greater potential importance is the possibility of structural gene defects caused by marihuana exposure. Since the cellular composition of the mature spermatozoon is a reflection of terminal gene germ cell action, such hypothetical defects could be manifested by alteration in sperm function, such as decreased motility, abnormal respiration and/or substrate utilization or altered acrosin content. These effects would be associated with altered fertility of the individual. Alternatively, gene defects could occur which would not affect the fertilizing capacity of the gamete, but would result in abnormal embryogenesis. The existence of both types of gene defects has been well established. Therefore, we evaluated several indirect indices of sperm function in these subjects, in addition to documenting the effect on total sperm production.

A brief review of the kinetics of human spermatogenesis is required to rationalize the experimental design employed and to interpret the findings. Germ cell development can be divided into three intratesticular phases: (1) spermatogonial mitotic divisions —28 days; (2) meiotic prophase—23 days; and (3) spermiogenesis—23 days, requiring a cycle length of 75 days for the production of a morphologically normal spermatozoon [7]. Transit through the male ductular system averages 12 days, with a range from 1–21 days. Effects on sperm production occurring during late spermiogenesis would be apparent 2 weeks after initial cannabinoid exposure. Alteration in sperm function may appear earlier if the cannabinoids directly affect sperm after their release from the Sertoli cell cytoplasm. If cannabinoids are able to interfere with stem cell (spermatogonial) renewal, such an effect could be manifested only during the second complete wave of spermatogenesis 3–6 months later.

The striking results observed suggest several possible mechanisms. The time course of the changes is consistent with an effect on spermiogenesis. During this period, gene activity gradually decreases as the spermatid chromatin is packaged within the dense matrix of the newly synthesized arginine-rich protamine. Interference with transcription, translation, or both, resulting in failure to synthesize the structural proteins required for axonemal development and the formation of the other specialized morphological elements of the mature spermatozoon, is likely to be associated with decreased sperm in the ejaculate 12–45 days later. Therefore, if it can be assumed that the decreased count noted reflected a specific perturbation of germ cell production 28 days earlier (at the beginning of period II), altered spermiogenesis best explains the observations. However, an effect resulting in altered epididymal transit or failure to complete meiosis cannot be excluded by these data. The constancy of semen volume speaks against an alteration of ejaculatory function, awareness of which was denied by each subject. In addition, ejaculatory frequency of every 24 hr for long periods is not associated with decreased sperm production or count [4]. Stress-associated decreases in sperm count have been reported, and appropriate in-hospital controls will be necessary to resolve this possibility, however unlikely.

The demonstration of a decrease in one or more of the cellular components of the mature spermatozoon would provide support for an intratesticular effect of marihuana on germ cell development. Increased sperm cyclic AMP levels, resulting from the dynamic equilibrium between adenyl cyclase and phosphodiesterase activities and, perhaps, after protein kinase activation, stimulate sperm motility in the absence of exogenous substrate. Based on the hypothesis of Lardy [5] and Hoskins [9], enhanced sperm motility should result in increased ATP hydrolysis, a lowered cellular "energy charge," and, thereby, stimulation of glycolysis. Potential dissociation between glycolysis and oxidative phosphorylation, cyclic AMP production, ATP hydrolysis, and motility could occur at many points as a result of decreased concentration of one or more cellular components.

At present, there is no clear understanding of the mechanism of theophylline stimulation on sperm motility. However, our studies have demonstrated that the extent of theophylline stimulation is inversely proportional to the initial sperm motility at which theophylline is added. In a small series of men with suspected infertility also studied in this laboratory, theophylline stimulation, at comparable motility, was significantly lower than that observed in donors of known fertility (14.0 ± 0.8 versus 37.9 ± 3.1). In 4 of 5 subjects in this study, theophylline stimulation correlated with motility changes or lack thereof. In only one case was an increase noted in the absence of a significant decrease in motility. Interpretation of these observations must await a more complete biochemical and enzymatic analysis of the relationship between the production and destruction of cyclic AMP and sperm motility.

REFERENCES

1. Bonati, B., P. Marrama, and L. Della Casa (1974) *The Endocrine Function of the Human Testis* (V. H. T. James, M. Serio, and L. Martini, eds.) Vol. 2. New York: Academic Press, p. 161.
2. Dyrenfurth, I., R. Jewelewicz, M. Warren, M. Ferin, and R. L. Vande Wiele (1974) *Biorhythms and Human Reproduction* (M. Ferin, F. Halberg, R. M. Richart, and R. Vande Wiele, eds.). New York: John Wiley & Sons, p. 171.
3. Edwards, R. G., P. C. Steptoe, and J. M. Purdy (1970) Fertilization and cleavage in vitro of preovulatory human oocytes. *Nature 227:* 1307.
4. Freund, M. (1963) Effect of frequency of emission on semen output and an estimate of daily sperm production in man. *J. Reprod. Fertil.* 6:269.
5. Garbers, D., N. L. First, and H. A. Lardy (1973) The stimulation of bovine epididymal sperm metabolism by cyclic nucleotide phosphodiesterase inhibitors. *Biol. Reprod.* 8:589.
6. Hansson, V., O. Trygstad, F. S. French, W. S. McLean, A. A. Smith,

D. J. Tindall, S. C. Weddington, P. Petrusz, S. N. Nayfeh, and E. M. Ritzen (1974) Androgen transport and receptor mechanisms in testis and epididymis. *Nature 250:*387.

7. Heller, Carl G. and Yves Clermont (1964) Kinetics of the germinal epithelium in man. *Recent Prog. Horm. Res. 20:*545.
8. Hembree, W. Unpublished data.
9. Hoskins, D. D. (1973) Adenine nucleotide mediation of fructolysis and motility in bovine epididymal spermatozoa. *J. Biol. Chem. 248:* 1135.
10. Jakubovic, A. and P. L. McGeer (1976) In vitro inhibition of protein and nucleic acid synthesis in rat testicular tissue by cannabinoids. *Marihuana: Chemistry, Biochemistry,* and *Cellular Effects* (G. Nahas *et al.,* eds.). New York: Springer Verlag, p. 223.
11. Johnsen, O. (1974) Effects of caffeine on the motility and metabolism of human spermatozoa. *Andrologia 6:*53.
12. Kolodny, R. C., W. H. Masters, R. M. Lolodner, and G. Toro (1974) Depression of plasma testosterone levels after chronic intensive marihuana use. *N. Engl. J. Med. 290:*872.
13. Leuchtenberger, L. and R. Leuchtenberger (1975) Cytological and cytochemical effects of whole smoke and of the gas vapour phase from marihuana cigarettes on growth and DNA metabolism of cultured mammalian cells. *Marihuana: Chemistry, Biochemistry,* and *Cellular Effects* (G. Nahas *et al.,* eds.). New York: Springer Verlag, p. 243.
14. Mendelson, J. H., Keuhnle, J. Ellingboe, and T. F. Babor (1974) Plasma testosterone levels before, during and after chronic marihuana smoking. *N. Engl. J. Med. 291:*1051.
15. Naftolin, F., H. L. Judd, and S. S. C. Yen (1973) Pulsatile pattern of gonadotropins and testosterone in man: the effects of clomiphene with and without testosterone. *J. Clin. Endocrinol. Metab. 36:*285.
16. Overstreet, J. W. and C. E. Adams (1971) Mechanisms of selective fertilization in the rabbit: sperm transport and viability. *J. Reprod. Fertil. 26:*219.
17. Overstreet, J. M. and W. C. Hembree (1976) Penetration of the zona pellucida of non-living human oocytes by human spermatozoa in vitro. Manuscript submitted.
18. Schaeffer, C. F., C. G. Gunn, and K. M. Dubowski (1975) Normal plasma testosterone concentrations after marihuana smoking. *Lancet 1:*867.
19. Steinberger, E., A. Root, M. Ficher, and K. D. Smith (1973) The role of androgens in the initiation of spermatogenesis in man. *J. Clin. Endocrinol. Metab. 37:*746.

43

Cellular Effects of Chronic Cannabis Use in Man

COSTAS N. STEFANIS AND
MARIETTA R. ISSIDORIDES

Introduction

Recent experimental research on cannabis yielded results indicating that use of this drug may lead to abnormalities of cellular metabolism with consequent functional aberrations potentially harmful to man's physical health, mental health, or both [6]. Yet however informative and eventually useful these findings may be in elucidating the drug's mode of action, they are not directly applicable to man. The adequately documented species differences in the action of cannabis [1] as well as the fact that animal experimental conditions hardly simulate cannabis smoking by man are but two of a series of factors to be considered when one attempts to extrapolate experimental findings from animals to man.

In the framework of these considerations, we extended the findings of a previous [1] long-term controlled investigation of the effects of chronic cannabis use on the clinical, behavioral, electrophysiological, and psychosocial level to a study of cannabis' effects on human cells at the macromolecular level.

In this chapter the findings obtained by the morphological, histochemical, and ultrastructural investigation of blood cells and spermatozoa of chronic cannabis users are presented.

Material and Methods

Clinical material

We studied 34 chronic cannabis users and 18 male control subjects. They were all paid volunteers recruited from a larger population that was used extensively in the collaborative study of chronic cannabis use in man cited above. Although the personal and family histories, smoking habits, and state of physical and mental health

Marihuana: Chemistry, Biochemistry, and Cellular Effects, edited by Gabriel G. Nahas, © 1976 by Springer-Verlag New York Inc.

of all subjects were already available, this information was reassessed before the subjects were admitted to the present study.

As in the initial study, inclusion criteria in the user's group were (1) age below 58 yr, (2) regular hashish use for more than 10 yr continuing up to the day of testing, (3) no use of other addictive substances except for tobacco smoking and irregular social alcohol drinking, and (4) absence of gross neurological disorder or incapacitating physical illness. Controls had to match the users with respect to age, place of upbringing and residence, education, and socioeconomic level. They had also to be regular tobacco smokers and could have never used any addictive substances other than alcohol (and this only irregularly or moderately).

The two groups in their final composition averaged 41.2 (SD 12.7) and 40.8 (SD 11.2) yr of age for the users and the control groups, respectively. They did not differ significantly with respect to the above-mentioned other matching criteria.

Data regarding hashish use by our group of users are shown in Table 43.1. The material the subjects smoked and classified as of average strength was revealed on analysis to contain 4–5 percent Δ^9-tetrahydrocannabinol (Δ^9-THC). Subjects were briefed before testing on the purpose and the conditions of this study, and their informed consent was obtained.

Users were allowed to smoke hashish *ad libidum* the day before the testing, but they were instructed not to smoke before blood drawing on the day of testing. They came to the laboratory in groups together with the controls at a fixed day and hour (usually at 9 AM), and blood was drawn 3 hr after their arrival. Cigarette smoking was allowed but on the condition that cigarettes would be offered by the social workers who occupied and entertained them. Blood was obtained by the medical staff of the hospital not otherwise related to the present study. All blood samples were coded and sent to the laboratory blind. The code was not broken until the final assessment of the laboratory material.

All 34 users and 18 controls were used for the morphological

Table 43.1 Data of hashish use

	Starting age	*Years of use*	*Past use*		*Current use*	
			Times/day	*Daily quant.*[a]	*Times/day*	*Daily quant.*[a]
Mean	16.3	25.1	6	8.2 gm	2.2	3.2 gm

[a] Estimated.

and the histochemical part of the study, but only 16 users and 10 controls adequately matched to age were used for the electron microscopic study. Fresh sperm was obtained by the standard procedures from 4 users and 4 controls. No other criteria but matching requirements and the subject's willingness to offer the material were considered for their selection from the larger group.

Cytological methods

Smears were made from peripheral capillary blood obtained by finger prick. The smears were stained by the routine May–Grünwald–Giemsa method for studying nuclear morphology.

We used the combined Luxol fast blue–periodic acid-Schiff technique (LFB–PAS) after which phospholipids stain blue and glycolipids stain red [20] for the histochemical study of membrane lipids.

We used the phosphotungstic acid–hematoxylin reagent (PTAH) of Mallory [28] to demonstrate nucleohistones [45]. This anionic stain shows a characteristic blue metachromasia in stained tissues when the concentration of amino, guanido, and imidazole groups is high, as in the basic proteins of the nucleus, the histones. The reagent was used at pH 1.8, the optimum for high protein binding [33,37]. When basic groups are not present or are neutralized by negative charges, such as the DNA phosphates, the nuclei remain pink. For this method, smears were fixed in 2.5 percent glutaraldehyde in 0.1 *M* cacodylate buffer (pH 7.2), rinsed in buffer, washed in distilled water, and stained by PTAH at room temperature for 24 hr. They were further washed in tap water, dehydrated in 95 percent and absolute ethanol, cleared, and mounted.

Acidic phosphoproteins of the nucleus were demonstrated by the cationic carbocyanin dye 1-ethyl-2-[3-(1-ethylnaphthol [1,2d] thiazolin-2-ylidene)-2-methyl-propenyl]-naphtho [1,2d] thiazolium bromide, which at pH 6.1 in sodium cacodylate buffer stains phosphoproteins blue and stains other cell constituents other colors [14].

Peripheral blood for electron microscopy was obtained on the same day and under the same conditions from users and controls by venipuncture. Ethylenediaminetetraacetic acid (EDTA) was used as an anticoagulant (1 drop/2 ml of blood). The red cells were permitted to sediment by gravity for about 1 hr at 37°C. The leukocyte-rich plasma was removed and centrifuged at 400 *g* for 10 min. The supernatant was discarded and the pellet of cells fixed for 24 hr at 4°C in 10 percent formalin neutralized with sodium acetate (2 gm/100 ml). The pellets were prepared for electron microscopic examination, according to the adaptation by MaCrae and Meetz [26] of the original ammoniacal silver reaction of Black and Ansley [5], which is specific for localizing nucleohistones—especially arginine-rich histones—in the light microscope. Thus, the ammoniacal silver reaction, which is carried out in bulk on the pellet, allows one to study Epon thick sections in the light microscope and correlate observations with the electron microscopic findings. Since the reaction products are colored under light, the localization of lysine-rich histones (yellow) and arginine-rich histones (brown-black) is sharper than in similarly stained smears of whole cells. The yellow stain for lysine in the light microscope has no dense product in the electron microscope; however, the brown-black stain for arginine has a dense deposit due to specific interaction of silver with reactive groups in the arginine molecule [27].

For the sperm study, the samples were treated as follows: 0.5 ml of ejaculate was added to 1 ml of isotonic sodium sulfate solution [7]; this mixture was kept at 30°C for 60 min, centrifuged, and then the pellet was fixed and processed for electron microscopy by the ammoniacal silver method as for the leukocytes.

Results

Membrane histochemistry

THC has a structural similarity to cholesterol [12]; it is insoluble in water and intensely soluble in fat. In the blood it is strongly bound and migrates in association with lipoproteins [46]. In tissues the lipid of cell membranes provides a major lipophilic sink. Investigators agree that the affinity of THC for membrane lipids may be an important factor in its molecular mode of action [31]. Since very little is known of the effect of THC on the histochemistry of membrane components in human users, the leukocytes of the two groups were investigated for phospholipids and glycolipids.

The LFB–PAS procedure revealed differences between controls and chronic users in the ratio of phospholipids to glycolipids. More specifically, a loss of phospholipids from the membrane and cortical cytoplasm and an increase in glycolipids in the cytoplasm of the users' neutrophils were noted. Although the loss of phospholipids from the membrane was uniform in the cells of all chronic users, the increase in glycolipids varied from subject to subject. In the controls, the cytoplasm of neutrophils was faintly PAS positive (Figure 43.1a); in the group of chronic users it was moderately to intensely PAS positive (Figure 43.1b), and in most of them the cytoplasm contained heavily stained granules—probably of a lysosomal nature—at the periphery, causing protrusions of the cell surface (Figure 43.1c). These cell surface deformities may result from the lowered content of membrane phospholipids, which are known to maintain the conformational and functional properties of membrane lipoproteins [35].

Nuclear morphology

The nuclei of adult human granulocytes are divided into lobes connected by fine filaments of nuclear membrane [29]. Unspecific nuclear projections have been described in several conditions including the terminal stages of malignancy and chronic illnesses. Such projections are seen rarely in normal cells and always in a very low percentage [4]. Specific extensions of the nucleus under normal conditions are the drumstick, containing compact chromatin and joined to the nucleus by a stalk, and the sessile nodules, appendages attached to the lobes by a broad base. The drumstick is characteristic of the female sex [8] and is found in 1–7 percent of the granulocytes of normal females. It is found in about 1 in every 500 normal males and in less than 1 percent of the total number of cells. Sessile nodules can also be seen under normal conditions in males, but only in a small percentage of cells [4], whereas in females the percentage is much higher [29].

Our observations of the May–Grünwald–Giemsa stained smears, based on counts of 200 cells per subject, indicated that 21 of the 34 chronic hashish users (61 percent; Table 43.2) displayed in their neutrophils nuclear appendages similar to the female drumstick (Figure 43.2). The frequency range was 8–16 percent of the polymorphonuclear leukocytes. That the "drumsticks" observed in the chronic users were actually extensions of nuclear chromatin and

Table 43.2 Drumstick in neutrophils of users and controls

	With drumstick		*Without drumstick*			
Subjects	*n*	%	*n*	%	χ^2	*p*
Cannabis users (*n*:34)	21	61	13	39	18.64	0.001
Controls (*n*:18)	0	0	18	100		

not vesicular formations of the nuclear envelope was established by electron microscopy of leukocyte pellets of the same subjects (Figure 44.2, inset). Sessile nodules (Figure 43.3) were found in up to 26 percent of the cells in the same subjects that displayed drumsticks in their neutrophils. In 3 of the 34 chronic users, small spherical chromatin bodies that were unattached to the nucleus were occasionally seen (Figure 43.4).

Histochemistry of the nucleus

In view of the morphological findings indicating altered structure of the nucleus, the histochemical investigation was directed mainly to chromosomal proteins. These histones maintain chromatin structure, whereas the nonhistone chromosomal proteins are involved in selective template activity.

Basic proteins

Histones, the major basic proteins of the chromatin, are rich in the basic amino acids lysine and arginine. They are divided into five principal classes, most of which are present in eukaryotic cells. Histones normally inhibit the capacity of the genes to be transcribed into RNA [43]. Their role in maintaining chromatin structure is as important as their ability to repress DNA-dependent RNA synthesis. The lysine-rich histone H1 is responsible for chromatin condensation [24], while the other histones interact more intimately with the DNA double helix [22].

Using the PTAH anionic metachromatic stain [45] specific for basic proteins [38], we observed the following. In all subjects in the control group and in all cells, the nuclear membrane of the neutrophils, patches of euchromatin in the nuclear lobes, and the lymphocyte nuclei were stained with a blue metachromatic reaction (Figure 43.5) indicative of a high concentration of basic groups. In contrast, in all cells of all users the reagent failed to bind to the nuclei, which thus appeared pale (Figure 43.6). This finding indicates that in the leukocytes of the chronic users no binding sites are available for the stain. Such a state may arise not from the absence of basic proteins, but from their binding to DNA phosphates, which results in a lower concentration of positive charges so that the metachromatic reaction cannot occur [45].

Acidic phosphoproteins

Under normal conditions, the nonhistone acidic proteins are known to be (1) mediators to target cells of gene activity–modulating stimuli like hormones [2], (2) activators, and (3) in certain